The ESC Handbook on Cardiovascular Pharmacotherapy

The ESC Handbook on Cardiovascular Pharmacotherapy

Editors

Juan Carlos Kaski

Molecular and Clinical Sciences Research Institute, St. George's, University of London; and Cardiology Clinical Academic Group, St George's University Hospitals NHS Foundation Trust, London, UK

Keld Per Kjeldsen

Department of Cardiology, Copenhagen University Hospital (Hvidovre-Amager), Copenhagen; and Department of Health Science and Technology, The Faculty of Medicine, Aalborg University, Aalborg, Denmark

Associate editors

Stefan Agewall
Basil S. Lewis

ESC Guidelines advisors

Heinz Drexel
Erland Erdmann
Xavier Garcia-Moll
Peter J. Schwartz
Udo Sechtem
Faiez Zannad

Section editors

Ljubica Vukelic Andersen
Dan Atar
Debasish Banerjee
Claudio Ceconi
Heinz Drexel
David Goldsmith
Birgitte Klindt Poulsen
Francesca Mantovani
Antoni Martínez-Rubio
Theresa McDonagh
Alexander Niessner
Joep Perk
Massimo Francesco Piepoli
Juan Tamargo
Sven Wassmann
Faiez Zannad

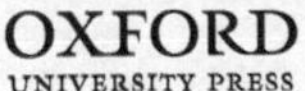

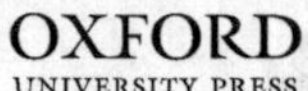

Great Clarendon Street, Oxford, OX2 6DP,
United Kingdom

Oxford University Press is a department of the University of Oxford. It furthers the University's objective of excellence in research, scholarship, and education by publishing worldwide. Oxford is a registered trade mark of Oxford University Press in the UK and in certain other countries

First Edition published in 2019

Published in the United States of America by Oxford University Press
198 Madison Avenue, New York, NY 10016, United States of America

British Library Cataloguing in Publication Data
Data available

Library of Congress Control Number: 2018951236

ISBN 978–0–19–875993–5

Printed and bound by
CPI Group (UK) Ltd, Croydon, CR0 4YY

Preface

Cardiovascular pharmacotherapy plays a truly major role in the management of cardiovascular disease across its whole spectrum. Drug therapy has been shown to be a life-saving or life-prolonging intervention in many cardiovascular conditions and a quality-of-life enhancer in others, as a result of its role in the improvement of otherwise debilitating symptoms. Over the past few years physicians have continued to witness and benefit from the arrival of large numbers of pharmacological agents objectively shown to have beneficial effects. Among the areas that have benefitted the most from this influx of newer pharmacological agents are dyslipidaemia, diabetes, coronary artery disease, heart failure, thrombosis and coagulation disorders, stroke prevention, and cardiac arrhythmias such as atrial fibrillation.

Albeit truly welcomed by the medical community, the relentless arrival of newer pharmacological agents represents a major challenge to the busy practising physician, for a variety of reasons. Health practitioners have to be conversant not only with the indications, absolute contraindications, and appropriate dosages of the new drugs but also—and very critically—with their adverse effects, their interactions with other cardiovascular and non-cardiovascular agents, and their effects on other organs and systems. Physicians are also expected to be aware of the basic pharmacological characteristics of the drugs they prescribe and to ensure that their therapeutic decisions are based on solid evidence.

Individual patient responsiveness, the impact of polypharmacy, subtle differences between agents grouped within drug classes, and the role of age and gender regarding drug efficacy and undesirable effects are also critically important.

An interesting phenomenon has emerged in recent years, namely that pharmacological knowledge and drug management of specific diseases is commonly devolved to 'disease-specific' experts, a fact that reduces the involvement of the general practitioner in everyday life patient management. The therapeutic challenge is compounded by the increasing complexity of the management guidelines emanating from different international cardiac societies in their attempt to make their recommendations more exhaustive and applicable to every clinical situation.

In view of all of the above, the ESC Working Group on Cardiovascular Pharmacotherapy has produced this handbook, *The ESC Handbook on Cardiovascular Pharmacotherapy*, which aims to assist physicians in their difficult task of prescribing wisely. The book is expected to facilitate access to practical information regarding cardiovascular diseases and their treatment, focusing on different aspects of pharmacotherapy as well as current recommendations for disease management. Previously published as *Drugs in Cardiology*, this fully revised handbook is aligned with the ESC Clinical Practice Guidelines.

In producing this handbook, the editors aimed at assisting several specific groups of health professionals who might find it useful to have access to up-to-date guidance on cardiovascular pharmacotherapy and disease management, all contained within a single volume, namely cardiologists, general practitioners, internal medicine specialists, anaesthetists, clinical pharmacologists, geriatricians, obstetricians, and nurse consultants. Junior doctors and trainees in all these specialties are also likely to find this book of help.

The content of this handbook is presented in nine sections. Sections 1 to 5 provide a brief description of all major cardiovascular conditions (including prevention, ischaemic heart disease, heart failure, arrhythmias, and structural heart disease) and recommendations for management, in accordance with current ESC Clinical Practice Guidelines. Section 6 deals with the important problem of cardiovascular pharmacotherapy in pregnancy. This section also covers important aspects of cardiovascular pharmacotherapy in patients with kidney or liver disease. Section 7 focuses on drug interactions, a topic of extreme importance in clinical practice and one which is not frequently addressed in management guidelines. Last but not least, sections 8 and 9 contain a comprehensive A–Z formulary of commonly and less commonly used cardiac and non-cardiac pharmacological agents, respectively, and both sections provide practical and accessible information on different aspects of pharmacology and pharmacotherapy. This will almost certainly help in streamlining drug prescribing and provide useful guidance for rational pharmacotherapy decision-making.

All chapters and sections of the book have been written and edited by international experts in their respective fields. Very importantly, to guarantee the accuracy of the therapeutic recommendations in the handbook, the content in every chapter has been carefully scrutinized by the editors as well as by ESC Guidelines advisors appointed by the editors on the basis of their outstanding expertise in cardiovascular pharmacotherapy and acquaintance with ESC Clinical Practice Guidelines.

The book's print edition comes with full access to its online version, allowing the reader to annotate and save chapters, download images, and follow links to references and guidelines. As cardiovascular pharmacotherapy is a rapidly evolving field, we will be reviewing the online content at yearly intervals to keep the book up to date for years to come, as appropriate. We also expect this handbook to represent an interactive, dynamic, bidirectional process among the book contributors and the readers and will hence welcome suggestions from the readership that can help improve the book content.

A substantial amount of time and effort has been put into the production of this work by all parties involved, often impacting on the professional, social, and family life of the authors who have contributed so generously to the project. The editors—like every individual taking part in the development of *The ESC Handbook on Cardiovascular Pharmacotherapy*—will however feel sufficiently rewarded if the content of this book succeeds in assisting health practitioners in their endeavours to serve better their patients.

JC Kaski and KP Kjeldsen on behalf of
the Associate editors, Section editors,
ESC Guidelines advisors and chapter authors

Contents

Note: Health professionals are encouraged to take the ESC Guidelines fully into account when exercising their clinical judgment, as well as in the determination and the implementation of preventive, diagnostic, or therapeutic medical strategies. However, the ESC Guidelines do not override in any way whatsoever the individual responsibility of health professionals to make appropriate and accurate decisions in consideration of each patient's health condition and in consultation with that patient or the patient's caregiver where appropriate and/or necessary. It is also the health professional's responsibility to verify the rules and regulations applicable to drugs and devices at the time of prescription.

Contributors

Stefan Agewall
Department of Cardiology, Oslo University Hospital and Institute of Clinical Medicine, Oslo University, Oslo, Norway

Aftab Ala
Gastroenterology Department, Royal Surrey County Hospital NHS Foundation Trust, Surrey, UK

Ljubica Vukelic Andersen
Department of Medicine, Randers Regional Hospital, and Department of Cardiology, Aalborg University Hospital, and Department of Biomedicine, Aarhus University, Denmark

Dan Atar
Oslo University Hospital Ulleval, Department of Cardiology, and Institute of Clinical Sciences, University of Oslo, Oslo, Norway

Anita Banerjee
Women's Health, Guy's and St Thomas' NHS Foundation Trust, London, UK

Debasish Banerjee
Renal and Transplantation Unit, St George's University Hospitals NHS Foundation Trust, Cardiology Clinical Academic Group, Molecular and Clinical Sciences Research Institute, St George's, University of London, London, UK

Giovanni Boffa
University of Padua, Padua, Italy

Martin Borggrefe
First Department of Medicine, University Medical Centre Mannheim (UMM), University of Heidelberg, Mannheim, Germany; German Center for Cardiovascular Research (DZHK), Partner Site Heidelberg/ Mannheim, Mannheim, Germany

Josep Brugada
Hospital Clinic, University of Barcelona, Barcelona, Spain

Haran Burri
Cardiology Department, University Hospital of Geneva, Geneva, Switzerland

Ricardo Caballero
Department of Pharmacology, School of Medicine, Universidad Complutense, Madrid, Spain

Claudio Ceconi
U.O. Cardiologia, Ospedale di Desenzano del Garda (BS), Italy

Gheorghe-Andrei Dan
'Carol Davila', University of Medicine, Colentina University Hospital, Bucharest, Romania

Antonio De Vita
Institute of Cardiology, Università Cattolica del Sacro Cuore, Fondazione Policlinico Universitario A Gemelli IRCCS, Rome, Italy

Eva Delpón
Department of Pharmacology, School of Medicine, Universidad Complutense, Madrid, Spain

Heinz Drexel
Division of Angiology, Swiss Cardiovascular Centre, University Hospital Bern, Bern, Switzerland; Vorarlberg Institute for Vascular Investigation and Treatment (VIVIT), Feldkirch, Austria

Erland Erdmann
Heart Center, University of Cologne, Cologne, Germany

João Pedro Ferreira
Cardiology and Centre d'Investigation Clinique, Centre Hospitalier Universitaire de Nancy, Nancy, France

Xavier Garcia-Moll
Cardiology Department, Santa Creu i Sant Pau Hospital, IIB-Sant Pau Research Institute, Universitat Autònoma de Barcelona, Spain

David Goldsmith
Cardiology Clinical Academic Group, Molecular and Clinical Sciences Research Institute, St George's, University of London, London, UK

Finn Gustafsson
The Heart Centre, Department of Cardiology, Rigshospitalet Copenhagen University Hospital, Copenhagen, Denmark

Maja Hellfritzsch Poulsen
Department of Public Health, Clinical Pharmacology and Pharmacy, University of Southern Denmark, Odense, Denmark

Nina Hojs
Cardiology Clinical Academic Group, Molecular and Clinical Sciences Research Institute, St George's, University of London, London, UK

Vivekanand Jha
The George Institute for Global Health, India; Professor of Nephrology and James Martin Fellow, University of Oxford, Oxford, UK; Adjunct Professor of Medicine, University of New South Wales, Sydney, Australia

Juan Carlos Kaski
Molecular and Clinical Sciences Research Institute, St. George's, University of London; and Cardiology Clinical Academic Group, St George's University Hospitals NHS Foundation Trust, London, UK

Keld Per Kjeldsen
Department of Cardiology, Copenhagen University Hospital (Hvidovre-Amager), Copenhagen; and Department of Health Science and Technology, The Faculty of Medicine, Aalborg University, Aalborg, Denmark

Birgitte Klindt Poulsen
Department of Clinical Pharmacology, Aalborg University Hospital, Aalborg, Denmark

Gaetano Antonio Lanza
Institute of Cardiology, Università Cattolica del Sacro Cuore, Fondazione Policlinico Universitario A Gemelli IRCCS, Rome, Italy

Basil S. Lewis
Lady Davis Carmel Medical Center and The Ruth and Bruce Rappaport School of Medicine, Technion-Israel Institute of Technology, Haifa, Israel

Marlene Lunddal Krogh
Department of Clinical Pharmacology, Aarhus University Hospital, Aarhus, Denmark

Alexander Lyon
Royal Brompton Hospital and Imperial College, London, UK

Brendan Madden
St George's University Hospitals NHS Foundation Trust, London, UK

Francesca Mantovani
Cardiology Department, Azienda Unità Sanitaria Locale, IRCCS di Reggio Emilia, Italy

Julio Martí-Almor
Department of Cardiology, Hospital del Mar, Barcelona; Associate Professor, Universitat Autònoma de Barcelona, Barcelona, Spain

Antoni Martínez-Rubio
Department of Cardiology, University Hospital of Sabadell, (University Autonoma of Barcelona), Sabadell, Barcelona, Spain

Theresa McDonagh
King's College Hospital, Denmark Hill, London, UK

Alexander Niessner
Department of Internal Medicine II, Division of Cardiology, Medical University of Vienna, Vienna, Austria

Elmir Omerovic
Department of Cardiology, Sahlgrenska University Hospital, Gothenburg University, Gothenburg, Sweden

Peter Ong
Department of Cardiology, Robert-Bosch Hospital, Stuttgart, Germany

Joep Perk
Faculty of Health and Life Sciences, Linnaeus University, Kalmar, Sweden

Sabine Perl
Department of Cardiology, Medical University Graz, Graz, Austria

Massimo Francesco Piepoli
Heart Failure Unit, Cardiac Unit, Gulielmo da Saliceto Hospital, AUSL Piacenza, Italy

Abhiram Prasad
Department of Cardiovascular Medicine, Mayo Clinic, Rochester, Minnesota, USA

Robin Ramphul
Renal and Transplantation Unit, St George's University Hospitals NHS Foundation Trust, London, UK

Claire Raphael
Department of Cardiology, Imperial NHS Foundation Trust, London, UK

Kasper Rossing
The Heart Centre, Department of Cardiology, Rigshospitalet Copenhagen University Hospital, Copenhagen, Denmark

Ricardo Ruiz-Granell
Arrhythmia Unit, Cardiology Department, Hospital Clinico Universitario and Hospital Quironsalud, Valencia, Spain

Kate Ryan
St George's University Hospitals NHS Foundation Trust, London, UK

Christoph H. Saely
Vorarlberg Institute for Vascular Investigation and Treatment (VIVIT), Academic Teaching Hospital Feldkirch, Feldkirch, Austria

Peter J. Schwartz
Center for Cardiac Arrhythmias of Genetic Origin, Istituto Auxologico Italiano IRCCS, Milan, Italy

Udo Sechtem
Cardiologicum and Department of Cardiology, Robert-Bosch Hospital, Stuttgart, Germany

Jan Steffel
University Heart Centre, Zurich, Switzerland

Mark Sweeney
Royal Brompton Hospital and Imperial College, London, UK

Juan Tamargo
Department of Pharmacology, School of Medicine, Universidad Complutense, Madrid, Spain

James Tonkin
St George's University Hospitals NHS Foundation Trust, London, UK

Erol Tülümen
First Department of Medicine, University Medical Centre Mannheim (UMM), University of Heidelberg, Mannheim, Germany; German Center for Cardiovascular Research (DZHK), Partner Site Heidelberg/Mannheim, Mannheim, Germany

Freek Verheugt
Onze Lieve Vrouwe Gasthuis (OLVG), Amsterdam, Netherlands

Sven Wassmann
Cardiology Pasing, Munich, Germany; University of the Saarland, Homburg/Saar, Germany

Faiez Zannad
Cardiology and Centre d'Investigation Clinique, Centre Hospitalier Universitaire de Nancy, Nancy, France

Robert Zweiker
Department of Cardiology, Medical University Graz, Graz, Austria

Symbols and Abbreviations

➲	cross-reference
α1AR	alpha-1 adrenoreceptor
AAD	antiarrhythmic drug
ABI	ankle–brachial index
ABPM	ambulatory blood pressure monitoring
ACC	American College of Cardiology
ACE	angiotensin-converting enzyme
ACEI	angiotensin-converting enzyme inhibitor
ACLS	advanced cardiac life support
ACR	acute cellular rejection
ACS	acute coronary syndrome
ACT	activated clotting time
ACTH	adrenocorticotrophic hormone
ADA	American Diabetes Association
ADH	antidiuretic hormone
ADHD	attention-deficit/hyperactivity disorder
ADP	adenosine diphosphate
ADPKD	autosomal dominant polycystic kidney disease
ADT	androgen deprivation therapy
AF	atrial fibrillation
AHA	American Heart Association
AHRE	atrial high-rate episode
AIDS	acquired immune deficiency syndrome
AKI	acute kidney injury
ALK	anaplastic lymphoma kinase
ALL	acute lymphoblastic leukaemia
ALT	alanine aminotransferase
AMR	antibody-mediated rejection
ANP	atrial natriuretic peptide
aPCC	activated prothrombin complex concentrate
APD	action potential duration
Apo B	apolipoprotein B
aPTT	activated partial thromboplastin time
AQP2	aquaporin-2
AR	aortic regurgitation
ARB	angiotensin receptor blocker
ARNI	angiotensin receptor–neprilysin inhibitor

ARVC	arrhythmogenic right ventricular cardiomyopathy
AS	aortic stenosis
ASA	acetyl salicylic acid
ASD	atrial septal defect
AST	aspartate aminotransferase
AT	atrial tachycardia
ATIII	antithrombin III
ATE	arterial thromboembolic event
ATG	anti-thymocyte globulin
ATP	adenosine triphosphate
AUC	area under the curve
AV	atrioventricular
AVB	atrioventricular block
AVN	atrioventricular node
AVNRT	atrioventricular nodal re-entrant tachycardia
AVR	aortic valve replacement
AVRT	atrioventricular re-entrant tachycardia
AZA	azathioprine
BCRP	breast cancer resistance protein
bd	twice daily
BMI	body mass index
BMPR2	bone morphogenetic type 2 receptor
BMS	bare-metal stent
BNP	brain natriuretic peptide
BP	blood pressure
bpm	beat per minute
BSEP	bile salt export pump
BUN	blood urea nitrogen
Ca^{2+}	calcium
CAAAA	centrally acting alpha-adrenergic agonist
CABG	coronary artery bypass graft
CAD	coronary artery disease
cAMP	cyclic adenosine monophosphate
CARDS	Collaborative Atorvastatin Diabetes Study
CAV	cardiac allograft vasculopathy
CCB	calcium channel blocker
CCM	cirrhotic cardiomyopathy
CCS	Canadian Cardiovascular Society
CDK	cyclin-dependent kinase
CETP	cholesteryl ester transfer protein

cGMP	cyclic guanosine monophosphate
CHD	coronary heart disease
CHF	congestive heart failure
CI	confidence interval
CK	creatine kinase
CKD	chronic kidney disease
Cl^-	chloride
CLL	chronic lymphocytic leukaemia
cm	centimetre
CME	Continuing Medical Education
cmH_2O	centimetre of water
CML	chronic myelogenous leukaemia
CMR	cardiac magnetic resonance
CMV	cytomegalovirus
CNI	calcineurin inhibitor
CNS	central nervous system
CO	cardiac output
COMT	catechol-*O*-methyltransferase
COPD	chronic obstructive pulmonary disease
COX	cyclo-oxygenase
CPK	creatine phosphokinase
CPVT	catecholaminergic polymorphic ventricular tachycardia
CR	controlled-release
CrCl	creatinine clearance
CRP	C-reactive protein
CRT	cardiac resynchronization therapy
CSA	chronic stable angina
CT	computed tomography
CTCA	computed tomography coronary angiography
CTEPH	chronic thromboembolic pulmonary hypertension
CTLA-4	cytotoxic T-lymphocyte antigen 4
CTPA	computed tomography pulmonary angiography
CV	cardiovascular
CVA	cerebrovascular accident
CVC	central venous catheter
CVRF	cardiovascular risk factor
CYP450	cytochrome P450
Da	dalton
DAPT	dual antiplatelet therapy
DBP	diastolic blood pressure

DC	direct current
DCA	dihydropyridine calcium channel antagonist
DCCV	direct current cardioversion
DCM	dilated cardiomyopathy
DDI	drug–drug interaction
DES	drug-eluting stent
DHA	docosahexaenoic acid
dL	decilitre
DLCO	diffusion of carbon monoxide
DNA	deoxyribonucleic acid
DOAC	dual oral anticoagulant
DPP-4	dipeptidyl peptidase 4
DRI	direct renin inhibitor
dTT	diluted thrombin time
DVT	deep vein thrombosis
EAD	early after-depolarization
ECG	electrocardiogram
ECT	ecarin clotting time
EECP	enhanced external counterpulsation
eGFR	estimated glomerular filtration rate
EHRA	European Heart Rhythm Association
EIF2AK4	eukaryotic translation initiation factor 2 α kinase 4
EMA	European Medicines Agency
ENaC	epithelial sodium channel
eNOS	endothelial nitric oxide synthase
EPA	eicosapentaenoic acid
ERA	endothelin receptor antagonist
ERP	effective refractory period
ESA	erythropoiesis-stimulating agent
ESC	European Society of Cardiology
ESH	European Society of Hypertension
ESR	erythrocyte sedimentation rate
ESRD	end-stage renal disease
ET1	endothelin 1
FDA	US Food and Drug Administration
FiO_2	fraction of inspired oxygen
FSH	follicle-stimulating hormone
g	gram
GABA	gamma-aminobutyric acid
G-CSF	granulocyte colony-stimulating factor

GFR	glomerular filtration rate
GH	growth hormone
GI	gastrointestinal
GIP	glucose-dependent insulinotropic polypeptide
GIST	gastrointestinal stromal tumour
GLP-1	glucagon-like peptide 1
GLP-1RA	glucagon-like peptide 1 receptor agonist
GM-CSF	granulocyte-macrophage colony-stimulating factor
GnRH	gonadotrophin-releasing hormone
GP	glycoprotein
G6PD	glucose-6-phosphate dehydrogenase
GRACE	Global Registry of Acute Coronary Events
GTN	glyceryl trinitrate
GTP	guanosine triphosphate
GTPCH-I	GTP-cyclohydrolase I
h	hour
H^+	hydrogen ion
HACA	human anti-chimeric antibody
HbA1c	glycated haemoglobin
HCL	hairy cell leukaemia
HCM	hypertrophic cardiomyopathy
HCO_3^-	bicarbonate
HCTZ	hydrochlorothiazide
HCV	hepatitis C virus
HDL	high-density lipoprotein
HF	heart failure
HFA	Heart Failure Association
HFmEF	heart failure with mid-range ejection fraction
HFpEF	heart failure with preserved ejection fraction
HFrEF	heart failure with reduced ejection fraction
HGFR	hepatocyte growth factor receptor
HIPAA	heparin-induced platelet activation assay
H-ISDN	hydralazine and isosorbide dinitrate
HIT	heparin-induced thrombocytopenia
HITTS	heparin-induced thrombocytopenia and thrombosis syndrome
HIV	human immunodeficiency virus
HLA	human leucocyte antigen
HMG CoA	hydroxyl-methyl-glutaryl coenzyme A
HoFH	homozygous familial hypercholesterolaemia

HOMA	homeostasis model assessment
HRT	hormone replacement therapy
hs-CRP	high-sensitivity C-reactive protein
HSV	herpes simplex virus
HVA	homovanillic acid
IABP	intra-aortic balloon pump
ICD	implantable cardioverter–defibrillator
ICU	intensive care unit
IDL	intermediate-density lipoprotein
Ig	immunoglobulin
IHD	ischaemic heart disease
IL	interleukin
IM	intramuscular
INR	international normalized ratio
INSTI	integrase inhibitor
IP3	inositol triphosphate
IPA	inhibition of platelet aggregation
IPAH	idiopathic pulmonary arterial hypertension
ISDN	isosorbide dinitrate
ISMN	isosorbide mononitrate
IUGR	intrauterine growth retardation
IV	intravenously
IVC	inferior vena cava
IVIG	intravenous immunoglobulin
IVUS	intravascular ultrasound
JVP	jugular venous pressure
K^+	potassium
kg	kilogram
L	litre
LBBB	left bundle branch block
LCSD	left cardiac sympathetic denervation
LDH	lactate dehydrogenase
LDL	low-density lipoprotein
LDL-C	low-density lipoprotein cholesterol
LDL-R	low-density lipoprotein receptor
LFT	liver function test
LGE	late gadolinium enhancement
LH	luteinizing hormone
LHRH	luteinizing hormone-releasing hormone
LMWH	low-molecular-weight heparin

LPL	lipoprotein lipase
LQTS	long QT syndrome
LV	left ventricular
LVAD	left ventricular assist device
LVEDP	left ventricular end-diastolic pressure
LVEF	left ventricular ejection fraction
LVH	left ventricular hypertrophy
LVOT	left ventricular outflow tract
m	metre
MACE	major cardiovascular event
MAO	monoamine oxidase
MAOI	monoamine oxidase inhibitor
mcg	microgram
MCL	mantle cell lymphoma
MDT	multidisciplinary team
MEK	mitogen-activated extracellular signal-regulated kinase
MELD	Model for End-stage Liver Disease
mEq	milliequivalent
MET	metabolic equivalent
MetS	metabolic syndrome
mg	milligram
Mg^{2+}	magnesium ion
MHC	major histocompatibility complex
MHV	metallic heart valve
MI	myocardial infarction
micromol	micromole
min	minute
mL	millilitre
MLC	myosin light chain
MM	multiple myeloma
MMF	mycophenolate mofetil
mmHg	millimetre of mercury
mmol	millimole
mPAP	mean pulmonary artery pressure
MR	mitral regurgitation; magnetic resonance
MRA	mineralocorticoid receptor antagonist
MRC	Medical Research Council
MRI	magnetic resonance imaging
ms	millisecond
MS	mitral stenosis

mTOR	mammalian target of rapamycin
mU	milliunit
MUGA	multigated acquisition scan
mV	millivolt
MVA	microvascular angina
MVO_2	myocardial oxygen consumption
6MWT	6-minute walk test
Na^+	sodium
NADPH	nicotinamide adenine dinucleotide phosphate
NAFLD	non-alcoholic fatty liver disease
NAPA	*N*-acetylprocainamide
NCCT	sodium chloride co-transporter
NCT	narrow complex tachycardia
NDCA	non-dihydropyridine calcium channel antagonist
NFAT	nuclear factor of activated T-cells
ng	nanogram
NG	nasogastric
NICE	National Institute for Health and Care Excellence
NIV	non-invasive ventilation
NK1	neurokinin 1
NMDA	*N*-methyl-*D*-aspartate
nmol	nanomole
NNRTI	non-nucleoside reverse transcriptase inhibitor
NO	nitric oxide
NOAC	new oral anticoagulant
NOS	nitric oxide synthase
NRTI	nucleoside reverse transcriptase inhibitor
NSAID	non-steroidal anti-inflammatory drug
NSCLC	non-small cell lung cancer
NSTE-ACS	non–ST-segment elevation acute coronary syndrome
NSTEMI	non-ST-segment elevation myocardial infarction
NSVT	non-sustained ventricular tachycardia
NTCP	sodium-dependent taurocholate co-transporting polypeptide
NT-pro-BNP	N-terminal prohormone brain natriuretic peptide
NVAF	non-valvular atrial fibrillation
NYHA	New York Heart Association
OAT	organic anion transporter
OCT	organic cation transporter
od	once daily

OR	odds ratio
PAD	peripheral artery disease
PAH	pulmonary arterial hypertension
PAI-1	plasminogen activator inhibitor-1
PAP	pulmonary artery pressure
PAR-1	protease-activated receptor-1
PARP	poly (ADP-ribose) polymerase
PBC	primary biliary cholangitis
PCH	pulmonary capillary haemangiomatosis
PCI	percutaneous coronary intervention
PCSK9	proprotein convertase subtilisin/kexin type 9
PCWP	pulmonary capillary wedge pressure
PD	pharmacodynamic
PD-1	programmed cell death-1
PDE	phosphodiesterase
PE	pulmonary embolism
PEA	pulseless electrical activity
PEEP	positive end-expiratory pressure
PET	positron emission tomography; pre-eclampsia
PGE1	prostaglandin E1
PGI2	prostacyclin
P-gp	P-glycoprotein
PI	protease inhibitor
PK	pharmacokinetic
PKA	protein kinase A
PO	orally
POMC	pro-opiomelanocortin
POST	Prevention of Syncope Trial
POTS	postural tachycardia syndrome
PPAR	peroxisome proliferator-activated receptor
PPCI	primary percutaneous coronary intervention
PPCM	peripartum cardiomyopathy
PPI	proton pump inhibitor
PRN	as required
PSI	proliferation signal inhibitor
PSVT	paroxysmal supraventricular tachycardia
PT	prothrombin time
PTCA	percutaneous transluminal coronary angioplasty
PVC	premature ventricular complex
PVOD	pulmonary veno-occlusive disease

PVR	peripheral vascular resistance
QTc	corrected QT interval
RA	rheumatoid arthritis
RAAS	renin–angiotensin–aldosterone system
RAS	renin–angiotensin system
RBBB	right bundle branch block
RCT	randomized controlled trial
rhuGM-CSF	recombinant human granulocyte–macrophage colony-stimulating factor
RNA	ribonucleic acid
ROPAC	Registry of Pregnancy and Cardiac Disease
RRR	relative risk reduction
RTK	receptor tyrosine kinase
rtPA	recombinant tissue plasminogen activator
RV	right ventricular
RVOT	right ventricular outflow tract
s	second
SA	sinoatrial
SAD	seasonal affective disorder
SaO_2	oxygen saturation
SARI	serotonin antagonist and reuptake inhibitor
SBP	systolic blood pressure
SC	subcutaneous
SCAD	stable coronary artery disease
SCD	sudden cardiac death
SCLC	small cell lung cancer
SCORE	Systematic COronary Risk Evaluation (chart)
SCS	spinal cord stimulation
SERCA	sarcoplasmic reticulum calcium pump
SERM	selective oestrogen receptor modulator
sGC	soluble guanylyl cyclase
SGLT2	sodium–glucose co-transporter 2
SGOT	serum glutamic-oxaloacetic transaminase
SGPT	serum glutamic-pyruvic transaminase
SIADH	syndrome of inappropriate antidiuretic hormone
SJS	Stevens–Johnson syndrome
SK	streptokinase
SLE	systemic lupus erythematosus
SNRI	serotonin noradrenaline reuptake inhibitor
SPAF	stroke prevention in atrial fibrillation

SPECT	single-photon emission computed tomography
SQTS	short QT syndrome
SR	sarcoplasmic reticulum
SSRI	selective serotonin reuptake inhibitor
STEMI	ST-segment elevation myocardial infarction
SVR	systemic vascular resistance
SVT	supraventricular tachycardia
t½	half-life
T3	triiodothyronine
T4	thyroxine
TAPSE	tricuspid annular plane systolic excursion
TAVI	transcatheter aortic valve implantation
T1DM	type 1 diabetes mellitus
T2DM	type 2 diabetes mellitus
TdP	torsades de pointes
tds	three times daily
TEN	toxic epidermal necrolysis
TG	triglyceride
TGF-β	transforming growth factor beta
THV	tissue heart valve
TIA	transient ischaemic attack
TIMI	Thrombolysis in Myocardial Infarction (score)
TKI	tyrosine kinase inhibitor
TnC	troponin C
TNF	tumour necrosis factor
TNFR	tumour necrosis factor alpha receptor
TOMHS	Treatment of Mild Hypertension Study
total-C	total cholesterol
TP	thromboxane (receptor)
tPA	tissue plasminogen activator
TPO	thrombopoietin
TR	tricuspid regurgitation
TRAP	thrombin receptor agonist peptide
TRL	triglyceride-rich remnant lipoprotein
TSH	thyroid-stimulating hormone
TT	thrombin time
TTR	time in therapeutic range
TTS	Takotsubo syndrome
TXA2	thromboxane A2
U	unit

UA	unstable angina
UFH	unfractionated heparin
UGT	uridine 5′-diphosphate glucuronosyltransferase
UKPDS	United Kingdom Prospective Diabetes Study
ULN	upper limit of normal
UV	ultraviolet
VA-ECMO	venous–arterial extra-corporeal membrane oxygenation
VASP	vasodilator-stimulated phosphoprotein
Vd	volume of distribution
VEGF	vascular endothelial growth factor
VEGFR	vascular endothelial growth factor receptor
VF	ventricular fibrillation
VHD	valvular heart disease
VKA	vitamin K antagonist
VKORC-1	vitamin K epoxide reductase complex-1
VLDL	very low-density lipoprotein
VLDL-C	very low-density lipoprotein cholesterol
VO_{2max}	maximal oxygen consumption
VPB	ventricular premature beat
V/Q	ventilation/perfusion
VSD	ventricular septal defect
VT	ventricular tachycardia
VTE	venous thromboembolism
VZV	varicella-zoster virus
WHO	World Health Organization
WPW	Wolff–Parkinson–White
WU	Wood unit
XL	extended-release

Classes of recommendations and levels of evidence

The present *ESC Handbook on Cardiovascular Pharmacotherapy* uses the scales predefined in ESC Clinical Practice Guidelines, 'Classes of recommendations' and 'Levels of evidence', to describe the strength of recommendations and levels of evidence of particular management options as outlined in Tables 1 and 2.

Table 1 Classes of recommendations

Classes of recommendations	Definition	Suggested wording to use
Class I	Evidence and/or general agreement that a given treatment or procedure is beneficial, useful, effective.	Is recommended/is indicated
Class II	Conflicting evidence and/or a divergence of opinion about the usefulness/efficacy of the given treatment or procedure.	
Class IIa	*Weight of evidence/opinion is in favour of usefulness/efficacy.*	Should be considered
Class IIb	*Usefulness/efficacy is less well established by evidence/opinion.*	May be considered
Class III	Evidence or general agreement that the given treatment or procedure is not useful/effective, and in some cases may be harmful.	Is not recommended

Table 2 Levels of evidence

Level of evidence A	Data derived from multiple randomized clinical trials or meta-analyses.
Level of evidence B	Data derived from a single randomized clinical trial or large non-randomized studies.
Level of evidence C	Consensus of opinion of the experts and/or small studies, retrospective studies, registries.

European Society of Cardiology publications

The ESC Textbook of Cardiovascular Medicine (Third Edition)
Edited by A. John Camm, Thomas F. Lüscher, Gerald Maurer, and Patrick W. Serruys
The ESC Textbook of Intensive and Acute Cardiovascular Care (Section Edition)
Edited by Marco Tubaro, Pascal Vranckx, Susanna Price, and Christiaan Vrints
The ESC Textbook of Cardiovascular Imaging (Second Edition)
Edited by Jose Luis Zamorano, Jeroen Bax, Juhani Knuuti, Patrizio Lancellotti, Luigi Badano, and Udo Sechtem
The ESC Textbook of Preventive Cardiology
Edited by Stephan Gielen, Guy De Backer, Massimo Piepoli, and David Wood
The EHRA Book of Pacemaker, ICD, and CRT Troubleshooting: Case-based learning with multiple choice questions
Edited by Harran Burri, Carsten Israel, and Jean-Claude Deharo
The EACVI Echo Handbook
Edited by Patrizio Lancellotti and Bernard Cosyns
The ESC Handbook of Preventive Cardiology: Putting prevention into practice
Edited by Catriona Jennings, Ian Graham, and Stephan Gielen
The EACVI Textbook of Echocardiography (Second Edition)
Edited by Patrizio Lancellotti, Jose Luis Zamorano, Gilbert Habib, and Luigi Badano
The EHRA Book of Interventional Electrophysiology: Case-based learning with multiple choice questions
Edited by Hein Heidbuchel, Matthias Duytschaever, and Harran Burri
The ESC Textbook of Vascular Biology
Edited by Robert Krams and Magnus Back
The ESC Textbook of Cardiovascular Development
Edited by Jose Maria Perez-Pomares and Robert G. Kelly
The ESC Textbook of Cardiovascular Magnetic Resonance
Edited by Massimo Lombardi, Sven Plein, Steffen Petersen, Emanuela R. Valsangiacomo, Chiara Bucciarelli-Ducci, Cristina Basso and Victor Ferrari

Forthcoming

The ESC Textbook of Sports Cardiology
Edited by Antonio Pelliccia, Hein Heidbuchel, Domenico Corrado, Mats Borjesson, and Sanjay Sharma

Section 1

Cardiovascular disease prevention

Section editors

Heinz Drexel
Massimo Francesco Piepoli

ESC Guidelines advisor

Heinz Drexel

Chapter 1.1

Hypertension

Robert Zweiker and Sabine Perl

Epidemiology, definition, and classification of hypertension

Epidemiology

Elevation of blood pressure (BP) shows a close correlation with stroke and cardiovascular (CV), peripheral artery, and end-stage renal disease (ESRD). Considering the global burden of diseases, hypertension contributes the most to disability-adjusted life years and has major impact on mortality.[1] Systemic BP represents a continuum of risk whereby CV mortality rates increase with increased BP levels. In the year 2000, in adults aged ≤30 years, two-thirds of stroke cases, 50% of ischaemic heart disease (IHD) cases, and 75% of hypertensive disease cases were associated with a mean systolic BP (SBP) of >115mmHg, which represents the nadir of BP level versus risk. Hypertension is the root cause of approximately 7.1 million deaths worldwide. The prevalence of hypertension varies in different countries. Around 35–40% of the adult population suffer from hypertension, and the disease shows a strong positive correlation with age.[2]

In the long run, hypertension is a risk factor for:

- Cerebrovascular disease.
- IHD.
- Left ventricular hypertrophy (LVH).
- Heart failure (HF) with preserved, moderately reduced, and reduced ejection fraction.
- Peripheral vascular disease.
- Hypertensive renal disease.
- Hypertensive retinopathy.

Definition and classification of hypertension

Systemic hypertension is defined as persistently elevated BP (see Fig. 1.1.1), i.e. based on office readings of SBP and/or diastolic BP (DBP) of ≥140 and 90mmHg, respectively. Hypertension can be classified according to degrees of severity, as shown in Table 1.1.1.

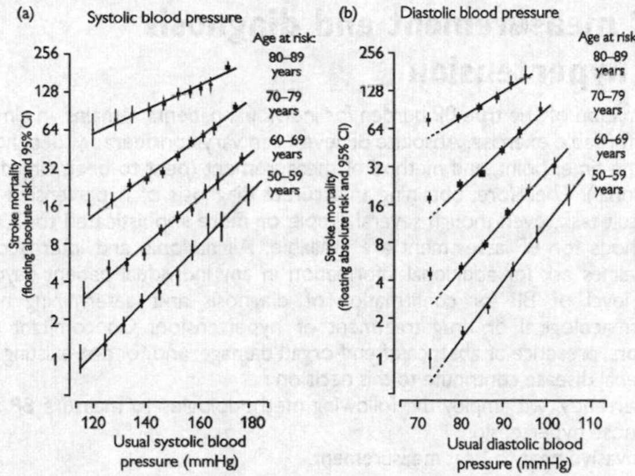

Fig. 1.1.1 Stroke mortality rate in each decade of age versus usual BP at the start of that decade. CI, confidence interval.

Reproduced from Prospective Studies Collaboration, Age-specific relevance of usual blood pressure to vascular mortality: a meta-analysis of individual data for one million adults in 61 prospective studies, *The Lancet*, Vol. 360, No 9349, Dec 2002, with permission from Elsevier.

Table 1.1.1 Definitions and classification of BP levels (mmHg)

Category	Systolic		Diastolic
Optimal	<120	and	<80
Normal	120–129	and/or	80–84
High normal	130–139	and/or	85–89
Grade 1 hypertension	140–159	and/or	90–99
Grade 2 hypertension	160–179	and/or	100–109
Grade 3 hypertension	≥180	and/or	≥110
Isolated systolic hypertension	≥140	and	≥90

The BP category is defined by the highest level of BP, whether systolic or diastolic. Isolated systolic hypertension should be graded 1, 2, or 3, according to systolic BP values in the ranges indicated.

Reproduced from Williams B, Mancia G, Spiering W *et al.* 2018 ESC/ESH Guidelines for the management of arterial hypertension. *Eur Heart J* 2018;**39**(33):3021–3104, with permission from Oxford University Press.

BP measurement and diagnosis of hypertension

Estimation of the true BP burden for individual patients remains an almost unaffordable exercise. Absolute BP levels can vary considerably, depending on the time, point, and method of measurement (beat-to-beat, circadian, seasonal). Therefore, obtaining an accurate diagnosis of hypertension is a difficult task, even though several simple or more sophisticated tools and methods for BP assessment are available. All national and international guidelines ask for additional information in any individual patient beyond the level of BP for confirmation of diagnosis and determining non-pharmacological or drug treatment of hypertension. Concomitant risk factors, presence or absence of end-organ damage, and/or pre-existing CV or renal disease contribute to this decision.[2]

Currently, we employ the following methodologies to measure BP and diagnose hypertension:

1. Invasive beat-to-beat measurement.
2. Non-invasive beat-to-beat measurement.
3. Office BP measurement—conventional.
4. Office BP measurement—automated.
5. Office BP measurement—automated and unattended.
6. Home BP monitoring.
7. Ambulatory BP monitoring (ABPM).
8. BP measurement during stress testing.

Invasive beat-to-beat measurement

This kind of BP assessment represents the gold standard. Due to its invasive nature, it is not suitable for routine use in the management of hypertension. It is considered an important tool for research on hypertension in experimental setups.

Non-invasive beat-to-beat measurement

Devices placed on a fingertip can perform non-invasive beat-to-beat measurement. They measure BP oscillometrically. For routine use, the advantages of beat-to-beat measurements are outweighed by the fact that hydrostatic pressure at the level of the site of measurement, compared to the reference which is the level of the heart, distorts the result. Today, these tools are restricted to research applications.

Office BP measurement—conventional

Nearly all evidence from epidemiologic studies that identified BP as an independent risk factor was gathered by conventional office BP measurement. The same holds true for almost all studies showing the beneficial effects of pharmacologic treatment of hypertension on morbidity and mortality. BP assessment by means of office BP measurement is based on the strongest evidence, but it lacks informative value and reproducibility in individual patients. In particular, BP variability and white-coat effects cannot be excluded.

High-quality standards for conventional office readings improve the result. The state-of-the-art measurement is defined by averaging three readings in an interval of 3–5min, which markedly improves the diagnosis, prognosis, and control of hypertension. According to recommendations of the European Society of Cardiology (ESC)/European Society of Hypertension (ESH), in most countries, the diagnosis of hypertension is based on conventional office BP readings with an average BP of >140mmHg systolic and/or >90mmHg diastolic.[2] By contrast, to confirm the presence or absence of hypertension, the scientific societies of Austria, Great Britain,[3] and Canada[4] have integrated the use of out-of-office BP measurements in their recommendations.

Office BP measurement—automated

Automated office BP measurements represent an improvement on the technique of taking conventional office BP readings by means of automated devices. The devices used measure BP oscillometrically, with cuffs attached to the upper arm. By taking an average of multiple readings, these devices reduce, according to some evidence, errors in measurement and increase the positive/negative predictive values.

Office BP measurement—automated and unattended

The main goal of this method is to avoid anxiety or white-coat effects during the assessment of BP. Patients should sit alone in a quiet room without talking for at least 5min. BP is taken by an automated oscillometric device, with the cuff attached to the upper arm. The device automatically calculates the average of three readings taken at intervals of at least 1min. This method of BP assessment gained publicity when it was used in the recent SBP intervention trial (SPRINT).[5] Despite its advantage of minimizing the white-coat effect, the scientific community discusses the fact that this method gives lower BP values in individual patients, compared to conventional office readings. Consequently, conclusions derived from studies using different methods of BP assessment are not transferable with respect to achieved BP levels and targets for treatment.

Home BP monitoring

Home BP monitoring has a long-standing tradition. It is a variant of the out-of-office BP assessment, which avoids the white-coat effect and facilitates long-term follow-up. Furthermore, this method empowers patients, as they actively participate in the management of their disease. It has been shown that this method improves control of hypertension due to better compliance and adherence to pharmacological therapy, as well as implementation of a healthier lifestyle. According to current recommendations, patients should use automated devices that measure BP oscillometrically, with the cuff attached to the upper arm.

Ambulatory BP monitoring (ABPM)

This method of BP assessment represents the gold standard of non-invasive measurement. It allows the recording of a large number of readings (every 15s during daytime, every 30s during night-time). The burden of BP in individual patients can be estimated reliably, with good reproducibility and close correlations with target organ damage (cross-sectional) or prognosis (longitudinal). The most important parameters calculated, based on 24h

ABPM, are the 24h mean BP, as well as the daytime and night-time means. Additionally, the circadian pattern of BP and its physiological or pathological variations are shown (normal dipping profile against abnormal non-dipping, extreme dipping, or inverse dipping). This method allows the calculation of early-morning surges of BP or BP variability. Furthermore, night-time BP readings are important to predict future events, if monitored in individuals without pharmacological therapy. However, BP values acquired by ABPM are not a substitute to office BP readings; they complement each other.

Regression to the mean causes a gap between office and ambulatory BP readings. The larger the gap, the higher office the BP values, and vice versa. On the other hand, if the office BP reading is low, the ambulatory BP reading might be higher than the office measurements. Ambulatory and home BP values show a closer correlation but are not interchangeable. Indeed, these technologies are complementary, and not competing.

An overview of BP levels corresponding to a correct diagnosis of hypertension and derived from different methods of measurement is provided in Table 1.1.2.

BP measurement during stress testing

The rise in BP during stress testing is considered physiological, but it can also contribute to the diagnosis or prognosis of hypertension and related issues. The maximum rise in BP during exercise should not exceed 10 ± 2mmHg per metabolic equivalent (MET). At peak exercise, SBP rises physiologically up to <210mmHg (male) or <190mmHg (female), and DBP up to <110mmHg (both sexes). Compared to baseline, the rise in SBP at peak exercise should not exceed 50–60mmHg (male) or 40–50mmHg (female). In higher age groups, these differences might also be more pronounced. Submaximal exercise, however, can yield more information on the prognosis of hypertension.

Several algorithms provide proposals to confirm the diagnosis of hypertension using out-of-office BP measurements. The very reasonable Canadian algorithm is shown in Fig. 1.1.2.

Table 1.1.2 Diagnosis of hypertension adjusted for the method of BP measurement used

Method	Hypertension (mmHg)
Office measurement—conventional	≥140/90
Office measurement—automatic, unattended	≥135/85
Home BP measurement	≥135/85
Ambulatory BP monitoring—24h mean	≥130/80
Ambulatory BP monitoring—daytime mean	≥135/85
Ambulatory BP monitoring—night-time mean	≥120/70

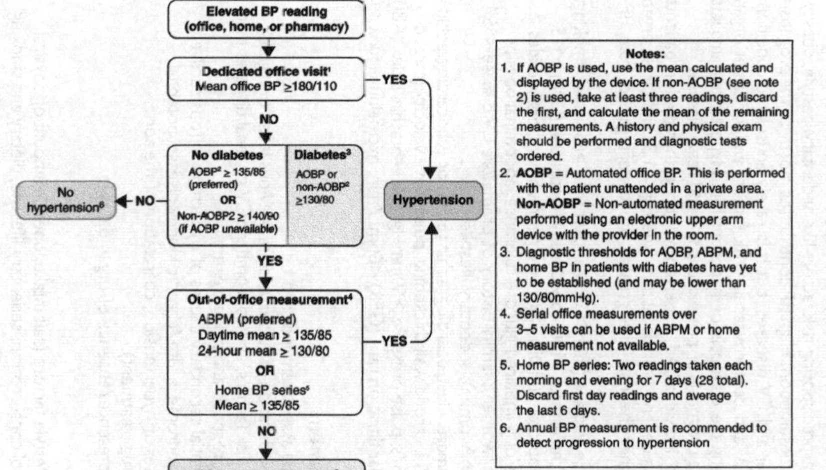

Fig. 1.1.2 Hypertension diagnostic algorithm, Canadian Society of Hypertension. ABPM, ambulatory blood pressure monitoring; AOBP, automated office blood pressure; BP, blood pressure.

Reproduced from Leung AA, Daskalopoulou SS, Dasgupta K, *et al.* Hypertension Canada's 2017 Guidelines for Diagnosis, Risk Assessment, Prevention, and Treatment of Hypertension in Adults. *Can J Cardiol* 2017;33:557–76, with permission from Elsevier.

Risk assessment and clinical evaluation

In >90% of cases, hypertension has no identifiable secondary/treatable causes. Essential (idiopathic, primary) hypertension is caused by polygenetic and environmental predisposing risk factors like sedentary lifestyle, obesity, and high alcohol consumption. High BP contributes mostly to the prognosis of cerebrovascular and CV diseases, but it is rarely an isolated condition. In many cases, CV and cerebrovascular risk factors and/or target organ damage accompany the diagnosis of hypertension. Hypertension impacts particularly on the prognosis of pre-existing CV and renal diseases.

Target BP and individualized hypertensive drug therapy for patients with hypertension depend on risk factors (see Fig. 1.1.3) and target organ damage. The higher the risk, the greater the benefit gained from BP-lowering therapy.

- *Risk factors*: male sex; age (men >55 years, women >65 years); smoking; dyslipidaemia [cholesterol >190, low-density lipoprotein (LDL) >115, high-density lipoprotein (HDL) <40/46 (men/women), triglycerides (TGs) >150mg/dL]; impaired glucose tolerance; abdominal obesity >88/102 (men/women); family history of premature CV disease <55/<65 years (men/women); sedentary lifestyle.
- *Target organ damage*: electrocardiographic (ECG) or echocardiographic evidence of LVH, carotid wall thickening, pulse wave velocity (carotid–femoral) >10m/s, pulse pressure >60mmHg, ankle–brachial index (ABI) <0.9; glomerular filtration rate (GFR) <60mL/min; microalbuminuria >30mg/24h.

Clinical assessment

The aims of clinical assessment include:

- Determining the duration of hypertension, previous levels of high BP, atherosclerotic risk factors, and concomitant CV or renal diseases that may affect the prognosis and guide treatment.
- Identifying potential secondary causes of hypertension (obstructive sleep apnoea syndrome, acute/chronic kidney disease, potential endocrine causes of hypertension, coarctation of the aorta, concomitant drug treatment).
- Detecting the presence/absence of organ damage.

Medical history

- Contributing lifestyle factors (salt intake, obesity, amount of physical exercise, alcohol consumption, sedentary lifestyle, dietary and smoking habits).
- Suggestion of secondary hypertension (hypertension in young age with sudden onset or worsening, especially in the absence of a family history of hypertension, organ damage disproportionate to the duration of hypertension, presentation as malignant hypertension, resistant hypertension—requiring ≤3 drugs).
- Family history of hypertension, kidney disease, and other CV risk factors.
- Concomitant drug treatment [e.g. non-steroidal anti-inflammatory drugs (NSAIDs), oral contraceptives, corticosteroids, mineralocorticoids, ciclosporin, amphetamines, erythropoietin, liquorice).

Hypertension disease staging	Other risk factors, HMOD, or disease	BP (mmHg) grading			
		High normal SBP 130–139 DBP 85–89	Grade 1 SBP 140–159 DBP 90–99	Grade 2 SBP 160–179 DBP 100–109	Grade 3 SBP ≥180 or DBP ≥110
Stage 1 (uncomplicated)	No other risk factors	Low risk	Low risk	Moderate risk	High risk
	1 or 2 risk factors	Low risk	Moderate risk	Moderate to high risk	High risk
	≥3 risk factors	Low to Moderate risk	Moderate to high risk	High risk	High risk
Stage 2 (asymptomatic disease)	HMOD, CKD grade 3, or diabetes mellitus without organ damage	Moderate to high risk	High risk	High risk	High to very high risk
Stage 3 (established disease)	Established CVD, CKD grade ≥4, or diabetes mellitus with organ damage	Very high risk	Very high risk	Very high risk	Very high risk

Fig. 1.1.3 Risk stratification in hypertensives according to BP level, presence/absence of concomitant risk factors, target organ damage, or established renal or cardio-/cerebrovascular disease. BP, blood pressure; CKD, chronic kidney disease; CV, cardiovascular; CVD, cardiovascular disease; DBP, diastolic blood pressure; HT, hypertension; OD, organ damage; RF, risk factor; SBP, systolic blood pressure.

Reproduced from Williams B, Mancia G, Spiering W *et al.* 2018 ESC/ESH Guidelines for the management of arterial hypertension. *Eur Heart J* 2018;39(33):3021–3104 with permission from Oxford University Press.

Examination

- Appropriate measurement of BP.
- Potential evidence of hypertensive target organ damage:
  - *Brain*: vertigo, transient ischaemic attack (TIA), stroke, neurological impairment, cognitive dysfunction.
  - *Eye*: optic fundi in hypertensive retinopathy.
  - *Heart*: shortness of breath, angina, history of myocardial infarction (MI), coronary revascularization, syncope, or HF, peripheral oedema, and fluid status, presence of atrial fibrillation (AF).
  - *Kidney*: examination of the abdomen for renal bruits, polyuria, nocturia, haematuria.
  - *Vessels*: carotid, abdominal, and femoral bruits, peripheral pulses in peripheral vascular disease.
- Calculation of body mass index (BMI) and waist circumference.

Investigations

- Laboratory examinations to assess for concomitant CV risk factors and potential underlying causes, i.e. renal or endocrine disease, initially with serum urea and electrolytes and creatinine, haemoglobin, fasting blood glucose, lipid profile, and urine dipstick (microalbuminuria).
- For detection of target organ damage, assessment by fundoscopy (hypertensive changes) and ECG and echocardiographic studies (LVH and strain, stress test). Assessment of blood vessels by ultrasound of carotid arteries. ABI and estimation of pulse wave velocity is also recommended.
- Assessment of other CV risk factors, according to the risk chart shown in Fig. 1.1.3, that may require aggressive management.
- Out-of-office BP (24h ABPM or home) measurements are especially indicated for the following: suspicion of white-coat, masked, and resistant hypertension, presence of unusual BP variability, symptomatic hypotension, and hypertension in pregnancy.

Secondary causes of hypertension

Identifiable causes of hypertension are present in 5–10% of patients. Screening should be based on raised pre-test likelihood. Factors that suggest secondary causes for hypertension are:[6]

- A course of disease with early onset of hypertension, severe or resistant, with sudden onset or worsening.
- Accelerated organ damage.
- Marginal or no family history of hypertension.

ABPM is of special relevance to identify hypertension rooted in secondary causes. ABPM can confirm truly resistant hypertension (= increased BP despite use of three antihypertensive drugs, including a diuretic, at optimal dosages) and reveal the cardiac BP pattern. If the cardiac BP pattern reveals a non-dipping course (lack of a nocturnal dip; normally –10 to –20%, compared to daytime BP), secondary hypertension (see Table 1.1.3) is more probable.

Table 1.1.3 Overview of most causes of secondary hypertension

Secondary cause	Prevalence (%)[a]	Prevalence (%)[b]	History	Screening	Clinical findings	Laboratory findings
Obstructive sleep apnoea	>5–15	>30	Snoring, daytime sleepiness, morning headache, irritability	Screening questionnaire, polysomnography	↑ neck circumference, obesity, peripheral oedema	Not specific
Renal parenchymal disease	1.6–8.0	2–10%	Loss of good BP control, diabetes, smoking, generalized atherosclerosis, previous renal failure, nocturia	Creatinine, ultrasound of the kidney	Peripheral oedema, pallor, loss of muscle mass	↑ creatinine, proteniuria; ↓ Ca^{2+}, ↑ K^+, ↑ PO_4
Renal artery stenosis	1.0–8.0	2.5–20	Generalized atherosclerosis, diabetes, smoking, previous renal failure, nocturia	Duplex or CT or MRI or angiography (drive by)	Abdominal bruits, peripheral vascular disease	Secondary aldosteronism: ARR ↔, ↓ K^+, ↓ Na^+
Primary aldosteronism	1.4–10	6–23	Fatigue, constipation, polyuria, polydipsia	ARR	Muscle weakness	↓ K^+, ARR ↑
Thyroid disease	1–2	1–3	*Hyperthyroidism*: palpitations, weight loss, anxiety, heat intolerance *Hypothyroidism*: weight gain, fatigue, constipation	TSH	*Hyperthyroidism*: tachycardia,AF, accentuated heart sounds, exophthalmos *Hypothyroidism*: bradycardia, muscle weakness, myxoedema	*Hyperthyroidism*: ↓ TSH, ↑ fT4 and/ or fT3 *Hypothyroidism*: ↑ TSH, ↓ fT4, ↑ cholesterol

Cushing's syndrome	0.5	<1.0	Weight gain, impotence, fatigue, psychological changes, polydipsia and polyuria	24h urinary cortisol, dexamethasone testing	Obesity, hirsutism, skin atrophy, striae rubrae, muscle weakness, osteopenia	↑ 24h urinary cortisol, ↑ glucose, ↑ cholesterol, ↓ K^+
Phaeochromo-cytoma	0.2–0.5	<1	Headache, palpitations, flushing, anxiety	Plasma metanephrines, 24h urinary catecholamine	The 5 'Ps'[c]: paroxysmal hypertension, pounding headache, perspiration, palpitations, pallor	↑ metanephrines
Coarctation of the aorta	<1	<1	Headache, nosebleed, leg weakness or claudication	Cardiac ultrasound	Different BP (≤20/10 mmHg) between upper and lower extremities and/or between right and left arms; ↓ and delayed femoral pulses, interscapular ejection murmur, rib notching on chest X-ray	Not specific

AF, atrial fibrillation; ARR, aldosterone–renin ratio; BP, blood pressure; Ca^{2+}, calcium; CT, computerized tomography; fT3, free triiodothyronine; fT4, free thyroxine; K^+, potassium; Na^+, sodium; PO_4, phosphate; TSH, thyroid-stimulating hormone.

[a] Prevalence in hypertensive patients.

[b] Prevalence in patients with resistant hypertension.

[c] *Kaplan's Clinical Hypertension*, tenth edition, 2010, Lippincott Williams & Wilkins, p. 363.

Reproduced from Rimoldi SF, Scherrer U, Messerli FH. Secondary arterial hypertension: when, who, and how to screen? *Eur Heart J* 2014;35(19):1245–54, with permission from Oxford University Press.

Treatment target

Initiation of antihypertensive therapy (see Fig. 1.1.4) has two main aims: reduction of *fatal* and *non-fatal* events of the cardiac, cerebral, and peripheral vasculature, kidneys, and eyes. In this regard, a considerable number of randomized controlled trials (RCTs) and a couple of subsequent meta-analyses confirmed the benefit of BP-lowering therapy in hypertensive patients. Treatment targets are dependent on BP levels and the overall CV risk as determined by risk charts such as the SCORE risk charts. Nevertheless, initiation and escalation of treatment strategies require an individualized approach, which is facilitated by several algorithms from different cardiology societies. The ESC/ESH guidelines recommend therapy in the presence of an increased CV risk, which is calculated by BP levels and by adding information on concomitant risk factors, the presence of (sub)clinical target organ damage, and pre-existing established CV or kidney disease.[2]

BP goals: the lower, the better?

According to the 2018 European guidelines, the goal of BP-lowering therapy is to achieve an SBP of 130–139mmHg in almost all settings. It is recommended for patients at low to moderate CV risk (class I-B), diabetics (class I-A), patients with previous stroke/TIA (class IIa-B), and patients with coronary artery disease (CAD) (class IIa-B) or with diabetic or non-diabetic chronic kidney disease (CKD) (class IIa-B). In patients aged <80 years, BP of 130–139mmHg remains the target (class I-A). In the very elderly (>80 years), the BP goal is defined as identical, but individual tolerability of low BP must be considered. The DBP goal is 70–79mmHg. In frail and/or elderly patients (>80 years of age), therapy should start if BP exceeds 160/90mmHg. Cautious treatment intensity (e.g. number of BP-lowering drugs) and BP targets should be considered, and clinical effects of treatment should be carefully monitored (Fig. 1.1.5).[7]

The recently published SPRINT (Systolic Blood Pressure Intervention Trial) might challenge these BP goals.[5] Treatment to achieve an SBP target of <120 versus <140mmHg in 9361 patients showed a statistically significant benefit in terms of a composite of MI, other acute coronary syndromes (ACS), stroke, HF, or death from CV causes, as well as all cause-mortality.

These results have two limitations. Firstly, the patients included had to have an increased CV risk, but patients with diabetes or previous stroke were excluded. Secondly, for BP estimation, the investigators used automated, unattended office BP measurements and averaged three readings obtained in a room without the presence of medical staff. BP levels obtained by this methodology have been shown to be lower than those gained by traditional office BP measurements. Based on office BP measurements, current guidelines have formulated actual BP targets. Therefore, assignment of new (definitely lower) BP goals coming from SPRINT faces some discussion within the scientific community.

One meta-analysis examined all evidence available up to the end of 2015, including results from SPRINT. The authors confirmed beneficial effects of more intense BP lowering to an SBP goal of <130mmHg, in terms of stroke, coronary heart disease (CHD), and CV death. At present, only Canadian hypertension guidelines have incorporated this evidence base into their recommendations.[4]

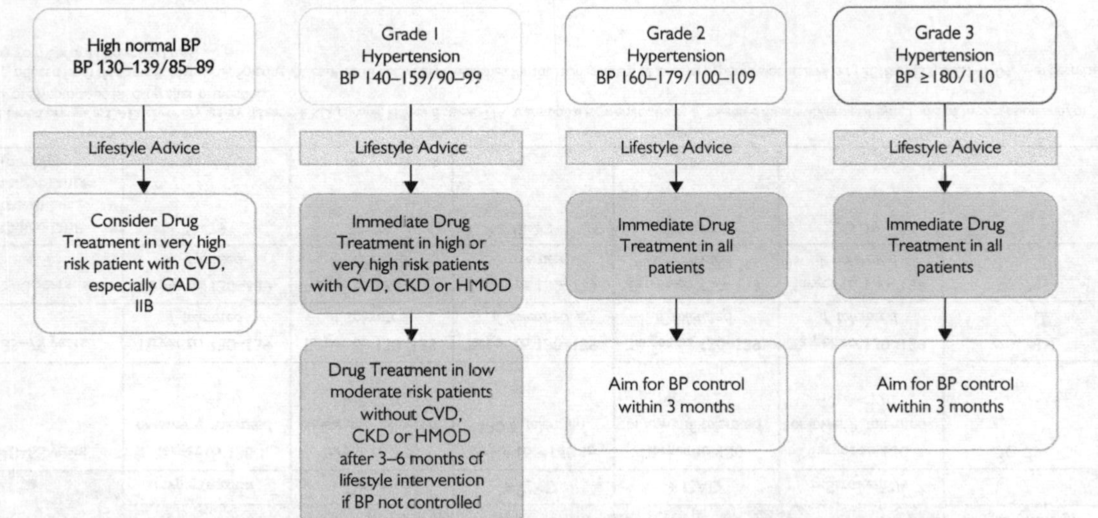

Fig. 1.1.4 Initiation of antihypertensive therapy, depending on individualized cardiovascular risk. BP, blood pressure; CKD, chronic kidney disease; CV, cardiovascular; CVD, cardiovascular disease; DBP, diastolic blood pressure; HT, hypertension; OD, organ damage; RF, risk factor; SBP, systolic blood pressure.

Reproduced from Williams B, Mancia G, Spiering W *et al.* 2018 ESC/ESH Guidelines for the management of arterial hypertension. *Eur Heart J* 2018;39(33):3021-3104 with permission from Oxford University Press.

Fig. 1.1.5 Office BP targets of antihypertensive therapy depending on age.

Age group	Office SBP treatment target ranges (mmHg)					Office DBP treatment target ranges (mmHg)
	Hypertension	+ Diabetes	+ CKD	+ CAD	+ Stroke/TIA	
18–65 years	**Target to 130** *or lower if tolerated* Not <120	**Target to 130** *or lower if tolerated* Not <120	**Target to <140 to 130** *if tolerated*	**Target to 130** *or lower if tolerated* Not <120	**Target to 130** *or lower if tolerated* Not <120	70–79
65–79 years	**Target to 130–139** *if tolerated*	**Target to 130–139** *if tolerated*	**Target to 130–139** *if tolerated*	**Target to 130–139** *if tolerated*	**Target to 130–139** *if tolerated*	70–79
≥80 years	**Target to 130–139** *if tolerated*	**Target to 130–139** *if tolerated*	**Target to 130–139** *if tolerated*	**Target to 130–139** *if tolerated*	**Target to 130–139** *if tolerated*	70–79
Office DBP treatment target ranges (mmHg)	70–79	70–79	70–79	70–79	70–79	

BP, blood pressure; CAD, coronary artery disease; CKD, chronic kidney disease; TIA, transitional ischaemic attack. *If tolerated* means absence of symptoms of hypotension and/or lack of symptomatic BP drop after orthostasis.

Reproduced from Williams B, Mancia G, Spiering W, *et al.* 2018 ESC/ESH Guidelines for the management of arterial hypertension. *Eur Heart J* 2018;39(33):3021–3104, with permission from Oxford University Press.

Pharmacological therapy

Numerous BP-lowering drugs have been developed and tested in many clinical trials. Antihypertensive drug therapy has been shown to produce significant reductions in CV morbidity and mortality. The main effects of pharmacological therapy are due to their antihypertensive properties, although several trials have claimed that certain combinations of medication are superior to others beyond the benefit of reduced BP. The extent of BP-lowering effects depends mostly on the initial BP. Law *et al.* published an informative epidemiologic meta-analysis by correlating antihypertensive effects of single- or combined-drug therapy with baseline BP levels and the potential for lowering the relative risks of CHD (see Fig. 1.1.6) and stroke in different age groups.[8]

Tailored antihypertensive therapy is feasible in special individual circumstances (e.g. planned pregnancy) and in the presence of concomitant risk factors, target organ damage, or overt CV or kidney disease. ESC/ESH guidelines recommend single or combination therapy, depending on initial BP levels and overall CV risk.[2] Different algorithms (see Fig. 1.1.7) for choosing first-line drugs, depending on age and/or the presence of concomitant renal disease or diabetes, are provided in the UK's National Institute for Health and Care Excellence (NICE) recommendations.

Several classes of antihypertensive drugs are suitable as first line, of which angiotensin-converting inhibitors (ACEIs), angiotensin receptor blockers (ARBs), calcium channel blockers (CCBs), diuretics (thiazides, chlortalidone, indapamide) are particularly recommended, with some caution with the use of β-blockers. Potential combination therapy regimens using different drug classes are shown in Fig. 1.1.8.

Antihypertensive drugs: an overview

Angiotensin-converting enzyme inhibitors

ACEIs are the most widely used drug class for the treatment of hypertension. Their effect rests upon blocking the conversion of angiotensin I to angiotensin II which has very strong vasoconstriction properties. Angiotensin II is also involved in vascular and left ventricular (LV) remodelling and in the development of LVH and intramyocardial fibrosis. Compelling indications for ACEIs are their beneficial action in chronic HF, atherosclerotic disease in any vascular bed, and CKD, especially by reducing proteinuria. ACE inhibition is an issue for women with childbearing potential, since they are linked to possible congenital malformations. In practice, ACE inhibition may cause an increase in potassium levels and a decrease in kidney function after the first dose and a few days of treatment.

Angiotensin receptor blockers

Their mechanism of action is blockade of the angiotensin II type I receptor. The effects are comparable to those of ACEIs; however, dry cough, one of the adverse effects of ACEIs, can be avoided with use of ARBs. Their indications, as well as contraindications, are comparable to those ACEIs. Combination therapy of ACEIs and ARBs has harmful effects and should be avoided. Both ACEIs and ARBs belong to the group of renin–angiotensin system (RAS)-blocking agents.

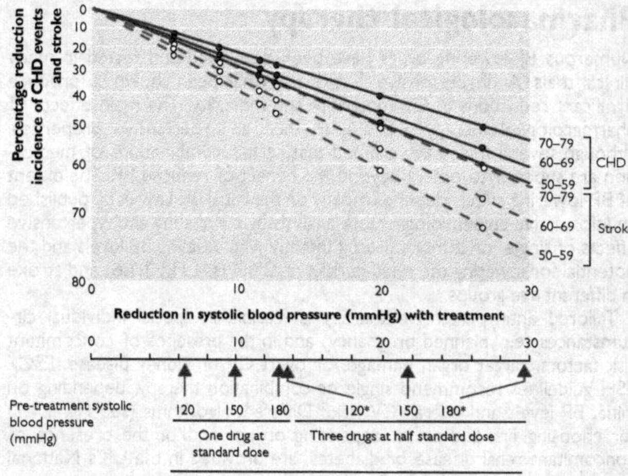

Fig. 1.1.6 Reduction in incidence of coronary heart disease (CHD) events and stroke in relation to reduction in systolic BP, according to the dose and combination of drugs, pre-treatment systolic BP, and age. Upper part: percentages of reductions in relative risk (*y*-axis) are shown for CHD and stroke, depending on the extent of BP lowering (*x*-axis). Blue lines refer to CHD and dotted red lines to stroke. Numbers on the right-hand side stratify data according to different ages. Lower part: drug-induced BP-lowering effects, depending on pre-treatment BP levels, are shown (horizontal line, mmHg). BP-lowering effects are more pronounced if pre-treatment BP is higher. Combination therapy (three drugs at half the standard dose) has stronger BP-lowering effects, compared to single drug strategies. For explanation: if pre-treatment BP is 180mmHg, one drug at the standard dose reduces BP by approximately 13mmHg, which results in a relative risk reduction for stroke of 45% and for CHD of 35% (in patients aged 50–59 years). If combination therapy is used, BP is lowered by 30mmHg, translating into −75% risk for stroke and −65% risk for CHD. * BP reductions are more uncertain and hence also reductions in disease incidence.

Reproduced from Law MR, Morris JK, Wald NJ. Use of blood pressure lowering drugs in the prevention of cardiovascular disease: meta-analysis of 147 randomised trials in the context of expectations from prospective epidemiological studies. *BMJ*. 2009 May 19;338:b1665. doi: 10.1136/bmj.b1665 with permission from BMJ.

Calcium channel blockers

CCBs have very good BP-lowering and some anti-atherosclerotic effects. Its high potential for prevention of stroke and regression of LVH has been demonstrated. Some concerns have been raised regarding their effects in overt HF. Reduction in the risk of new-onset HF has been shown, compared to placebo, but to a lesser extent compared to diuretics, ACEIs, or β-blockers.

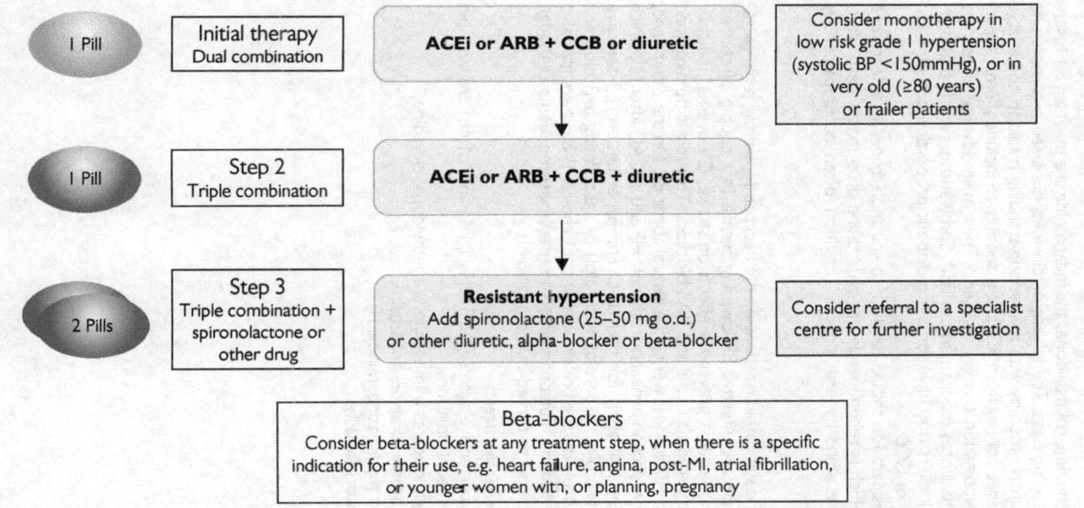

Fig. 1.1.7 Algorithm for antihypertensive therapy, as suggested by the 2018 ESC/ESH guidelines. BP, blood pressure.

Reproduced from Williams B, Mancia G, Spiering W *et al.* 2018 ESC/ESH Guidelines for the management of arterial hypertension. *Eur Heart J* 2018;39(33):3021–3104, with permission from Oxford University Press.

Diuretics

Hydrochlorothiazide, chlortalidone, and indapamide are the main representatives of this drug class. The advent of diuretics has been a cornerstone in antihypertensive therapy with a very long-standing tradition and a large body of evidence coming from RCTs. It is sensible to include diuretics, particularly in combination therapy regimens. Their main adverse effects are electrolyte imbalances (sodium, potassium). Some authors argue that diuretics and β-blockers may have some pro-diabetic properties, compared to ACEIs, ARBs, or CCBs.

Special consideration should be given to spironolactone, an aldosterone antagonist, which is recommended as a third-line drug that is particularly effective in resistant hypertension, a condition often accompanied by aldosteronism.

Beta-blockers

By blocking the sympathetic actions on the heart and lowering renin secretion, β-blockers are effective BP-lowering agents. In a couple of studies, β-blockers showed less preventive effects on stroke, CV events, and total mortality, compared to CCBs and RAS blockers. This might be explained by their lower efficacy in lowering the central aortic BP. On the other hand, β-blockers have proven beneficial in chronic HF and in CAD after MI, which is a compelling indication for their use. For hypertension, β1-selective blockers (metoprolol, bisoprolol, nebivolol) or vasodilating α-β-blockers, such as carvedilol, are the preferred agents of choice. β-blockers may also facilitate pro-diabetic metabolic effects in predisposed patients (although this does not apply to carvedilol and nebivolol).

Other antihypertensive agents

Several antihypertensive agents (see Tables 1.1.4a and 1.1.4b) are available as standby in special situations.

- Centrally acting agents (rilmenidine, α-methyldopa, clonidine).
- α-blocking agents (urapidil, doxazosin).
- Vasodilators (hydralazine, minoxidil).
- Renin inhibitors (aliskiren).

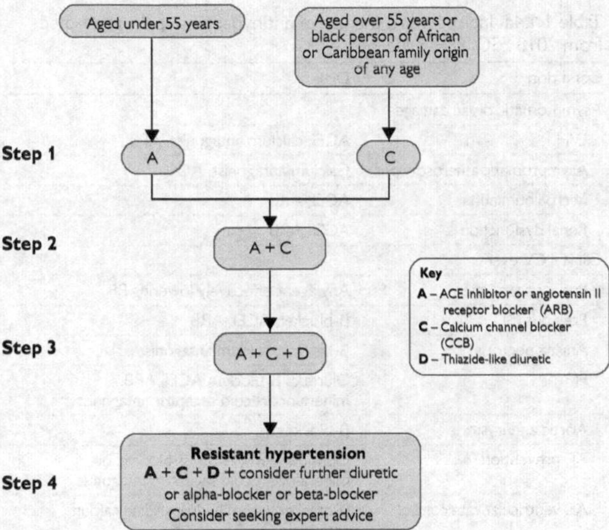

Fig. 1.1.8 First-line agents for treatment of hypertension and their potential use in combination therapy, as shown in UK NICE guidelines.

Source data from McCormack T, Krause T, O'Flynn N. Management of hypertension in adults in primary care: NICE guideline. *Br J Gen Pract* 2012;62(596):163–4.

Table 1.1.4a Indications to the use of antihypertensive drugs adapted from 2018 ESC/ESH guidelines

Condition	Drug
Asymptomatic organ damage	
LVH	ACEI, calcium antagonist, ARB
Asymptomatic atherosclerosis	Calcium antagonist, ACEI
Microalbuminuria	ACEI, ARB
Renal dysfunction	ACEI, ARB
Clinical CV event	
Previous stroke	Any agent effectively lowering BP
Previous MI	β-blocker, ACEI, ARB
Angina pectoris	β-blocker, calcium antagonist
HF	Diuretic, β-blocker, ACEI, ARB, mineralocorticoid receptor antagonist
Aortic aneurysm	β-blocker
AF, prevention	Consider ARB, ACEI, β-blocker, or mineralocorticoid receptor antagonist
AF, ventricular rate control	β-blocker, non-dihydropyridine calcium antagonist
ESRD/proteinuria	ACEI, ARB
Peripheral artery disease	ACEI, calcium antagonist
Other	
ISH (elderly)	Diuretic, calcium antagonist
MetS	ACEI, ARB, calcium antagonist
Diabetes mellitus	ACEI, ARB
Pregnancy	Methyldopa, β-blocker, calcium antagonist
Blacks	Diuretic, calcium antagonist

ACEI, angiotensin-converting enzyme inhibitor; AF, atrial fibrillation; ARB, angiotensin receptor blocker; BP, blood pressure; CV, cardiovascular; ESRD, end-stage renal disease; HF, heart failure. ISH, isolated systolic hypertension; LVH, left ventricular hypertrophy; MI, myocardial infarction.

Reproduced from Williams B, Mancia G, Spiering W et *al*. 2018 ESC/ESH Guidelines for the management of arterial hypertension. *Eur Heart J* 2018;39(33):3021–3104, with permission from Oxford University Press.

Table 1.1.4b Contrandications to the use of antihypertensive drugs adapted from 2018 ESC/ESH guidelines

Drug	Compelling	Possible
Diuretics (thiazides)	Gout	Metabolic syndrome Glucose intolerance Pregnancy Hypercalcaemia Hypokalaemia
β-blockers	Asthma Sinuaricular or AV block (grade 2 or 3, bradycardia <60beats/min)	Metabolic syndrome Glucose intolerance Athletes and physically active patients
Calcium antagonists (dihydropyridines)		Tachyarrhythmia Heart failure Severe leg oedema
Calcium antagonists (verapamil, diltiazem)	AV block (grade 2 or 3, trifascicular block) Severe LV dysfunction Heart failure	
ACE inhibitors	Pregnancy Angioneurotic oedema Hyperkalaemia Bilateral renal artery stenosis	Women with childhearing potential and without reliable contraception
Angiotensin receptor blockers	Pregnancy Hyperkalaemia Bilateral renal artery stenosis	Women with childbearing potential and without reliable contraception
Mineralocorticoid receptor antagonists	Acute or severe renal failure (eGFR <30mL/min) Hyperkalaemia	

ACE, angiotensin-converting enzyme; AV, atrioventricular; eGFR, estimated glomerular filtration rate; LV, left ventricular.

Reproduced from Williams B, Mancia G, Spiering W *et al.* 2018 ESC/ESH Guidelines for the management of arterial hypertension. *Eur Heart J* 2018;**39**(33):3021–3104, with permission from Oxford University Press.

Non-pharmacological therapy and lifestyle

Lifestyle changes are recommended for all patients with high-normal and high BP—with or without therapy. It should always be the first step of BP treatment but should not delay the initiation of medical BP-lowering therapy in high-risk patients. The greatest and most sustained BP benefit is obtained when multiple lifestyle interventions are incorporated simultaneously. Appropriate lifestyle changes may delay or prevent hypertension in non-hypertensives, delay or prevent medical therapy in grade 1 hypertensive individuals, and contribute to BP reduction in hypertensive individuals already on medical treatment, allowing a decrease in the number and doses of antihypertensive agents.[9]

Recommended lifestyle measures known to lower BP and CV risk are:

- Salt restriction.
- Moderation of alcohol consumption.
- High consumption of vegetables and fruits and low-fat and dairy products.
- Weight reduction and maintenance.
- Regular physical exercise.

Salt restriction

The average daily salt intake is between 9 and 12g/per day. Salt restriction <5g (e.g. one small teaspoon) is recommended. A meta-analysis showed that a reduction of 1.75g sodium/day (4.4g salt/day) was associated with a mean 4.2/2.1mmHg reduction in SBP/DBP, with a more pronounced effect (-5.4/-2.8mmHg) in people with hypertension. The effect of sodium restriction on BP was greater in blacks and older people, as well as in individuals with diabetes, metabolic syndrome (MetS), and CKD, i.e. groups that have a less responsive renin–angiotensin–aldosterone system (RAAS). To reduce salt intake, processed and oversalted food should be avoided; meals should be cooked from fresh ingredients, and salt could be substituted for herbs. As 80% of salt consumption involves hidden salt, it has been calculated that salt reduction in the manufacturing processes of bread, processed meat and cheese, margarine, and cereals will result in an increase in quality-adjusted life years.

Moderation of alcohol consumption

A linear relationship between alcohol consumption, BP levels, and the prevalence of hypertension has been demonstrated. Regular alcohol consumption raises BP, and increased alcohol intake attenuates the effects of antihypertensive drug therapy, which is mostly reversible within 1 or 2 weeks.

Hypertensive men should be advised to limit their consumption of alcohol to 14 and women to 8 units per week (1 unit = 125ml of wine or 250ml of beer). There should be alcohol-free days during the week and binge drinking must be avoided.

Other dietary changes

All hypertensive patients should be advised to eat a healthy balanced diet containing vegetables, legumes, fresh fruits, low-fat dairy products, whole grains, fish, and unsaturated fatty acids (especially olive oil). Low consumption of red meat and saturated fatty acids is recommended (DASH- and Mediterranean diet). Significant reductions in ambulatory BP, blood glucose, lipids, cardiovascular risk, and stroke have been shown.

Weight reduction

Body weight seems to be directly associated with BP, and excess body fat predisposes to increased BP and hypertension. Weight reduction lowers BP in obese patients and has beneficial effects on associated risk factors such as insulin resistance, diabetes, hyperlipidaemia, LVH, and obstructive sleep apnoea. In a meta-analysis, an average weight loss of 5.1kg resulted in a mean SBP and DBP reduction of 4.4 and 3.6mmHg, respectively. Maintenance of a health body weight (BMI of about 25kg/m^2) and waist circumference (<94cm for men and <80cm for women) is recommended for non-hypertensive individuals to prevent hypertension and for hypertensive patients to reduce BP. A multidisciplinary approach could be helpful.

Physical exercise

Studies indicated that physical activity was inversely related to mortality in hypertensive patients, meaning that patients with hypertension who were more active showed lower CV and all-cause mortality. A meta-analysis of RCTs showed that dynamic aerobic endurance, exercise resistance, and isometric training reduce SBP and DBP in the general population, but only endurance training reduces BP in hypertensive patients. Therefore, moderate-intensity dynamic aerobic exercise (walking, jogging, cycling, or swimming) is recommended for at least 30min 5–7 days/week. Additionally, resistance exercise can be advised two to three times per week.

Smoking cessation

Smoking triggers an acute increase in BP and heart rate, persisting for >15min after smoking a cigarette, through stimulation of the sympathetic nervous system. Smoking cessation is reported to be the single most effective lifestyle measure for prevention of a many CV diseases, including stroke and MI. Even in motivated patients, programmes to stop smoking after 1 year are only successful in 2–23%. To support smoking cessation, nicotine replacement therapy, bupropion, or varenicline can be prescribed.

Structured educational programmes in multidisciplinary teams (MDTs) can help improve adherence to lifestyle intervention and medical treatment, leading to sustained, adequate BP control.

Hypertension in special situations

White-coat hypertension

In white-coat hypertensives, BP is elevated in office BP measurements and normal in ambulatory BP measurements. There is no clear evidence that administration of BP-lowering drugs leads to a reduction in CV events. In high-risk individuals, who have dysmetabolic risk factors or asymptomatic organ damage, drug treatment could be considered. Both lifestyle changes and drug treatment may be considered when normal ambulatory BP values are accompanied by abnormal home BP levels. Lifestyle intervention can be recommended to all patients with white-coat hypertension.

Masked hypertension

In cases of masked hypertension, clinic BP is normal, but ambulatory BP measurements show hypertensive BP levels. When this condition is identified, both lifestyle measures and drug treatment should be considered, because patients are at an elevated risk for CV disease.

The elderly

The Hypertension in the Very Elderly Trial (HYVET) reported significant reductions in CV events and all-cause deaths in octogenarians by aiming for an SBP of <150mmHg. There is no evidence that different classes of antihypertensive drugs are differently effective in younger versus older patients.

Young adults

In young hypertensives with isolated elevation of DBP and other CV risk factors, BP should be reduced to <140/90mmHg. Young individuals in whom brachial SBP is elevated and DBP is normal, central SBP is sometimes normal; these patients can be managed with lifestyle measures only.

Women

A subgroup analysis by sex of 31 RCTs found similar BP reductions in men and women and no evidence that different antihypertensive drugs were more effective in one sex or the other.[10] Use of older oral contraceptives with a higher oestrogen content resulted in an increase in BP. A study on low-dose oestrogen and second- or third-generation progestins did not find that use of oral contraceptives increased the risk of MI. Current recommendations indicate that oral contraceptives should be selected and their use initiated by weighing the risks and benefits for each individual person. It is not recommended for oral contraceptives to be used in women with uncontrolled hypertension.

Pregnancy

Severe hypertension in pregnancy (SBP >160mmHg or DBP >110mmHg) should be treated immediately with antihypertensive drugs, whereas the benefit of antihypertensive drug therapy in mildly to moderately elevated BP is uncertain. Methyldopa, labetalol, and nifedipine have been tested in pregnancy and their safety profile confirmed. β-blockers should not be given in early pregnancy (potentially causing fetal growth retardation), while diuretics should be used with caution (causing reduction in plasma volume). All agents interfering with the RAS should be avoided.

Diabetes and metabolic syndrome

Hypertension is a common comorbidity in diabetic patients. There are clear recommendations for BP goals and antihypertensive treatment (see Table 1.1.5). In patients with MetS, lifestyle changes, particularly weight loss and physical exercise, are recommended and BP should be maintained at 130–120/80–70mmHg.

Obstructive sleep apnoea

Obstructive sleep apnoea seems to be responsible for considerable BP elevation and a non-dipping pattern. Ambulatory BP measurement and oximetry confirm the diagnosis. Weight loss and exercise should be recommended in obese patients with sleep apnoea. A successful therapy for obstructive sleep apnoea is continuous positive airway pressure, although a meta-analysis showed only minimal effects on BP reduction (1–2mmHg) as a result.

Nephropathy

Studies showed a direct relationship between BP and progression of CKD and incident ESRD. A meta-analysis of studies in patients with ESRD undergoing dialysis showed a reduction in CV events, CV death, and all-cause mortality by lowering SBP and DBP. Therapeutic strategies in patients with nephropathy are given in Table 1.1.6.

Table 1.1.5 Treatment strategies in patients with diabetes (adapted from ESC/ESH Guidelines 2013 and 2018)

Recommendations	Class[a]	Level[b]
While initiation of antihypertensive drug treatment in diabetic patients whose SBP is >160mmHg is mandatory, it is strongly recommended to start drug treatment also when SBP is >140mmHg	I	A
An SBP goal of 130mmHg is recommended in patients with diabetes	I	A
The DBP target in patients with diabetes is recommended to be 70–79mmHg	I	A
All classes of antihypertensive agents are recommended and can be used in patients with diabetes; RAS blockers may be preferred, especially in the presence of proteinuria or microalbuminuria	I	A
It is recommended that individual drug choice takes comorbidities into account	I	C
Simultaneous administration of two blockers of the RAS is not recommended and should be avoided in patients with diabetes	III	B

DBP, diastolic blood pressure; RAS, renin–angiotensin system; SBP, systolic blood pressure.

[a] Class of recommendation.

[b] Level of evidence.

Reproduced from Mancia G, Fagard R, Narkiewicz K *et al*; 2013 ESH/ESC Guidelines for the management of arterial hypertension. The Task Force for the management of arterial hypertension of the European Society of Hypertension (ESH) and of the European Society of Cardiology (ESC). *Eur Heart J* 2013; **34**: 2159–2219, and from Williams B, Mancia G, Spiering W *et al*. 2018 ESC/ESH Guidelines for the management of arterial hypertension. *Eur Heart J* 2018;39(33):3021–3104, with permission from Oxford University Press.

Atrial fibrillation

Hypertension is the most prevalent concomitant condition in patients with AF. Even high-normal BP is associated with the development of AF. The consequences of AF include overall mortality, stroke, HF, and hospitalizations. Therefore, prevention of, or delaying, new-onset AF is desirable. ARBs (losartan, valsartan) were found to prevent a first occurrence of AF better than β-blockers (atenolol) or CCBs (amlodipine). However, trials in high-risk patients (PRoFESS, TRANSCEND) did not confirm these findings. Because of data heterogeneity, it has been suggested that beneficial effects of ARBs may be limited to the prevention of incident AF in hypertensive patients with structural heart disease such as LVH or dysfunction or at high risk in general, but with no history of AF.

Table 1.1.6 Therapeutic strategies in patients with nephropathy (adapted from ESC/ESH Guidelines 2013 and 2018)

Recommendations	Class[a]	Level[b]
Lowering SBP to 130–139mmHg should be considered	IIa	B
RAS blockers are more effective in reducing albuminuria than other antihypertensive agents and are indicated in hypertensive patients in the presence of microalbuminuria or overt proteinuria	I	A
Reaching BP goals usually requires combination therapy, and it is recommended to combine RAS blockers with other antihypertensive agents	I	A
Combination of two RAS blockers, though potentially more effective in reducing proteinuria, is not recommended	III	A
Aldosterone antagonists cannot be recommended in CKD, if eGFR is <45mL/min/1.72 m² or baseline Kp > -4.5mmol/L especially in combination with a RAS blocker, because of the risk of excessive reduction in renal function and of hyperkalaemia	III	C

BP, blood pressure; CKD, chronic kidney disease; eGFR, estimated glomerular filtration rate; RAS, renin–angiotensin system; SBP, systolic blood pressure.

[a] Class of recommendation.

[b] Level of evidence.

Reproduced from Mancia G, Fagard R, Narkiewicz K *et al*; 2013 ESH/ESC Guidelines for the management of arterial hypertension. The Task Force for the management of arterial hypertension of the European Society of Hypertension (ESH) and of the European Society of Cardiology (ESC). *Eur Heart J* 2013; **34**: 2159–2219, and from Williams B, Mancia G, Spiering W *et al.* 2018 ESC/ESH Guidelines for the management of arterial hypertension. *Eur Heart J* 2018;**39**(33):3021–3104, with permission from Oxford University Press.

References

1 Lim SS, Vos T, Flaxman AD, *et al*. A comparative risk assessment of burden of disease and injury attributable to 67 risk factors and risk factor clusters in 21 regions, 1990–2010: a systematic analysis for the Global Burden of Disease Study 2010. *Lancet* 2012;**380**:2224–60.

2 Williams B, Mancia G, Spiering W *et al*. 2018 ESC/ESH Guidelines for the management of arterial hypertension. *Eur Heart J* 2018;**39**(33):3021–3104.

3 National Institute for Health and Care Excellence (2011). *Hypertension in adults: diagnosis and management*. Clinical guideline [CG127]. Available at: https://www.nice.org.uk/guidance/cg127/resources/hypertension-in-adults-diagnosis-and-management-pdf-35109454941637 [accessed 25 October 2018].

4 Leung AA, Daskalopoulou SS, Dasgupta K, *et al*. Hypertension Canada's 2017 guidelines for diagnosis, risk assessment, prevention, and treatment of hypertension in adults. *Can J Cardiol* 2017;**33**:557–76.

5 SPRINT Research Group, Wright JT Jr, Williamson JD, Whelton PK, *et al*. A randomized trial of intensive versus standard blood-pressure control. *N Engl J Med* 2015;**373**:2103–16.

6 Rimoldi SF, Scherrer U, Messerli FH. Secondary arterial hypertension: when, who, and how to screen? *Eur Heart J* 2014;**35**:1245–54.

7 Piepoli MF, Hoes AW, Agewall S, *et al*. European Guidelines on cardiovascular disease prevention in clinical practice: the Sixth Joint Task Force of the European Society of Cardiology and Other Societies on Cardiovascular Disease Prevention in Clinical Practice. *Eur J Prev Cardiol* 2016;**23**:NP1–96.

8 Law MR, Morris JK, Wald NJ. Use of blood pressure lowering drugs in the prevention of cardiovascular disease: meta-analysis of 147 randomised trials in the context of expectations from prospective epidemiological studies. *BMJ* 2009;**338**:b1665.

9 He FJ, Macgregor GA. Effect of longer-term modest salt reduction on blood pressure. *Cochrane Database Syst Rev* 2013;**4**:CD004937.

10 Estruch R, Ros E, Salas-Salvado J, *et al*. PREDIMED Study Investigators. Primary prevention of cardiovascular disease with a Mediterranean diet. *N Engl J Med* 2013;**368**:1279–90.

Chapter 1.2

Dyslipidaemia

Heinz Drexel

General introduction to pharmacotherapy of dyslipidaemia

Ever since it was recognized that cholesterol is present in atherosclerotic plaques, this has fostered interest in lipid metabolism in blood and tissues. Because the main lipids found in blood—cholesteryl esters and TGs—are apolar, i.e. hydrophobic, they are not soluble in blood like, for example, glucose or urea.

Lipid solubility in the aqueous medium of blood is facilitated by molecules that have both hydrophilic (water-soluble) and hydrophobic (water-insoluble) properties, including phospholipids, unesterified cholesterol, and specific proteins—the so-called apolipoproteins. These amphiphilic molecules form a monomolecular surface layer around the apolar lipid droplet, so building the core of a spherical particle; thus, the lipid droplet and surface layer together become a lipoprotein (see Fig. 1.2.1).

The amount of lipids carried by lipoproteins determines their specific mass, and hence their density. Fig. 1.2.1 illustrates the larger the lipid core, the lower the density of the lipoprotein. This is explained by the lower density of the core lipid droplet, as compared to that of the surface layer.

Lipoprotein research has been instrumental in elucidating the association between cholesterol and atherosclerosis. For a risk factor to become useful in preventive medicine, it is important to prove causality. The mandatory prerequisites for a risk factor to be useful in preventive pharmacotherapy are:

- A strong association.
- An independent association.
- A dose-dependent association.

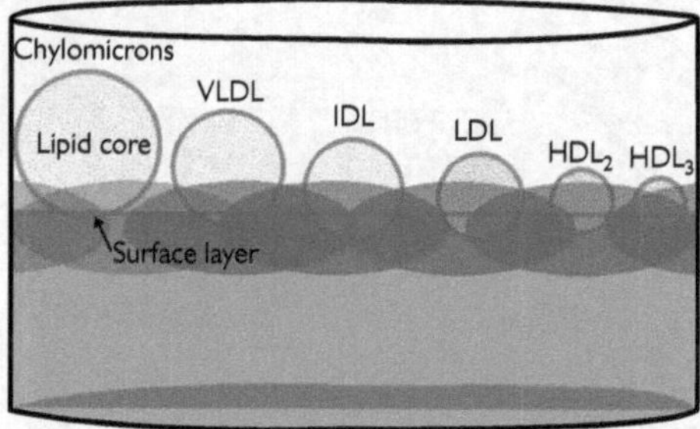

Fig. 1.2.1 Density classes of lipoprotein particles. The lipid core contains low-density hydrophobic molecules and is surrounded by an amphiphilic surface monolayer with high density. Therefore, the rule is that the larger the lipid core, the lower the density of the lipoprotein particle. The lipid core consists mainly of triglycerides and cholesteryl esters. The figure depicts triglycerides in white and cholesteryl esters in yellow. Therefore, the lipoprotein classes are depicted as a mixture of white and yellow, i.e. of triglycerides and cholesteryl esters, respectively.

- The predictive value.
- Consistent data.
- A coherent mechanism.
- Reversibility upon therapy.

LDL is the major transport particle of cholesteryl esters in blood. Its physiological role is to deliver cholesterol to tissues with high cholesterol demands, e.g. the adrenal glands. Given its physico-chemical properties, LDL is also predestined to be deposited in the subendothelial layer of the arterial wall. Therefore, its cholesterol content becomes a primary constituent of an atherosclerotic plaque. The knowledge of this now called 'LDL principle' first came from animal experiments and was subsequently expanded in human epidemiological studies. Recent Mendelian randomization studies corroborated the link between LDL and atherogenesis by proving that life-long elevation of LDL particle mass in blood is strongly associated with atherothrombotic events, as exemplified by MI and stroke.

Three molecules involved in the removal of plasma LDL from blood have been important contributors to understanding how drugs not only lower LDL, but also protect against atherosclerosis. LDL binds to the cell surface (e.g. on hepatocytes) via a specific apolipoprotein—apoprotein B100. On the cell surface, the LDL receptor (LDL-R) is the molecule that binds the LDL particle. The resulting LDL-R complex is taken up into the cell;

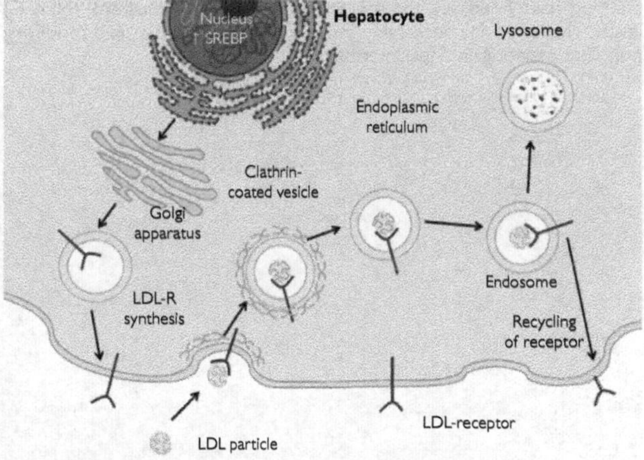

Fig. 1.2.2a LDL uptake from plasma and recycling of the LDL receptor. The uptake of an LDL particle from plasma is facilitated by its specific LDL receptor. In the endosome, the LDL particle and the receptor are separated; the LDL particle undergoes 'digestion' in the lysosome, and the unaltered LDL receptor is recycled to the cell surface, ready to bind the next LDL particle. This is an ideal situation in the absence of PCSK9.[1]

LDL is degraded, and the LDL-R is recycled back to the cell surface (see Fig. 1.2.2a).[1] High functional activity of this uptake increases the cellular concentration of cholesterol, which, in turn, inhibits, via negative feedback, the *de novo* synthesis of cholesterol by the cell itself. The cell meets its cholesterol demands by importing LDL from blood, thereby obviating the need for *de novo* cholesterol synthesis.

This ideal situation is modified by proprotein convertase subtilisin/kexin type 9 (PCSK9) which prevents the intracellular separation of LDL from the LDL-R, consequently leading to the degradation of both the receptor and its ligand. This results in the loss of LDL-Rs available for recycling towards the cell surface. Inherited defects of Apo B and LDL-Rs, and gain-of-function mutations in the *PCSK9* gene all lead to impaired removal of LDL from plasma, as demonstrated in Mendelian randomization studies. This makes it reasonable to therapeutically target cellular LDL uptake by enhancing the receptor number and function.

In brief, the 'LDL principle' explains that high receptor-mediated uptake of LDL from plasma into cells reduces plasma levels of LDL and prevents their incorporation into the arterial wall. By contrast, low LDL uptake, as occurs with low receptor activity or with high PSCK9 levels, results in LDL accumulating in blood and thus attacking the arterial wall (see Figs. 1.2.2b and c).

Given the above explanation, the role of other lipoproteins in atherogenesis becomes less relevant. Indeed, this view is strongly influenced by the evidence that LDL-lowering drugs reduce atherosclerotic events. Other attempts have failed, e.g. the concept of raising HDL cholesterol (HDL-C) levels. This does not necessarily mean that in future other lipid-modifying principles cannot gain equal interest.

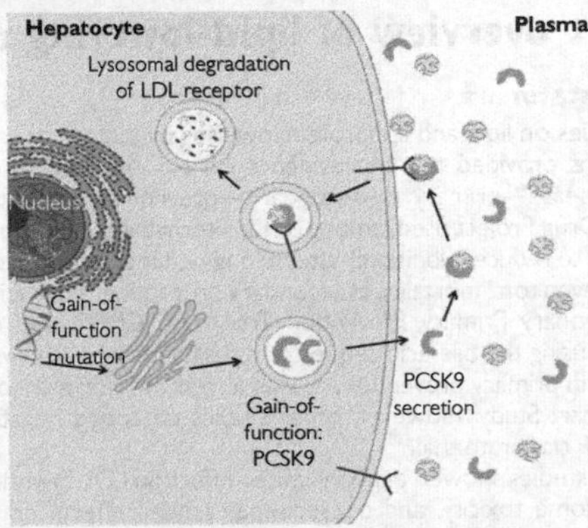

Fig. 1.2.2b Gain-of-function mutation in the *PCSK9* gene → high plasma levels of LDL → high risk for atherosclerosis. In the case of a high PCSK9 plasma level, e.g. as a result of gain-of-function mutations, PCSK9 assembles a binding complex with both the LDL particle and the LDL receptor. PCSK9 acts like glue, such the LDL particle and its receptor cannot be separated in the endosome but are degraded together in the lysosome. Consequently, the recycling of LDL receptors to the cell surface is reduced; LDL particles are not taken up by the cell and thus accumulate in blood. This results in high LDL levels in the plasma, and therefore a high risk for atherosclerosis. Thus, in brief, high PCSK9 levels lead to high LDL levels—in other words, PCSK9 is a 'bad guy'.

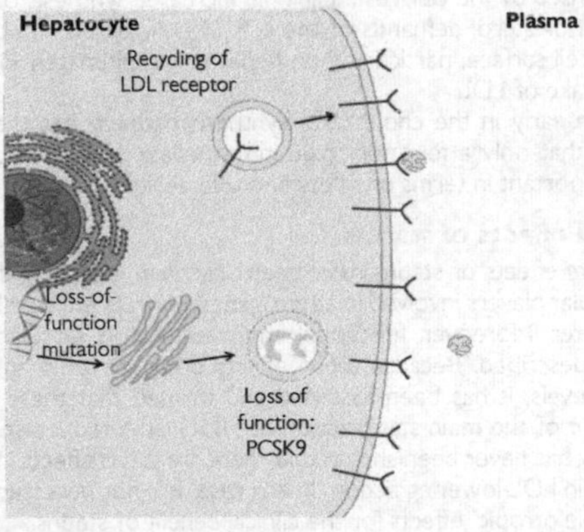

Fig. 1.2.2c Loss-of-function mutation in the *PCSK9* gene → low plasma levels of LDL → atheroprotection. Conversely, in a loss-of-function state of PCSK9, LDL receptors are recycled correctly to the cell surface. A loss-of-function mutation in the *PCSK9* gene therefore leads to a high rate of cellular uptake of LDL and therefore lowers LDL plasma levels, ultimately resulting in atheroprotection.

A short overview of lipid-lowering drugs

The pre-statin era

Earlier studies on lipid and lipoprotein lowering by dietary, as well as drug, interventions provided the first evidence of a positive effect on atherosclerotic disease—primary or secondary—prevention. For example, the Coronary Drug Project used, among other alternatives, nicotinic acid which was proved to reduce (albeit only after a long lag time) atherosclerotic morbidity, and even total mortality, in secondary prevention. The Lipid Research Clinics Coronary Primary Prevention Trial (LRC-CPPT) trial of primary prevention using the bile acid sequestrant resin colestipol showed its positive effects in primary prevention, as was also shown for gemfibrozil in the Helsinki Heart Study. However, other studies described negative effects, e.g. the BHF clofibrate trial.

All these studies showed either a limited effect on LDL lowering or demonstrated some toxicity, and consequently limited effects on preventing clinical endpoints such as MI or stroke. Therefore, this led to an intensive search for more potent and safer agents to lower blood lipids, in particular LDL cholesterol (LDL-C).

The main breakthrough came with the so-called statins which have proved very effective in lowering LDL-C.

Statins: mode of action

These drugs have a unique mode of action—they competitively inhibit the enzyme hydroxyl-methyl-glutaryl coenzyme A (HMG CoA) reductase, which catalyses an early step in the biosynthesis of cholesterol (see Fig. 1.2.3). Statins therefore lower the intracellular level of cholesterol, which is sensed by the cell, resulting in an increased synthesis of LDL-Rs to meet the cholesterol demands of the cell. The increased number of LDL-Rs on the cell surface, particularly on hepatocytes, ultimately increases the cellular uptake of LDL.

Inhibition early in the cholesterol synthesis pathway has the additional advantage that only a few non-toxic intermediate molecules accumulate, which is important in terms of safety and tolerability.

Non-lipid effects of statins

Many *in vitro* effects of statins have been described, including their actions on key cellular players involved in atherogenesis such as endothelial cells and thrombocytes. Moreover, functional improvements in vascular tone have also been described. Because these effects occur earlier than reductions in LDL-C levels, it has been assumed and claimed that these effects are independent of the main statin action of HMG CoA reductase inhibition.[2] However, it has never been shown that there are statin effects independent of their main LDL-lowering action. In any case, it is not necessary to postulate such 'pleiotropic' effects for the clinical benefit of statins.

Statins—the evidence

The main breakthrough for statins came with the publication of the Scandinavian Simvastatin Survival Study (4S) in 1994. This randomized, placebo-controlled, double-blind trial was performed in a high risk

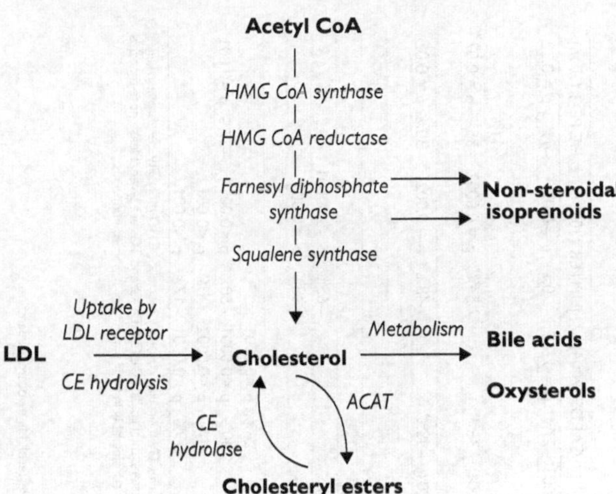

Fig. 1.2.3 Overview of the metabolic and transport pathways that control cholesterol levels in mammalian cells.

population of 4444 patients with high LDL-C and a prior CV event and was stopped at a predefined number of 444 deaths in both the simvastatin arm and the placebo arm. Significant effects were demonstrated for all-cause mortality, atherosclerotic mortality, major and any coronary events, and myocardial revascularization procedures.

Although the 4S was a breakthrough trial, the community waited for a second study corroborating the 4S results. This was accomplished by the CARE study, which showed similar effects in a somewhat lower-risk population. A large number of randomized clinical trials were to follow. To mention just a few, the Long-Term Intervention with Pravastatin in Ischaemic Disease (LIPID) trial was a very large study, as was the Heart Protection Study (HPS). The Collaborative Atorvastatin Diabetes Study (CARDS)[3] focused specifically on patients with diabetes mellitus and even had to be stopped prematurely because of a clear benefit. More recently, the Justification for the Use of Statins in Prevention: an Intervention Trial Evaluating Rosuvastatin (JUPITER) and the Heart Outcomes Prevention Evaluation (HOPE)-3 trials also corroborated the evidence for statins.

For examples of statin trials, see Table 1.2.1a.

The randomized trials have been performed in both primary and secondary prevention settings. It is the merit of the Cholesterol Treatment Trialists' Collaboration (CTTC) to include all available study data in a set of meta-analyses. Moreover, levels were expressed in absolute terms (mmol/L), and not as percentages. The ordinate depicts the percentage reduction in CV events. In the CTTC analysis, the percentage reduction of events was plotted against the absolute reduction in LDL-C. Using this

Table 1.2.1a Examples of statin trials

Endpoint	4S (1994)		CARE (1996)		LIPID (1998)		HPS (2002)		CARDS (2004)		JUPITER (2008)		HOPE-3 (2016)	
Total mortality	–30%	p = 0.0003	–9%	p = 0.37	–22%	p <0.001	–13%	p = 0.0003	–27%	p = 0.059	–20%	p = 0.02	–7%	p = 0.32
Specific mortality														
Cardiovascular	–35%				–25%	p <0.001							–11%	
Coronary/MI	–42%		–37%	p = 0.07	–29%*	p <0.001	–27%	p <0.0001	–36%*		–54%*	p = 0.0002	–35*	p = 0.02
CHD			–20%	p = 0.10	–24%	p <0.001								
Cerebrovascular	–30%*	p = 0.024	–31%	p = 0.03	–19%*	p <0.048	–25%	p <0.0001	–48%*		–48%*	p = 0.002	–30%*	p = 0.02
Non-fatal events														
Any coronary	–27%	p <0.00001												
Major coronary	–34%	p <0.00001												
Non-fatal MI	–37%		–23%	p = 0.01			–38%				–65%	p <0.00001		
Cerebrovascular							–27%				–48%	p = 0.003		
Surrogate parameters														
Total lipids	–25%§		–20%	p <0.0001	–18%+	p <0.001	–20%		–26%	p <0.0001				
LDL-C	–35%§		–28%	p <0.0001	–25%+	p <0.001	–29%		–40%	p <0.0001	–50%‡	p <0.001	–27%	p <0.001
HDL-C	+8%§		+5%	p <0.0001	+5%+	p <0.001	+3%		+1%	p <0.0002	+4%‡	p <0.001		
Triglycerides	–10%§		–14%	p <0.0001	–11%+	p <0.001	–14%		–19%	p <0.0001	–17%‡	p <0.001		

Relative risk reductions by statin therapy and *p*-values are depicted for different endpoint categories: total mortality, CV mortality, coronary mortality, CHD mortality, cerebrovascular mortality, any and major coronary events, non-fatal MI, and non-fatal cerebrovascular events. For surrogate markers, total lipids, LDL-C, HDL-C, and TGs are given. Please note that this compilation does not attempt to comprehensively include all randomized studies performed. Also studies differ considerably in their patterns of reported endpoints.

* Fatal and non-fatal MI/cerebrovascular events.

§ Change from baseline.

\+ Average over first 5 years.

‡ First 12 months.

CHD, coronary heart disease; HDL-C, high-density lipoprotein cholesterol; LDL-C, low-density lipoprotein cholesterol; MI, myocardial infarction.

approach to trial data analysis, it was derived that many interpretations and guidelines focused on the absolute reduction of LDL-C achieved by the investigational drug versus the comparator.[2]

Until then, randomized trials of statins focused on the effects of statins versus placebo. Because the number of residual events in these trials was high—only about one-third of the rate of events in the placebo arm was reduced—later trials tested more intensive statin regimens to reduce LDL-C levels further, with a view to further protect against CV events. Indeed, trials such as Pravastatin or Atorvastatin Evaluation and Infection Therapy (PROVE-IT) and Treating New Targets (TNT) demonstrated additional benefits in reducing events (see Table 1.2.1b). A detailed look at the results reveals clear and significant effects on non-fatal events for which the studies were powered. In contrast to the placebo-controlled trials, these new trials were not powered to demonstrate further mortality reductions. Nevertheless, even trends to lower mortality rates were observed, albeit not significant. This observation should be kept in mind when interpreting trial results on the effects of non-statin lipid-lowering drugs (see Table 1.2.1b).

Moreover, the CTTC performed a further meta-analysis of trials comparing more intensive statin interventions versus standard statins. This

Table 1.2.1b Examples of statin trials: intensive versus moderate lipid-lowering therapy

Endpoint	PROVE-IT (2004)		TNT (2005)	
Total mortality	–28%	p = 0.07	0	p = NS
Specific mortality				
Coronary/MI	–13%*		–20%	p = 0.09
CHD	–30%		–25%*	p = 0.02
Cerebrovascular	+9% (stroke, NS)			
Events				
Major cardiovascular			–22%	p <0.001
Any cardiovascular			–19%	p <0.001
Major coronary			–20%	p = 0.002
Any coronary			–21%	p <0.001
Cerebrovascular			–23%	p = 0.007
Surrogate parameters				
Total lipids LDL-C HDL-C Triglycerides	–10% (P) versus 42% (A)	p <0.001	–49% (A 80) versus 34% (A 20)	

* Fatal and non-fatal MI/cerebrovascular events.

A, atorvastatin; A 80, atorvastatin 80mg; A 20, atorvastatin 20mg; CHD, coronary heart disease; HDL-C, high-density lipoprotein cholesterol; LDL-C, low-density lipoprotein cholesterol; MI myocardial infarction; NS, not significant.; P, pravastatin.

clearly revealed additional benefit in outcome with further lowering of LDL-C. Ever since, for statin trials, one conclusion was drawn for LDL-C: the lower, the better.

Other CTTC publications focused on statin trials in diabetes mellitus and low-risk cohorts, particularly in women.[4] From all these, it emerged that statins provide a very consistent benefit in the prevention of CV events. A similar meta-analysis has recently been published by Silverman *et al.* (2016),[5] which agreed with the concept of 'the lower, the better'. The authors also made a further interesting comment that all lipid interventions that 'ultimately predominantly' increase the activity or number of LDL-Rs improve outcome. In contrast, other lipid interventions [e.g. inhibition of cholesteryl ester transfer protein (CETP)] were deemed not to improve outcomes.

Problems with statins

Ever since the first studies in animals, as well as in humans, there was close attention on untoward statin effects and adverse events. Over the course of treatment with statins, symptoms and conditions of ageing were observed, a paradigm of which was the formation of cataracts. However, when compared to untreated or placebo-treated controls, it soon emerged that there was no increased risk for cataracts in statin users. Therefore, only rates above those for controls were of further interest when the causality of statins for a particular condition was investigated. In line with this concept, cataracts are no longer considered an adverse event caused by statins, but simply a consequence of ageing over the observational periods.

Neurocognitive changes in the early studies of statins were of interest because a positive effect of statins due to cerebrovascular protection seemed possible. Both positive and negative effects of statins were claimed, which sparked a long-standing debate. At present, the view of most experts and in the literature is that statins probably have no consistently measurable effects on mental function. However, it is recognized that better methods than the currently used functional tests are needed to reach a definite answer (see also ➔ PCSK9 inhibitors, pp. 45–6).

The main clinical problem with statins is myopathy. Like cataracts, muscle-related problems were detected very early on with statin treatment. At present, we have excellent data on muscle toxicity both from randomized clinical trials and from registries. Similar to the issue with cataracts, demonstration of muscle symptoms truly caused by statins is mandatory both qualitatively and quantitatively.

A helpful example to study the incidence of statin-induced muscle symptoms is the Heart Protection Study (HPS) trial. Here, the protocol included repeated evaluations of muscle problems, which showed that 32.9% of patients receiving statins developed muscle symptoms. However, due to the double-blind design of the trial, patients in the placebo group also underwent the same repeated scrutiny. A rate of 33.2% of placebo-treated patients with muscle complaints was reported. Thus, no excess rate of muscle symptoms as a result of statin use was detected. This notion is often used in Continuing Medical Education (CME) seminars given by the author. When asked about muscle pain in the preceding 3 months, most physicians not taking statins concede that there have been at least episodes of muscle

Table 1.2.2 Definition of myalgia, myositis, and rhabdomyopathy, after Stroes *et al.* (2015)

Term	CK	Incidence (%)
Myalgia	Normal	2–11*
Myositis	>10 times ULN	1:10,000**
Rhabdomyolysis	>40 times ULN	1:100,000**

* Observational.

** Randomized clinical trials.

CK, creatinine kinase; ULN, upper limit of normal.

discomfort. A recent review by Collins *et al.* (2016)[6] summarized that the incidence of myopathies caused by statins is <1%. Stroes *et al.* (2015) recently reviewed the topic of statin myopathy and gave precise definitions of the terms myalgia, myositis, and rhabdomyopathy, which are detailed in Table 1.2.2.

The clinical picture of statin myopathy is typically characterized by muscle pain and weakness in the proximal extremities.

One major problem encountered by CV pharmacotherapists is statin intolerance, a state defined as an inability or unwillingness to take the drug. Statin intolerance is partly, but not totally, related to muscle problems.

An increase in liver enzymes can be induced by statin therapy. However, no clinical liver disease development has ever been described. Indeed, statins are now considered even for the treatment of some liver diseases such as non-alcoholic fatty liver disease. Current guidelines do not recommend laboratory screening for creatine kinase (CK) or liver enzymes.

One side effect of statins was detected only after many years of randomized studies. For the first time, an increased incidence of physician-reported diabetes mellitus was described in the JUPITER trial. This study investigated the use of rosuvastatin in primary prevention for patients with normal LDL-C but elevated (high-sensitive) C-reactive protein (CRP). From the same study, it was nevertheless clear that CV protection was maintained, as well as strong, also in cohorts with newly detected diabetes. In addition, a meta-analysis of other studies also found an increased diabetes incidence with statins of about 9%, with an absolute incidence of 4.89% in statin-treated patients versus 4.5% in the placebo group or of 3.97% and 4.42% in patients receiving moderate-intensity and high-intensity statin regimens, respectively. By contrast, the magnitude of outcome benefit was approximately 44%. Moreover, a detailed analysis revealed that diabetes onset occurred only a few weeks earlier in patients receiving statins than in placebo-treated patients and that the problem occurred only in patients with high risk for developing diabetes such as those with the metabolic syndrome, but not in patients without such risk factors. From genetic studies and other data, it appears that the mechanism for the increased diabetes incidence includes, perhaps among other factors, the lowering of LDL. This would imply that this effect is not confined to statins only but also can be expected with other LDL-lowering drugs.

Ezetimibe

Among the lipid-lowering drugs, this compound is unique in that its action was detected before its molecular target was known. In terms of evidence for its benefit in reducing CV endpoints, it also happened serendipitously.

Mode of action

Ezetimibe is a competitive inhibitor of the Niemann-Pick C1-like 1 (NPC1L1) protein, which is a sterol transporter in the small intestine. It lowers serum cholesterol and LDL-C levels by about 15% and 18.5%, respectively. Effects on HDL-C and TG levels are small, with an increase of <5% for HDL-C and a reduction of serum TGs by about 8%.

Outcome studies

In the Ezetimibe and Simvastatin in Hypercholesterolemia Enhances Atherosclerosis Regression (ENHANCE) study, ezetimibe was used on a population of heterozygous familial hypercholesterolaemia patients. The study failed to prove an outcome benefit. Next, the Simvastatin and Ezetimibe in Aortic Stenosis (SEAS) study investigated the drug's effects in a population with aortic valve stenosis. Again, no significant outcome benefit was observed. Even worse, an increase in the incidence of carcinoma was obtained. However, when these findings were combined with interim data from the IMProved Reduction of Outcomes: Vytorin Efficacy International Trial (IMPROVE-IT), there was no evidence of an increased incidence of carcinoma. Therefore, the IMPROVE-IT study was continued. In the meantime, the Study of Heart and Renal Protection (SHARP) study demonstrated a combination of simvastatin with ezetimibe to be beneficial in patients with impaired kidney function,[7,8] e.g. the incidence of non-haemorrhagic stroke was reduced significantly in comparison with the placebo group. However, criticism was raised that there was no statin-only comparison group.

The breakthrough for ezetimibe was achieved in the IMPROVE-IT study where a total of 18,144 patients were randomized post-ACS to either simvastatin 40 mg/day alone or ezetimibe 10 mg/day plus simvastatin 40 mg/day. The primary endpoint was a combination of CV death, MI, stroke, hospitalization for unstable angina (UA), and coronary revascularization. The follow-up period was 2.5–7 years. Study termination was endpoint-driven after 5250 events had occurred. The combination therapy of ezetimibe plus simvastatin resulted in an improved outcome. In particular, the incidence of new MIs and ischaemic strokes was reduced significantly. The effect was especially evident in very high-risk patients such as those with diabetes mellitus or those above 65 years of age. In a further more detailed analysis, it was shown that these subpopulations with a high absolute risk for CV events benefitted most from ezetimibe addition.

Recommendations

The 2016 ESC guidelines on dyslipidaemias recommend ezetimibe as follows. The first-line treatment includes use of statins up to the highest recommended or highest tolerated dose[9] (see ➔ Statins—the evidence, pp. 38–42). The next step is ezetimibe with a Class IIa recommendation and level of evidence B (stemming from IMPROVE-IT) (see Table 1.2.3).

Table 1.2.3 Recommendations for pharmacological treatment of hypercholesterolaemia

Recommendations	Class[a]	Level[b]
Prescribe statin up to the highest recommended dose or highest tolerable dose to reach the goal	I	A
In the case of statin intolerance, ezetimibe or bile acid sequestrants, or these combined, should be considered	IIa	C
If the goal is not reached, statin combination with a cholesterol absorption inhibitor should be considered	IIa	B
If the goal is not reached, statin combination with a bile acid sequestrant may be considered	IIb	C

[a] Class of recommendation.
[b] Level of evidence.
Reproduced from Catapano AL, Graham I, De Backer G *et al.* 2016 ESC/EAS Guidelines for the management of dyslipidaemias. *Eur Heart J* 2016; 37: 2999–3058, with permission from Oxford University Press.

International approval

Ezetimibe is approved in most countries for treatment of elevated serum cholesterol and LDL-C, in particular by the US Food and Drug Administration (FDA) and the European Medicines Agency (EMA). Moreover, at the time of writing, ezetimibe is also approved for use in the treatment of ACS by the EMA, but not by the FDA.

PCSK9 inhibitors

Mode of action

PCSK9 binds to the LDL-R and induces intracellular proteolysis of the receptor, predominantly in the liver. Consequently, hepatocellular uptake of LDL by the LDL-R is decreased and LDL blood levels increase. Accordingly, gain-of-function mutations in the *PCSK9* gene have been shown to increase LDL levels and lead to premature atherosclerosis. In contrast, observed loss-of-function mutations in the *PCSK9* gene correlate with low LDL levels and protection from atherosclerotic disease.[1]

It is therefore desirable to lower PCSK9 levels in plasma. Different approaches have been investigated, of which only humanized monoclonal antibodies have entered clinical use. Three monoclonal antibodies have been developed to date: evolocumab, alirocumab, and bococizumab.

In phase I, II, and III studies, these antibodies have been shown to be very effective in lowering LDL-C levels, with a 50–60% reduction achieved. In contrast to alirocumab and evolocumab which lead to sustained reductions of LDL-C, bococizumab also induces inactivating antibodies, which thus diminishes its effects. This is because bococizumab is not a fully humanized antibody, in contrast to alirocumab and evolocumab.

Recently, two outcome studies were published. In the Further Cardiovascular Outcomes Research with PCSK9 Inhibition in Subjects with Elevated Risk (FOURIER) study, the incidence of CV events was significantly reduced in patients with established atherosclerotic coronary, cerebrovascular, or peripheral vascular disease. Importantly, the incidence of both MI and ischaemic stroke was significantly reduced. Crucially, there was an excellent safety profile, with no increase in the incidence of myopathy, cataracts, diabetes, or neurocognitive events reported. However, somewhat disappointingly, CV mortality, and accordingly total mortality, was not reduced. The study was discontinued earlier than expected because trial termination was event-driven by design. The composite primary endpoints included relatively soft endpoints like coronary revascularization and hospitalization for UA, and not mortality only, which meant that the study design did not allow for mortality to be assessed (nor did the study have the statistical power for such assessment).

On the other hand, the FOURIER study showed that reductions in LDL-C even to very low levels (which were not observed in earlier outcome studies) are safe. This finding was supported by the Evaluating PCSK9 Binding Antibody Influence on Cognitive Health in High Cardiovascular Risk Subjects (EBBINGHAUS) study that investigated, in particular, neurocognitive events in patients in whom very low LDL-C levels were achieved. No neurocognitive problems were reported.

In the Studies of PCSK9 Inhibition and the Reduction of Vascular Events (SPIRE) studies to evaluate the efficacy of bococizumab, the FOURIER findings were essentially confirmed. However, the studies were terminated before outcome trials could be completed, because bococizumab was withdrawn from further development by the pharmaceutical company for reasons outlined earlier.

The third monoclonal outcome trial has recently been completed. ODYSSEY OUTCOMES recruited patients at an age of ≥40 with an ACS 1–12 months before inclusion (*n*=18924; medium follow-up of 2.8 years). The main difference to FOURIER is that all these patients had had ACS, thus ODYSSEY OUTCOMES investigated a homogeneous population. The outcome of morbidity events was similar as in FOURIER (−14% reduction in MI, −12% coronary revascularization, −27% ischaemic strokes). In addition, CV mortality and total mortality were significantly reduced but because of a hierarchical stepwise evaluation this was only a nominal endpoint. Both trials also showed excellent safety whereby the relative short duration has to be taken into account.

Interesting news was also found on omega-3 fatty acids, which up to 2018 had not shown clear outcome benefits. In the REDUCE-IT trial 8179 patients were included who received, on top of statins, icosapent ethyl. A significant reduction of the primary endpoint (composite of CV death, non-fatal MI, non-fatal stroke, coronary revascularization, or unstable angina) by 25% was observed; this is a major breakthrough and, because patients were selected on the basis of elevated triglycerides, brings triglycerides back to modern cardiological science. However, in the marine omega-3 fatty acids VITAL trial simple supplementation by omega-3 fatty acids in the nutrition did not significantly improve outcome. Therefore, it is not clear whether the good result of REDUCE-IT is only specific for the compound used or only specific for this population. Further mechanistic studies are needed.

A practical guide to treatment of dyslipidaemia

A major cornerstone in the prevention of atherosclerosis in dyslipidaemia is a healthy lifestyle, including healthy nutrition. The prudent diet in the management of dyslipidaemia is also beneficial to people without dyslipidaemia, and therefore, the cooking approach in every household should consider the principles detailed in the prevention guidelines. Dietary recommendations include, among others, whole grains, raw and cooked vegetables, fresh or frozen fruit, non-caloric sweeteners, lean and oily fish, poultry without skin, and skimmed milk and yogurt.[9] Because this chapter focuses on pharmacotherapy, lifestyle changes are not covered in detail here.

A logical stepwise approach to pharmacotherapy in dyslipidaemia ideally follows the guidelines.[9]

The first step involves estimating a patient's risk using the score tables or, if known CV risk is present, from the patient's past medical history and clinical records. From this, a risk category can thus be defined for the patient, as described in Table 1.2.4, which also details the target LDL-C levels for each CV risk group. If desired, as a secondary target, non-HDL-C levels can also be selected, which is always approximately 30mg/dL higher than LDL-C levels[9] (not shown in the table).

Once the target LDL-C level is established, according to the ESC guidelines, a sequential approach to pharmacotherapy is indicated (see Table 1.2.3). The first step is prescription of a statin at the highest tolerated, or necessary, dose according to the target LDL-C level.

If the target goal is not achieved, the next step is to prescribe ezetimibe. An alternative is a bile acid sequestrant resin, of which colesevelam has found recent interest because it also improves glucose tolerance.

Table 1.2.4 Recommendations for treatment goals for low-density lipoprotein cholesterol

Recommendations	Class[a]	Level[b]
In patients at VERY HIGH CV risk, an LDL-C goal of <1.8mmol/L (70mg/dL) or a reduction of at least 50% if the baseline LDL-C is between 1.8 and 3.5mmol/L (70 and 135mg/dL) is recommended	I	B
In patients at HIGH CV risk[d], an LDL-C goal of <2.3mmol/L (100mg/dL), or a reduction of at least 50% if the baseline LDL-C[e] is between 2.6 and 5.2mmol/L (100 and 200mg/dL) is recommended	I	B
In subjects at LOW or MODERATE risk[d], an LDL-C goal of <3.0mmol/L (<115mg/dL) should be considered	IIa	C

[a] Class of recommendation.
[b] Level of evidence.
Reproduced from Catapano AL, Graham I, De Backer G *et al.* 2016 ESC/EAS Guidelines for the management of dyslipidaemias. *Eur Heart J* 2016; **37**: 2999–3058, with permission from Oxford University Press.

Only if the target goal is still not achieved with statins alone or a combination of statin plus ezetimibe are further combinations necessary or can the novel class of PCSK9 inhibitors be added. In the ESC 2016 guidelines, the addition of PCSK9 inhibitors was given a level of evidence C. However, since publication of the FOURIER study findings, this should be reconsidered as a level of evidence B.

Monitoring of liver enzymes or CK levels is not generally recommended. However, if muscle pain arises, CK levels should be measured. The rationale is to obtain baseline levels of liver enzymes and CK.

The lipid-lowering effect of pharmacotherapy reaches a new steady state after about 12 weeks of treatment. However, an evaluation after only 6 weeks would inform the clinician whether the target goal is achievable or not. In the case of PCSK9 inhibitors, the new target level is reached much sooner, i.e. about 2 weeks, after treatment initiation, so this is an exception to the rule of 6–12 weeks that are required before reaching a new steady state.

References

1 Catapano AL, Papadopoulos N. The safety of therapeutic monoclonal antibodies: implications for cardiovascular disease and targeting the PCSK9 pathway. *Atherosclerosis* 2013;**228**:18–28.

2 Baigent C, Keech A, Kearney PM, *et al.*; Cholesterol Treatment Trialists' (CTT) Collaborators. Efficacy and safety of cholesterol-lowering treatment: prospective meta-analysis of data from 90,056 participants in 14 randomised trials of statins. *Lancet* 2005;**366**:1267–78.

3 Colhoun HM, Betteridge DJ, Durrington PN, *et al.*; CARDS investigators. Primary prevention of cardiovascular disease with atorvastatin in type 2 diabetes in the Collaborative Atorvastatin Diabetes Study (CARDS): multicentre randomised placebo-controlled trial. *Lancet* 2004;**364**:685–96.

4 Fulcher J, O'Connell R, Voysey M, *et al.*; Cholesterol Treatment Trialists' (CTT) Collaboration. Efficacy and safety of LDL lowering therapy among men and women: meta-analysis of individual data from 174,000 participants in 27 randomised trials. *Lancet* 2015;**385**:1397–405.

5 Silverman MG, Ference BA, Im K, *et al.* Association between lowering LDL-C and cardiovascular risk reduction among different therapeutic interventions: a systematic review and meta-analysis. *JAMA* 2016;**316**:1289–97.

6 Collins R, Reith C, Emberson J, *et al.* Interpretation of the evidence for the efficacy and safety of statin therapy. *Lancet* 2016;**388**:2532–61.

7 Baigent C, Landray MJ, Reith C, *et al.*; SHARP Investigators. The effects of lowering LDL cholesterol with simvastatin plus ezetimibe in patients with chronic kidney disease (Study of Heart and Renal Protection): a randomized placebo-controlled trial. *Lancet* 2011;**377**:2181–92.

8 Baigent C, Landray M, Reith C, *et al.*; SHARP Collaborative Group. Study of Heart and Renal Protection (SHARP): randomized trial to assess the effects of lowering low-density lipoprotein cholesterol among 9,438 patients with chronic kidney disease. *Am Heart J* 2010;**160**:785–94.

9 Catapano AL, Graham I, De Backer G, *et al.* 2016 ESC/EAS Guidelines for the management of dyslipidaemias. *Eur Heart J* 2016;**37**:2999–3058.

Chapter 1.3

Metabolic syndrome and diabetes

Christoph H. Saely

The metabolic syndrome, diabetes, and cardiovascular disease

Pathophysiology and definitions

Overweight and obesity, together with a lack of physical exercise, lead to insulin resistance, which, when pancreatic β-cells no longer maintain the high insulin requirement caused by insulin resistance, may lead to type 2 diabetes mellitus (T2DM). Clinically, insulin resistance typically is associated with central obesity, indicated by a large waist circumference, dyslipidaemia characterized by high TGs and low HDL-C, elevated blood glucose levels, and high BP.[1] This cluster of CV risk factors associated with insulin resistance is referred to as the metabolic syndrome (MetS). As a clinical entity, the MetS can be diagnosed when at least three of the five stigmata—large waist circumference, high TGs, low HDL-C, elevated blood glucose levels, or high BP—are present. However, most clinicians currently use the MetS as a pathophysiological concept, rather than as a diagnostic entity.

Diabetes is diagnosed when fasting plasma glucose is ≥126mg/dL, post-challenge plasma glucose after an oral load of 75g of glucose is ≥200mg, or glycated haemoglobin (HbA1c) is ≥6.5%.[2] However, it is important to consider that the pathophysiological development of T2DM is continuous, rather than dichotomous, and that the MetS is not categorically different from T2DM regarding its pathophysiology and partly also regarding its CV consequences.

Cardiovascular consequences

All components of the MetS, as well as the syndrome itself, strongly indicate an increased risk of CV disease, and insulin resistance, as measured by the homeostasis model assessment (HOMA) index, indicates an increased CV risk independently from the clinical diagnosis of the MetS. CV risk further increases when diabetes becomes manifest—partly because overt diabetes indicates a later time point within the cardiodiabetic continuum that leads from insulin resistance over diabetes to CV disease, and partly because high glucose directly damages the artery wall.

In this respect, it is important to consider that not all patients with diabetes are equal. Whereas previously diabetes simply was considered a CHD risk equivalent, we now know that some patients with diabetes are at a higher risk than others and that diabetes mellitus per se does not confer the same amount of CV risk as established CV disease. CV risk is extremely high in patients with diabetes who already have developed end-organ damage.

Given the crucial role of insulin resistance in the development of T2DM, it is clear that T2DM is not merely a disease of increased glucose levels. Other manifestations of insulin resistance or the MetS, particularly dyslipidaemia and arterial hypertension, are also characteristic for T2DM.[1] Moreover, CV risk in the MetS is carried by dyslipidaemia, rather than by elevated blood glucose values. Therefore, it cannot be expected that lowering blood glucose will solve the problem of elevated CV risk in patients with diabetes.

Glucose lowering

Micro- versus macrovascular diabetes complications

Diabetes is diagnosed based on elevated glucose values, and an increasing HbA1c is associated with an increasing risk of CV events in epidemiological observations.[2] Lowering elevated blood glucose therefore appears as a plausible target to reduce the elevated CV risk of patients with diabetes. However, things are not that easy. While microvascular diabetes complications, such as diabetic retinopathy, diabetic nephropathy, or diabetic neuropathy, are specific to diabetes, macrovascular diabetes complications, i.e. manifestations of atherosclerotic CV disease, are not specific to diabetes; however, the risk of atherosclerotic CV disease is increased by a factor of 2–3 in patients with diabetes. CV disease is the most important cause of death in patients with diabetes.

Type 1 diabetes

Type 1 diabetes (T1DM) is pathophysiologically very different from T2DM. It is caused by autoimmune destruction of pancreatic β-cells, and much more than T2DM, it can be regarded primarily as a high glucose disease. Because T1DM in the long term is associated with an increased risk of CV disease, a causal link between high glucose and CV risk appears plausible.

The Diabetes Control and Complications Trial (DCCT) investigated the impact of intensive glucose lowering on diabetes outcomes in T1DM over 6.5 years. Microvascular diabetes complications were significantly reduced, while macrovascular diabetes complications were not significantly reduced during the original trial. However, in the Epidemiology of Diabetes Interventions and Complications (EDIC) study, the long-term open-label follow-up study of DCCT patients, a strong reduction of CV events was observed over a follow-up period of 17 years in those patients who had previously been randomized to more intensive blood glucose-lowering therapy. It thus appears possible that lowering glucose eventually will translate into a reduction of CV events, but only after very long periods of time, and this assumption is not based on the primary evaluation of a randomized trial.

Does lowering glucose lower cardiovascular risk in T2DM?

This concept is supported by observations in patients with T2DM. In the United Kingdom Prospective Diabetes Study (UKPDS), >4000 patients with newly diagnosed T2DM were randomized to what was then considered intensive versus less intensive glucose-lowering therapy, reaching HbA1c values of 7.0% and 7.9%, respectively. Like in the T1DM patients in DCCT, lowering glucose with insulin or sulfonylurea in T2DM patients in UKPDS over 10 years significantly lowered the risk of microvascular complications, but not the risk of macrovascular events such as MI, stroke, or peripheral arterial disease (PAD). However, a long-term follow-up of UKPDS patients again found that previous randomization to more intensive glucose lowering was associated with a reduction of CV events in the long term.

Mean HbA1c values in UKPDS were 7.9% in the less intensive, and 7.0% in the more intensive, treatment arm. Subsequently, it was hypothesized that lowering HbA1c values further may yield further benefits. This was investigated in three large trials—Action to Control Cardiovascular Risk in Diabetes (ACCORD), Action in Diabetes and Vascular Disease: Preterax and Diamicron MR Controlled Evaluation (ADVANCE), and Veterans Affairs Diabetes Trial (VADT). However, the results of these trials were not very convincing.

In ACCORD, high-risk patients with T2DM were randomized to aggressive glucose treatment aiming for an HbA1c of <6.0% versus less intensive glucose lowering according to standard therapy targeting an HbA1c of 7.0–7.9%. The primary endpoint of non-fatal MI, non-fatal stroke, or death from CV causes was not reduced. Most importantly, the trial had to be terminated early because of an increased mortality risk in the more intensely treated patients.

Indeed, overly aggressive glucose lowering may lead to serious consequences, particularly to weight gain and an increased incidence of hypoglycaemia. Hypoglycaemia, in turn, is strongly associated with an increased risk of CV events. Epidemiological studies cannot prove a causal relationship between hypoglycaemia and CV event risk. However, such a causal link is plausible—hypoglycaemia increases the duration of the myocyte action potential and leads to myocyte calcium overload, which are the two most important mechanisms causing cardiac arrhythmia.

Similarly, in the ADVANCE trial, randomization to more intensive glucose lowering aiming for an HbA1c of <6.5%, compared with standard treatment, did not reduce macrovascular events whereas, like in UKPDS, microvascular diabetes complications were significantly reduced. Also in VADT, macrovascular events were not reduced during the original trial with lowering HbA1c to 6.9% versus 8.4%. Again, in the long-term follow-up, the incidence of CV events was lower in those previously randomized to more aggressive blood glucose control in VADT.

Taken together, it appears that lowering blood glucose may reduce CV events in the long term, but not over the time spans typically covered by clinical trials. Lowering blood glucose does not solve the problem of macrovascular disease in patients with diabetes. Current American Diabetes Association (ADA) guidelines recommend an HbA1c of <7.0% primarily for the prevention of microvascular diabetes complications.[2] Because intensive glucose lowering was associated with a lower long-term CV event risk in DCCT, UKPDS, and VADT, and because in subgroup analyses from ACCORD and VADT, more intense glucose control reduced the risk of CV events in healthier individuals without established CV disease or with lower coronary artery calcium scores, a lower HbA1c target for these patients should be considered.[3]

Specific advantages of particular glucose-lowering drugs

Whereas the case is not too strong for CV risk reduction by glucose lowering per se, trials have shown clear CV benefits for some antidiabetic drugs in patients with T2DM at very high CV risk. These results are extremely important for the management of diabetes in patients with established CV disease.

Current guideline recommendations

Current ESC guidelines recommend a target HbA1c of <7.0% for the reduction in risk of CV disease and microvascular complications in diabetes for the majority of non pregnant adults with either T1DM or T2DM and state that a target HbA1c of ≤6.5% should be considered at diagnosis or early in the course of T2DM in patients who are not frail and do not have CV disease.[3] For patients with a long duration of diabetes, the elderly, those who are frail, or those with existing CV disease, a relaxing of the HbA1c targets should be considered,[3] e.g. to a target of <8.0% that is suggested as an option for these patients by the ADA.[2] Also, the European Association for the Study of Diabetes states that the usual HbA1c goal is <7.0%, but that instead of a one-size-fits-all approach, personalization is necessary to balance the benefits of glycaemic control against its potential risks, taking into account, among other considerations, patient age as well as health status and the risk of hypoglycaemia with overly aggressive blood glucose lowering.[4]

Lipid therapy

Lipid therapy is discussed in ➔ Chapter 1.2. In brief, LDL-C is causally responsible for the development of atherosclerosis, and the more LDL-C is reduced, the more the CV risk is also reduced. This holds true for MetS patients, as well as for subjects without the MetS, and for patients with T2DM as well as for non-diabetic patients. In a large meta-analysis of statin-treated patients, the relative risk of CV events was reduced by 22% per mmol (i.e. per 37.8mg/dL) of LDL-C reduction with statins in patients with diabetes, compared to 19% in non-diabetic subjects. The CARDS study already prior to the publication of this meta-analysis had shown that statin treatment reduces CV risk in high-risk primary prevention patients with T2DM. In the large IMPROVE-IT trial, the cholesterol absorption inhibitor ezetimibe in ACS patients significantly reduced CV risk also in patients with diabetes enrolled in this trial.

Current ESC guidelines on lipid management in patients at very high risk recommend LDL-C lowering to <70mg/dL or at least a 50% reduction in LDL cholesterol, when untreated baseline LDL-C is 70–135mg/dL.[3,5] Patients with diabetes who already have end-organ damage, such as diabetic nephropathy or retinopathy, those with diabetes plus another main risk factor for CV events, and those with established CV disease, such as a history of MI or stroke, but also those with atherosclerotic plaques, e.g. at carotid artery imaging, fall into the category of very high-risk patients. This includes the majority of patients with T2DM and all patients with the combination of T2DM and CV disease. Most of the remaining patients with diabetes fall in the category of high CV risk; for them, guidelines recommend an LDL-C of <100mg/dL or a 50% reduction in LDL-C when untreated baseline cholesterol is between 100 and 200mg/dL.

No specific LDL-C targets exist for patients with the MetS. In the presence of risk factors putting MetS patients in the ESC risk categories of very high or high CV risk, the respective LDL-C goals demanded for these risk categories should be attained. For other MetS patients, the 10-year risk of fatal CV risk should be estimated, based on Systematic COronary Risk Evaluation (SCORE) charts; their LDL-C targets depend on this risk estimation.

Unfortunately, most very high-risk patients, and even most patients with the combination of T2DM and CV disease, are not at the recommended LDL-C goal.

Antihypertensive therapy

Antihypertensive therapy in detail is discussed in ➲ Chapter 1.1. The management of hypertension, according to current guidelines, does not differ significantly between patients with the MetS and those who do not have the MetS or between patients with diabetes and non-diabetic individuals.[3]

For all subjects with high-normal BP and for all those with hypertension, lifestyle measures, including weight control, increased physical activity, alcohol moderation, sodium restriction, and increased consumption of fruits, vegetables, and low-fat dairy products, are recommended. In patients with grade 3 hypertension, as well as in those with grade 1 or grade 2 hypertension who are at very high CV risk, drug treatment for arterial hypertension is recommended; drug treatment, according to current guidelines, should also be considered in patients with grade 1 or grade 2 hypertension who are at high CV risk. Given their usually very high or at least high CV risk, drug treatment thus is warranted in hypertensive patients with T2DM.

Blood pressure treatment targets

Irrespective of the presence of the MetS and irrespective of the diabetes status, current guidelines recommend a treatment target of SBP of <140mmHg and DBP of <90mmHg in patients <60 years of age; in patients aged ≥60 years, an SBP target of 150–160mmHg is recommended.[3] The ADA suggests an optional lower BP target of 130/80mmHg in diabetic patients at high risk of CV disease tolerating intensive BP lowering without undue treatment burden.[2]

A meta-analysis addressing outcomes with antihypertensive treatment in T2DM depending on baseline SBP found that total and CV mortality, as well as CAD events, were significantly reduced only with a baseline BP of ≥140mmHg; in contrast, strokes, as well as the development of albuminuria and retinopathy, were reduced also when the baseline BP was <140mmHg.[6]

Choice of blood pressure-lowering medications

Regarding the choice of antihypertensive medications, guidelines provide a class IA statement that all major BP-lowering drug classes (i.e. diuretics, ACEIs, calcium antagonists, ARBs, and β-blockers) do not differ in their BP-lowering potency and thus are recommended as BP-lowering treatment.[3] For patients with diabetes, a weak recommendation is made that ACEIs or ARBs should be preferred.

However, data supporting the superiority of these classes of hypertensive drugs over other BP-lowering options to reduce CV events or the incidence of new nephropathy are not strong. In patients with diabetes who have albuminuria, ACEIs and ARBs probably have specific advantages. Treatment of patients with diabetic kidney disease with an ACEI or an ARB reduces the risk of progressing to ESRD; however, strong evidence is available only for patients with albuminuria of ≥300mg/g of creatinine.

In MetS patients at high risk of developing diabetes, β-blockers and thiazide diuretics are not recommended as primary medications to lower BP because these medications further increase the risk of developing T2DM.[3] These agents, however, are not contraindicated in MetS patients or in diabetes patients, and especially diuretics are frequently used in antihypertensive combination therapy in these patients.

Indeed, most patients with T2DM require antihypertensive combination therapy to achieve BP goals. Initial combination therapy is recommended in patients with markedly elevated baseline BP or at high CV risk, which includes most patients with T2DM. The current guidelines also suggest considering single-pill combinations because of improved patient adherence.[3]

From this background, it is an important question of which antihypertensive combination therapy is best in MetS or diabetes patients. In the Avoiding Cardiovascular Events in Combination Therapy in Patients Living with Systolic Hypertension (ACCOMPLISH) trial, 11,506 patients with arterial hypertension and a high risk of CV events were randomized to receive the ACEI benazepril together with hydrochlorothiazide or together with amlodipine. Over a mean follow-up of 3 years, the primary endpoint of severe CV events was significantly reduced with the ACEI/amlodipine combination, when compared to the ACEI/hydrochlorothiazide combination. This result specifically was also obtained in patients with diabetes; among high-risk diabetic patients, the number needed to treat to prevent one CV event over 3 years was as low as 28.

Antiplatelet therapy

Antiplatelet therapy is discussed in detail in ➲ Chapter 1.4. The MetS, and in particular T2DM, is associated with platelet hyper-reactivity; this contributes to the particularly high risk of atherothrombotic events in T2DM patients with established CV disease. In secondary prevention, aspirin is clearly indicated in patients with the MetS, as well as in those with T2DM, similarly as in patients without these metabolic disorders.[2]

In individuals without CV disease, current ESC guidelines do not recommend antiplatelet therapy due to the increased risk of major bleeding, irrespective of the presence of the MetS and diabetes.[3] Indeed, the efficacy of aspirin to reduce CV events in primary prevention patients with T2DM could not be demonstrated in a dedicated trial. Still, however, the ADA recommends aspirin in men and women with diabetes ≥50 years of age with at least one additional CV risk factor if the bleeding risk is not high.[2] Two ongoing trials—A Study of Cardiovascular Events iN Diabetes (ASCEND) and Aspirin and Simvastatin Combination for Cardiovascular Events Prevention Trial in Diabetes (ACCEPT-D)—investigating the benefits and risks of antiplatelet therapy specifically in patients with diabetes will help to resolve this controversial issue.

Conclusion

A multifactorial approach is required to reduce CV risk in patients with the MetS or diabetes. Glucose control is essential to reduce microvascular diabetes complications and, over long periods of time, may also lower the risk of CV events in patients with diabetes. As in other patient populations, lowering LDL-C and treating arterial hypertension are paramount interventions to reduce CV event risk in patients with the MetS and diabetes. Most patients with diabetes must be considered at very high risk of CV events, which qualifies them for low LDL-C targets. Antiplatelet therapy is recommended for patients with the MetS or diabetes who already have established CV disease. Because the MetS or diabetes confers an extremely high risk of CV events once CV disease is established, it is extremely important to intervene early to prevent these patients from developing CV disease.

References

1 Eckel RH, Grundy SM, Zimmet PZ. The metabolic syndrome. *Lancet* 2005;**365**:1415–28.
2 Standards of medical care in diabetes—2017: summary of revisions. *Diabetes Care* 2017;**40**(Suppl 1):S4–5.
3 Piepoli MF, Hoes AW, Agewall S, *et al.*; ESC Scientific Document Group. 2016 European Guidelines on cardiovascular disease prevention in clinical practice: The Sixth Joint Task Force of the European Society of Cardiology and Other Societies on Cardiovascular Disease Prevention in Clinical Practice (constituted by representatives of 10 societies and by invited experts)Developed with the special contribution of the European Association for Cardiovascular Prevention & Rehabilitation (EACPR). *Eur Heart J* 2016;**37**:2315–81.
4 Inzucchi SE, Bergenstal RM, Buse JB, *et al.* Management of hyperglycaemia in type 2 diabetes, 2015: a patient-centred approach. Update to a position statement of the American Diabetes Association and the European Association for the Study of Diabetes. *Diabetologia* 2015;**58**:429–42.
5 Catapano AL, Graham I, De Backer G, *et al.* 2016 ESC/EAS guidelines for the management of dyslipidaemias. *Eur Heart J* 2016;**37**:2999–3058.
6 Emdin CA, Rahimi K, Neal B, Callender T, Perkovic V, Patel A. Blood pressure lowering in type 2 diabetes: a systematic review and meta-analysis. *JAMA* 2015;**313**:603–15.

Chapter 1.4

Thrombosis

Freek Verheugt

Primary prevention of cardiovascular disease with antithrombotic therapy

Benefit and risk of warfarin in the primary prevention of acute myocardial infarction

The efficacy and safety of warfarin in the primary prevention of ischaemic heart disease (IHD) were studied in the placebo-controlled Thrombosis Prevention Trial in general practices in the United Kingdom in 2540 high-risk men.[1] After 6 years, incident IHD was reduced by 24%, from 13.3% with placebo to 10.3% with warfarin [odds ratio (OR) 0.76, 95% confidence interval (CI) 0.56–1.02; $p = 0.07$]. However, major bleeding occurred in nine cases in the warfarin group, compared to four in the placebo group. Given the complexity of warfarin and the increased risk of bleeding, warfarin is not used in primary prevention.

Benefit and risk of aspirin in the primary prevention of acute myocardial infarction

Six large-scale trials on primary prevention of MI were carried out, including 660,000 person-years in over 95,000 individuals.[2] Coronary heart disease (CHD) mortality and non-fatal MI were reduced by 18% with aspirin, but with an increase of 54% in major extracranial bleeding. Each two major coronary events were prevented by prophylactic aspirin at the cost of one major extracranial bleed. These clinical trials were carried out in general practices, in hypertension clinics, in both, or in neither (see Fig. 1.4.1). Cardiovascular (CV) disease can also be prevented by the use of statins. Although there has never been a randomized trial performed to evaluate the benefit of aspirin relative to that of statins, it is likely that both are effective, given their different modes of action. In fact, observations from statin randomized trials suggest that they potentiate each other. Since the bleeding risk of aspirin is strongly related to the ischaemic risk, the benefit of aspirin may be overshadowed by the bleeding hazard. Even worse, if aspirin is combined with other strategies that halve the risk of a major ischaemic event, like statins do, the benefit of aspirin is almost completed annihilated theoretically (see Table 1.4.1), as shown in the meta-analysis mentioned above.[2] Thus, the efficacy of aspirin in primary prevention should be considered by weighing the risk of ischaemic events against the risk of bleeding. The 2016 ESC guidelines on prevention consider the role of aspirin in patients without CV disease to be unproven[3]—not only because of its suggested cardioprotective effects, but also because there is increasing evidence of chemoprotection of aspirin against cancer.[4]

Table 1.4.1 Five-year benefit and harm of aspirin in the primary prevention of vascular disease

Risk category	Five-year risk of CVD*	Benefit per 1000	Benefit per 1000 with other prevention**	Harm per 1000***	Net benefit per 1000****	Net benefit per 1000 with other prevention
Low	<5%	2	1	1	1	Nil
Medium	5–10%	14	8	4	10	4
High	>10%	20	10	10	10	Nil

* CV disease (CV death, MI, or stroke).

** Theoretical situation in which the risk is halved by statins and other primary prevention measures.

*** Non-fatal GI or extracranial bleeding.

**** Benefit minus harm.

Reproduced from Verheugt FWA. The role of the cardiologist in the primary prevention of cardiovascular disease with aspirin. *J Am Coll Cardiol* 2014;**65**:122–124 with permission from Elsevier.

Study (Ref. #)	Clinical Setting
British Male Doctor Study (7)	5,139 male U.K. physicians invited from the medical directory
Physician's Health Study (8)	22,071 male AMA-registered physicians in the United States invited by letter
Thrombosis Prevention Trial (9)	5,499 high-risk male subjects in 108 general group practice in the United Kingdom
HOT (10)	18,790 male and female hypertensive patients in hypertension clinics worldwide
Primary Prevention Project (11)	4,495 male and female subjects in general practices in Italy
Women's Health Study (12)	39,876 female health professionals in the United States

Fig. 1.4.1 Clinical setting of six major randomized controlled trials of aspirin in the primary prevention of cardiovascular disease. AMA, American Medical Association; HOT, Hypertension Optimal Treatment trial.

Reproduced from Verheugt FWA. The role of the cardiologist in the primary prevention of cardiovascular disease with aspirin. *J Am Coll Cardiol* 2014;**65**:122–124 with permission from Elsevier.

Secondary prevention of cardiovascular disease with antithrombotic therapy

IHD may be clinically silent over many years but usually becomes apparent either as chronic stable angina pectoris or as acute coronary syndrome (ACS).

Antithrombotic therapy in chronic stable ischaemic heart disease

Given the pathophysiology of chronic IHD and its complications, antithrombotic therapy is warranted. The types of pharmacotherapy for conservative and invasive management of chronic CHD will be discussed in ➲ Chapter 2.3.

Antithrombotic therapy in acute coronary syndromes and thereafter

Since coronary thrombosis is pivotal in these syndromes, immediate initiation of antithrombotic therapy is mandated, whether an early invasive strategy is applied or not. After stabilization, long-term antithrombotic therapy is necessary for secondary prevention. The types of pharmacotherapy in the acute phase of ACS and the stages thereafter will be dealt with in ➲ Chapters 2.1 and 2.2.

Stroke prevention in atrial fibrillation

Palpitations, fatigue, and dyspnoea are the common consequences of AF, the commonest heart arrhythmia, especially in the elderly. Thromboembolic stroke is a devastating complication which occurs in 1–5% of patients per year, largely depending on age and any underlying heart or systemic disease. Ischaemic stroke can be effectively prevented by antithrombotic therapy, mostly oral anticoagulation. Pharmacotherapy for this purpose will be discussed in ➲ Chapter 4.1.

Antithrombotic therapy in patients with artificial heart valves

Putting artificial valves in the pulmonary and/or systemic circulation can be complicated by thrombosis of the prostheses and subsequent thromboembolism, which can be prevented by antithrombotic therapy. Both mechanical and biological valves are used, the latter being implanted surgically or percutaneously. Pharmacotherapy to prevent valve thrombosis and thromboembolic complications are described in ➲ Chapter 5.1.

Antithrombotic therapy in patients with heart failure

Patients with heart failure (HF) with reduced left ventricular ejection fraction (LVEF) run a significant risk of stroke. This is probably based on thromboembolism from the dilated left ventricle. Antithrombotic protection for these patients is described in ➲ Chapter 3.1.

Antithrombotic therapy in patients with peripheral artery disease

Peripheral artery disease (PAD) is part of systemic atherosclerotic disease, which includes carotid artery disease and PAD in the lower extremities. Therefore, preventive measures like antithrombotic therapy are similar to that in CHD. Current guidelines give a strong recommendation for antiplatelet therapy. The Antithrombotic Trialists' Collaboration meta-analysis combined results from 42 randomized controlled studies including 9706 patients with intermittent claudication and/or peripheral arterial bypass or angioplasty.[5] In that meta-analysis, vascular death, non-fatal MI, and non-fatal stroke at follow-up were significantly decreased by 23% by antiplatelet drugs, mostly aspirin. In the Clopidogrel versus Aspirin in Patients at Risk of Ischaemic Events (CAPRIE) trial, aspirin 325mg daily was compared head-to-head with the P2Y12 antagonist clopidogrel 75mg daily in 6652 patients diagnosed with PAD. Here clopidogrel showed a relative risk reduction of 24%, compared with aspirin (p = 0.0028), with a 25% reduction in gastrointestinal (GI) bleeding (p = 0.0024).[6] Therefore, clopidogrel monotherapy seems preferable to aspirin 325mg daily monotherapy in the management of symptomatic PAD, but whether this is also true for low-dose aspirin (75–100mg daily) remains questionable.

The 2017 ESC guidelines on peripheral vascular disease recommend dual antiplatelet therapy with aspirin and clopidogrel for at least 1 month only after percutaneous or surgical revascularization.[7] For all situations, single antiplatelet therapy (aspirin or clopidogrel) is recommended. Use of oral anticoagulation, such as vitamin K antagonists (VKAs), has been popular after peripheral artery bypass surgery but proved to be not superior to aspirin—the reason why routine VKAs are no longer often used for this indication.

Antithrombotic therapy in patients after a transient ischaemic attack or an ischaemic stroke

For secondary prevention after a TIA or an ischaemic stroke, mainly either aspirin monotherapy or a combination of aspirin plus dipyridamole and clopidogrel monotherapy have been studied. Aspirin did not perform better than clopidogrel in the CAPRIE trial and showed more GI bleeding.[6] Other options are mainly based on the outcomes of the largest trial in this field [Prevention Regimen for Effectively Avoiding Second Strokes (PRoFESS)].[8] This study, including 20,332 patients, showed that aspirin plus dipyridamole caused significantly more intracranial haemorrhage than clopidogrel (see Fig. 1.4.2) and also significantly more headache and dizziness, but without a reduction in total stroke. Long-term combination of aspirin and clopidogrel should be avoided, because it increases the risk of intracranial haemorrhage, but may be effective and safe if it is given only in the first 3 months after the event. More studies are needed on this combination.

The problem with clopidogrel is that it is a prodrug and needs metabolization into an active metabolite. Only 15% of the drug ends up as an active metabolite. Studies with the stronger platelet P2Y12 blockers like prasugrel and ticagrelor, which are not prodrugs, were welcome in this field. But a new large study [Acute Stroke or Transient Ischaemic Attack Treated with Aspirin or Ticagrelor and Patient Outcomes (SOCRATES)] compared ticagrelor with low-dose aspirin in 13,369 patients and did not show a significant benefit with ticagrelor in stroke, death, or MI (see Fig. 1.4.3).[9] Major bleeding with ticagrelor (0.5%) was similar as with aspirin (0.6%), with no differences in intracranial haemorrhage. Thus, clopidogrel monotherapy seems to offer optimal antithrombotic protection for patients after a TIA or an ischaemic stroke.

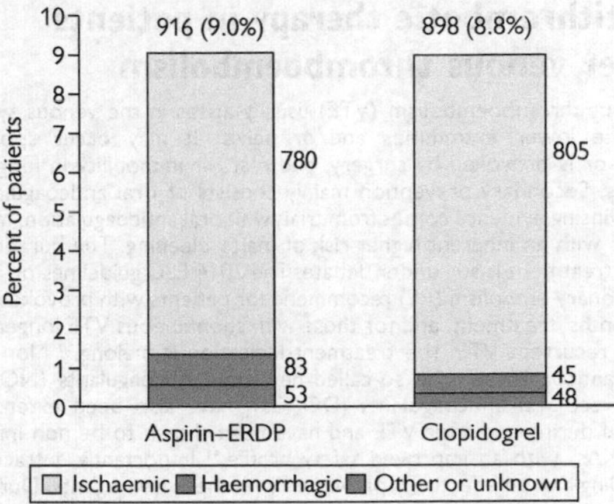

Fig. 1.4.2 Frequency of types of recurrent stroke in PRoFESS. ERDP, extended-release dipyridamole.

Reproduced from Sacco RL, Diener HC, Yusuf S, *et al*. Aspirin and extended-release dipyridamole versus clopidogrel for recurrent stroke. *N Engl J Med*. 2008;359:1238–1251 with permission from Massachusetts Medical Society.

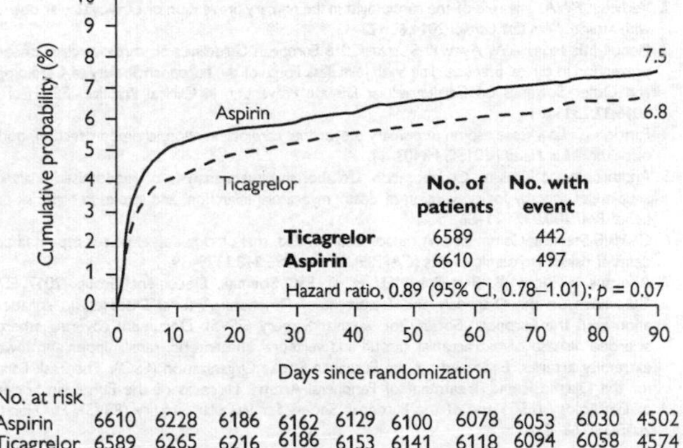

Fig. 1.4.3 Stroke, death, or myocardial infarction in SOCRATES.

Reproduced from Johnston SC, Amarenco P, Albers GW, *et al*. Ticagrelor versus Aspirin in Acute Stroke or Transient Ischemic Attack. *N Engl J Med* 2016;375:35–43 with permission from Massachusetts Medical Society.

Antithrombotic therapy in patients after venous thromboembolism

Venous thromboembolism (VTE) usually arises in the venous system of the lower extremities and/or pelvis. It may occur spontaneous or is provoked by surgery, bed rest, or immobility in long-haul flights. Secondary prevention mainly consists of oral anticoagulation. Convincing evidence comes from trials with oral anticoagulation, mainly VKAs with an inherent higher risk of major bleeding. The duration of VKA treatment is still under debate. The 2014 ESC guidelines on acute pulmonary embolism (PE) recommend for patients with provoked VTE 3 months' treatment, and for those with spontaneous VTE longer, and after recurrent VTE, the treatment indication is lifelong.[10] Non-VKA oral anticoagulants [the so-called new oral anticoagulants (NOACs) or direct oral anticoagulants (DOACs)] have also been extensively tested during and after VTE and have been shown to be non-inferior to VKAs, with an improved safety profile.[11] Importantly, intracranial bleeding can be effectively prevented with these new agents. Duration of treatment is probably similar as with VKAs but may be longer in the future because of the better safety profile and ease of administration. Thus, secondary prevention after VTE can be optimally achieved by oral anticoagulation.

References

1 MRC General Practice Research Framework. Thrombosis prevention trial: randomised factorial comparison of low intensity oral anticoagulation with warfarin and low dose aspirin in the primary prevention of ischaemic heart disease in high risk men. *Lancet* 1998;**351**: 233–41.

2 Verheugt FWA. The role of the cardiologist in the primary prevention of cardiovascular disease with aspirin. *J Am Coll Cardiol* 2014;**65**:122–4.

3 Piepoli MF, Hoes AW, Agewall S, *et al*. 2016 European Guidelines on cardiovascular disease prevention in clinical practice: The Sixth Joint Task Force of the European Society of Cardiology and Other Societies on Cardiovascular Disease Prevention in Clinical Practice. *Eur Heart J* 2016;**37**:2315–81.

4 Patrono C. Low-dose aspirin in primary prevention: cardioprotection, chemoprotection, both, or neither? *Eur Heart J* 2013;**34**:3403–11.

5 Antithrombotic Trialists' Collaboration. Collaborative meta-analysis of randomised trials of antiplatelet therapy for prevention of death, myocardial infarction, and stroke in high risk patients. *BMJ* 2002;**324**:71–86.

6 CAPRIE Steering Committee. A randomised, blinded, trial of clopidogrel versus aspirin in patients at risk of ischaemic events (CAPRIE). *Lancet* 1996;**348**:1329–39.

7 Aboyans V, Ricco JB, Bartelink MEL, *et al*.; ESC Scientific Document Group. 2017 ESC Guidelines on the Diagnosis and Treatment of Peripheral Arterial Diseases, in collaboration with the European Society for Vascular Surgery (ESVS): Document covering atherosclerotic disease of extracranial carotid and vertebral, mesenteric, renal, upper and lower extremity arteries. Endorsed by: the European Stroke Organization (ESO), The Task Force for the Diagnosis and Treatment of Peripheral Arterial Diseases of the European Society of Cardiology (ESC) and of the European Society for Vascular Surgery (ESVS). *Eur Heart J* 2018;**39**:763–816.

8 Sacco RL, Diener HC, Yusuf S, *et al*. Aspirin and extended-release dipyridamole versus clopidogrel for recurrent stroke. *N Engl J Med* 2008;**359**:1238–51.
9 Johnston SC, Amarenco P, Albers GW, *et al*. Ticagrelor versus aspirin in acute stroke or transient ischemic attack. *N Engl J Med* 2016;**375**:35–43.
10 Konstantinides SV, Torbicki A, Agnelli G, *et al*. 2014 ESC Guidelines on the diagnosis and management of acute pulmonary embolism. *Eur Heart J* 2014;**35**:3033–80.
11 Van der Hulle T, Kooiman J, den Exter PL, Dekkers OM, Klok FA, Huisman MV. Effectiveness and safety of novel oral anticoagulants as compared with vitamin K antagonists in the treatment of acute symptomatic venous thromboembolism: a systematic review and meta-analysis. *J Thromb Haemost* 2014;**12**:320–8.

Section 2

Ischaemic heart disease

Section editors

Alexander Niessner
Sven Wassmann

ESC Guidelines advisor
Udo Sechtem

Chapter 2.1

Acute coronary syndrome: STEMI and NSTEMI

Abhiram Prasad and Claire Raphael

Background

ACS encompasses a spectrum of disorders resulting from acute myocardial ischaemia. Rupture or erosion of an unstable atheromatous plaque leads to acute intracoronary thrombosis, platelet activation, release of acute inflammatory mediators, and coronary vasoconstriction.[1]

Two major clinical presentations have been identified that require emergent/urgent and effective treatment:

- ST-segment elevation MI (STEMI).
- UA and non-ST-segment elevation MI (NSTEMI).

Despite a broadly common pathophysiological background, differences exist between these two forms of ACS regarding treatment, mainly in relation to the timing of reperfusion therapy.

The clinical presentation and chest pain characteristics are important for defining the likelihood that a patient has an ACS and also for risk stratification[2] (see Fig. 2.1.1).

- Typical chest pain is characterized by a retrosternal sensation of pressure or heaviness ('angina') radiating to the left arm (less frequently to both arms or to the right arm), neck, or jaw, which may be intermittent (usually lasting several minutes) or persistent.
- Additional symptoms may be present, e.g. sweating, nausea, abdominal pain, dyspnoea, and syncope.
- Atypical presentations include epigastric pain, indigestion-like symptoms, and dyspnoea—more often in the elderly, women, and patients with diabetes, chronic renal disease, or dementia.
- The resting 12-lead electrocardiogram (ECG) should be performed within 10min of arrival to the emergency room in patients suspected of ACS, in order to promptly diagnose STEMI or severe ischaemia (see Fig. 2.1.1).
- Troponin levels are helpful in the diagnosis, risk stratification, and management of patients with suspected NSTEMI.

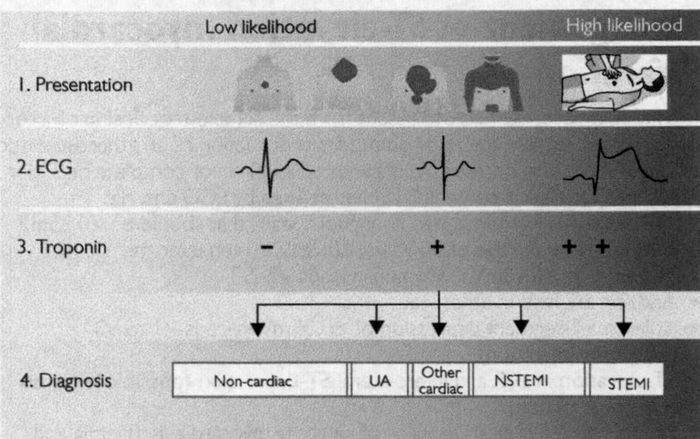

Fig. 2.1.1 Initial assessment of patients with suspected acute coronary syndromes. The initial assessment is based on the integration of low-likelihood and/or high-likelihood features derived from clinical presentation (i.e. symptoms and vital signs), 12-lead ECG, and cardiac troponin levels. The proportion of the final diagnoses derived from the integration of these parameters is visualized by the size of their respective boxes. 'Other cardiac' includes, among others, myocarditis, Takotsubo cardiomyopathy, or tachyarrhythmias. 'Non-cardiac' refers to thoracic diseases such as pneumonia or pneumothorax. Cardiac troponin should be interpreted as a quantitative marker—the higher the level, the higher the likelihood for the presence of myocardial infarction. In patients presenting with cardiac arrest or haemodynamic instability of presumed cardiovascular origin, echocardiography should be performed/interpreted by trained physicians, immediately following a 12-lead ECG. If the initial evaluation suggests aortic dissection or pulmonary embolism, D-dimers and multi-detector computed tomography angiography are recommended, according to dedicated algorithms. NSTEMI, non-ST-elevation myocardial infarction; STEMI, ST-elevation myocardial infarction; UA, unstable angina.

Management of ST-elevation myocardial infarction

In STEMI, myocardial necrosis results from the complete occlusion of a coronary vessel, usually due to thrombus from disruption of an atherosclerotic plaque. Myocardial necrosis occurs within 15–30min of complete occlusion.

In a proper clinical context, STEMI is defined by ECG criteria:

- ST-segment elevation in two contiguous leads that should be ≥0.25mV in men below the age of 40 years, ≥0.2mV in men over the age of 40 years, or ≥0.15mV in women in leads V2–V3.
- And/or ≥0.1mV in other leads.
- Isolated ST-segment depression of ≥0.05mV in leads V1 to V3 (posterior infarction).
- ST-elevation in aVR and inferolateral ST-depression (possible left main stem obstruction).
- Patients with a clinical suspicion of ongoing myocardial ischaemia and left bundle branch block (LBBB) should be managed in a way similar to STEMI patients, regardless of whether the LBBB was previously known. Primary percutaneous coronary intervention (PPCI) should be considered when persistent ischaemic symptoms occur in the presence of right bundle branch block (RBBB).

These ECG changes are associated with a rise in cardiac troponins, but it is important to note that, if suspected, STEMI should be treated immediately, even before the result of cardiac troponins is available.

For STEMI, the goal is restoration of coronary perfusion. This is most commonly achieved via PPCI, as it is the preferred reperfusion therapy for the treatment of STEMI. However, fibrinolysis may be used within 12h of symptom onset if the anticipated time between STEMI diagnosis and reperfusion (wire-crossing) would be >120min. The management algorithm for STEMI patients is shown in Fig. 2.1.2.[3] PPCI is indicated even if symptoms may have started >12h beforehand if there is evidence of ongoing ischaemia or if pain and ECG changes have been stuttering. PPCI is indicated for patients with severe acute heart failure (HF) or cardiogenic shock.

In addition to reperfusion therapy (PPCI or thrombolysis), the following pharmacological treatments should be administered (see Table 2.1.1).

General measures for patient stabilization

- Oxygen—for hypoxia and acute HF.
- Morphine and nitrates for pain relief.
- NSAID analgesics should not be used.
- Atropine may be required for treatment of bradycardia.

Antiplatelet therapy

- Aspirin.
- P2Y12 inhibitor:
  - Prasugrel or ticagrelor (PPCI).
  - Clopidogrel (PPCI or fibrinolysis).
  - Cangrelor.
- Glycoprotein IIb/IIIa receptor inhibitors (abciximab, eptifibatide, tirofiban): administered during PPCI if angiographic evidence of a massive thrombus, slow or no reflow, or a thrombotic complication.

Anticoagulants

Typically administered during PPCI/fibrinolysis. Options are:

- Unfractionated heparin (UFH) (PPCI/fibrinolysis).
- Low-molecular-weight heparin (LMWH)/enoxaparin (PPCI/fibrinolysis).
- Direct thrombin inhibitors (bivalirudin, PPCI).
- Factor Xa inhibitor/fondaparinux (fibrinolysis).

Fibrinolytics

- Tenecteplase, alteplase, reteplase (see Table 2.1.1 for contraindications).

Secondary prevention medications

- Aspirin—for patients who are intolerant of aspirin, clopidogrel is an alternative.
- DAPT with a combination of aspirin and prasugrel or aspirin and ticagrelor is recommended (over aspirin and clopidogrel) in patients treated with percutaneous coronary intervention (PCI).
- β-blockers: oral treatment with β-blockers is indicated in patients with HF and/or LVEF ≤40%, unless contraindicated. Routine oral treatment with β-blockers should be considered in all patients without contraindications.

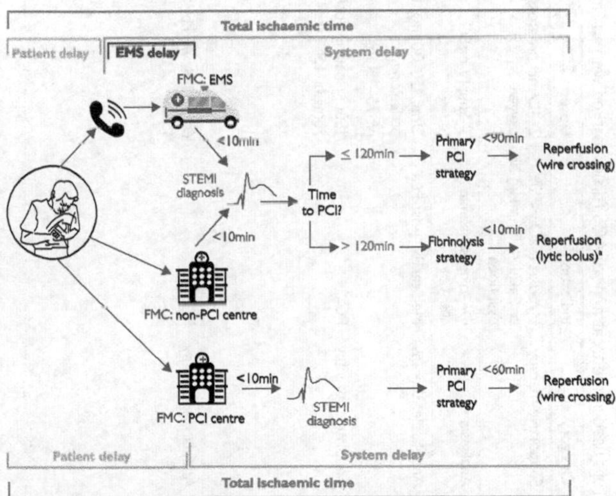

Fig. 2.1.2 Prehospital and in-hospital management and reperfusion strategies within 24h of first medical contact. FMC, first medical contact.

Reproduced from Neumann FJ, Sousa-Uva M, Ahlsson A. 2018 ESC/EACTS Guidelines on myocardial revascularization. *Eur Heart J* 2019;40(2):87–165, with permission from Oxford University Press.

Table 2.1.1 Drugs used in the treatment of ACS (drugs marked with an * are only considered in STEMI)

Therapy	Category	Indication	Dose	Contraindications	Cautions
Oxygen	Supportive therapy	Hypoxia (SaO_2 <90% or PaO_2 <60mmHg) or dyspnoea	2–4L/min progressing to high-flow oxygen	–	COPD
Morphine	Analgesia	Ongoing ischaemic chest pain	3–5mg IV or SC	Opioid allergy	Respiratory depression, bradycardia
Aspirin	Antiplatelet therapy	Medical Rx/post-PCI	Oral: 150–300mg, then 75–100mg od lifelong IV: 75–150mg	Aspirin/NSAID hypersensitivity	Asthma, allergic disease, history of severe bleeding, severe hepatic impairment
Ticagrelor	Antiplatelet therapy	PCI	180mg loading dose, followed by 90mg bd for 1 year	Anaphylactic reaction to drug in the past, previous intracranial haemorrhage or ongoing bleeding, severe hepatic impairment	Increased bleeding risk, oral anticoagulant therapy
Prasugrel	Antiplatelet therapy	PCI	60mg, followed by 10mg od for 1 year	Anaphylactic reaction to drug in the past, previous intracranial haemorrhage, ischaemic stroke or TIA or ongoing bleeding, severe hepatic impairment	Increased bleeding risk, age ≥75 years, body weight <60kg. In case prasugrel is used in these patients, a reduced dose (5mg) is recommended.

Clopidogrel	Antiplatelet therapy	Medical Rx/PCI	600mg, followed by 75mg od for 1 year	Anaphylactic reaction to drug in the past, ongoing bleeding	Increased risk of bleeding
Cangrelor	Antiplatelet therapy	PCI	30 mcg/kg IV bolus prior to PCI, then 4mcg/kg/min IV infusion for at least 2h or for the duration of PCI	Anaphylactic reaction to drug in the past, ongoing bleeding	History of bleeding/ predisposition to bleeding
Nitrates	Anti-ischaemic therapy	Angina	Sublingual GTN every 5min for 15min, then IV GTN	Recent use of type 5 phosphodiesterase inhibitor (e.g. sildenafil)	Hypotension
UFH	Anticoagulant	PCI	70–100U/kg IV bolus when no glycoprotein IIb/IIIa inhibitor is planned; 50–70U/kg IV bolus with glycoprotein IIb/IIIa inhibitors. Titrate to ACT	HIT, heparin allergy	History of bleeding, recent cerebral haemorrhage, haemophilia
		Fibrinolytics	60U/kg IV bolus with a maximum of 4000U, followed by an IV infusion of 12U/kg with a maximum of 1000U/h for 24–48h. Target aPTT: 50–70s or 1.5–2.0 times that of control		

(Continued)

Table 2.1.1 (*Contd.*)

Therapy	Category	Indication	Dose	Contraindications	Cautions
Enoxaparin	Anticoagulant	PCI	0.5mg/kg IV bolus	HIT, heparin allergy	History of bleeding, recent cerebral haemorrhage, haemophilia
		Anticoagulant for ACS treatment	1mg/kg administered SC bd, reduce to 1mg/kg od if eGFR <30mL/min/1.73m^2	LMWH should not be administered in patients with eGFR <15mL/min/1.73m^2	
		Fibrinolytics	In patients aged <75 years: 30mg IV bolus, followed 15min later by 1mg/kg SC every 12h until hospital discharge for a maximum of 8 days. The first two doses should not exceed 100mg In patients aged >75 years: no IV bolus; start with first SC dose of 0.75mg/kg with a maximum of 75mg for the first two SC doses In patients with creatinine clearance (CrCl) of <30mL/min, regardless of age, the SC doses are given once every 2h		
Bivalirudin	Anticoagulant	PCI	0.75mg/kg IV bolus, then infusion of 1.75mg/kg/h during procedure and for up to 4h after procedure	Anaphylactic reaction to drug in the past, ongoing bleeding	History of bleeding, recent cerebral haemorrhage, haemophilia
Fondaparinux	Anticoagulant	Fibrinolytics	2.5mg IV bolus, followed by an SC dose of 2.5mg od up to 8 days or hospital discharge	Do not give if the patient is scheduled for immediate angiography	

Glycoprotein IIb/IIIa antagonist	Antiplatelet therapy	PCI: high thrombus load, reduced coronary flow, potential for malabsorption of oral antiplatelet medications, mechanical complications of PCI (e.g. dissection)	Abciximab: bolus of 0.25mg/kg over 1min, followed by an IV infusion of 0.125mcg/kg/min Tirofiban: bolus of 25mcg/kg over 3min, then infusion of 0.15mcg/kg/min for up to 18h Eptifibatide: double bolus of 180mcg/kg IV (given at 10-min interval), followed by an infusion of 2.0mcg/kg/min for 18h	Active bleeding, recent trauma, severe untreated hypertension (>200 systolic), thrombocytopenia	Renal impairment, pregnancy, history of bleeding/predisposition to bleeding
Fibrinolytic agent	Reperfusion therapy	See text	Alteplase: 15mg IV bolus, then 0.75mg/kg over 30min (max 50mg), then 0.5mg/kg over 1h (max 35mg) with IV heparin Reteplase: 10U IV over 1–2min, then additional 10U after 30min Tenecteplase: 30–50mg IV (dosing chart by body weight) over 10s	Previous intracranial haemorrhage or stroke of unknown origin Ischaemic stroke in last 6 months Major head trauma in last 3 weeks Aortic dissection Non-compressible punctures in past 24h, e.g. lumbar puncture Bleeding disorders GI bleed in last month	TIA in last 6 months Oral anticoagulant therapy Pregnancy or within 1 week postpartum Refractory hypertension (SBP >180mmHg) Advanced liver disease Active peptic ulcer Prolonged or traumatic resuscitation

ACT, activated clotting time; aPTT, activated partial thromboplastin time; eGFR, estimated glomerular filtration rate; GTN, glyceryl trinitrate; TIA, transient ischaemic attack.

Table 2.1.2 Contraindications to fibrinolytic therapy

Absolute
Previous intracranial haemorrhage or stroke of unknown origin at any time
Ischaemic stroke in the preceding 6 months
Central nervous system damage or neoplasms or arteriovenous malformation
Recent major trauma/surgery/head injury (within the preceding month)
Gastrointestinal bleeding within the past month
Known bleeding disorder (excluding menses)
Aortic dissection
Non-compressible punctures in the past 24h (e.g. liver biopsy, lumbar puncture)
Relative
Transient ischaemic attack in the preceding 6 months
Oral anticoagulant therapy
Pregnancy or within 1 week postpartum
Refractory hypertension (SBP >180mmHg and/or DBP >110mmHg)
Advanced liver disease
Infective endocarditis
Active peptic ulcer
Prolonged or traumatic resuscitation

Reproduced from Ibanez B, James S, Agewall S, et *al.* 2017 ESC Guidelines for the management of acute myocardial infarction in patients presenting with ST-segment elevation. *Eur Heart J* 2018;39 (2):119–177 with permission from Oxford University Press.

- ACEIs or ARBs are indicated in patients with evidence of acute HF, LV systolic dysfunction, diabetes, or an anterior infarction. ACEIs should be considered in all patients in the absence of contraindications.
- Lipid-lowering drugs (high-intensity statins, started early after admission, regardless of initial cholesterol values). An LDL-C goal of <1.8mmol/L (70mg/dL) or a reduction of at least 50% if the baseline LDL-C is between 1.8 and 3.5mmol/L (70–135mg/dL) is recommended. Consider adding a non-statin treatment to patients at high risk who do not reach treatment targets after STEMI despite the maximum tolerated dose of statin.
- Aldosterone antagonists are indicated in patients with an ejection fraction of ≤40% and HF or diabetes, provided there is no renal failure or hyperkalaemia.

Management of non-ST-elevation myocardial infarction and unstable angina

In NSTEMI, myocardial necrosis is caused by plaque instability with a non-occlusive thrombus or embolization of micro-thrombi from larger vessels. ECG changes associated with NSTEMI and UA include:

- Persistent or transient ST-depression.
- T-wave changes (inversion, flattening, pseudo-normalization).

UA is diagnosed when there is new-onset severe angina, angina occurring at rest, or—in the case of previously diagnosed angina—angina which is increasing in frequency or with reduced exertion, in the absence of troponin elevation. The incidence of UA has decreased with the use of high-sensitivity troponin assays, resulting in more patients being diagnosed with NSTEMI.

Although patients presenting with NSTEMI have lower immediate and short-term mortality than those with STEMI, long-term mortality is significantly increased, and so NSTEMI should also be managed aggressively.

Fig. 2.1.3 describes the diagnostic approach and early risk stratification using GRACE (Global Registry of Acute Coronary Events) risk score and high-sensitivity troponin. High-risk patients are managed with an early invasive strategy:

- Very high risk criteria include haemodynamic instability or cardiogenic shock, recurrent or ongoing chest pain refractory to medical treatment, life-threatening arrhythmias or cardiac arrest, mechanical complications of MI, acute HF, and recurrent dynamic ST–T wave changes.
- High risk criteria include rise or fall in cardiac troponin compatible with MI, dynamic ST- or T-wave changes (symptomatic or silent), and GRACE score of >140.
- Intermediate risk criteria include diabetes mellitus, LVEF of <40% or congestive heart failure (CHF), early post-infarction angina, prior PCI or coronary artery bypass graft (CABG), and GRACE risk score of 110–139.

General measures for patient stabilization

- Oxygen—for hypoxia and acute HF.
- Morphine and nitrates for pain relief.
- NSAID analgesics should not be used.
- Atropine may be required for treatment of bradycardia.

Anti-ischaemic medications

- Nitrates (at presentation).
- β-blockers (at presentation and in chronic secondary prevention).

Antiplatelet therapy

- Aspirin (at presentation).
- P2Y12 inhibitor (at presentation)—options include:
  - Prasugrel (only for patients who are proceeding to PCI).
  - Ticagrelor.
  - Clopidogrel (for patients who cannot receive ticagrelor or prasugrel or who require oral anticoagulation).
- Glycoprotein IIb/IIIa receptor inhibitors (abciximab, eptifibatide, tirofiban): considered for bailout situations or thrombotic complications during PCI.

Anticoagulants

Options include:
- UFH (at presentation).
- Fondaparinux (at presentation).
- Bivalirudin (initiated at the time of PCI).
- Enoxaparin (at presentation). Crossover between UFH and enoxaparin is not recommended.

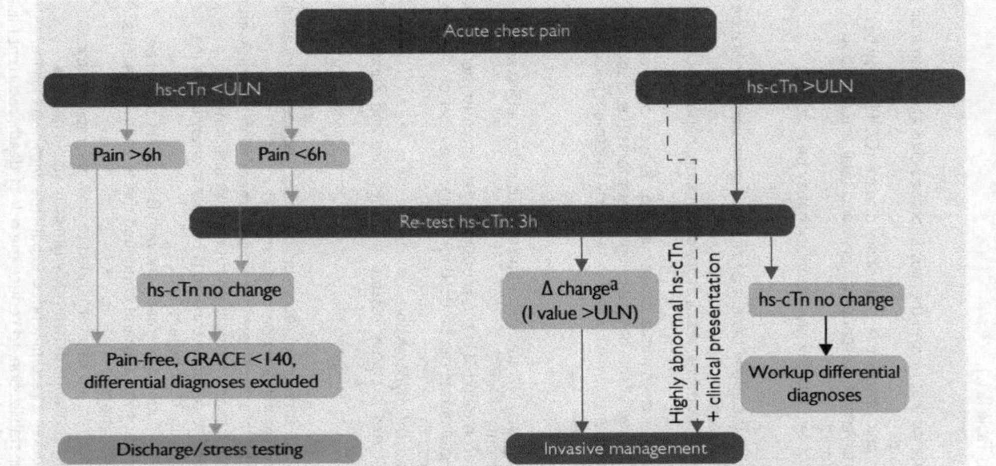

Fig. 2.1.3 The 3-hour rule-out algorithm of non-ST-segment elevation acute coronary syndromes using high-sensitivity cardiac troponin assays. GRACE, Global Registry of Acute Coronary Events score; hs-cTn, high-sensitivity cardiac troponin; ULN, upper limit of normal, 99th percentile of healthy controls. [a]Δ change, dependent on assay. Highly abnormal hsTn defines values beyond 5-fold the upper limit of normal.

Reproduced from Roffi M, Patrono C, Collet J-P, *et al.* 2015 ESC Guidelines for the management of acute coronary syndromes in patients presenting without persistent ST-segment elevation. *Eur Heart J.* 2016;37(3):267–315, with permission from Oxford University Press.

Pharmacological agents

Choice of drugs and indications may vary between STEMI and NSTEMI and are summarized in Table 2.1.1.

Oxygen

- There is no evidence that oxygen therapy improves clinical outcome or reduces infarct size.
- Patients with chronic obstructive pulmonary disease (COPD) may be given high-flow oxygen at presentation, provided their arterial blood gases are monitored.
- In severe cases of hypoxia, invasive ventilation may be required.

Morphine

- Alleviating pain has the added benefit of reduced sympathetic activation and myocardial oxygen demand.
- Side effects: nausea, vomiting, respiratory depression, hypotension, and bradycardia.
- Morphine use is associated with a slower uptake, delayed onset of action, and diminished effects of oral antiplatelet agents (i.e. clopidogrel, ticagrelor, and prasugrel), which may lead to early treatment failure in susceptible individuals.

Nitrates

Nitrates are vasodilators. Nitrates should be used to relieve angina and prevent/relieve symptoms of HF.

- IV nitrates are recommended in the acute management of ischaemic episodes. Sublingual nitrate can be used for immediate relief of ischaemia/angina.
- Side effects: headache, hypotension.

Tolerance to nitrates is closely related to drug dose and duration of treatment.

Beta-blockers

Administration of β-adrenergic receptor blockers reduces myocardial workload and increases the duration of diastole.

- Early initiation of β-blocker treatment is recommended in patients with ongoing ischaemic symptoms and without contraindications.
- It is recommended to continue chronic β-blocker therapy unless the patient is in Killip class III or higher.
- In STEMI patients, routine oral treatment with β-blockers should be considered during hospital stay and continued thereafter in all patients without contraindications.
- Intravenous β-blockers are recommended to slow the rapid ventricular response to atrial fibrillation in haemodynamically stable patients.
- Long-term β-blocker is recommended in patients with heart failure/LVEF ≤40% after stabilization, to reduce the risk of death, recurrent MI, and hospitalization for HF.
- Side effects: bradycardia, HF, hypotension, conduction disturbances, peripheral artery vasoconstriction, bronchospasm, headaches, and fatigue.

Antiplatelet agents

Aspirin: aspirin is a cyclo-oxygenase (COX) inhibitor, preventing the production of thromboxane A_2 and thereby reducing platelet aggregation and thrombus formation. Aspirin should be given to all patients with suspected ACS, unless contraindicated.

- 150–300mg chewable, non-enteric-coated aspirin, followed by 75–100mg once daily (od) indefinitely.
- May be given IV or via a nasogastric (NG) tube in patients who cannot swallow.
- Side effects: GI bleeding, rarely bronchospasm in patients with the syndrome of asthma, rhinitis, and nasal polyps, and anaphylactic shock in aspirin-allergic patients.

A proton pump inhibitor (PPI), in combination with DAPT, is recommended in patients at higher-than-average risk of GI bleeds (i.e. history of GI ulcer/haemorrhage, anticoagulant therapy, chronic NSAID/corticosteroid use, or two or more of the following: age ≥65 years, dyspepsia, gastro-oesophageal reflux disease, *Helicobacter pylori* infection, chronic alcohol use). More recently, a more liberal use of PPIs for all patients on DAPT has been recommended.[4]

$P2Y_{12}$ (ADP) receptor inhibitors (clopidogrel, prasugrel, ticagrelor): $P2Y_{12}$ receptor antagonists further reduce platelet aggregation and should be used in conjunction with aspirin.[4]

- In patients with stent implantation, DAPT with a P2Y12 inhibitor on top of aspirin is recommended for 12 months, unless there are contraindications such as excessive risk of bleeding (e.g. PRECISE-DAPT ≥25).
- In patients with stent implantation who are at high risk of bleeding (e.g. PRECISE-DAPT ≥25), discontinuation of P2Y12 inhibitor therapy after 6 months should be considered.
- In patients with ACS who have tolerated DAPT without a bleeding complication, continuation of DAPT for longer than 12 months may be considered.
- Lifelong single antiplatelet therapy should be continued thereafter, usually aspirin.

Clopidogrel

- First P2Y12 receptor antagonist to be used in ACS treatment.

Clopidogrel may be used when prasugrel or ticagrelor are not available or are contraindicated, including those with prior intracranial bleeding or indication for oral anticoagulants.

- Absorption and onset of action are longer than of prasugrel or ticagrelor.

A small number of patients are clopidogrel-resistant, and if this is suspected, an alternative agent should be used.

- Side effects: bleeding, skin rash, GI intolerance.

Prasugrel

- A prodrug that irreversibly blocks the P2Y12 platelet receptor. Shorter time of onset and more potent platelet inhibition than clopidogrel.
- Side effects: bleeding

Ticagrelor

- Reversible P2Y12 inhibitor. Shorter time of onset and more potent platelet inhibition than clopidogrel.
- Side effects: bleeding, dyspnoea, ventricular pauses.

Cangrelor

- Potent IV reversible P2Y12 inhibitor with a rapid onset and offset of action.
- May be considered in patients not pre-treated with oral P2Y12 receptor inhibitors at the time of PCI or in those who are considered unable to absorb oral agents.

Key facts

- If cardiac or non-cardiac surgery is indicated, ticagrelor, clopidogrel, and prasugrel should be stopped for 3, 5, and 7 days, respectively, prior to the intervention, when possible, to minimize the risk of excessive bleeding.
- There is a theoretical concern regarding the concomitant use of clopidogrel and PPIs; however, there are minimal data to suggest an effect on clinical outcomes. ESC guidelines suggest newer PPIs, such as pantoprazole, may be preferable; however, they do not discourage the use of omeprazole.

Glycoprotein IIb/IIIa antagonists

These include abciximab, eptifibatide, and tirofiban. These agents block the final pathway of platelet aggregation by inhibiting the cross-linking of platelets. Abciximab is a monoclonal antibody, eptifibatide a cyclic peptide, and tirofiban a peptidomimetic inhibitor.

They may be used in ACS patients undergoing PCI, predominantly in the situation of a high thrombus load, reduced coronary flow, and mechanical complications of PCI (e.g. dissection).

Key facts

- Not recommended for routine use in PCI.
- Must be combined with anticoagulant therapy (heparin).
- Inherent risk of bleeding by virtue of their mode of action.
- Thrombocytopenia may occur rarely, and platelet counts need regular monitoring during prolonged infusion (infrequent in current practice). Thrombocytopenia can last for up to 5 days after termination of infusion.
- In contemporary practice, therapy is often limited to the procedure, or a few hours thereafter, to reduce bleeding risk and cost.
- Intracoronary administration is not superior to IV use.

Anticoagulant agents

Anticoagulants should be administered to all patients with ACS. During PCI, if UFH is given, activated clotting time (ACT) is maintained between 250 and 300s.

Indications in STEMI

- Prior to coronary revascularization with PPCI:
  - Routine use of UFH is recommended.
  - Bivalirudin, a direct thrombin inhibitor, is recommended in patients with a history of heparin-induced thrombocytopenia (HIT). Routine use should be considered (Class IIa).
  - Routine use of IV enoxaparin should be considered (Class IIa).
  - Fondaparinux is contraindicated.
- With fibrinolytic administration (alteplase, reteplase, tenecteplase):
  - Enoxaparin IV followed by subcutaneously (SC) (preferred over UFH).
  - UFH.
  - Fondaparinux (in patients treated with streptokinase).
- In patients in whom fibrinolysis is contraindicated and if PCI is unavailable within 2h (UFH, IV enoxaparin, or fondaparinux).

Indications in NSTEMI

- Fondaparinux (2.5mg SC daily) is recommended as having the most favourable efficacy–safety profile regardless of the management strategy.
- Patients on fondaparinux (2.5mg SC daily) undergoing PCI, a single IV bolus of UFH (70–85 IU/kg, or 50–60 IU/kg in the case of concomitant use of GPIIb/IIIa inhibitors) is recommended during the procedure.
- Enoxaparin or UFH are recommended in patients undergoing PCI when fondaparinux is not available.
- Bivalirudin, a direct thrombin inhibitor, is recommended in patients with a history of HIT. Bivalirudin is recommended as an alternative to UFH plus glycoprotein IIb/IIIa inhibitors during PCI.

Fibrinolytic therapy

- Fibrinolytic therapy allows plasminogen to be converted to plasmin, which causes lysis of the fibrin-rich clot to allow coronary reperfusion.
- This is a valid treatment option in patients with STEMI only. It may be used if time since symptom onset is <12h and PPCI cannot be performed within 120min of STEMI diagnosis. It may also be considered in early presenters (<2h since symptom onset) with a large infarction and low bleeding risk if time from first medical contact to PPCI will be >90min (see contraindications in Table 2.1.2).
- Time plays an important role regarding the benefit of thrombolysis. The greatest benefit of fibrinolytic treatment is seen within the first 2h. Twelve hours after the onset of chest pain, fibrinolysis is not recommended and is associated with an increased incidence of serious complications such as cardiac rupture.
- Fibrin-specific lytic agents (tenecteplase, alteplase, reteplase) are recommended over non-fibrin-specific agents such as streptokinase.
- PCI with coronary stenting produces better results in STEMI patients than fibrinolytic therapy and should be considered as the first-line management option.
- Anticoagulation is recommended in patients treated with lytics until revascularization (if performed) or for the duration of hospital stay up to 8 days.
- Clopidogrel is indicated, in addition to aspirin; 48h after fibrinolysis, a switch to prasugrel/ticagrelor may be considered in PCI-treated patients.

Side effects

- Haemorrhage: intracranial haemorrhage is the most serious.
- Reperfusion arrhythmias may occur.
- Allergic reaction, particularly with streptokinase, which may require treatment with 100mg of IV hydrocortisone and antihistamines (e.g. diphenhydramine).
- Hypotension.

Drugs for secondary prevention therapy after ACS

A variety of drugs are useful in the long-term management of CAD following ACS, and it is important that both primary and secondary care services work together to ensure that the patient is on optimal medical therapy, with respect to the combination and dose of pharmacological agents, to minimize morbidity and mortality. Drugs used in secondary prevention are summarized in Table 2.1.3.

References

1 Neumann FJ, Sousa-Uva M, Ahlsson A, *et al.* 2018 ESC/EACTS Guidelines on myocardial revascularization. *Eur Heart J* 2019;40(2):87–165.
2 Roffi M, Patrono C, Collet J-P, *et al.* 2015 ESC Guidelines for the management of acute coronary syndromes in patients presenting without persistent ST-segment elevation. *Eur Heart J* 2016;37:267–315.
3 Ibanez B, James S, Agewall S, *et al.* 2017 ESC Guidelines for the management of acute myocardial infarction in patients presenting with ST-segment elevation. *Eur Heart J* 2018;39:119–77.
4 Valgimigli M, Bueno H, Byrne RA, *et al.* 2017 ESC focused update on dual antiplatelet therapy in coronary artery disease developed in collaboration with EACTS. *Eur Heart J* 2018;39:213–54.

Table 2.1.3 Drugs used post-STEMI and NSTEMI for secondary prevention

Therapy	Category	Dose	Contraindications	Cautions
Aspirin	Antiplatelet therapy	75–100mg od lifelong	Aspirin/NSAID hypersensitivity	Asthma, allergic disease, history of severe bleeding, severe hepatic impairment
Clopidogrel/ prasugrel/ ticagrelor	Antiplatelet therapy: see recommendations for STEMI and NSTEMI separately	Dosing as in Table 2.1.1	Anaphylactic reaction to drug in the past, ongoing bleeding	Increased risk of bleeding
ACEI	Inhibition of renin–angiotensin–aldosterone system (RAAS)	Start at low dose and titrate to maximum tolerated dose	Hypersensitivity/angio-oedema with ACEI, pregnancy	Hypotension, renal disease, severe aortic stenosis, renal artery stenosis, hyperkalaemia
ARB (if ACEI contraindicated)		Start at low dose and titrate to maximum tolerated dose	Pregnancy	
β-blockers	Anti-ischaemic therapy	Start at low dose and titrate upwards	Acute heart failure (pulmonary oedema), atrioventricular block, cardiogenic shock, hypotension	Asthma with history of bronchospasm, breastfeeding
HMG CoA reductase inhibitors (statins)	Cholesterol lowering	High-intensity statin: atorvastatin 40–80mg, rosuvastatin 20–40mg daily	Anaphylactic reaction	Liver impairment, previous myopathy/rhabdomyolysis with statins
Ezetimibe		10mg daily	Anaphylaxis, moderate to severe hepatic impairment	Caution in pregnancy (no safety data available)
PCSK9 inhibitors (alirocumab, evolocumab)		Alirocumab: 75mg or 150mg every 2 weeks. Evolocumab: 140mg every 2 weeks	Treatment of primary hypercholesterolaemia (heterozygous familial and non-familial) or mixed dyslipidaemia	Prescribe under the supervision of a specialist lipid clinic. Avoid in severe renal or hepatic impairment

Chapter 2.2

Chronic stable angina

Gaetano Antonio Lanza
and Antonio De Vita

Overview of chronic stable angina

Epidemiologic features

The term chronic stable angina (CSA) identifies a clinical picture characterized by episodes of angina pectoris that show the same frequency and characteristics of presentation and resolution for at least the 2 previous months.

The prevalence of CSA in the population is around 4–5% but increases with ageing. Thus, the prevalence is around 4–7% in men aged 45–54 years, whereas it is 12–14% in men aged 65–84 years. Furthermore, the incidence and prevalence of CSA (as of other forms of IHD) are higher in men than in women. The difference between the two sexes is greater below the age of 50–55 years, likely due to the protective effects of oestrogens, but persists at older ages.

Importantly, the prevalence of chronic IHD is much higher than CSA, due to the frequent absence of angina symptoms in stable or stabilized patients with known or unknown IHD. The therapeutic approach to patients with stable forms of IHD is similar, independent of the presence of angina symptoms. Accordingly, the content of this chapter is entirely applicable to all patients with known or suspected stable IHD.

Characteristics and pathophysiologic substrate

The term angina pectoris describes the typical symptom caused by myocardial ischaemia. In its classical presentation, angina pectoris is described by patients as a constrictive or an oppressive chest pain or discomfort localized in the retrosternal area, which often variably radiates towards the neck, the left shoulder, and the medial side of the left arm, the jaw, and the epigastrium. Furthermore, in CSA, the pain is most frequently triggered by exertion and slowly disappears within 2–5min of rest or following the administration of sublingual nitrates. Other conditions able to increase myocardial oxygen consumption (MVO_2) (e.g. emotional and psychological stresses, heavy meals, hypertensive episodes), however, may also trigger angina attacks.

In some patients, myocardial ischaemia manifests as angina equivalents, i.e. symptoms different from chest pain, mainly including shortness of breath and arrhythmias. Moreover, most spontaneous episodes of transient myocardial ischaemia (up to 70–80%) are silent (i.e. not associated with either angina or angina equivalents), which has the same clinical implications of symptomatic ischaemia.

Elicitation of chest pain during myocardial ischaemia is due to excitation of chemo-sensitive and mechano-sensitive receptors in neural endings in the heart. An important chemical algogenic stimulus is adenosine, which is released by cardiomyocytes during ischaemia and also exerts a major role in the metabolic regulation of myocardial blood flow through its powerful vasodilator effect on arterioles.

The pathologic substrate of myocardial ischaemia in CSA is typically constituted by the presence of flow-limiting stenoses in epicardial coronary arteries, which do not allow an adequate increase in coronary blood flow during increased MVO_2 due to exhaustion of coronary flow reserve. Typically, myocardial ischaemia in CSA is limited to subendocardial layers, which, on the ECG, is usually manifested by ST-segment depression (most often in leads V4–V6).

In most patients, chest pain occurs at a predictable and reproducible level of exertion or conditions that increase MVO_2, because of the presence of fixed stenoses. However, in many cases, the ischaemic threshold (i.e. the level of MVO_2 at which ischaemia appears) is variable due to vasomotor phenomena at the site of pliable stenoses that modify their severity (dynamic stenoses). Vasomotor changes in the coronary microcirculation or collateral vessels, or even significant changes in cardiac preload and/or afterload, may also contribute to variability of the ischaemic threshold.

Diagnostic workflow

In patients presenting with recurrent episodes of chest pain, alternative diagnoses to CSA, both CV and non-CV, are to be accurately excluded by careful assessment of the clinical history and adequate diagnostic investigation.

ECG exercise stress test (by treadmill or bicycle) and stress tests (either exercise or pharmacological) in combination with imaging methods (i.e. radionuclide scans, echocardiography, cardiovascular magnetic resonance) are variably used to detect myocardial ischaemia in patients with suspected CSA, depending on patient characteristics and the availability and expertise at single centres.

Computed tomography coronary angiography (CTCA) now allows adequate non-invasive assessment of the coronary anatomy in most cases and has been advocated as a valid first-line alternative to stress tests for the diagnostic assessment of patients with suspected CSA. Controlled studies, however, failed to show tangible advantages of CTCA over functional stress tests.

By definition, obstructive CAD, as the cause of CSA, is ultimately diagnosed by invasive coronary angiography. The latter, however, is indicated in specific subsets of patients only, including those with a high probability of needing myocardial revascularization (due to potential prognostic benefits), those at high risk because of resuscitated sudden death or life-threatening arrhythmias, and those who continue to be symptomatic despite optimal medical therapy.

Risk stratification of CSA patients

Severity of angina symptoms [as typically assessed by the Canadian Cardiovascular Society (CCS) class], symptoms of acute LV dysfunction during angina attacks, reduced LVEF, low effort tolerance, and evidence of severe myocardial ischaemia on stress tests all constitute negative prognostic factors in CSA and should prompt for full investigation. Composite scores that combine multiple prognostic variables have also been proposed to better predict outcome. The Duke treadmill score is perhaps the most commonly used and is based on exercise capacity (exercise duration), severity of myocardial ischaemia (maximal ST-segment depression), and limiting or non-limiting angina during the exercise stress test. A Duke score of –11 or less is associated with a high risk, with a 4-year survival rate of 79% only.

Treatment of chronic stable angina

Treatment of patients with CSA has two main objectives: to improve prognosis, by reducing mortality and the rate of acute coronary events, and abolish or minimize angina symptoms. Control of cardiovascular risk factors (CVRFs), antithrombotic and anti-ischaemic drug therapy, and coronary revascularization procedures variably contribute to achieve these goals.

Also, clinical conditions that may facilitate or exacerbate myocardial ischaemia (e.g. anaemia, tachyarrhythmias, fever, thyroid disease, hypoxaemia) should always be recognized and appropriately treated.

Control of cardiovascular risk factors

Correct management of CSA patients includes tight control of CVRFs, which can be achieved by adequate lifestyle modification and pharmacological therapy, and significantly reduces the risk of CV events (see ➲ Section 1).

Lifestyle modification

Lifestyle changes, including smoking cessation, weight loss, physical exercise, and dietary control, play a crucial role in the management of CSA. They may indeed modify the atherosclerotic process by 'stabilizing' coronary plaques and prevent acute coronary events by also reducing platelet activation, the inflammatory state, and vascular dysfunction.

Diet should include adjustment of calorie intake to avoid overweight, increased consumption of fruit, vegetables, fish, lean meat, and low-fat dairy products, reduction in total fats to <30% of the total calorie intake, and reduction of salt intake if BP is high.

Physical activity should be done by practising 30min of moderate to vigorous aerobic exercise for at least three times a week. In symptomatic patients, however, strenuous physical activities should be avoided because of the risk of atherosclerotic plaque complications. Stress management may represent a useful strategy in some clusters of patients.

Pharmacological control of cardiovascular risk factors

BP should be kept at values of <130/80mmHg, although values of up to <140/90mmHg are acceptable. Due to their anti-ischaemic effects, β-blockers and CCBs may be preferred over other antihypertensive agents to achieve these BP targets in CSA patients.

Management of hypercholesterolaemia should be based on the use of appropriate doses of statins, with the objective to achieve LDL-C levels of <70mg/dL or to reduce them by >50%. The addition of ezetimibe (10mg od) should be considered in cases of intolerance to increasing doses of statins. In patients intolerant of any dose of statins or with persistently high levels of LDL-C despite optimal statin therapy, the use of anti-PCSK9 monoclonal antibodies should be considered.

Adequate control of glycaemic values in patients with diabetes mellitus is also recommended, with the aim to achieve HbA1c levels of <7%. Although benefits on CV outcome have long been controversial, recent trials have shown significant beneficial CV effects with the use of glucagon-like peptide-1 analogues (liraglutide) and sodium-glucose co-transporter 2 inhibitors (empagliflozin, canagliflozin).

In patients who do not manage to quit smoking spontaneously and with the help of psychological/motivational interventions, pharmacological treatment with nicotine replacement therapy, varenicline, or bupropion should be considered. All these drugs have indeed been shown effective for smoking cessation. However, whether and how their effects on smoking translate into improved clinical outcome is not known at present.

Pharmacological therapy for chronic stable angina

Table 2.2.1 summarizes the current ESC and American College of Cardiology (ACC)/American Heart Association (AHA) guidelines of pharmacological treatment of CSA and of chronic IHD in general. Some minor differences exist between the two documents, the most relevant concerning the use of long-acting nitrates in the prevention of angina and the absence of some anti-ischaemic drugs (unavailable in the United States) in the American guidelines.

Table 2.2.2 summarizes the pharmacological and clinical characteristics of the main kinds of drugs used in CSA patients.

Finally, Fig. 2.2.1 shows a flow diagram of a practical stepwise approach to the treatment of these patients, reflecting a synthesis from international guidelines and personal clinical experience.

Drugs that improve prognosis

Antiplatelet drugs

Low-dose aspirin (75–100mg daily) should be used in all patients with CSA who have no specific contraindications. Aspirin indeed improves long-term outcome in these patients. In the Swedish Angina Pectoris Aspirin Trial (SAPAT), aspirin reduced the rate of acute MI by 39% ($p < 0.01$) and showed a trend towards survival improvement ($p = 0.10$). Aspirin irreversibly inhibits platelet thromboxane A2 synthesis, which has pro-aggregating and vasoconstrictive properties by inhibiting the COX-1 enzyme, and therefore, its antiplatelet effects last for the entire lifespan of the platelet (9–10 days). GI side effects, including bleeding, are the most frequent unwanted effects of aspirin. Use of antacid agents (mainly PPIs) improves the GI tolerance of the drug.

In patients with contraindications or intolerance to aspirin, clopidogrel (75mg daily) should be prescribed as an antiplatelet drug. Clopidogrel is a thienopyridine that acts as a non-competitive adenosine diphosphate (ADP) receptor antagonist. It has been found to have clinical effects comparable to those of aspirin in patients with stable forms of IHD, and it is better tolerated at the GI level. In CSA patients undergoing PCI with drug-eluting stents (DES) or bare-metal stents (BMS), clopidogrel should be combined with aspirin for a period of 6 months to prevent coronary stent thrombosis and restenosis, independently of the stent type. The dual antiplatelet regimen, however, can be prolonged (in particular with DES and usually to 12 months) or shortened (usually to 3 months) based on the thrombotic and bleeding risk of the patient.

In patients needing a thienopyridine drug but who have intolerance to clopidogrel, ticlopidine (250mg bd) can be administered. Ticlopidine has similar pharmacological properties and clinical effects to those of clopidogrel, but its use has been limited by the higher risk of serious adverse effects, including neutropenia and thrombocytopenia.

New ADP receptor antagonists, i.e. the thienopyridine prasugrel and the triazol-pyrimidine ticagrelor, that have been found to present some clinical advantages over clopidogrel in patients with ACS, do not have specific indications in CSA patients at present, as they have not been tested as an alternative to aspirin or clopidogrel and may not have a favourable cost-effective profile in CSA patients.

Table 2.2.1 Summary of the main indications of pharmacological therapy for patients with chronic stable angina/ischaemic heart disease according to international guidelines

	ESC guidelines (2013)	ACC/AHA guidelines (2012)
Event prevention		
Low-dose aspirin	In all chronic CSA patients (Class IA)	In all chronic CSA patients (Class IA)
Clopidogrel	If intolerance to aspirin (Class IB)	If intolerance to aspirin (Class IB)
Aspirin + clopidogrel	–	In high-risk patients with CSA (Class IIb B)
β-blockers	–	If LVEF <40%, HF, or prior MI (Class I B)
ACEIs	If LVEF <40%, hypertension, diabetes (Class IA)	If LVEF <40%, hypertension, diabetes, or CKD (Class IA)
ARBs	In patients intolerant of ACEIs (Class IA)	In patients intolerant of ACEIs (Class IA)
Statin	In all CSA patients (Class IA)	In all CSA patients (Class IA)
Angina/ischaemia relief		
Short-acting nitrates	Immediate relief of angina (Class I B)	Immediate relief of angina (Class I B)
β-blockers	First-line treatment (Class I A)	First-line treatment (Class I A)
Dihydropyridine CCBs	As alternative or associated with β-blockers (Class I A)	As alternative or associated with β-blockers (Class I B)
Non-dihydropyridine CCBs	As alternative to β-blockers (Class I A)	As alternative with β-blockers (Class IIa B)
Long-acting nitrates	Second-line treatment (Class IIa B)	As alternative or associated with β-blockers (Class I B)
Ranolazine	Second-line treatment (Class IIa B)	Associated with β-blockers (Class IIa A) As alternative to β-blockers (Class IIa B)
Ivabradine	Second-line treatment (Class IIa B)	–
Nicorandil	Second-line treatment (Class IIa B)	–
Trimetazidine	Second-line treatment (Class IIb B)	–

ACC/AHA, American College of Cardiology/American heart Association; ACEI, angiotensin-converting enzyme inhibitor; ARB, angiotensin receptor blocker; CCB, calcium channel blocker; CKD, chronic kidney disease; CSA, chronic stable angina; ESC, European Society of Cardiology; MI, myocardial infarction.

Table 2.2.2 Main anti-anginal medications for chronic stable angina

Drug	Dosage	Action	Main side effects	Observations
Short-acting nitrates		Systemic venodilatation, with decrease in preload, wall tension, and MVO_2	Hypotension Headache	Interaction with phosphodiesterase-5 inhibitors may cause life-threatening hypotension Caution in patients with severe aortic stenosis or HOCM
Glyceryl trinitrate	0.3–0.4mg SL			
Isosorbide dinitrate	5mg SL			
Long-acting nitrates		Systemic and coronary artery vasodilatation, with decrease in afterload and improvement of myocardial perfusion		
Isosorbide dinitrate	10mg tds			
Isosorbide mononitrate	20mg bd			
Glyceryl trinitrate	5–10mg od			
β-blockers		Decrease in MVO_2 by reduction in HR, myocardial inotropism, and BP	Bradyarrhythmias Fatigue Libido disorders	Should be avoided in asthma, variant angina, and bradyarrhythmias Caution in peripheral vascular disease
Metoprolol	25–100mg bd			
Bisoprolol	1.25–10mg od			
Atenolol	25–100mg od			
Nebivolol	2.5–10mg od			
NDH-CCBs		Reduction in MVO_2 by systemic vasodilatation (all CCBs) and reduction in HR and myocardial contractility (NDH-CCBs) Improvement of myocardial perfusion (coronary dilatation)	*All CCBs:* Hypotension Ankle oedema *NDH-CCBs:* Bradyarrhythmias Stipsis *DH-CCBs:* Tachycardia Flushing Headache	NDH-CCBs to be used with caution in combination with β-blockers Avoid DHP-CCBs in severe aortic stenosis or HOCM NDH-CCBs contraindicated in patients with bradyarrhythmias or depressed LV function
Verapamil	40–120mg tds			
Diltiazem	60–120mg tds			
DHP-CCBs				
Nifedipine (SR)	20–30mg bd			
Amlodipine	5–10mg od			
Felodipine	2.5–10mg od			
Barnidipine	10–20mg od			
Lercanidipine	10–20mg od			

Ranolazine	375–1000mg bd	Inhibition of the late sodium current of cardiomyocytes, with prevention of calcium overload in ischaemic myocardium Decrease in diastolic wall tension, with decrease in MVO_2 and improvement of myocardial perfusion		Contraindicated in patients with prolonged QT interval, use of other drugs that prolong QT interval, hepatic failure, and use of drugs that inhibit liver enzymes (such as verapamil and diltiazem)
Ivabradine	2.5–7.5mg bd	Selective inhibition of the I_f current of the sinus node, resulting in HR slowing, with reduced MVO_2 and improvement of myocardial perfusion	Visual disturbances	Contraindicated in patients with sick sinus syndrome Drug interaction with certain liver enzyme inhibitors
Nicorandil	10–20mg bd	Potassium channel opener with nitrate-like effects Coronary and systemic vasodilatation, with decrease in preload and afterload and improvement of coronary flow Possible preconditioning effects	Headache Oral ulceration	Avoid in patients with severe aortic stenosis and HOCM
Metabolic agents Trimetazidine	20mg tds	Inhibition of fatty acid oxidation by promoting glucose utilization, with increased efficiency of cardiac metabolism during ischaemia	Tremor Muscle disorders Gastro-oesophageal burning	Contraindicated in Parkinson's disease and severe renal failure Reduce dose to 20mg bd in moderate renal failure

CCB, calcium channel blocker; DHP, dihydropyridine; HOCM, hypertrophic obstructive cardiomyopathy; HR, heart rate; LV, left ventricular; MVO_2, myocardial oxygen consumption; NDHP, non-dihydropyridine; SR, slow release.

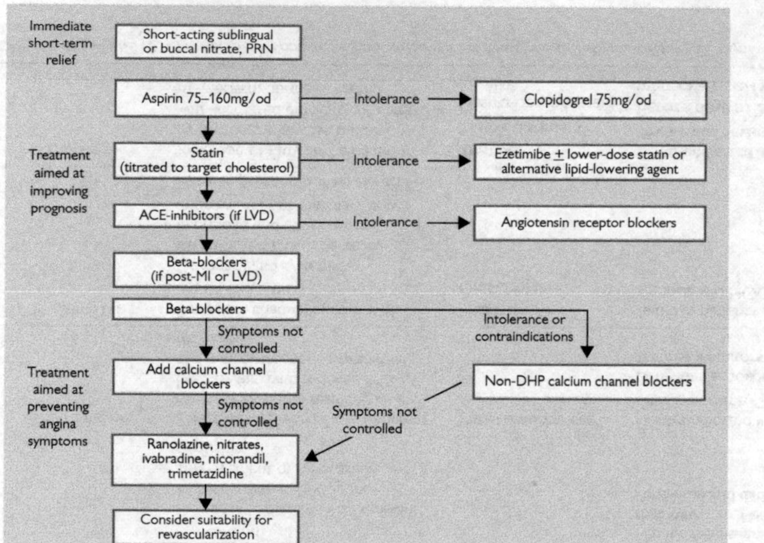

Fig. 2.2.1 Scheme of therapeutic pharmacological approach to patients with chronic stable angina. ACEI, angiotensin-converting enzyme inhibitor; LVD, left ventricular dysfunction; MI, myocardial infarction; non-DHP, non-dihydropyridine.

Other antiplatelet agents (e.g. dipyridamole, indobufen, picotamide) are not recommended in this setting, as there is no clear evidence of their benefits. Dipyridamole, in particular, has the potential risk of worsening angina symptoms and should therefore be avoided.

Anti-cholesterolaemic drugs

Statins, which inhibit the enzyme HMG CoA reductase, reduce endogenous cholesterol synthesis but have also anti-inflammatory and antithrombotic properties that likely contribute to the improved survival benefits seen with these drugs. Statins are indicated for all patients with documented CAD, irrespective of their plasma cholesterol levels, although their clinical benefits are greater in those with elevated levels of cholesterol. As mentioned previously, the addition of ezetimibe to statins, which inhibits the absorption of cholesterol from the small intestine, and the use of PCSK9 inhibitors, which increase LDL-C removal from blood by liver cells, should be considered in patients with various degrees of intolerance to statins.

Beta-blockers

A β-blocker should be considered in all patients with chronic IHD who experienced an acute MI. They are recommended in patients with an impairment of LV function. Furthermore, possible beneficial effects have been reported in patients with episodes of silent myocardial ischaemia during daily life. Notably, β-blockers remain the first-line therapy for the prevention of angina episodes (see ➔ Chronic treatment/prophylaxis, p. 102).

β-blockers counteract the negative effects of adrenergic activation on the ischaemic heart. They reduce MVO_2 by reducing the heart rate, BP, and myocardial contractility, with improvement of LV remodelling; perfusion of subendocardial ischaemic areas may also be improved by prolongation of diastole. Furthermore, in cases of acute coronary complications, β-blockers limit the infarct size and reduce life-threatening ventricular arrhythmias.

Anti-β-1 selective agents should be preferred, as evidence of efficacy has mainly been obtained with this kind of β-blockers; furthermore, they have lower rates of side effects and are better tolerated, compared to non-selective agents. β-blockers with intrinsic sympathomimetic activity are not recommended, due to their overall lower efficacy and a lack of prognostic benefits. Carvedilol, a combined α- and β-blocker agent, can be used in patients with LV dysfunction.

Side effects of β-blockade include fatigue, cold extremities, symptomatic bradycardia, and sexual dysfunction. Of note, non-cardioselective β-blockers should not be prescribed to patients with asthma or COPD. According to recent evidence, instead, when indicated, cardioselective β-blockers can be prescribed safely in these patients, with the recommendation to start with a low dose and gradually up-titrate to the optimal dose.

Anti-renin–angiotensin–aldosterone drugs

An ACEI is recommended in patients with CSA who present with a reduced LVEF (≤40%), with or without a previous MI, and with or without signs of HF. ACEIs indeed prevent LV remodelling and improve survival in these patients by counteracting the deleterious effects of RAAS activation. It is also appropriate to consider an ACEI in patients with coexisting diabetes mellitus, hypertension, and/or CKD. Patients who do not tolerate an ACEI should be given an ARB.

Anti-aldosterone agents (spironolactone) should also be considered in post-MI patients who have a reduced LVEF, in the absence of renal failure and hyperkalaemia.

Drugs to improve angina symptoms

Drugs effective in relieving symptoms of angina act via different mechanisms that result in a reduction in myocardial work and oxygen requirements, an improvement of coronary blood flow and myocardial perfusion, or a combination of both. A combination of drugs that act via different mechanisms may result in better control of myocardial ischaemia and angina than simply increasing the dose of single anti-ischaemic agents.

Acute treatment of angina

Short-acting formulations of nitrates [glyceryl trinitrate or isosorbide dinitrate (ISDN)] provide rapid and effective relief of angina pectoris. The anti-ischaemic effect is mainly related to reduced LV preload caused by peripheral venous dilatation, which reduces MVO_2 and favours subendocardial perfusion; furthermore, coronary artery dilatation may also contribute. Short-acting nitrates might also be taken as a preventive therapy a few minutes before performing an activity known to usually trigger angina pain.

Chronic treatment/prophylaxis

Classically, the prophylactic treatment of CSA was based on the use of β-blockers, CCBs, and long-acting nitrates, but other anti-ischaemic drugs, with peculiar mechanisms, have recently become available (see Table 2.2.2).

Beta-blockers

β-blockers should be considered the first-line treatment for the prevention of angina. Their main effect is to reduce MVO_2 at various levels of physical activity. The main goal of β-blocker therapy should be to maintain a heart rate of <60bpm at rest and <110–115bpm at peak exercise.

Calcium channel blockers

CCBs cause peripheral and coronary vasodilatation. Furthermore, non-dihydropyridine CCBs (verapamil, diltiazem) also reduce the heart rate and myocardial contractility and are the first alternative to β-blockers for angina prevention, in particular in slow-release formulations, when the latter cannot be used.

Dihydropyridine CCBs (e.g. nifedipine, amlodipine, felodipine, barnidipine, lercanidipine) have greater vasodilator properties, with no appreciable effects on myocardial contractility and the cardiac conduction system. They may cause, however, hypotension and reflex sympathetic activation, with an increase in heart rate, which may limit their anti-ischaemic action. Long-acting dihydropyridine CCBs (e.g. amlodipine) or sustained-release formulations of short-acting compounds (e.g. nifedipine, felodipine) are preferred, as they cause less hypotension and adrenergic activation.

Side effects of CCBs include headache, flushing, and ankle oedema, which are more frequent with dihydropyridine agents. Verapamil and diltiazem, on the other hand, may cause bradycardia and constipation.

Both types of CCBs can be added to β-blockers when symptoms persist. A combination of non-dihydropyridine CCBs and β-blockers, however, needs careful monitoring, because of possible excessive bradycardia. Accordingly, dihydropyridine CCBs are considered the first choice to add to β-blockers when a second anti-anginal drug is indicated (see Fig. 2.2.1).

Long-acting nitrates

Although long-acting nitrates (in oral or transdermal formulations) have been used for many years for angina prevention, there are no robust data on their effectiveness. As mentioned previousy, the main anti-anginal effect of nitrates is exerted by reducing myocardial work through reduction in cardiac preload (see ➔ Drugs to improve angina symptoms, p. 102). Tolerance is believed to be a major limitation to the chronic anti-anginal effect of nitrates. Nitrate-free intervals or modified delivery systems to provide a period of low blood nitrate concentrations have been recommended to restore sensitivity to their action. Of note, administration of nitrates might be scheduled in a way that would cover, when applicable, periods of the day with the highest probability of occurrence of angina attacks. Adverse effects include headache and occasionally postural hypotension.

Other anti-anginal drugs

Ranolazine is a selective inhibitor of the late sodium current of cardiomyocytes. This effect results in a reduction in intracellular sodium-dependent calcium overload during myocardial ischaemia, which improves myocardial relaxation, with possible improvement of diastolic perfusion, as well as reduction in preload and MVO_2. Ranolazine has been demonstrated to improve angina symptoms and exercise-related myocardial ischaemia in some clinical trials, in addition to β-blockers and/or CCBs. In the recent Ranolazine in patients with Incomplete Revascularisation after Percutaneous Coronary Intervention (RIVER-PCI) trial, however, ranolazine failed to significantly improve angina status at long-term follow-up in patients undergoing incomplete coronary revascularization by PCI. This study, however, is biased by the expected favourable anti-anginal effects of PCI in the whole population of enrolled patients. The dose of ranolazine is 375–1500mg bd or 750–1000mg bd for a sustained-release formulation. The most commonly reported adverse effects with ranolazine are constipation, dizziness, nausea, and asthenia.

Ivabradine is a specific inhibitor of I_f, the primary pacemaker current of the sinus node. Ivabradine exerts its anti-ischaemic effects by lowering resting and exercise heart rate without affecting BP or myocardial contractility. This results in lower MVO_2 and improved coronary perfusion due to prolonging of diastolic time. Some controlled studies have shown favourable effects of ivabradine on angina symptoms, as well as exercise tolerance and exercise-induced myocardial ischaemia. The drug can be used to lower heart rate in patients in whom β-blockers cannot be used, or even in association with β-blockers to achieve resting and exercise heart rate targets. In IHD patients with LV dysfunction and a heart rate of >70bpm, ivabradine has been found to reduce hospitalization for HF and therefore should be considered in this setting. However, in the Study assessInG the morbidity-mortality beNefits of the If inhibitor ivabradine in patients with coronarY artery disease (SIGNIFY) trial, ivabradine was associated with a worse clinical outcome (CV death or acute MI) in stable IHD patients without HF with activity-limiting angina, suggesting caution in its broader use. The dose of ivabradine is 2.5–5mg bd. The main side effect is represented by visual disturbances that are related to the presence in the retina of ion channels similar to those mediating I_f and that subside after drug withdrawal.

Nicorandil is a hybrid compound, available in some European countries only, that comprises an adenosine triphosphate (ATP)-sensitive potassium channel opener and a nitrate moiety. It reduces both cardiac preload and afterload. Angiographic studies have shown that nicorandil also dilates both stenotic and non-stenotic coronary arteries. Finally, some studies have shown that the drug may mimic ischaemic preconditioning (pharmacological preconditioning). Unlike classical nitrates, chronic administration of nicorandil does not seem to induce tolerance. In the Impact Of Nicorandil in Angina (IONA) trial, nicorandil, compared to placebo, significantly reduced major coronary events in CSA patients; the early prognostic benefit, however, was lost at follow-up, although the reduction in hospital admissions for angina pain persisted. The usual dose of nicorandil is 20mg bd. Headache is the commonest side effect, but it tends to subside with chronic dosing; furthermore, oral and distal GI ulceration have been reported in some patients.

Trimetazidine is available in some European countries only. The mechanisms of its anti-ischaemic effects are not fully known. The drug, however, seems to improve energy utilization during myocardial ischaemia, stimulating glucose oxidation and partially inhibiting fatty acid oxidation, with modulatory effects on intracellular calcium. Both immediate-release [20mg three times a day (tds)] and modified-release (35mg od) formulations of trimetazidine have been found to improve angina symptoms in small studies of CSA patients. The most commonly reported adverse effects with clinical doses are fatigue and drowsiness.

Other drugs

Some other compounds have been proposed as anti-anginal medications, including *molsidomine* [a nitric oxide (NO) donor with vasodilator action similar to that of organic nitrates] and *perhexiline* (a metabolic agent that favours glucose oxidation in ischaemic myocardium), but they are available in some countries only, and evidence of their benefits is limited.

Oral *anticoagulants* have long been considered not indicated in CSA patients, except in the presence of associated specific conditions in which they are known to improve clinical outcome (e.g. patients with AF, cardiac prosthetic valves, or pulmonary thromboembolism). In these cases, the choice between classical VKAs and NOACs should be made according to the clinical context and characteristics of individual patients.

The recent Cardiovascular Outcomes for People Using Anticoagulation Strategies (COMPASS) trial, however, has shown that the addition of low-dose rivaroxaban (2.5mg bd) to acetylsalicylic acid (ASA) (100mg) in patients with stable CAD significantly reduced CV events (death, MI, stroke) at 2-year follow-up. The net benefit, however, seemed limited (about 0.5% per year) and occurred at the expense of increased major bleeding. Thus, further assessment of this combined therapy seems indicated to better establish its benefit–cost/risk ratio.

Finally, it is worth noting that some drugs should be avoided or used with caution in CSA patients, due to their potential adverse CV effects, including

NSAIDs, selective COX-2 inhibitors, including diclofenac, and long-term oestrogens (in women).

Myocardial revascularization for chronic stable angina

Coronary revascularization can be achieved by either PCIs or CABG surgery. In CSA patients, CABG surgery is indicated for prognostic purposes in well-defined categories of patients, including those with left main disease, three-vessel disease with reduced LV function, and proximal stenosis of the left anterior descending coronary artery in the presence of multivessel disease, and those with extensive myocardial ischaemia, whereas there is little or no advantage of CABG surgery over optimal medical therapy in other subgroups of patients.

On the other hand, no study has, until now, demonstrated prognostic benefits of PCIs over optimal medical therapy in CSA patients. In patients with left main disease and low coronary atherosclerotic burden, however, PCIs seem comparable to CABG surgery for medium-term survival. Myocardial revascularization is indicated, regardless of its effect on the outcome, in patients who remain symptomatic in spite of optimal medical treatment. Clinical conditions and coronary anatomy should be considered in making the choice between the two options.

Of note, optimal medical therapy has been found to improve clinical outcome in patients who underwent coronary revascularization by either CABG or PCIs.

Management of refractory angina

Refractory angina pectoris is defined as the occurrence of frequent episodes of angina, significantly limiting daily activities (usually CCS classes III–IV), which cannot be sufficiently controlled by optimal drug therapy and, at the same time, are not treatable with coronary revascularization procedures due to a coronary anatomy judged unsuitable for both PCI and CABG surgery.

Among various alternative therapies proposed for this condition, two main forms of treatment are presently advised to be considered, i.e. spinal cord stimulation (SCS) and enhanced external counterpulsation (EECP), due to some evidence of a favourable risk:benefit ratio.

SCS consists of electrical stimulation of the dorsal horns of the spinal cord via an electrode placed in the epidural space at C7–T5. The neural stimulation would reduce transmission of angina pain stimuli to the cortex by activating inhibitory neurons (gate theory) but would also improve myocardial blood flow by modulating the sympathetic drive to the heart. SCS has been reported to improve symptoms in refractory angina patients in multicentre registries and some small controlled studies. No life-threatening complications related to SCS have been reported, while local infections or catheter dislodgement requiring a reimplant occur in a minority of patients.

EECP consists of cyclic inflation/deflation of pneumatic cuffs placed on the lower legs, which increase arterial BP and retrograde aortic/coronary blood flow during diastole, but reduced afterload during systole, resulting in reduced MVO_2 and improved coronary flow. The favourable effects of EECP in refractory CSA have been shown in some registries and a small trial. Some conditions represent contraindications to EECP, however, including severe impairment of LV function, uncontrolled hypertension, aortic disease, aortic regurgitation, peripheral venous disease, and anti-coagulant therapy.

Further reading

Neumann FJ, Sousa-Uva M, Ahlsson A, *et al.* 2018 ESC/EACTS Guidelines on myocardial revascularization. *Eur Heart J* 2019;40:87–165.

Fihn SD, Gardin JM, Abrams J, *et al.* 2012 ACCF/AHA/ACP/AATS/PCNA/SCAI/STS Guideline for the diagnosis and management of patients with stable ischemic heart disease: a report of the American College of Cardiology Foundation/American Heart Association Task Force on Practice Guidelines, and the American College of Physicians, American Association for Thoracic Surgery, Preventive Cardiovascular Nurses Association, Society for Cardiovascular Angiography and Interventions, and Society of Thoracic Surgeons. *J Am Coll Cardiol* 2012;**60**:e44–164.

Piepoli MF, Hoes AW, Agewall S, *et al.* 2016 European Guidelines on cardiovascular disease prevention in clinical practice: The Sixth Joint Task Force of the European Society of Cardiology and Other Societies on Cardiovascular Disease Prevention in Clinical Practice (constituted by representatives of 10 societies and by invited experts) Developed with the special contribution of the European Association for Cardiovascular Prevention & Rehabilitation (EACPR). *Eur Heart J* 2016;37:2315–81.

Task Force Members, Montalescot G, Sechtem U, *et al.* 2013 ESC guidelines on the management of stable coronary artery disease: the Task Force on the management of stable coronary artery disease of the European Society of Cardiology. *Eur Heart J* 2013;34:2949–3003.

Valgimigli M, Bueno H, Byrne RA, *et al.* 2017 ESC focused update on dual antiplatelet therapy in coronary artery disease developed in collaboration with EACTS: The Task Force for dual antiplatelet therapy in coronary artery disease of the European Society of Cardiology (ESC) and of the European Association for Cardio-Thoracic Surgery (EACTS). *Eur Heart J* 2018;39:213–60.

Clinical trials/reference articles

Eikelboom JW, Connolly SJ, Bosch J, *et al.* Rivaroxaban with or without aspirin in stable cardiovascular disease. *N Engl J Med* 2017;377:1319–30.

Fox K, Ford I, Steg PG, Tendera M, Ferrari R; BEAUTIFUL Investigators. Ivabradine for patients with stable coronary artery disease and left-ventricular systolic dysfunction (BEAUTIFUL): a randomised, double-blind, placebo-controlled trial. *Lancet* 2008;372:807–16.

Heidenreich PA, McDonald KM, Hastie T, *et al.* Meta-analysis of trials comparing beta-blockers, calcium antagonists, and nitrates for stable angina. *JAMA* 1999;**281**:1927–36.

Lanza GA. Alternative treatments for angina. *Heart* 2007;93:544–6.

Sendón JL, Lee S, Cheng ML, *et al.* Effects of ranolazine on exercise tolerance and angina frequency in patients with severe chronic angina receiving maximally-tolerated background therapy: analysis from the Combination Assessment of Ranolazine In Stable Angina (CARISA) randomized trial. *Eur J Prev Cardiol* 2012;19:952–9.

Yusuf S, Hawken S, Ounpuu S, *et al.* Effect of potentially modifiable risk factors associated with myocardial infarction in 52 countries (the INTERHEART study): case-control study. *Lancet* 2004;364:937–52.

Chapter 2.3

Coronary artery spasm and microvascular angina

Peter Ong and Udo Sechtem

Clinical presentation and diagnosis of coronary artery spasm

Clinical presentation

Classically, patients with coronary artery spasm report resting angina that promptly responds to short-acting nitrates. Such patients have a preserved exercise capacity, and transient ST-segment elevation can be recorded in a 12-lead ECG during a chest pain attack. This pattern is known as Prinzmetal's angina or variant angina. Initially, occlusive spasm of one or several non-obstructed epicardial coronary arteries is seen angiographically in such patients. However, patients with epicardial spasm may also share other features such as exercise-related angina or a combination of rest and effort angina. Moreover, epicardial coronary spasm may also occur clinically silent or may cause MI. In addition, arrhythmias and syncope have been described in patients with epicardial vasospasm. Smoking is an established predisposing risk factor and is often found in male patients.

Another form of coronary spasm is microvascular spasm. It is frequently observed in patients (especially women) with resting angina despite normal epicardial coronary arteries. ST-segment elevation is very uncommon during an attack, but ST-segment depression is often seen.

This form of coronary spasm is often unresponsive to short-acting nitrates. Treatment of coronary microvascular spasm is difficult and often empiric, due to the fact that different structural and functional abnormalities may be present in the coronary microcirculation. In addition, patients with microvascular spasm and angina at rest often complain of dyspnoea with non-strenuous exertion. The differentiation between vasospastic angina (a term which has been reserved for angina at rest caused by epicardial spasm) and resting angina caused by microvascular spasm can only be made during invasive provocation testing.

Diagnosis

The current ESC guidelines on the management of stable CAD recommend recording a 12-lead ECG during episodes of chest pain in patients with suspected coronary spasm to assess ischaemic ECG changes associated with the chest pain. In patients with characteristic resting angina and ST-segment shifts that resolve with nitrates and/or calcium antagonists, coronary angiography is useful to determine the extent of the underlying coronary disease. In addition, intracoronary provocative spasm testing (using acetylcholine or ergonovine) should be performed in patients with normal or unobstructed coronary arteries by coronary angiography and the clinical picture of coronary spasm to diagnose the site and mode of spasm (see Fig. 2.3.1). A frequently used definition of epicardial spasm is transient total or subtotal coronary artery occlusion (≥90% narrowing) with angina and ischaemic ECG shifts either spontaneously or in response to a provocative stimulus. The definition of coronary microvascular spasm usually comprises ischaemic ST-segment changes and angina during acetylcholine testing, in the absence of epicardial spasm.

Focal spasm pattern

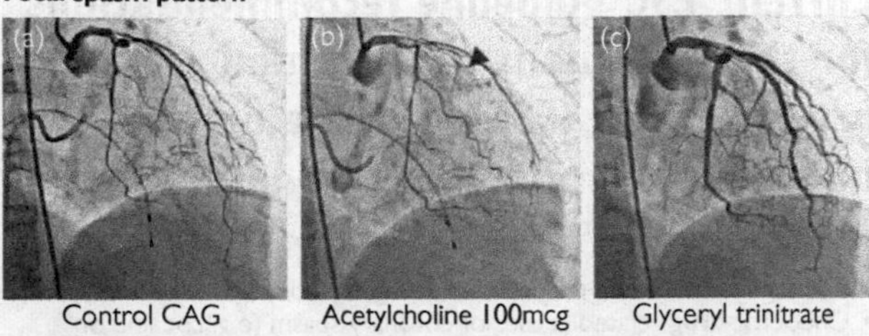

Diffuse spasm pattern

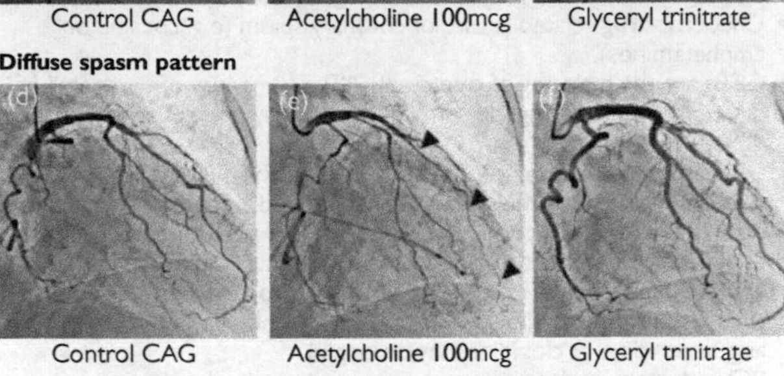

Fig. 2.3.1 Visualization of different types of epicardial coronary spasm (focal versus diffuse). Acetylcholine (ACh)-induced focal and diffuse spasm patterns. (a–c) Focal spasm pattern. (b) Injection of 100mcg of ACh into the left coronary artery induced focal spasm in the proximal site of the left anterior descending artery. (d–f) Diffuse spasm pattern. (e) Injection of 100mcg of ACh into the left coronary artery induced diffuse spasm in the whole left coronary artery, including the left circumflex artery. CAG, coronary angiography.

Reproduced from Sato, K., *et al*, Coronary Vasomotor Response to Intracoronary Acetylcholine Injection, Clinical Features, and Long-term Prognosis in 873 Consecutive Patients With Coronary Spasm: Analysis of a Single-Center ± Study Over 20 Years, *Journal of the American Heart Association*, 2013, with permission from Wiley.

Special care should be taken to record ischaemic ECG changes during simultaneous 12-lead-ECG recording and to interrogate the patient about any known or unknown symptoms occurring during spasm testing. Angiographically, coronary spasm may appear in a proximal, mid-vessel, or distal portion of the epicardial artery. Moreover, spasm can be focal or diffuse and can involve multiple epicardial arteries (i.e. multivessel spasm). Epicardial spasm can occur in normal, unobstructed, or stenosed coronary arteries. Coronary spasm can also be found during provocative testing in patients with angina persisting following successful PCI. Focal epicardial coronary spasm identified during intracoronary provocative testing carries a worse prognosis than diffuse epicardial spasm.

Current ESC guideline recommendations for the treatment of epicardial coronary artery spasm (ESC guideline on the management of stable coronary artery disease)

- Risk factor control, in particular smoking cessation and aspirin.
- Check for drug-related causes of coronary spasm (e.g. cocaine or amphetamines).
- CCBs are the mainstay of treatment; 240–360mg/day of verapamil or diltiazem and 40–60mg/day of nifedipine usually prevent spasm in about 90% of patients.
- Long-acting nitrates can be added to improve the efficacy of treatment.
- Avoid β-blockers, as they can aggravate epicardial spasm by leaving α-mediated vasoconstriction unopposed by β-mediated vasodilatation.
- In patients with refractory angina due to coronary artery spasm (i.e. approximately 10% of those with proof of coronary spasm and under standard treatment with CCBs and nitrates), anti-adrenergic drugs such as guanethidine or clonidine may be helpful.
- PCI with stent implantation at the site of spasm (in the absence of significant stenosis) is not recommended.

Proposed management of patients with coronary artery spasm

First of all, management of patients with coronary spasm consists of lifestyle and risk factor modification, as well as the avoidance of potential vasospastic agents. Pharmacological treatment is based on CCBs and short-acting nitrates as first-line drugs and a selection of second-line drugs such as long-acting nitrates, statins, and nicorandil. Third-line drugs are guanethidine, clonidine, and magnesium, and oestrogens in post-menopausal women. In patients with refractory spasm and proof of ischaemia-related life-threatening arrhythmias, implantation of an automatic cardioverter–defibrillator or of a pacemaker is indicated (see Fig. 2.3.2).

Lifestyle and risk factor modifications

- Smoking cessation.
- BP control.
- Maintenance of ideal body weight.
- Correction of impaired glucose tolerance.
- Correction of lipid abnormalities.
- Avoidance of excessive fatigue and mental stress.
- No or moderate alcohol consumption.

Avoidance of potential vasospastic agents

Certain medications may precipitate a vasospastic episode and should be used with caution:

- β-blockers.
- Ergot compounds (e.g. migraine treatment or obstetric preparations).
- Sympathomimetic agents such as adrenaline or cocaine.
- Serotonergic compounds (anti-migraine, antidepressant medication).
- Chemotherapeutic agents such as fluorouracil, capecitabine, or sorafenib.
- Alcohol ingestion debatable.

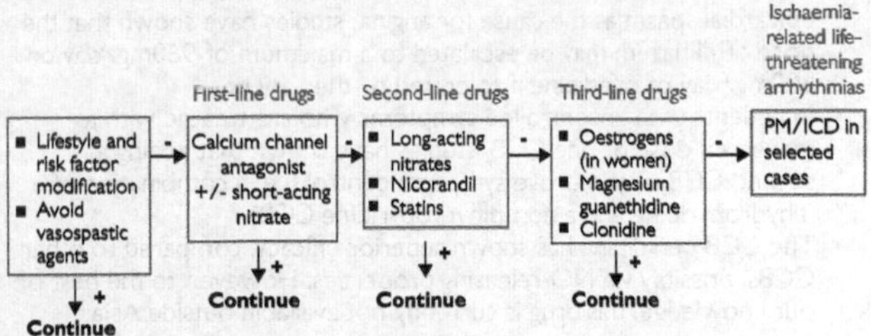

Fig. 2.3.2 Proposed treatment algorithm for patients with coronary spasm. ICD, implantable cardioverter–defibrillator; PM, pacemaker.

Suggested pharmacological treatment for coronary spasm

Acute chest pain attack

Acute chest pain attacks in patients with coronary spasm require prompt treatment with sublingual nitrates such as 0.4mg of glyceryl trinitrate or 5–10mg of ISDN. In patients without improvement of symptoms, the latter may be repeated after 5–10min. In patients resistant to sublingual nitrates, sublingual CCBs are often effective such as nifedipine 5–10mg or nitrendipine 5mg. Patients with ongoing symptoms, despite the above-mentioned treatments, should present to an emergency department for further treatment (e.g. IV nitrates) and evaluation of other potential underlying causes.

Long-term treatment

Calcium channel blockers

- *Indications*: CCBs are the first-line drugs in patients with proof of epicardial coronary spasm. Dihydropyridine CCBs, such as, for example, amlodipine (maximum dose 10mg/day) or nifedipine (maximum dose 60mg/day), can be used, as well as non-dihydropyridine CCBs (e.g. verapamil up to 480mg/day or diltiazem up to 360mg/day). Which drug is chosen in the individual patient remains to the decision of the treating physician. CCBs should be individually titrated to a dose that achieves adequate symptom control and ideally avoids any adverse effects.
- *Common side effects*:
  - Dihydropyridine CCBs: headache, ankle swelling, fatigue, flushing, reflex tachycardia.
  - Non-dihydropyridine CCBs: bradycardia, heart conduction abnormalities, negative inotropic effects, constipation, gingival hyperplasia.
- *Common contraindications*:
  - Dihydropyridine CCBs: cardiogenic shock, severe aortic stenosis, hypertrophic obstructive cardiomyopathy.
  - Non-dihydropyridine CCBs: bradycardic heart rhythm disorder, sick sinus syndrome, CHF, hypotension.
- *Practical notes*:
  - In patients with uncontrolled symptoms but with clear proof of epicardial spasm as the cause for angina, studies have shown that the dose of diltiazem may be escalated to a maximum of 960mg/day or 100mg/day of nifedipine if tolerated by the patient.
  - In patients with uncontrolled symptoms who are treated with a maximum dose of one CCB, studies have shown that adding a second CCB may improve symptom control (i.e. a combination of a dihydropyridine and a non-dihydropyridine CCB).
  - The CCB benidipine has shown superior efficacy, compared to other CCBs, possibly via NO-releasing properties. However, to the best of our knowledge, this drug is currently not available outside Asia.

Nitrates

- *Indications*: the addition of long-acting nitrates to CCB treatment for coronary spasm has been debated in the literature. Older studies have shown a favourable effect of long-acting nitrates in suppressing angina due to coronary spasm with, for example ISDN 20–120mg/day.

However, more recently, it has become clear that chronic nitrate therapy does not improve the long-term prognosis. We recommend long-acting nitrates as second-line drugs, in addition to CCBs, if symptoms are uncontrolled.

- *Common side effects*: headache, flushing, tachycardia, hypotension, dizziness.
- *Common contraindications*: cardiogenic shock, prolonged hypotension (<90mmHg SBP), severe anaemia, severe hypovolaemia, concomitant use of phosphodiesterase type 5 (PDE-5) inhibitors, e.g. sildenafil.
- *Practical notes*:
  - A nitrate-free interval of 12–14h between the evening dose and morning dose should be utilized to reduce the formation of superoxides and prevent nitrate tolerance.
  - In countries where molsidomine is available, this coronary artery dilator may be used in the nitrate-free interval to suppress coronary spasm.

Nicorandil

- *Indications*: nicorandil is a potassium channel opener, with additional nitrate-like properties. Although it is not available in all countries (e.g. not in Germany and not in the United States), it can be used as a second-line drug in the treatment of coronary spasm. The starting dose is 10mg/day, with uptitration to a maximum of 40mg/day if symptoms are not controlled.
- *Common side effects*: dizziness, fatigue, tachycardia, flush, nausea, vomiting.
- *Common contraindications*: cardiogenic shock, CHF, hypotension, acute pulmonary oedema, concomitant use of PDE-5 inhibitors (e.g. sildenafil), concomitant use of soluble guanylate cyclase stimulators (e.g. riociguat).
- *Practical notes*:
  - In patients with known cephalgia, the starting dose should be 5mg bd, rather than 10mg od, in the first 7 days.
  - Hyperkalaemia has rarely been reported during nicorandil treatment. However, in patients with simultaneous intake of drugs which enhance the potassium concentration or with moderate to severe renal insufficiency, it should be used with caution.

Statins

- *Indications*: patients with evidence of coronary plaques have a clear indication for statin treatment. The same is true for patients who have a very high CV risk, even without atherosclerosis demonstrated by imaging. Even if risk factor assessment does not indicate a need for statin treatment in a patient with coronary spasm, such a drug should be considered, in addition to CCB treatment. Studies have shown that up to 30mg/day of fluvastatin significantly decreased the coronary spasm frequency. Other studies used 20mg/day of pravastatin, in addition to a CCB. The reasons for these findings are likely to be multiple. It has been speculated that, apart from LDL-C-lowering, pleiotropic effects of statins, especially suppression of inflammation and inhibition of the Rho-kinase pathway, could be responsible for the observed effect.

- *Common side effects (fluvastatin)*: insomnia, cephalgia, nausea, dyspepsia, arthralgia.
- *Common contraindications (fluvastatin)*: patients with active liver disease or persistent elevation of serum transaminases of unknown origin, pregnancy, and lactation.
- *Practical notes*: myopathy with fluvastatin is rare. Myositis and rhabdomyolysis are extremely rare. If muscular pain occurs, patients should be investigated for potential causes.

Others

- In patients with refractory symptoms, despite individually titrated doses and combinations of the aforementioned substances, other drugs that have been investigated in coronary spasm may be tried. However, due to scarce data, no general recommendations can be made and every patient's individual situation has to be taken into account. These substances include magnesium, clonidine, and guanethidine, and oestrogen replacement therapy in post-menopausal women. In patients with ischaemia-related life-threatening tachyarrhythmias or bradyarrhythmias, respectively, when coronary spasm presents a poor or an uncertain response to medical therapy, implantation of an automatic cardioverter–defibrillator or of a pacemaker is indicated.

Clinical presentation and diagnosis of microvascular angina

Clinical presentation

Angina due to coronary microvascular dysfunction can clinically be divided into primary stable and primary unstable microvascular angina. The latter includes clinical conditions such as Takotsubo syndrome. This chapter will focus on primary stable microvascular angina (MVA), characterized by coronary microvascular dysfunction in patients with (usually exertional) angina pectoris (or dyspnoea as an angina equivalent) and proof of myocardial ischaemia in the absence of significant epicardial coronary disease and without myocardial disease (type 1, according to Crea and Camici).

The clinical presentation of patients with MVA is often indistinguishable from that in patients with obstructive CAD. However, one distinguishing feature is that patients with primary stable MVA frequently have exertional angina which persists after physical exercise. Most patients with MVA also report shortness of breath that can be the leading complaint. Moreover, patients with MVA and those with HF with preserved ejection fraction (HFpEF) share several similarities, pointing towards a potential common pathophysiological background. Many patients with MVA additionally report angina at rest of variable duration. In some cases this may resemble an ACS and can be caused by coronary microvascular spasm. Because patients with microvascular spasm often have mild chronic troponin elevations, coronary angiography is often performed when these patients present to the emergency department complaining of angina at rest. Usually, no epicardial abnormality explaining this constellation, which resembles NSTEMI, is found. Although symptoms in women and men with MVA may be comparable, it has been shown that patients with MVA are more often female (most often post-menopausal).

Diagnosis

Non-invasive assessments

If the patient's history is suggestive of MVA (e.g. exertional dyspnoea as the main complaint, angina often after physical exercise, often prolonged angina without improvement by sublingual nitrates, frequently attacks of dyspnoea at rest or resting angina, discrete ST-segment depressions on a resting ECG), the combination of CTCA and measurement of the myocardial flow reserve using positron emission tomography (PET) represents the ideal non-invasive way to establish the diagnosis. MVA can be diagnosed if CTCA shows no coronary stenosis and the coronary flow reserve is <2.5 or <2.0. Alternatively to PET, coronary flow reserve can also be measured using transthoracic Doppler echocardiography, although this investigation may prove difficult in patients with lung disease or increased body weight. If non-invasive ischaemia testing is performed, suspecting MVA as the diagnosis depends on the methodology used. Patients with MVA rarely have a pathological stress echocardiography, whereas single-photon emission computed tomography (SPECT) and cardiac stress magnetic resonance imaging may be abnormal. In such cases, visualization of the coronary arteries is mandatory to exclude relevant epicardial disease. If, however, the imaging tests do not show ischaemia, MVA can nevertheless be present in patients with a consistent clinical presentation.

Invasive assessments

If invasive coronary angiography is performed, it is usually necessary to exclude relevant epicardial atherosclerotic disease in order to establish the diagnosis of MVA. A purely visual assessment of epicardial stenoses is often inaccurate in determining the haemodynamic relevance. Thus, fractional flow reserve or instantaneous wave-free ratio measurements should be performed in patients with borderline epicardial stenoses (approximately 30–70% of diameter reduction) to assess the haemodynamic relevance of such lesions. Invasive techniques for demonstrating microvascular dysfunction are measurement of coronary flow reserve using a Doppler or thermodilution wire after adenosine injection or infusion. An indirect proof of MVA is the demonstration of microvascular spasm using intracoronary acetylcholine provocation testing. Acetylcholine testing can reveal that the resting angina reported by such patients is due to microvascular spasm. One would then assume that the exercise-related symptoms may also be caused by a microvascular abnormality if coronary angiography does not show epicardial disease. Studies have shown that approximately 50% of women with angina and unobstructed coronary arteries have a reduced coronary flow reserve of <2.5 on invasive coronary flow reserve measurements with adenosine. In addition, coronary microvascular dysfunction manifesting itself as microvascular spasm provoked by acetylcholine can be detected in approximately 30% of patients with stable angina without obstructed coronary arteries (see Fig. 2.3.3).

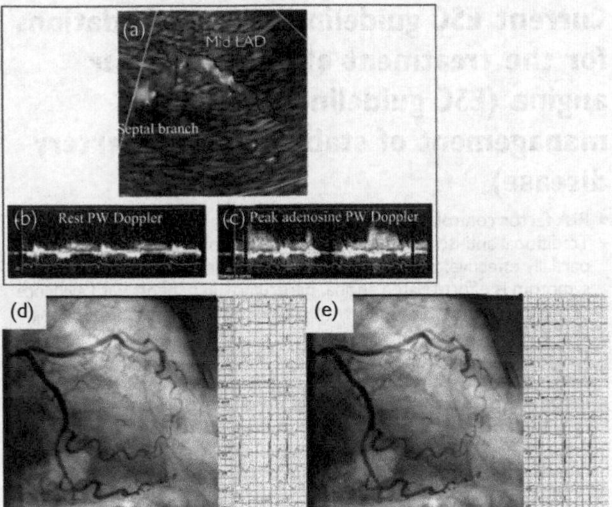

Fig. 2.3.3 Microvascular angina is frequently diagnosed by impaired coronary flow reserve (a–c) or by intracoronary acetylcholine testing (d–e). (a) Colour Doppler image of the mid-left anterior descending artery and a septal branch. Pulse wave (PW) Doppler velocity spectrum at rest (b) and at peak adenosine infusion (c). Coronary flow reserve was 2.3 as a result of the ratio between 0.35m/s flow velocity at peak adenosine infusion and 0.15m/s flow velocity at rest. Panels (d) and (e) show an example of a patient with microvascular spasm. During acetylcholine infusion, the patient had reproduction of chest pain and ischaemic ECG changes, but no epicardial vasoconstriction (d). After intracoronary glyceryl trinitrate, chest pain and ECG changes resolved (e).

(a–c) Reproduced from Galiuto L, Sestito A, Barchetta S, *et al*., Noninvasive evaluation of flow reserve in the left anterior descending coronary artery in patients with cardiac syndrome X, *The American Journal of Cardiology*, Volume **99**, Issue 10, 15 May 2007, Pages 1378–1383 with permission from Elsevier. (d–e) Reproduced from Ong, P., *et al*, High Prevalence of a Pathological Response to Acetylcholine Testing in Patients With Stable Angina Pectoris and Unobstructed Coronary Arteries The ACOVA Study (Abnormal COronary VAsomotion in patients with stable angina and unobstructed coronary arteries), *J Am Coll Cardiol* 2012;**59**:with permission from Elsevier.

Current ESC guideline recommendations for the treatment of microvascular angina (ESC guideline on the management of stable coronary artery disease)

- Risk factor control.
- Traditional anti-ischaemic drugs: short-acting nitrates are often only partially effective; β-blockers are recommended because the dominant symptom is effort-related angina, particularly in patients with evidence of increased adrenergic activity (e.g. high heart rate at rest or during low-workload exercise).
- Calcium antagonists, however, can be the first-line therapy in patients with a significant variable threshold of effort angina.
- In patients with persisting symptoms, despite optimal anti-ischaemic drug therapy, several other treatments have been proposed. ACEIs (and possibly ARBs) may improve microvascular function by counteracting the vasoconstrictor effects of angiotensin II.
- α-adrenergic antagonists may decrease sympathetic-mediated vasoconstriction and may be considered in individual patients.
- Refractory patients: nicorandil, oestrogen replacement in post-menopausal women, and xanthine derivatives (aminophylline, bamifylline) can be added to anti-ischaemic treatment to reduce angina by adenosine receptor blockade; adenosine is indeed a major mediator of cardiac ischaemic pain.
- Newer anti-ischaemic drugs, such as ranolazine or ivabradine, have shown effects in some patients with MVA.

Proposed management of patients with microvascular angina

In patients with MVA, a strict control of CVRFs is recommended. Therefore, most patients receive a statin and an ACEI. β-blockers are the first-line treatment. If this treatment does not achieve sufficient relief of symptoms or is not tolerated, CCBs can be useful, especially if patients also report symptoms at rest, suggesting a vasoconstrictor component. In patients with refractory symptoms, anti-anginal drugs, such as ranolazine, nicorandil, or ivabradine, can be tried, depending on local availability. Imipramine and/or bamifylline are alternative options in patients with refractory symptoms, despite the aforementioned anti-anginal treatments. SCS should be considered in patients refractory to pharmacological treatment. A suggested algorithm is shown in Fig. 2.3.4.

Beta-blockers

- *Indications*: β-blockers are recommended as first-line drugs in the treatment of MVA. An early study reported favourable effects regarding symptoms and exercise stress test parameters in MVA patients with up to 100mg/day of atenolol. More recently, there have been reports assessing the effect of nebivolol in such patients, showing beneficial effects in doses of up to 5mg/day.
- *Common side effects (nebivolol and other β-blockers)*: headache, dizziness, paraesthesiae, dyspnoea, obstipation, nausea, diarrhoea, fatigue, oedema, bradycardia, heart conduction abnormalities.
- *Common contraindications (nebivolol and other β-blockers)*: cardiogenic shock, acute decompensated HF, sick sinus syndrome, atrioventricular block (AVB) grades 2 and 3, hepatic insufficiency, bronchial asthma, hypotension (SBP <90mmHg), heart rate <60bpm before treatment.
- *Practical note*: β-blockers may be especially effective in patients with a high resting heart rate or an increased sympathetic tone, whereas they should be avoided in patients with concomitant epicardial vasospastic disorders.

Calcium channel blockers

- *Indications*: CCBs have been shown to improve symptoms and exercise stress test parameters in patients with MVA. Studies have

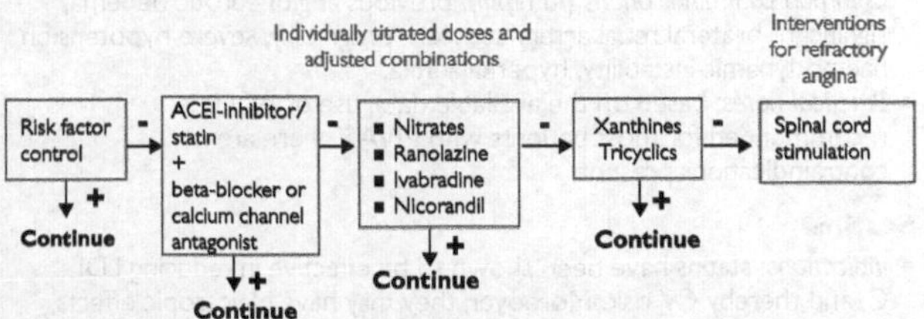

Fig. 2.3.4 Proposed treatment algorithm for patients with microvascular angina.

used verapamil (non-dihydropyridine CCB, 40–160mg, four times per day) and nifedipine (dihydropyridine CCB, 10–30mg, four times per day). Other studies have shown beneficial effects for nisoldipine (dihydropyridine CCB, 5mg bd) and diltiazem (non-dihydropyridine CCB, 90mg/day).

- *Common side effects*:
  - Dihydropyridine CCBs: headache, ankle swelling, fatigue, flushing, reflex tachycardia.
  - Non-dihydropyridine CCBs: bradycardia, heart conduction abnormalities, negative inotropic effects, constipation, gingival hyperplasia.
- *Common contraindications*:
  - Dihydropyridine CCBs: cardiogenic shock, severe aortic stenosis, hypertrophic obstructive cardiomyopathy.
  - Non-dihydropyridine CCBs: bradycardic heart rhythm disorder, sick sinus syndrome, CHF, hypotension.
- *Practical notes*:
  - Non-dihydropyridine CCBs can be first-line drugs in patients with concomitant vasospastic disorders.
  - CCBs are recommended in patients with mainly exercise-related symptoms if β-blockers are not effective or tolerated.
  - Some patients may paradoxically experience worsening of symptoms on CCBs, necessitating withdrawal of treatment.

Angiotensin-converting enzyme inhibitors

- *Indications*: available studies assessing the effects of ACEIs in patients with MVA have generally shown beneficial results. Early studies by Kaski and Nalbantgil demonstrated improvement of exercise stress test parameters in patients with microvascular dysfunction with enalapril (10mg/day) and cilazapril (2.5mg bd). Other studies used ramipril 2.5mg daily or a combination of ramipril 10mg/day and atorvastatin 40mg/day. More recently, quinapril (80mg od) has been shown to improve coronary flow reserve in response to adenosine, as well as angina pectoris symptoms, compared to placebo.
- *Common side effects (ramipril)*: dry cough, hyperkalaemia, headache, dizziness, orthostatic hypotension, syncope, bronchitis, dyspnoea, dyspepsia, abdominal pain, nausea, diarrhoea, myalgia, exanthema, fatigue.
- *Common contraindications (ramipril)*: previous angioneurotic oedema, significant bilateral renal artery stenosis, pregnancy, severe hypotension, haemodynamic instability, hyperkalaemia.
- *Practical notes*: based on the available data, use of ACEIs is recommended for most patients with MVA if there are no contraindications present.

Statins

- *Indications*: statins have been shown to be effective in reducing LDL-C, and thereby CV risk. Moreover, they may have pleiotropic effects, including a reduction in vascular inflammation and an improvement of endothelial function. There are three studies available showing a beneficial effect in patients with MVA regarding improvement in exercise duration and ischaemic markers on treadmill testing. These studies used pravastatin 40mg/day, or simvastatin 20mg/day, or fluvastatin 40mg/day.

- *Common side effects (fluvastatin)*: insomnia, cephalgia, nausea, dyspepsia, arthralgia.
- *Common contraindications (fluvastatin)*: patients with active liver disease or persistent elevation of serum transaminases of unknown origin, pregnancy, and lactation.
- *Practical notes*: for myalgia and myopathy, see ➔ Statins under Suggested pharmacological treatment for coronary spasm, pp. 113–14. Based on the available studies, use of statins is recommended for most patients with MVA if there are no contraindications present.

Others

- *Nitrates*: studies on long-acting nitrates have generally shown no positive effect and are thus not recommended as first-line drugs in these patients. This has recently been highlighted in a study by Russo *et al.*, showing that ISDN was effective in relieving symptoms and in improving exercise stress test results in patients with stable epicardial coronary disease, but ISDN was not helpful in patients with coronary microvascular dysfunction. Short-acting nitrates are often effective in relieving chest pain symptoms in patients with MVA, especially when administered on a background of β-blocker or CCB treatment. Long-acting nitrates, however, only rarely ameliorate symptoms in MVA patients, although some patients may react favourably to such agents.
- Several other drugs have been investigated in patients with MVA. However, due to scarce data, no general recommendations can be made and every patient's individual situation has to be taken into account. These substances include ranolazine and ivabradine, metformin, trimetazidine, nicorandil, oestrogen replacement therapy in post-menopausal women, imipramine, and xanthine antagonists. Ongoing studies, especially regarding ivabradine and ranolazine, may provide more robust data for future therapeutic recommendations.

Further reading

The following articles provide further information on the pharmacological treatment of patients with coronary artery spasm and MVA, respectively. They are suggested for further reading.

Agewall S, Beltrame JF, Reynolds HR, *et al.*; WG on Cardiovascular Pharmacotherapy. ESC working group position paper on myocardial infarction with non-obstructive coronary arteries. *Eur Heart J* 2017;**38**:143–53.

Bairey Merz CN, Handberg EM, Shufelt CL, *et al.* A randomized, placebo-controlled trial of late Na current inhibition (ranolazine) in coronary microvascular dysfunction (CMD): impact on angina and myocardial perfusion reserve. *Eur Heart J* 2016;**37**:1504–13.

Beltrame JF, Crea F, Kaski JC, *et al.*; Coronary Vasomotion Disorders International Study Group (COVADIS). The who, what, why, when, how and where of vasospastic angina. *Circ J* 2016;**80**:289–98.

Beltrame JF, Crea F, Kaski JC, *et al.*; Coronary Vasomotion Disorders International Study Group (COVADIS). International standardization of diagnostic criteria for vasospastic angina. *Eur Heart J* 2017;**38**:2565–8.

Camici PG, Crea F. Coronary microvascular dysfunction. *N Engl J Med* 2007;**356**:830–40.

Crea F, Bairey Merz CN, Beltrame JF, *et al.*; Coronary Vasomotion Disorders International Study Group (COVADIS). The parallel tales of microvascular angina and heart failure with preserved ejection fraction: a paradigm shift. *Eur Heart J* 2017;**38**:473–7.

Lanza GA, Crea F. Primary coronary microvascular dysfunction: clinical presentation, pathophysiology, and management. *Circulation* 2010;**121**:2317–25.

Marinescu MA, Löffler AI, Ouellette M, Smith L, Kramer CM, Bourque JM. Coronary microvascular dysfunction, microvascular angina, and treatment strategies. *JACC Cardiovasc Imaging* 2015;**8**:210–20.

Murthy VL, Naya M, Taqueti VR, *et al.* Effects of sex on coronary microvascular dysfunction and cardiac outcomes. *Circulation* 2014;**129**:2518–27.

Ong P, Athanasiadis A, Borgulya G, *et al.* Clinical usefulness, angiographic characteristics, and safety evaluation of intracoronary acetylcholine provocation testing among 921 consecutive white patients with unobstructed coronary arteries. *Circulation* 2014;**129**:1723–30.

Ong P, Athanasiadis A, Sechtem U. Pharmacotherapy for coronary microvascular dysfunction. *Eur Heart J Cardiovasc Pharmacother* 2015;**1**:65–71.

Piepoli MF, Hoes AW, Agewall S, *et al.*; ESC Scientific Document Group. 2016 European Guidelines on cardiovascular disease prevention in clinical practice: The Sixth Joint Task Force of the European Society of Cardiology and Other Societies on Cardiovascular Disease Prevention in Clinical Practice (constituted by representatives of 10 societies and by invited experts) Developed with the special contribution of the European Association for Cardiovascular Prevention & Rehabilitation (EACPR). *Eur Heart J* 2016;**37**:2315–81.

Takahashi J, Nihei T, Takagi Y, *et al.* Prognostic impact of chronic nitrate therapy in patients with vasospastic angina: multicenter registry study of the Japanese coronary spasm association. *Eur Heart J* 2015;**36**:228–37.

Task Force Members, Montalescot G, Sechtem U, *et al.* 2013 ESC guidelines on the management of stable coronary artery disease. *Eur Heart J* 2013;**34**:2949–3003.

Takotsubo syndrome

Alexander Lyon, Mark Sweeney, and Elmir Omerovic

Introduction

Takotsubo syndrome (TTS) is characterized by acute-onset, reversible regional ventricular dysfunction in the absence of flow-limiting lesions in coronary arteries. It was described initially by Sato and colleagues in Japan in 1990, and its presentation has commonly been linked to a stressful emotional or physical event.

TTS mimics an ACS, presenting with symptoms of chest pain or breathlessness, ST-segment changes on the ECG, and troponin elevation. In the era of urgent coronary angiography for presentations with acute chest pain, TTS is being increasingly recognized as a cause of acute cardiac chest pain, ECG changes, and biomarker elevation.

The original name 'Takotsubo' comes from the classical appearance of the left ventricle during ventriculography, which demonstrates extensive akinesia in the apical segments of the left ventricle and basal hypercontractility during end-systole. This resembles a traditional Japanese fishing pot, with a wide base and a narrow neck, which was used to catch octopuses. Multiple names and descriptions have been used since this first description to describe this presentation, including 'apical ballooning syndrome' related to the classical anatomical appearances of the left ventricle, 'stress-related cardiomyopathy', or 'broken heart syndrome' related to its common association with stressful life events or bereavement. More rarely, there are reports of positive emotional stress resulting in TTS, giving rise to the name 'happy heart syndrome'.

Recently, the term 'Takotsubo syndrome' has been adopted as the preferred terminology, rather than cardiomyopathy, due to emerging evidence that other organ systems are also involved.

The ESC's Heart Failure Association (HFA) has recently published a position statement on TTS[1] to provide an expert consensus on approaching the diagnosis, risk stratification, and management of this syndrome, to help optimize and standardize the management of an increasingly commonly recognized condition.

Prognosis

The prognosis of TTS varies dramatically. Previously, it was thought that TTS carries an almost universally good prognosis, due to the perceived recovery of LV function on resting echocardiography and the fact that more severe life-threatening cases likely were not identified as TTS presentations. The majority of patients with TTS have a self-limiting illness, with complete resolution of LV function. However, minor and major complications occur in over 50% of cases, which results in significant morbidity and mortality. The in-hospital mortality of between 2% and 5% is comparable to that of STEMI, and the all-cause mortality at 5 years is significantly worse, approaching 25% in some registries.[2] In addition, 10–20% of TTS patients experience ongoing exertional chest pain, breathlessness, or arrhythmias at long-term follow-up.

Epidemiology

Incidence

- TTS accounts for approximately 2% of all presentations with suspected ACS, and 7–10% of women presenting with acute chest pain.
- There are approximately 100,000 new cases per year in the United States and similar numbers in European registries.[1]
- These are conservative estimates, and the incidence has been growing in recent years due to improved recognition, but perhaps also a real increase in the incidence. There is also a subset of subclinical cases which do not present to hospital, meaning that overall the incidence is almost certainly higher than is currently reported.

Age

- TTS typically presents in older adults, with a mean age of presentation of 66.8 years.
- Cases have been reported across all age ranges, including children.

Gender

- TTS is commoner in post-menopausal females, with almost 90% of cases occurring in women over 50 years old.
- Less than 10% of patients presenting with TTS are men.
- Men tend to have a less favourable prognosis, with higher long-term mortality, and it is unclear if this excess mortality is related to the severity of the underlying illness or the Takotsubo presentation.

Geographical distribution

Although initially described in Japan, cases have been reported worldwide. While significant geographical preponderance cannot be excluded, there is no firm evidence that the incidence of TTS differs between different countries and regions. Some evidence suggests that some ethnic groups may be more prone to develop TTS.[3]

Aetiology

TTS presentations can be divided clinically into two main categories—primary TTS where cardiac symptoms are the primary cause for presentation to medical services, and secondary TTS where the primary reason for contact with medical services is another medical condition and TTS develops as a secondary complication of the underlying illness.

Primary Takotsubo syndrome

This encompasses the classical stress-related cardiomyopathy, as primary TTS most commonly presents as a result of emotional stress. There are a wide variety of reported emotional stressors; however, the commonest ones are:

- Recent bereavement of a loved one.
- Interpersonal conflict.
- Severe anger or frustration.
- Financial or employment difficulties.
- Panic attacks or severe anxiety.
- Winning the lottery.

Patients presenting with TTS commonly have a much higher prevalence of chronic neuropsychiatric disorders, including epilepsy, stroke, depression, anxiety, and adjustment disorder.

Secondary Takotsubo syndrome

Secondary TTS caused by a physical trigger, including neurological and psychiatric disorders, is the commonest cause of TTS and carries a less favourable prognosis than primary emotional triggers. There are a wide range of medical conditions and procedures reported to be associated with developing secondary TTS, the commonest of which are the following:

- Acute respiratory failure.
- Post-surgery.
- Acute neuromuscular failure, autonomic disturbances, or neurosurgical emergencies, e.g. subarachnoid haemorrhage.
- Infection.
- Malignancy.
- Endocrine—thyrotoxicosis, phaeochromocytoma.
- Iatrogenic—exogenous administration of catecholamines, such as adrenaline, noradrenaline, or dobutamine, during intensive care admission or cardiac stress testing.
- Stroke (ischaemic or haemorrhagic brain damage).
- Head injury.
- Internal bleeding.

Management of presentations of secondary TTS must deal with both TTS and the underlying cause.

Presentation and diagnosis

TTS has a wide spectrum of presentations. The classical presentation of TTS is with acute chest pain or shortness of breath related to a triggering event. Patients are typically admitted to hospital as a suspected acute MI. There is also a subset of subclinical presentations with patients who experience self-limiting chest pain in response to a triggering event but who do not seek medical attention. In patients already hospitalized for other reasons, TTS may present in less classical ways such as haemodynamic disturbances on induction of an anaesthetic or in the operating theatre or intensive care unit (ICU). Approximately 10% of presentations of TTS is with acute LV failure and cardiogenic shock, requiring urgent inotropic or mechanical support.[4]

The recent consensus statement on TTS from the ESC's HFA proposed seven diagnostic criteria which indicate a diagnosis of TTS. (see Box 2.4.1).

Box 2.4.1 Heart Failure Association's diagnostic criteria for Takotsubo syndrome

1. Transient regional wall motion abnormalities of the LV or RV myocardium which are frequently, but not always, preceded by a stressful trigger (emotional or physical).
2. The regional wall motion abnormalities usually extend beyond a single epicardial vascular distribution and often result in circumferential dysfunction of the ventricular segments involved.
3. The absence of culprit atherosclerotic CAD, including acute plaque rupture, thrombus formation, and coronary dissection or other pathological conditions, to explain the pattern of temporary LV dysfunction observed [e.g. hypertrophic cardiomyopathy (HCM), viral myocarditis].
4. New and reversible ECG abnormalities (ST-segment elevation, ST-depression, LBBB, T-wave inversion, and/or QTc prolongation) during the acute phase (3 months).
5. Significantly elevated serum natriuretic peptide (BNP or NT-pro-BNP) during the acute phase.
6. Positive, but relatively small, elevation in cardiac troponin measured with a conventional assay (i.e. disparity between the troponin level and the amount of dysfunctional myocardium present).
7. Recovery of ventricular systolic function on cardiac imaging at follow-up (3–6 months).

Source data from Lyon AR, Bossone E, Schneider B, *et al.* Current state of knowledge on Takotsubo syndrome: a Position Statement from the Taskforce on Takotsubo Syndrome of the Heart Failure Association of the European Society of Cardiology. *Eur J Heart Fail* 2016;**18**:8–27.

Pathogenesis

The mechanisms underlying TTS are yet to be conclusively defined. There are several possible theories, and most relate to a surge of catecholamines which occurs in response to acute emotional or physical stress, which has a variety of potential effects on the myocardium and vasculature. This hypothesis was reinforced by the finding that the levels of circulating catecholamines in patients with TTS are significantly higher than in similar individuals presenting with acute left anterior descending artery occlusion and in animal models where TTS is induced by overstimulation of the adrenergic system.

Coronary artery spasm

One possible mechanism is the presence of multivessel coronary spasm in response to high circulating levels of catecholamines. This has been postulated to cause widespread transient ischaemia, resulting in regional wall motion abnormalities. However, in the majority of cases, no coronary spasm is observed, and although spasm can be provoked in some patients, it is not clear if spasm is a cause or a consequence of the syndrome.

Transiently increased afterload

High levels of circulating catecholamines have also been postulated to cause an acute transient increase in afterload either via extreme peripheral vasoconstriction or acute left ventricular outflow tract obstruction (LVOTO). The high intra-cardiac pressures may contribute to the regional wall motion abnormalities, as the wall stress will be reduced by apical dysfunction. This is often followed by significant peripheral vasodilatation in the setting of a low cardiac output (CO) which contributes to the hypotension.

Catecholamine-mediated myocardial stunning

Pre-clinical studies have demonstrated a gradient of β-adrenergic receptors throughout the myocardium, with higher concentrations of β2-adrenergic receptors at the apex and higher concentrations of β1-adrenoreceptors (β1ARs) at the base. At higher concentrations of adrenaline, β2-adrenoreceptors (β2ARs) switch from a stimulatory and positively inotropic Gs protein-coupling to a negatively inotropic Gi inhibitory signal. This molecular switching acutely has a negative inotropic effect on the myocardium, more marked at the apex, which may be a cardioprotective response to inhibit apoptosis and ventricular arrhythmias in the setting of high circulating catecholamines. This is also in keeping with the modest elevation seen in cardiac troponin and minimal or absent areas of infarction seen on cardiac magnetic resonance imaging (MRI). Experimental studies have shown that overstimulation of both β1ARs and β2ARs causes a TTS-like condition.

Investigations

Electrocardiogram

A 12-lead ECG is almost always abnormal in TTS. The commonest ECG findings are:

- ST-elevation/depression.
- T-wave inversion.
- New LBBB.
- Pathological Q waves.
- Prolongation of the corrected QT interval (QTc).
- AF.
- Ventricular arrhythmias.

In over 50% of cases, the ECG will demonstrate significant ST-segment elevation or depression. This is seen most commonly in the precordial leads V2–V4; however, this can occur in any leads.

Cardiac biomarkers

- Troponin is elevated on admission in the majority of patients.
- Some patients may be troponin-negative.
- The peak troponin elevation is relatively mild, in comparison to the degree of wall motion abnormality, and is significantly lower than would be seen in a similar STEMI presentation.
- N-terminal pro-B-type natriuretic peptide (NT-pro-BNP) or brain natriuretic peptide (BNP) are usually very significantly raised in TTS, to a much higher degree than is expected in STEMI.
- Low levels of BNP predict a more favourable prognosis; however, persistent elevation of biomarkers, following the recovery of LV function, is associated with persistent cardiac symptoms.

Echocardiography

- Urgent echocardiographic assessment of cardiac function is essential for the diagnosis of TTS and to permit risk stratification of these patients.
- The classical echocardiographic findings and the anatomical variants are described in Box 2.4.2.
- The area of hypokinesis is usually not limited to a single coronary territory, and the overall LV function can appear very significantly impaired.
- Measures of LVEF are <45% in over 50% of patients presenting with TTS.
- LVEF correlates poorly with invasive or non-invasive measures of CO, which are often higher than the LVEF would suggest.
- The majority of patients with acute TTS have a normal or near-normal CO, despite lower SBP.
- Right ventricular (RV) involvement occurs in approximately 20% of patients with TTS.
- Early echocardiography is also important to identify complications associated with TTS, including apical thrombus, LV free wall rupture, ventricular septal defect (VSD) formation, new mitral regurgitation, or LVOTO.

Cardiac magnetic resonance imaging

Cardiac MRI is a useful imaging modality in TTS to confirm the diagnosis, determine the extent of myocardial dysfunction, and rule out alternative causes, and it has a number of advantages over echocardiography:

- It has greater precision at imaging the apical myocardium.
- It is more sensitive than transthoracic echocardiography at detecting RV involvement, which can be seen in up to a third of cases and carries a less favourable prognosis.
- It is particularly useful for differentiating between TTS and myocarditis. The areas of wall motion abnormality in TTS demonstrate myocardial oedema with high T2 signal. The distribution of oedema is usually transmural, which distinguishes it from a myocarditic pattern which is typically subepicardial.
- Late gadolinium enhancement (LGE) is rarely observed in TTS, and its presence suggests an alternative diagnosis. It is occasionally present as small patchy areas of LGE during the acute phase, reflecting oedema, but resolves at follow-up, in contrast to the permanent non-ischaemic epicardial LGE pattern seen following viral myocarditis.

Box 2.4.2 Anatomical variants of Takotsubo syndrome

The anatomical variants of TTS are significantly less common than the typical morphology. These appear to have similar long-term outcomes as the apical variant and require a similar approach to management.

- *Classical variant (75–80%)*—akinetic apical and mid-ventricular regions with a hypercontractile base. This gives rise to the name 'Takotsubo' after the appearance of the Japanese fishing pot.
- *Mid-left ventricular variant (10–15%)*—the apical and basal regions are preserved, and the mid-left ventricle is the only affected region. This gives the appearance of an 'ace of spades' on ventriculography.
- *Inverted variant (5%)*—the inverted phenotype is characterized by hypercontractility of the apex, with hypokinesis of the basal segments. This appearance is often referred to as the 'nutmeg heart' or 'artichoke heart'.
- *Regional variants (<1%)*—there are several other variants which have been reported much less commonly, including RV, global, and focal variants.

Acute complications

The high level of in-hospital mortality is due to serious haemodynamically significant complications, which occur in up to 52% of patients either at presentation or during the acute hospital admission.[1]

Heart failure and cardiogenic shock

- Acute HF occurs in 12–45% of patients.
- Cardiogenic shock is present in up to 10% of patients due to profound impairment of LV function.
- Early escalation to intensive care for inotropic support and consideration of mechanical support are essential, as the mortality in this setting is significantly elevated.

Left ventricular outflow tract obstruction

- LVOTO is very common, occurring in up to 25% of cases.
- It is caused by basal hypercontractility, leading to impingement of the outflow tract, which, combined with dysfunction of the mitral valve apparatus due to apical akinesis, causes systolic anterior motion of the mitral valve leaflet and obstruction of the outflow tract.
- There can be large gradients within the mid-ventricular cavity, and gradients of >40mmHg carry a poor prognosis.
- Avoidance of intravascular volume depletion is important to prevent exacerbating the LVOTO.
- β-blockers may be helpful if significant LVOTO is present.

Mitral regurgitation

- New moderate to severe mitral regurgitation occurs in up to 25% of presentations.
- Usually caused by dysfunction of the mitral valve apparatus and systolic anterior motion of the anterior leaflet, rather than a primary mitral valve problem.
- Acute mitral regurgitation causes pulmonary oedema in the acute phase; however, as the LV function improves, mitral regurgitation tends to improve also.

Ventricular septal defect and free wall rupture

- An uncommon, but serious, complication which occurs in <1% of cases.
- Areas of contraction band necrosis which form after severe episodes of TTS and are vulnerable to rupture up to day 10 post-presentation.

Apical thrombus

- Apical thrombus is present in 2–8% of patients.
- It is usually found in the apex due to the profound akinesis of this segment.
- High risk of systemic embolization, as the LV function recovers.

Arrhythmia

- AF is seen in up to 15% of patients, which is very poorly tolerated due to already significant LV impairment.
- Ventricular tachyarrhythmias occur in up to 9% of cases and contribute to significant early mortality with TTS.
- Bradyarrhythmias and conduction blocks have also been reported.

Long-term complications

Mortality

Long-term mortality at 1 and 5 years have recently been demonstrated to be significantly higher than previously thought and has dispelled the notion that Takotsubo is a single acute benign presentation.

- The 5-year all-cause mortality is 25%, compared to a mortality rate of 15% in age-matched patients presenting with STEMI.[2]
- The rates of CV death are similar in both groups.
- The excess mortality is accounted for by non-cardiac causes, which was 10% in TTS patients, compared with 3% in STEMI patients.[2]

This suggests that the underlying acute illness contributing to initial hospital admission and subsequent presentation with TTS plays a significant role in long-term mortality. In keeping with this is the finding that TTS presenting because of physical stressors have an increased mortality rate, in comparison to cases presenting following emotional stressors. Ensuring optimal management of the underlying condition therefore is a vital step in improving long-term outcomes.

Recurrence

- The risk of recurrence of TTS is commoner than has been anticipated previously.
- Five to 22% of cases have a second presentation, with an approximately 10–15% recurrence rate reported in the largest series.[1,5]
- The timing of recurrence can vary from a few months to many years after the index presentation.
- This carries a similar risk of in-hospital morbidity and mortality as the initial presentation and suggests that, despite macroscopic resolution of myocardial function, there remains an underlying predisposition to developing TTS.

Persisting symptoms

There are a significant proportion of patients (15–20%) who continue to have cardiac symptoms, despite macroscopic recovery of ventricular function. The commonest symptoms include:

- Chest pain.
- Dyspnoea.
- Fatigue.
- Palpitations due to atrial or ventricular arrhythmias.

It is likely these symptoms have a true cardiac origin, and this should prompt a thorough investigation for causes, including arrhythmias, diastolic dysfunction, and microvascular dysfunction. These patients will often have subtle objective signs of ongoing cardiac disease, including impaired global longitudinal strain, persistent elevation of cardiac biomarkers, and a commoner incidence of atrial arrhythmias on ambulatory monitoring.

Risk stratification

Effectively risk-stratifying patients to identify those at significant risk of serious complications is vital. Box 2.4.3 highlights the important major and minor criteria for stratifying patients proposed by the HFA Takotsubo syndrome Taskforce in 2016.

In conjunction with the management algorithm in Fig. 2.4.1, these risk factors act as a tool to recommend appropriate levels of monitoring and management for patients presenting with TTS.

The presence of one major criteria or two minor criteria is sufficient to be considered high risk.

Box 2.4.3 Heart Failure Association risk stratification in TTS

Major risk factors

- Age >75 years
- SBP <110mmHg
- Clinical pulmonary oedema
- LVEF <35%
- Unexplained syncope, ventricular tachycardia (VT), or ventricular fibrillation (VF)
- LVOTO gradient >40mmHg
- New moderate to severe mitral regurgitation
- VSD or LV wall rupture

Minor risk factors

- Age 70–75 years
- Physical stressor
- Bystander coronary disease
- LVEF 35–40%
- Biventricular involvement
- ECG:
    - QTc >500ms
    - Pathological Q waves
    - Persistent ST-elevation
- Natriuretic peptide:
    - BNP >600pg/mL
    - NT-pro-BNP >2000pg/mL

Source data from Lyon AR, Bossone E, Schneider B, *et al.* Current state of knowledge on Takotsubo syndrome: a Position Statement from the Taskforce on Takotsubo Syndrome of the Heart Failure Association of the European Society of Cardiology. *Eur J Heart Fail* 2016;**18**:8–27.

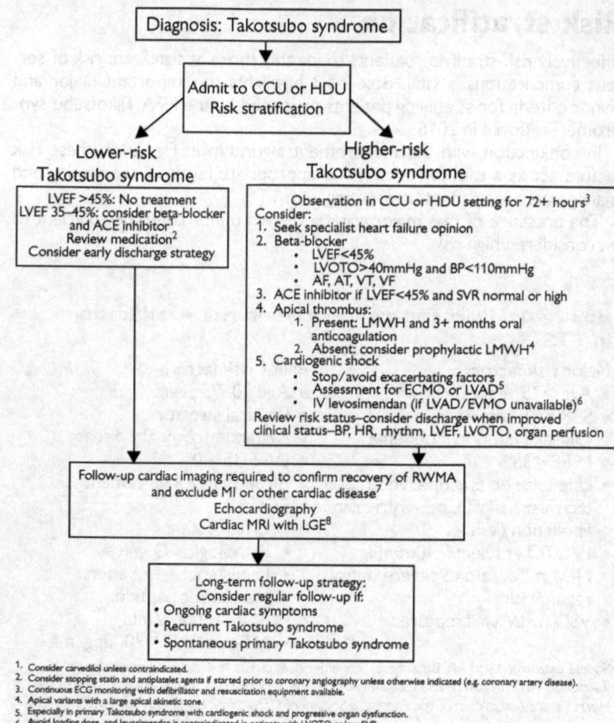

Fig. 2.4.1 European Society of Cardiology Takotsubo Syndrome Management Algorithm. ACE inhibitor, angiotensin-converting enzyme inhibitor; AF, atrial fibrillation; AT, atrial tachycardia; BP, blood pressure; CCU, coronary care unit; ECMO, extra-corporeal membrane oxygenation; HDU, high-dependency unit; HR, heart rate; LGE, late gadolinium enhancement; LMWH, low-molecular-weight heparin; LVAD, left ventricular assist device; LVEF, left ventricular ejection fraction; LVOTO, left ventricular outflow tract obstruction; MRI, magnetic resonance imaging; VF, ventricular fibrillation; VT, ventricular tachycardia.

Reproduced from Lyon AR, Bossone E, Schneider B, Sechtem U, Citro R, Underwood SR, *et al.* Current state of knowledge on Takotsubo syndrome: a Position Statement from the Taskforce on Takotsubo Syndrome of the Heart Failure Association of the European Society of Cardiology. *Eur J Heart Fail* 2016;**18**(1):8–27 with permission from Wiley.

Management

General considerations

The management of TTS is not informed by any prospective RCTs to date, and the treatment is largely supportive, with vigilant monitoring for the development of any significant complications to enable initiation of prompt management. The HFA TTS Taskforce has developed an algorithm (see Fig 2.4.1) to guide the acute management of patients with TTS.

- Patients should be monitored in a high-dependency environment or on a coronary care unit for at least 24h following admission.
- Continuous ECG monitoring is important due to the risk of ventricular tachyarrhythmias.
- Frequent reassessment for haemodynamic deterioration is important to enable a rapid response to life-threatening complications.

Low-risk patients

- Low-risk patients typically have an uneventful recovery and good long-term prognosis with or without medical intervention.
- Monitoring for 24h in a high-dependency environment with continuous ECG monitoring is important to accurately identify high-risk features.
- If uncomplicated, they can be moved to a ward after 24h.
- Consider early discharge when their symptoms have abated.
- All patients must be followed up with outpatient echocardiography after 3–6 months to confirm recovery of ventricular function.

Low-risk patients—mild systolic impairment

- Low-risk patients with mild systolic impairment should have a conservative approach to treatment.
- Patients usually recover well in this subset without intervention.
- There is little evidence to guide interventions and there is significant risk of iatrogenic harm in this setting.

Low-risk patients—moderate systolic impairment

- Introduction of β-blockers and ACEIs may be beneficial in this setting; however, they must be weighed against the risks of therapy.
- Often treatments are introduced after the patient has become haemodynamically stable and the LV function has started to improve.

High-risk patients

- Prolonged monitoring in a high-dependency environment with continuous ECG monitoring is important for at least 72h.
- Treatment is mainly supportive, with careful monitoring for acute complications, which carry significant mortality if not addressed early.
- The advice of HF specialists is invaluable in this setting.
- Discussion with specialist centres should be undertaken early if mechanical CV support is likely to be required.

ACE inhibitors and angiotensin receptor blockers

The role of ACEIs and ARBs is extrapolated from their role in systolic HF and small observational studies. Therefore, treatment with ACEIs is typically initiated in those patients who have a significant impairment of LVEF.

- Vasodilatory effects of ACEIs may limit the elevation of BP and afterload related to surges of catecholamines.
- The myocardial remodelling properties may help to improve LV function in the long term.
- A retrospective analysis of patients presenting with TTS found that the use of ACEIs or ARBs was associated with improved survival at 1 year.[5]

ACE inhibitors in left ventricular outflow tract obstruction

- ACEIs can worsen the gradient across the outflow tract in LVOTO by causing peripheral vasodilatation, which increases flow velocities across the outflow tract, causing worsening of the systolic anterior motion of the mitral valve.
- ACEIs should be avoided in this setting.

ACE inhibitors in low systemic vascular resistance

- The HFA TTS position statement suggests considering an ACEI in most low-risk patients with moderate LV impairment.
- A subset of patients with TTS have paradoxically low systemic vascular resistance (SVR), due to altered peripheral sympathetic activity. Vasodilating agents in this setting may cause significant harm, particularly in patients with a low CO. In patients with a higher risk of complications, calculation of the SVR is suggested before introducing ACEIs which should be avoided in the subset of patients with low SVR.

ACE inhibitors/angiotensin receptor blockers in the prevention of recurrence

- A systematic review of retrospective studies of patients presenting with TTS found that use of ACEIs/ARBs was associated with a lower risk of recurrence of TTS.[5]

Mineralocorticoid receptor antagonists

Evidence is lacking regarding any role for mineralocorticoid receptor antagonists (MRAs) in the treatment of TTS. Although robust evidence exists in patients with HF with reduced ejection fraction, extrapolation to use in this setting is difficult.

In patients who have incomplete recovery with persisting impairment of ventricular function with reduced LVEF, this class of drugs could be considered.

Beta-blockers

High-quality evidence is lacking to guide the role of β-blockade in TTS. Recommendations are based predominantly on extrapolation from the role of β-blockers in systolic HF, pre-clinical studies, and basic mechanistic principles.

- β-blockers are a logical approach to manage a presumed hypercatecholaminergic state. They aim to reduce adrenergic signalling, in an attempt to reverse or limit the pathological mechanism.
- Antiarrhythmic properties may help to reduce the high rates of malignant ventricular arrhythmias seen with TTS.
- Animal studies demonstrated improvement of LV function following administration of metoprolol in primates and that non-selective β-blockers, such as carvedilol, are beneficial in rats.
- A retrospective analysis of patients admitted with TTS found no improvement in TTS recurrence or survival at 1 year for patients taking β-blockers.[2,5]

Risks of beta-blocker therapy

- β-blockers can potentially cause significant harm in the acute phase of TTS, particularly in patients with severe LV impairment, due to their negative inotropic effects.
- TTS is typically a self-resolving condition; therefore, the decision to use β-blockers in this setting needs to be considered carefully.

Beta-blockers in left ventricular outflow tract obstruction

- β-blockers should be considered in patients with LVOTO with a gradient of >40mmHg and SBP of <110mmHg.
- β-blockade will increase diastolic filling time and end-diastolic volume which reduces the gradient across the LVOT.
- Short-acting IV β-blockers, such as metoprolol, should be preferred acutely due to the risk of worsening HF.
- In pre-clinical studies, non-selective β-blockers, such as carvedilol and propranolol, were shown to more effectively reduce basal hypercontractility, which may help reduce LVOTO, but at the expense of worsening the apical hypokinesis.
- α-agonists, such as phenylephrine, can be used as an alternative to increase afterload in LVOTO if BP is insufficient to permit the use of β-blockers.

Beta-blockers in the prevention of recurrence

- β-blockers would be expected to protect against catecholamine surges, and abrupt withdrawal of β-blockers can precipitate TTS.
- A meta-analysis of preventative strategies found no reduction in recurrence rates in patients taking β-blockers.[5] However, this did not compare non-selective β-blockers, such as carvedilol [inhibits α-1 adrenoreceptors (α1ARs), β1ARs, and β2ARs], with more β1AR-selective β-blockers (e.g. bisoprolol), which theoretically may have less protective effects.
- In selected patients with high levels of sympathetic tone, anxiety, or recurrent TTS, prophylactic use of β-blockers is a reasonable strategy to reduce the rate of recurrence.

Inotropes and vasopressors

Catecholamine-based inotropes

- Noradrenaline, adrenaline, milrinone, and dobutamine should be avoided in patients with TTS.
- These increase adrenergic stimulation and are likely to worsen the clinical picture, contribute to an increased gradient across the LVOT, and delay spontaneous recovery.
- Inotropes, such as dobutamine, used for stress echocardiography and adrenaline used in intensive care have been known to trigger episodes of TTS and should be avoided.

Levosimendan

- Enhances binding between actin and myosin filaments by sensitizing these molecules to calcium, therefore, unlike other inotropes, improves contractility without raising intracellular calcium levels.
- Levosimendan may be considered in Takotsubo patients in cardiogenic shock and with multi-organ failure, in whom mechanical support is not immediately available.
- Pre-clinical studies in rodents suggest that levosimendan reduces mortality associated with TTS.
- Levosimendan causes peripheral vasodilatation at higher doses and therefore may not be suitable for patients who are already haemodynamically compromised.

Anticoagulation and antiplatelets

- LV thrombus is common because of the profound akinesis of significant portions of the LV wall.
- LV thrombus found on echocardiography should prompt therapeutic anticoagulation initially with LMWH, followed by oral anticoagulation with VKAs such as warfarin. This should be continued until resolution of the thrombus and wall motion abnormalities have been proven by echocardiography.
- In patients with severely akinetic segments, prophylactic LMWH should be considered to prevent future thromboembolic events until the LV function has recovered.
- Many patients with TTS will receive antiplatelet therapy due to suspected MI on admission. Once MI has been excluded, P2Y12 inhibitors, such as clopidogrel, prasugrel, and ticagrelor, can be discontinued.

Mechanical support

Patients with cardiogenic shock who are developing multi-organ failure should be considered early for mechanical circulatory support.

- Intra-aortic balloon pumps are not recommended, due to poor outcomes in cardiogenic shock trials and the risk of worsening LVOTO.
- Use of LV assist devices (LVADs) or venous–arterial extra-corporeal membrane oxygenation (VA-ECMO) as a short-term bridge to recovery should be considered in these patients.
- Consideration needs to be taken of the prognosis of the comorbidities, particularly if this was triggered by acute illness.
- Good recovery of native LV function is very likely, and therefore, there is a strong likelihood of successfully weaning off mechanical support without needing to resort to heart transplantation.

Follow-up

All TTS patients should be followed up after 3–6 months with:

- A clinical review regarding symptoms.
- Repeat ECG.
- Repeat cardiac biomarkers.
- Repeat echocardiography to confirm recovery of LV function.
- Cardiac MRI to confirm the diagnosis.
- Spontaneous cases—consider screening for phaeochromocytoma.

Persistence of ECG changes and elevation of biomarkers at this stage highlight patients who are at risk of persistent symptoms or recurrence of TTS in the future.

Longer-term follow-up should be offered to patients with:

- Ongoing cardiac symptoms, despite resolution of ventricular function, to consider prophylactic therapy to prevent recurrence.
- Recurrent episodes of TTS.
- Episodes with no clear triggering event.

Conclusion

TTS is an increasingly commonly recognized medical entity, and recently, there have been significant advances in the understanding of the pathophysiology and potential therapeutic strategies. The diagnosis and management are currently guided by expert opinion, and the HFA TTS position statement has provided clarity in a number of areas. Currently, prospective clinical trial evidence is lacking, and management is based on clinical opinion. At present, optimal supportive care and avoidance of catecholamines are the mainstay of treatment.

References

1 Lyon AR, Bossone E, Schneider B, *et al.* Current state of knowledge on Tako-tsubo syndrome: a Position Statement from the Taskforce on Takotsubo Syndrome of the Heart Failure Association of the European Society of Cardiology. *Eur J Heart Fail* 2016;**18**:8–27.

2 Stiermaier T, Moeller C, Oehler K, *et al.* Long-term excess mortality in takotsubo cardiomyopathy: predictors, causes and clinical consequences. *Eur J Heart Fail* 2016;**18**:650–6.

3 Schultz T, Shao Y, Redfors B, *et al.* Stress-induced cardiomyopathy in Sweden: evidence for different ethnic predisposition and altered cardio-circulatory status. *Cardiology* 2012;**122**:180–6.

4 Templin C, Ghadri JR, Diekmann J, *et al.* Clinical features and outcomes of Takotsubo (stress) cardiomyopathy. *N Engl J Med* 2015;**373**:929–38.

5 Singh K, Carson K, Usmani Z, Sawhney G, Shah R, Horowitz J. Systematic review and meta-analysis of incidence and correlates of recurrence of takotsubo cardiomyopathy. *Int J Cardiol* 2014;**174**:696–701.

Section 3

Heart failure

Section editors

Theresa McDonagh
Faiez Zannad

ESC Guidelines advisor
Faiez Zannad

Chapter 3.1

Heart failure

Faiez Zannad, João Pedro Ferreira, and Theresa McDonagh

Introduction

Heart failure (HF) is a complex condition that results from cardiac functional and/or structural abnormalities that affect the ability of the heart to pump blood, potentially leading to inadequate organ perfusion and/or systemic congestion. The commonest manifestations of HF are dyspnoea and fatigue.

The HF syndrome can result from both impaired systolic and/or diastolic function. Up to 50% of HF cases occur in the presence of a preserved systolic function (LVEF ≥45–50%), currently referred to as HF with preserved ejection fraction (HFpEF), in contrast to HF with reduced ejection fraction (HFrEF). This division is mainly made on the basis of trial results, since HF treatments only reduced mortality in HFrEF. More recently, an 'intermediate' class was created. This class refers to HF with mid-range ejection fraction (HFmEF) for patients with LVEF of 40–50%. However, this division is based on 'expert opinion' and does not reflect trial results. Hence, for the purposes of HF management, we will refer only to HFpEF or HfrEF, as just described.

HF can also be classified as acute or chronic, depending on how quickly symptoms and signs develop, and 'right' versus 'left' HF indicating whether symptoms predominantly suggest RV failure with peripheral oedema, raised jugular venous pressure (JVP), and hepatomegaly, or predominantly LV failure with pulmonary oedema and/or hypoperfusion. HF can also be classified has high- versus low-output, depending on conditions that may increase or decrease the CO.

Ejection fraction can be assessed objectively with echocardiography, cardiac magnetic resonance (CMR), or nuclear imaging. Independently of the used method, LVEF has been used systematically as a major inclusion criterion in HF trials, and, as stated earlier, it has become one of the most commonly used measurements for the assessment of the severity of LV dysfunction and for treatment indication. Although the severity of LV dysfunction does not necessarily correlate with HF severity and symptoms, useful grading systems exist in the clinical setting that are based on symptoms and cardiac function, i.e. the New York Heart Association (NHYA) classification for symptoms and the ACC/AHA classification for symptoms in the context of cardiac structure and function (see Table 3.1.1). Note that the ACC/AHA classification is much different to the NYHA functional classification system, in that there is no moving backwards to prior stages. Once symptoms develop, stage C overt HF is present and stage B will never again be achieved. In the NYHA classification, in contrast, patients can move between class I and class IV relatively quickly, as these are all designated on symptoms alone.

The present chapter discusses, separately, three subgroups of HF patients:

- Chronic HF with reduced LVEF (HFrEF).
- Chronic HF with preserved LVEF (HFpEF).
- Acute HF.

Table 3.1.1 New York Heart Association (NHYA) classification for symptoms and the American College of Cardiology/American Heart Association (ACC/AHA) classification for symptoms in the context of cardiac structure and function

NYHA classification I–IV	
Class	Symptoms
I	No limitation to physical activity. Ordinary physical activity does not cause fatigue, breathlessness, or palpitations (asymptomatic HF)
II	Slight limitation to physical activity. Such patients are comfortable at rest. Ordinary physical activity results in fatigue, palpitations, breathlessness, or angina pectoris (mildly symptomatic HF)
III	Marked limitation of physical activity. Although patients are comfortable at rest, less than ordinary physical activity will lead to symptoms (symptomatically 'moderate' HF)
IV	Inability to carry out any physical activity without discomfort. Symptoms are even present at rest (symptomatically 'severe' HF)
ACC/AHA classification A–D	
Stage	Cardiac structure and function
A	Patients at risk for HF who have not yet developed structural heart changes (i.e. those with diabetes, those with coronary disease without prior infarct)
B	Patients with structural heart disease (i.e. reduced ejection fraction, LVH, chamber enlargement) who have not yet developed HF symptoms
C	Patients who have developed clinical HF
D	Patients with refractory HF requiring advanced intervention (i.e. biventricular pacemakers, LVAD, transplantation)

Source data from http://www.heart.org/HEARTORG/Conditions/HeartFailure/AboutHeartFailure/Classes-of-Heart-Failure_UCM_306328_Article.jsp#.WxEoFDQvyUk

Chronic heart failure with reduced LVEF (HFrEF)

Incidence and prognosis

HF is a common condition, with an increasing incidence with age. Due to demographic trends of an ageing population, its prevalence is also increasing.

There are an estimated 934,000 people over the age of 45 years who have diagnosed or suspected HF in the United Kingdom.

Mortality has been quoted as high as 30% at 1 year after diagnosis, but survival has improved with newer HF treatments.

Aetiology

The commonest HF causes are:

- IHD—the commonest cause in developed countries (50–70% of cases).
- Arterial hypertension, which often causes HF with preserved LVEF.
- The cardiomyopathies, including dilated cardiomyopathy, hypertrophic cardiomyopathy, restrictive cardiomyopathy, peripartum cardiomyopathy, and arrhythmogenic cardiomyopathy.
- Other common causes include: alcohol consumption, treatments/drugs (i.e. chemotherapy), valvular heart disease (VHD), infiltrative disorders (amyloid and sarcoid), and rhythm disturbances such as chronic uncontrolled tachycardia.
- High-output HF is a less common form of presentation and can be caused by thyrotoxicosis, beriberi, Paget's disease, sepsis, anaemia, and some arrhythmias.
- The commonest causes for an acute decompensation in a patient with chronic HF include myocardial ischaemia or infarction, arrhythmias, inappropriate or insufficient drug therapy, infection, anaemia, etc.

Symptoms and signs of heart failure

The cardinal symptoms of HF are dyspnoea at rest or on exertion, orthopnoea, paroxysmal nocturnal dyspnoea, and fatigue. Signs of HF include those attributable to LV failure, such as pulmonary oedema, cold extremities, hypotension, and a third heart sound, and those of right HF such as a raised JVP, peripheral oedema, hepatomegaly, and ascites.

Useful investigations

Blood tests

- In addition to routine blood tests, including blood count, urea, creatinine, electrolytes, fasting glucose, lipids, liver function tests (LFTs), and thyroid function tests, the measurement of natriuretic peptides is relevant. Natriuretic peptides can help not only in the diagnosis and prognosis of patients with HF, but also in the assessment of response to treatment. A normal BNP concentration in an untreated patient makes the diagnosis of HF unlikely, whereas a high BNP level, despite maximal medical treatment, often indicates a poor prognosis. Conditions other than HF that can lead to a raised BNP level include: sepsis, renal dysfunction, LV hypertrophy (LVH), myocardial ischaemia, and advanced age.
- The resting 12-lead ECG may show signs of IHD, such as an old infarction or LBBB, LVH, conduction disturbances [important to note that a QRS of >120ms is one of the criteria for cardiac resynchronization therapy (CRT)], or cardiac arrhythmias. Holter monitoring might be considered to look for VT in high-risk patients.
- The chest X-ray provides evidence for cardiomegaly, pulmonary venous congestion, pulmonary oedema, pleural effusion, and lung disease.
- Transthoracic echocardiography is essential in the assessment of patients with symptoms/signs of HF. LVEF is used to classify HF as diastolic or systolic, and the echocardiogram may establish the aetiology of HF in the individual patient, e.g. VHD, MI, LVH, or global LV dysfunction associated with dilated cardiomyopathy (DCM). Stress echocardiography can be used to detect reversible myocardial ischaemia and to assess for myocardial hibernation, valvular abnormalities, and the response to CRT.
- Coronary angiography should be performed in patients presenting with HF who have angina or significant myocardial ischaemia on non-invasive testing. Controlled trials have not addressed the issue of whether coronary revascularization can improve clinical outcomes in patients with HF who do not have angina pectoris.
- MRI is the gold standard for evaluating ventricular dimensions, as it has a high degree of reproducibility. It is also extremely useful for the assessment of ventricular function and wall motion abnormalities, myocardial viability, and scar tissue. It can also be useful for detecting RV dysplasia and identifying the presence of pericardial disease.
- Maximal oxygen consumption (VO_{2max}) exercise testing can give useful information in patients presenting with HF who may be candidates for cardiac transplantation or device implantation.

Pharmacological management of chronic heart failure

The recommendations that follow are based on NICE, ESC, and AHA guidelines. Of importance, the NICE guidelines apply only to patients who already have HF. AHA guidelines take into account patients without HF but who have risk factors for HF, including known CAD, hypertension, diabetes mellitus, and a family history of cardiomyopathy. These high-risk patients require treatment with disease-modifying agents. There is substantial trial evidence for the treatment of HF, but one should acknowledge that women, blacks, and the very elderly are not well represented in these trials.

Pharmacological treatment

This can be divided into:

- Treatments that prolong life in patients with HFrEF and should be prescribed to all patients with HfrEF, unless contraindicated, i.e. ACEIs, ARBs, angiotensin receptor–neprilysin inhibitor (ARNI) (i.e. sacubitril/valsartan), aldosterone antagonists (i.e. spironolactone and eplerenone), and β-blockers.
- Treatments that improve symptoms only (i.e. diuretics and digoxin).
- Ivabradine which can be used to decrease hospitalizations in HFrEF patients with high heart rate.

See the flow chart in Fig. 3.1.1 for a summary of the pharmacological management of chronic systolic HF.

ACE inhibitors or angiotensin receptor blockers (class I, level of evidence A)

ACE inhibitors

ACEIs are recommended as first-line therapy (unless contraindicated) in all patients with LVEF of <40%, irrespective of symptoms. Multiple trials have shown that ACEIs reduce mortality and morbidity in patients with HFrEF. However, many patients are excluded from these trials, such as those with hypotension, CKD (stage ≥4), normal ejection fraction, and the very elderly. ACEIs should be uptitrated to the maximum tolerated dose, in order to achieve adequate inhibition of the RAAS. However, there is evidence that, in clinical practice, the majority of patients receive suboptimal doses of ACEIs. Some patients improve within a few days of starting ACEI therapy, but most patients only get benefit after several weeks or months of treatment. Below we present some data from cornerstone trials with ACEIs in HFrEF.

- The Survival and Ventricular Enlargement (SAVE) trial was the first large trial of ACEIs in LV dysfunction following MI. Over 2000 patients with an ejection fraction of <40% 3–16 days following MI were randomized to either placebo or captopril. All-cause mortality was 19% lower in the ACEI group. There was also a 37% reduction in the development of severe HF.
- Cooperative North Scandinavian Enalapril Survival Study (CONSENSUS) and Studies of Left Ventricular Dysfunction (SOLVD) randomized patients with mild to severe HF to treatment with placebo or enalapril. There was a reduction in mortality of 27% in CONSENSUS and 16% in SOLVD.

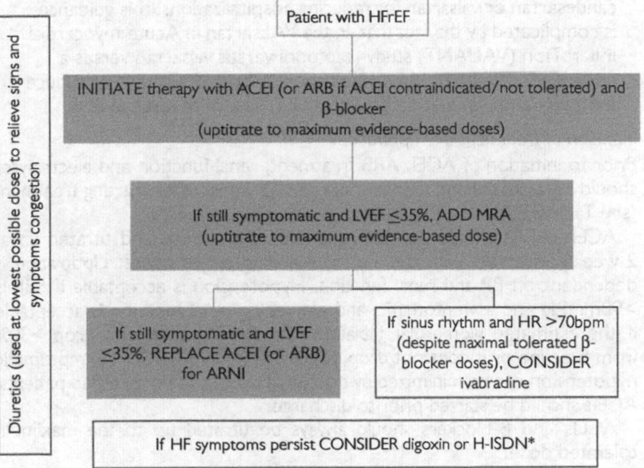

Fig. 3.1.1 Summary of pharmacological treatment for HFrEF. ACEI, angiotensin-converting enzyme inhibitor; ARB, angiotensin receptor blocker; ARNI, angiotensin receptor–neprilysin inhibitor; HFrEF, heart failure with reduced ejection fraction; H-ISDN, hydralazine and isosorbide dinitrate; HR, heart rate; LVEF, left ventricular ejection fraction. Green boxes = mortality benefit. White boxes = no mortality benefit. * Device therapy or heart transplant are beyond the scope of this schema.

- The SOLVD-Prevention trial showed that patients with low ejection fraction, but no symptoms, benefited from ACEI with a 20% relative risk reduction (RRR) in death or hospitalization with HF. This emphasizes the importance of starting ACEI therapy in patients with HF, even before they become symptomatic.

Angiotensin receptor blockers

ACEIs are generally preferred to ARBs, because there is more clinical experience and weight of trials behind their use, compared to ARBs. It is reasonable to use an ARB when a patient is intolerant to ACEIs (e.g. develops significant ACEI-induced cough). The combination of an ACEI plus an ARB is not generally recommended due to increased adverse events (e.g. symptomatic hypotension and worsening renal function) without mortality benefit. In the context of adding another RAAS blocker, an MRA should be preferred. Below we present some data from cornerstone trials with ARBs in HFrEF.

- Candesartan in Heart failure: Assessment of Reduction in Mortality and morbidity (CHARM)-Alternative was a placebo-controlled trial with candesartan in patients with LVEF of <40%, who were intolerant to ACEIs. Candesartan resulted in an RRR of death from a CV cause or hospital admission for worsening HF of 23%.
- Despite some evidence [CHARM–Added and Valsartan Heart Failure Trial (Val-HeFT)] that HFrEF patients in NYHA class III or IV, despite ACEI and β-blocker therapy, do benefit from the addition of

candesartan or valsartan for reducing hospitalizations, this guidance is complicated by the fact that, in the VALsartan In Acute myocardial iNfarcTion (VALIANT) study (captopril versus valsartan versus a combination of both), the combination of both drugs did not reduce mortality and was associated with an increase in adverse events.

Initiation of treatment and uptitration

Prior to initiation of ACEI/ARB treatment, renal function and electrolytes should be assessed and then rechecked 1–2 weeks after starting treatment (see Table 3.1.2).

ACEIs/ARBs should be commenced at a low dose and titrated up at 2-weekly intervals, with the aim of reaching target doses. Uptitration is dependent on BP and renal function. Hypotension is acceptable if SBP is >90mmHg and asymptomatic, and worsening renal function is acceptable if the estimated glomerular filtration rate (eGFR) does not drop >30% from baseline or it does not drop below 30mL/min/1.73m^2. Symptomatic hypotension can be minimized by nocturnal dosing. In hospitalized patients, ACEIs should be started prior to discharge.

ACEIs and β-blockers should always be titrated up to the maximum tolerated dose.

Contraindications

History of angio-oedema, bilateral renal artery stenosis, serum potassium >5mmol/L, eGFR <30mL/min/1.73m^2, severe aortic stenosis.

Side effects

- Cough: a dry cough related to the use of ACEIs is the commonest reason for the withdrawal of long-term treatment. It occurs in 5–10% of white patients and up to 50% of Chinese patients. It usually appears within the first month of treatment and disappears within 1–2 weeks of discontinuing treatment. Given the known benefits of ACEIs, it is important to try and persist with treatment, unless the cough is severe, particularly since the cough may be coincidental, as found in many studies. If a significant and persistent cough does develop on an ACEI, then an ARB should be used instead.

Table 3.1.2 Doses of ACEIs and ARBs with the largest evidence in HF trials

	Starting dose	Target dose
ACEI		
Captopril	6.25mg tds	50–100mg tds
Enalapril	2.5mg od	10–20mg bd
Lisinopril	2.5mg od	20–35mg od
Ramipril	1.25–2.5mg od	10mg od
ARB		
Candesartan	4–8mg od	32mg od
Valsartan	40mg bd	160mg bd

- Hypotension: if a patient develops symptomatic hypotension, reduce the dose of any other antihypertensives before reducing the dose of the ACEI.
- Hyperkalaemia: may be managed by stopping potassium supplements or potassium-sparing diuretics. If the potassium level still rises above 5.5mmol/L, halve the dose of the ACEI. If the potassium level rises above 6.0mmol/L, then stop the ACEI.
- Deterioration in renal function: some increase in urea and creatinine levels can be expected after starting an ACEI. A decrease of up to 30% in the eGFR may be acceptable but must be carefully monitored.
- Angio-oedema is a very serious side effect, and if this occurs, then the ACEI must be stopped immediately.

Beta-blockers (class I, level of evidence A)

β-blockers should be used (unless contraindicated) in all patients with LVEF of <40%, irrespective of symptoms. Like ACEIs, they have been shown to reduce mortality and morbidity. Evidence to support the use of β-blockers derives from the following trials.

- Cardiac Insufficiency Bisoprolol Study II (CIBIS II) (bisoprolol), Carvedilol Prospective Randomized Cumulative Survival (COPERNICUS) (carvedilol), and Metoprolol CR/XL Randomised Intervention Trial in Congestive Heart Failure (MERIT-HF) (sustained-release metoprolol). These trials randomized nearly 9000 patients with HF to either placebo or β-blocker therapy; 90% of these patients were on an ACEI or ARB. Each of these trials showed that β-blockers reduced mortality (RRR of about 34% in each trial) and hospital admissions for worsening HF (RRR 28–36%).
- There are very few trials in HF that included elderly patients. The Study of the Effects of Nebivolol Intervention on Outcomes and Rehospitalisation in Seniors with Heart Failure (SENIORS) trial was an RCT in elderly (>70 years old) patients with HF. Treatment with nebivolol resulted in an RRR of 14% in the primary composite endpoint of death or hospital admissions for a CV reason.

Of note, not all β-blockers have the same effect. Metoprolol tartrate (as opposed to sustained-release metoprolol succinate) does not confer as much benefit as carvedilol [Carvedilol Or Metoprolol European Trial (COMET)]. There is no evidence of benefit for bucindolol (increases death in African Americans), and xamoterol has been found to be harmful. As such, the only recommended β-blockers for management of HF patients are bisoprolol, carvedilol, nebivolol, and sustained-release metoprolol (not available in the United Kingdom).

Commencing therapy and uptitration

β-blockers should be commenced at a low dose and titrated up to target doses at 2- to 4-weekly intervals (see Table 3.1.3). They should usually be initiated in stable patients and only with caution in recently decompensated patients. Do not increase the dose if signs of worsening HF or symptomatic hypotension appear, or if the heart rate is <50bpm.

In patients admitted with a decompensation of HF and hypotension, β-blockers may need to be discontinued temporarily. However, a recent study has shown increased mortality in HF patients who have their β-blockers stopped during hospital stay.

Table 3.1.3 Doses of β-blockers with the largest evidence in HF trials

β-blockers	Starting dose	Target dose
Bisoprolol	1.25mg od	10mg od
Carvedilol	3.125mg bd	25–50mg bd
Metoprolol succinate	12.5mg od	200mg od
Nebivolol	1.25mg od	10mg od

Contraindications

- Second- or third-degree heart block.
- Sinus bradycardia (<50bpm).
- Symptomatic hypotension.
- Peripheral vascular disease: relative contraindication as benefits may outweigh a potential deterioration in symptoms of peripheral vascular disease.
- Obstructive airways disease (not COPD per se): relative contraindication as benefits may outweigh risks, and respiratory symptoms should be assessed during β-blocker uptitration.

Side effects

Symptomatic hypotension is relatively common but often improves over time. If hypotension appears, it may require β-blocker dose reduction. Asymptomatic hypotension does not require intervention.

Symptomatic bradycardia (<50bpm) may also require β-blocker dose adaptation.

Mineralocorticoid receptor antagonists (class I, level of evidence A)

MRAs should be used (unless contraindicated) in all HFrEF patients (with mild or severe symptoms) with an LVEF of <35%, in combination with ACEIs, β-blockers, and diuretics. MRAs have demonstrated to reduce mortality and morbidity in these patients and also in post-MI patients with systolic dysfunction (eplerenone).

MRA therapy has been evaluated in three large RCTs:

- Randomized Aldactone Evaluation Study (RALES).
- Eplerenone in Patients with Systolic Heart Failure and Mild Symptoms (EMPHASIS).
- Eplerenone Post-Acute Myocardial Infarction Heart Failure Efficacy and Survival Study (EPHESUS).

These trials showed that MRAs reduce the mortality and morbidity rate from 15% (EPHESUS) to 35% (RALES and EMPHASIS), compared to placebo (see Table 3.1.4).

Table 3.1.4 Doses of MRAs with the largest evidence in HF trials

β-blockers	Starting dose	Target dose
Spironolactone	12.5mg od	50mg od
Eplerenone	12.5mg od	50mg od

Cautions/contraindications

Cautions for starting treatment include hyperkalaemia and renal impairment. Check renal function prior to starting therapy and again at 1 and 4 weeks after starting treatment. Increase the dose after 4–8 weeks. Recheck renal function and potassium levels at 1 and 4 weeks after each dose increase and 3-monthly thereafter.

MRAs should not be prescribed if a patient is receiving combined treatment with an ACEI and an ARB.

In the case of intolerance (e.g. gynaecomastia, hyperkalaemia, worsening renal function, or sexual dysfunction), clinicians should assess all possible causes, including medication interactions, and consider other agents of the MRA class before stopping treatment.

Side effects

- Hyperkalaemia: if the potassium level rises to >5.5mmol/L, the dose of the MRA should be halved and potassium levels monitored. If the potassium level rises to 6.0mmol/L, stop spironolactone or eplerenone and monitor carefully.
- Worsening renal function: if the eGFR drops below 50mL/min/1.73m^2, halve the MRA dose. If the eGFR drops below 50mL/min/1.73m^2 or deteriorates >30% relative to the baseline value, then stop spironolactone or eplerenone and resume carefully after renal function recovery.
- Gynaecomastia: occurs in about 10% of patients given spironolactone. These patients should be switched to eplerenone.

Angiotensin receptor–neprilysin inhibitor (class I, level of evidence B)

A new therapeutic class of agents acting on the RAAS and the neutral endopeptidase system has been developed (ARNI). LCZ696 is a molecule that combines the moieties of valsartan and sacubitril (the neprilysin inhibitor) in a single substance. By inhibiting neprilysin, the degradation of natriuretic peptides, bradykinin, and other peptides is slowed. Hence, high circulating levels of natriuretic peptides enhance diuresis, natriuresis, myocardial relaxation, and anti-remodelling, on top of the ARB effects of valsartan.

Sacubitril/valsartan reduced mortality and morbidity by 20%, compared to enalapril, in the Prospective Comparison of ARNI with ACEI to Determine Impact on Global Mortality and Morbidity in Heart Failure (PARADIGM-HF) trial that included symptomatic HFrEF patients with an LVEF of <40% (changed to <35% during the study), elevated plasma natriuretic peptide levels, and eGFR of >30mL/min/1.73m^2, who were able to tolerate separate treatments periods with enalapril (10mg bd) and sacubitril/valsartan (97/103mg bd) during a run-in period. Sacubitril/valsartan is therefore recommended in patients with HFrEF who fit this profile.

Cautions/contraindications

In the PARADIGM-HF trial, symptomatic hypotension was more often present in the sacubitril/valsartan group.

The risk of angio-oedema in the trial was reduced by recruiting only those who tolerated therapy with enalapril and sacubitril/valsartan during an active run-in phase. Moreover, the number of African American patients, who are at a higher risk of angio-oedema, was relatively small in this study. To minimize the risk of angio-oedema caused by overlapping ACE and neprilysin inhibition, the ACEI should be withheld for at least 36h before initiating sacubitril/valsartan.

Combined treatment with an ACEI (or ARB) and sacubitril/valsartan is contraindicated.

There are additional concerns about its effects on the degradation of β-amyloid peptide in the brain, which could theoretically accelerate amyloid deposition, but this is yet to be proven in humans and long-term safety needs to be addressed.

Side effects

The side effects for this combined agent are the same as those reported earlier for ACEIs/ARBs. However, symptomatic hypotension is more frequent with sacubitril/valsartan (see Table 3.1.5).

Ivabradine (class IIa, level of evidence B)

Ivabradine slows the heart rate through inhibition of the I_f channel in the sinus node and therefore should only be used for patients in sinus rhythm.

Ivabradine reduced by 18% the combined endpoint of mortality or hospitalization for HF in patients with symptomatic HFrEF in sinus rhythm and with a heart rate of >70bpm who had been hospitalized for HF within the previous 12 months in the Systolic Heart Failure Treatment with the *I*(f) Inhibitor Ivabradine Trial (SHIFT). Hence, it can be used in patients with these characteristics.

Cautions/contraindications/side effects

Patients taking ivabradine (see Table 3.1.6) may experience symptomatic bradycardia in nearly 5% of cases. Visual side effects (phosphenes) can also occur in <3% of cases.

Digoxin (class IIa, level of evidence B for reducing hospital admissions)

Digoxin is of particular benefit in patients with AF and HF. It slows down the ventricular rate, leading to increased filling time, and has a positive inotropic effect. If a patient is in sinus rhythm, digoxin can still be beneficial if symptoms persist despite maximum treatment, by reducing hospital admissions, although there is no effect on mortality.

Loading doses are not generally required in stable patients. A daily dose of 125–250mcg is appropriate in the context of normal renal function. In the elderly and those with renal failure, a smaller dose may be required.

Contraindications

Digoxin is contraindicated in second- or third-degree heart block and pre-excitation syndromes. Caution is required in patients with renal dysfunction.

Table 3.1.5 Sacubitril/valsartan doses

Sacubitril/valsartan	Starting dose	Target dose
Sacubitril/valsartan	49/51mg bd	97/103mg bd

Table 3.1.6 Ivabradine doses

Ivabradine	Starting dose	Target dose
Ivabradine	5mg bd	7.5mg bd

Diuretics (symptomatic improvement only)

Diuretics are used in HF to alleviate symptoms by reducing fluid overload but have not been shown to improve mortality (see Table 3.1.7). Diuretics reduce hospital admissions for worsening HF and improve exercise capacity. Commonly used diuretics include loop diuretics and thiazides. Thiazide diuretics may be preferred in hypertensive patients with HF.

Patients who are in decompensated HF can develop resistance to oral diuretics due to reduced drug absorption. These patients often require admission to hospital for IV diuretics.

Side effects

- Hypokalaemia, hyponatraemia, hypocalcaemia, hypomagnesaemia.
- Hypotension.
- Ototoxicity.
- Hyperuricaemia.

Combination of hydralazine and isosorbide dinitrate (H-ISDN) (class IIa, level of evidence A)

Recommendations for the use of a combination of nitrates and hydralazine (H-ISDN) differ between NICE and AHA/ESC. NICE guidelines recommend, under specialist supervision, that this combination may be used in patients intolerant of ACEIs or ARBs but do not suggest using it in combination with ACEIs/ARBs.

There is some evidence that patients who still have moderate to severe symptoms, despite ACEIs or ARBs and β-blockers, may benefit from the addition of hydralazine and a nitrate, and this is recommended in the AHA/ESC guidelines. Evidence is strongest in those of African American background.

- Veterans Administration Cooperative Vasodilator—Heart Failure Trial (V-HeFT I) trial: 642 men were randomized to placebo, prazosin, or H-ISDN. No patients were on β-blockers or ACEIs. With H-ISDN, there was a trend to a reduction in all-cause mortality (RRR 22%). H-ISDN increased exercise capacity and LVEF, compared with placebo.
- African-American Heart Failure Trial (A-HeFT): 1050 African American men and women in NYHA class III or IV were randomized to either placebo or H-ISDN. Patients were already on ACEIs (70%), ARBs (17%), or β-blockers (74%). The trial was terminated prematurely at 10 months because of a significant reduction in mortality (RRR 43%).

Table 3.1.7 Diuretics used in the management of heart failure

Diuretics	Usual dose (mg)	Up to (mg)
Loop diuretics		
Furosemide	20–40	240
Bumetanide	0.5–1	5
Thiazide diuretics		
Metolazone	2.5	10
Bendroflumethiazide	2.5	10

Contraindications

Symptomatic hypotension, 'lupus syndrome' (in V-HeFT I and II, there was a sustained increase in antinuclear antibody in 2–3% of patients, but lupus-like syndrome was rare), and severe renal failure.

Side effects

The commonest side effects are headache, dizziness, hypotension, and nausea.

Anticoagulation in heart failure

RCTs have shown a reduction in the risk of stroke in patients on warfarin who have HF and AF. The non-vitamin K anticoagulants may also be effective in patients with HF and AF.

There is no good evidence for warfarin in HF patients with intra-cardiac thrombus or an LV aneurysm, but the consensus is that this group of patients probably benefits from anticoagulation.

There is no evidence to support the use of oral anticoagulants in HF patients in sinus rhythm.

Calcium channel blockers in heart failure

Amlodipine can be used to treat hypertension and angina in patients with HF. The use of verapamil, diltiazem, or short-acting dihydropyridines can cause clinical deterioration and should be avoided.

Renin inhibitors

Aliskiren (a direct renin inhibitor) failed to improve outcomes in HF and is not recommended as an alternative to ACEIs or ARBs.

Management of atrial fibrillation in heart failure

AF is common in patients with HF. Some people may benefit from restoration of sinus rhythm, but this decision should be made on an individual basis, with specialist input. There are no RCTs demonstrating that restoration of sinus rhythm in patients with AF and HF improves mortality.

A review of large RCTs of β-blockers in HF showed that the benefits of these agents are the same whether the patient is in sinus rhythm or AF.

Non-pharmacological management of chronic heart failure

Description of the non-pharmacological management of HF is beyond the scope of this book, and the following section therefore represents just a brief summary.

Weight monitoring

Patients should weigh themselves regularly, and if they have sudden weight gain (approximately 2kg in 3 days), they should know how to increase their diuretic therapy. They should also be aware of the risk of volume depletion if their weight falls rapidly.

Fluid restriction

Restricting the volume intake to 1.5–2L of fluid in patients with severe HF may be considered but does not seem to help patients with mild to moderate HF.

Sodium restriction

Reducing salt intake may help to reduce fluid retention.

Alcohol

Patients suffering from alcohol-induced cardiomyopathy should completely abstain from alcohol. All other patients should not drink excessively, as alcohol has a negative inotropic effect, may increase BP, and can be cytotoxic.

Smoking

Smoking cessation should be strongly recommended, as it is associated with dismal prognosis.

Vaccination

Vaccination against influenza (annual) and *Pneumococcus* (once) should be considered.

Myocardial reperfusion

Reperfusion should be performed if there is evidence of myocardial ischaemia. Routine coronary angiography in all patients with HF is not recommended. Conduct angiography in patients with angina, and perform viability studies in selected patients.

Cardiac resynchronization therapy/implantable cardioverter–defibrillator

CRT is recommended if QRS is ≥130ms in the presence of LBBB (in sinus rhythm). CRT should/may be considered if QRS is ≥130ms with non-LBBB (in sinus rhythm) or in patients with AF, provided a strategy to ensure biventricular capture is in place (individualized decision).

An Implantable cardioverter–defibrillator (ICD) is recommended to reduce the risk of sudden death and all-cause mortality in patients with symptomatic HF (NYHA classes II–III) and an LVEF of ≤35%, despite ≥3 months of optimal medical therapy, provided they are expected to survive substantially longer than 1 year, with good functional status, and they have:

- IHD (unless they had an MI in the previous 40 days).
- DCM.

An ICD should be used for secondary prevention in patients who have recovered from a ventricular arrhythmia causing haemodynamic instability and who are expected to survive for >1 year with good functional status.

Transplantation

Specialist assessment for transplantation should be considered for patients with severe refractory symptoms or refractory cardiogenic shock.

Indications

Objective evidence of cardiopulmonary limitation, e.g. peak VO_{2max} of <10mL/min/kg and patient dependent on inotropes.

Cautions/contraindications

Alcohol or drug abuse, severe renal failure (eGFR <30mL/min). Fixed high pulmonary vascular resistance [pulmonary artery pressure (PAP) >60mmHg], significant liver impairment.

Left ventricular assist devices

This needs specialist assessment. LVADs may provide an alternative to transplantation in advanced HF.

Chronic heart failure with preserved LVEF (HFpEF)

HF is most simply defined as the presence of symptoms and/or signs in the presence of cardiac dysfunction. Those with an LVEF of ≤40% are now more usually referred to as having HFrEF. Patients with an LVEF of >50% (in the normal range) are classified, according to the ESC 2016 guideline, as having HFpEF.[1] The latter body has created a new category for those with an intermediate LVEF of 41–49% (HFmEF). In practice, this makes little difference to management, as no specific disease-modifying therapy exists for both categories.

The diagnosis of HFpEF or HFmEF by echocardiography is less clear-cut, with many abnormalities having been described in diagnostic algorithms. However, criteria for relevant structural heart disease such as LVH (LV mass index >115g/m^2 for men and >95g/m^2 for women) or an increased left atrial volume (left atrial volume index >34mL/m^2) make the diagnosis more likely. Many of these patients have 'diastolic dysfunction'. Tissue Doppler measures of raised filling pressures have emerged as useful predictors of diastolic abnormalities. Useful cut points to indicate 'diastolic dysfunction' are: an E/e′ average of ≥13 or an e′ average (lateral–septal) of <9cm/s.

The main echocardiographic abnormalities used for confirming the diagnosis of the HF syndrome and categorizing it into HFrEF, HFpEF, and HFmEF, according to the ESC 2016 guideline, are summarized in Table 3.1.8. For those with HFpEF or HFmEF, in addition to symptoms and/or signs of HF, raised natriuretic peptide levels are also required and at least one other criterion reflecting structural heart disease or 'diastolic dysfunction'.

Prevalence and prognosis

HFpEF is present in up to 50% of patients presenting with HF. It is commoner in elderly people and those with hypertension or diabetes. Ageing is associated with decreases in the elastic properties of the heart and great vessels. The prognosis has been shown to be similar to that of systolic HF. The proportion of HFpEF patients dying from non-CV causes is higher than in HFrEF.

Table 3.1.8 Classification of heart failure according to the ESC 2016 Heart Failure Guideline

HFrEF	HFpEF	HFmEF
Symptoms/signs	Symptoms/signs	Symptoms/signs
LVEF ≤40%	LVEF ≥50%	LVEF = 41–49%
–	1. Increased NP 2. At least one additional criteria of: relevant structural heart disease, e.g LAE, LVH, or diastolic dysfunction	1. Increased NP 2. At least one additional criteria of: relevant structural heart disease, e.g LAE, LVH, or diastolic dysfunction

HFpEF: heart failure with preserved ejection fraction; HFmEF, heart failure with mid-range ejection fraction; HFrEF, heart failure with reduced ejection fraction; LAE, left atrial enlargement; LVEF, left ventricular ejection fraction; LVH, left ventricular hypertrophy; NP, natriuretic peptide.

Aetiology

The commonest causes of HFpEF are:

- Hypertension.
- CAS.
- VHD.

HFpEF is the predominant type of HF found in hypertrophic cardiomyopathy. Comorbidities are very common in HFpEF, particularly AF, diabetes, obesity, and CKD.

Treatment

No disease-modifying therapies are available, to date, for HFpEF. Results of large outcome trials with ACEIs/ARBs and MRAs have been disappointing. Treatment is therefore directed towards two goals:

1. Management of symptoms and signs of fluid retention.
2. Treatment of the underlying cardiac disease.

In practice, this means that many HFpEF patients end up on much the same therapy as HFrEF patients.

Results of major trials in HFpEF

- *Perindopril in Elderly People with Chronic Heart Failure (PEP-CHF) trial*: among patients aged ≥70 years with clinical HF and preserved LV systolic function, treatment with perindopril did not differ from placebo in the primary endpoint of death or unplanned hospitalizations for HF.[2]
- *Candesartan in Patients with Chronic Heart Failure and Preserved Left Ventricular Ejection Fraction (CHARM-Preserved) trial*: candesartan in patients with preserved LVEF did not show a significant reduction in the composite endpoint of death from CV causes or admissions with HF but did show a significant reduction in the risk of investigator-reported admissions for HF.[3]
- *Irbesartan in Heart Failure with Preserved Ejection Fraction Study (I-PRESERVE)*: investigated patients who were mostly NYHA class III (77%) with normal LVEF. The trial confirmed that angiotensin receptor blockade with irbesartan is not associated with a reduction in CV mortality and morbidity in patients with HF and a normal ejection fraction. In fact, there was an increase in the incidence of observed adverse effects, including hyperkalaemia.[4]
- *SENIORS trial*: this trial of nebivolol in older patients with HF also included patients with an LVEF of >40%. All-cause mortality was reduced overall in the trial with nebivolol. There was no indication that patients treated with nebivolol who had HFpEF behaved differently from those with HFrEF, although the trial was not powered sufficiently to definitively comment on a reduction in outcomes for HFpEF.[5] It does show that β-blockers are not harmful in HFpEF.
- *Digitalis Investigation Group (DIG) trial*: the outcome trial with digoxin for those with HF and in sinus rhythm, also included patients with HFpEF. There was a neutral effect on mortality overall.[6]
- *Treatment of Preserved Cardiac Function Heart Failure with an Aldosterone Antagonist (TOPCAT) trial*: this trial investigated the use of spironolactone in 3445 patients with HFpEF, compared to placebo. There was no significant reduction in the primary composite endpoint of CV death,

HF hospitalization, or resuscitated cardiac arrest. A reduction in hospitalization for HF was seen.[7] There was significant regional variation in outcomes between patients recruited in the Americas who did seem to benefit, compared to those recruited in Russia and Georgia.

Useful points for treating HFpEF

1. Give loop diuretics to relieve symptoms and signs of congestion, i.e. peripheral and pulmonary oedema. Use the minimum dose necessary to achieve euvolaemia.
2. Treat the underlying cause of HFpEF:
   a) For CAD: statin, ACEIs/ARBs, and β-blockers are useful. Revascularize, as appropriate.
   b) Hypertension: aim for a BP of <130/80mmHg—use thiazides, ACEIs/ARBs, and CCBs. Spironolactone and eplerenone are useful in resistant hypertension.
   c) Control the ventricular rate in patients with AF with β-blockers (and rate-limiting CCBs, as necessary).

Acute heart failure

Acute HF is characterized by a rapid onset of signs and symptoms of HF, requiring urgent treatment. Acute HF may present as a first occurrence (*de novo*) or, more frequently, as a consequence of acute decompensation of chronic HF and may be caused by primary cardiac dysfunction or precipitated by extrinsic factors, often in patients with chronic HF. In most cases, patients with acute HF present with either 'normal' (90–140mmHg) or 'high' (>140mmHg; hypertensive acute HF) SBP. Only 5–8% of all patients present with low BP (i.e. <90mmHg; hypotensive acute HF), which is associated with poor prognosis, particularly when hypoperfusion is also present. Therefore, there are several possible presentations, and an overlap of these presentations can occur:

- Acute pulmonary oedema with severe respiratory distress.
- Cardiogenic shock, defined as tissue hypoperfusion—associated with high in-hospital mortality, i.e. 40–60%.
- Hypertensive HF, with evidence of vasoconstriction and tachycardia—there is often a relatively normal LVEF in these patients, and in-hospital mortality is relatively low.
- Progressive worsening of chronic HF, with a gradual increase in systemic and pulmonary congestion.
- Isolated right HF characterized by raised venous pressure, absence of pulmonary congestion, and a low output state due to low LV filling pressures.

Aetiology

The commonest aetiologies for acute HF are:

- Ischaemia/MI.
- Arrhythmias.
- Infection/sepsis.
- Hypertensive crisis.
- Anaemia.
- Lack of adherence to treatment.
- Renal dysfunction.
- Thyrotoxicosis.
- Valve dysfunction.
- Endocarditis.
- Aortic dissection.
- Pericardial disease.
- PE.
- Asthma and COPD.
- Alcohol and drug abuse.

Diagnosis

The diagnosis of acute HF should be both rapid and accurate, in order to initiate treatment/interventions as soon as possible. A possible workup algorithm is depicted in Fig. 3.1.2. The diagnosis of acute HF in patients presenting with acute dyspnoea should be performed, including a clinical history, physical examination, 12-lead ECG, and natriuretic peptide levels. An echocardiography can be useful in '*de novo*' HF (e.g. for excluding cardiac tamponade). After acute HF confirmation, the appropriate treatment should be initiated and adapted to each patient's presentation and comorbidities.

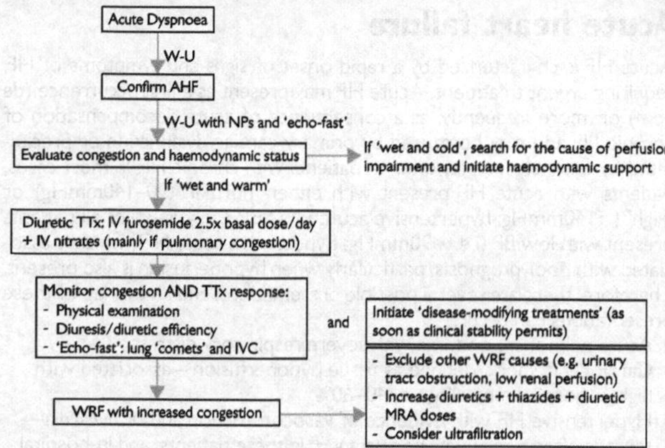

Fig. 3.1.2 Heart failure algorithm. IVC, inferior vena cava; MRA, mineralocorticoid receptor antagonist; TTx, treatment; WRF, worsening renal function; W-U, workup.

Treatment

In the published trials of acute HF, most agents have been shown to improve CV haemodynamics, but no agent has been shown to reduce mortality. The following recommendations are from expert consensus, and therefore, the level of evidence is C, unless otherwise stated.

Diuretics (class I, level of evidence B)

IV loop diuretics have never been evaluated in an RCT but are universally accepted to be beneficial and are recommended for all patients with acute HF admitted with signs/symptoms of fluid overload, to improve symptoms. It is recommended to regularly monitor symptoms, urine output, renal function, and electrolytes during use of IV diuretics.

- An initial dose of 20–40mg of furosemide (or equivalent, e.g. bumetanide 0.5–1mg) can be tried and adjusted afterwards, according to patients` response (higher initial doses may be needed if the patient has renal failure or is receiving chronic diuretic therapy).
- The highest dose of a diuretic that should really be used is as an infusion of 240mg in 24h (in exceptional circumstances, 480mg in 24h).
- A combination of a loop diuretic with either a thiazide-type diuretic or spironolactone may be considered in patients with resistant oedema or persistent signs and symptoms. If diuresis cannot be restored, patients may need renal specialist treatment.

Oxygen

Administer to maintain oxygen saturation of 94–98% (88–92% in COPD if evidence of carbon dioxide retention has been obtained).

Non-invasive ventilation

Early non-invasive ventilation (NIV) with positive end-expiratory pressure (PEEP) improves LV function by reducing LV afterload. NIV should be used with caution in cardiogenic shock and RV failure. Intubation should not be delayed for a trial of NIV. Three recent meta-analyses found that early application of NIV reduces the need for intubation and reduces short-term mortality. However, in the Three Interventions in Cardiogenic Pulmonary Oedema (3CPO) trial, a large RCT, NIV improved clinical parameters, but not mortality. Start with a PEEP of 5–7.5cmH_2O, and titrate up to 10cmH_2O. Use a fraction of inspired oxygen (FiO_2) of >40%.

Morphine

Morphine is good for treating restlessness, dyspnoea, anxiety, and chest pain. It also acts as a vasodilator. Use boluses of 2.5–5mg IV.

Use with great caution in patients with carbon dioxide retention due to reduced consciousness level, in sedated patients, and in hypotension.

Vasodilators (class I, level of evidence B)

IV nitrates decrease left and right filling pressures and SVR, i.e. GTN continuous infusion of 1–10mg/h. They are recommended early in acute HF if SBP is >110mmHg and may be used with caution if SBP is between 90 and 110mmHg. They are particularly useful in hypertensive HF. It is important to monitor BP levels and to avoid acute drops in BP. Use with caution in patients with aortic stenosis, as they may lead to marked hypotension. Patients develop tolerance to vasodilators with continuous use (see Table 3.1.9).

Side effects

- Headache, hypotension.

Inotropic agents

- They may acutely improve haemodynamics, but they increase oxygen consumption and may worsen myocardial ischaemia/necrosis. No evidence for improved mortality. Initiated as early as required, but stopped as soon as no longer needed.
- Continuous ECG monitoring is advised. BP should be monitored closely.
- Dose should be titrated according to BP, organ perfusion, clinical condition, and diuresis. When weaning off inotropes, do this gradually.
- Indications: low SBP in the presence of hypoperfusion if the patient has not responded to correction of preload with fluids or when there is a poor response to diuretics/nitrates due to hypotension.
  (See Table 3.1.10.)

Side effects

Increased risk of ventricular and atrial arrhythmias. Caution is needed in patients with a resting heart rate of over 100bpm.

Additional interventions

If the measures listed earlier fail to treat cardiogenic shock, the following mechanical interventions can be considered: IABP, intubation, and LVADs as a bridge to transplantation. If ACS is the underlying cause of acute HF, then coronary reperfusion with PCI or surgery may improve prognosis. Urgent surgery can be indicated in patients with mechanical complications after MI.

Table 3.1.9 Intravenous vasodilators used to treat acute heart failure

Vasodilator	Dosing
Glyceryl trinitrate	Start with 10–20mcg/min, increase up to 200mcg/min
Isosorbide dinitrate	Start with 1mg/h, increase up to 10mg/h
Nitroprusside	Start with 0.3mcg/kg/min, increase up to 5mcg/kg/min
Nesiritide	Bolus of 2mcg/kg + infusion of 0.01mcg/kg/min

Table 3.1.10 Inotropic treatment in acute heart failure

Inotrope	Bolus	Infusion rate
Dobutamine	No	2–20mcg/kg/min
Dopamine	No	3–5mcg/kg/min: inotropic >5mcg/kg/min: vasopressor
Milrinone	25–75mcg/kg over 10–20min	0.375–0.75mcg/kg/min
Enoximone	0.5–1.0mg/kg over 5–10min	5–20mcg/kg/min
Levosimendan	12mcg/kg over 10min (optional)	0.1mcg/kg/min, which can be decreased to 0.05mcg/kg/min or increased up to 0.2mcg/kg/min
Noradrenaline	No	0.2–1.0mcg/kg/min
Adrenaline	Bolus: 1mg can be given IV during resuscitation, repeated every 3–5min	0.05–0.5mcg/kg/min

References

1 Ponikowski P, Voors AA, Anker SD, *et al.* 2016 ESC Guidelines for the diagnosis and treatment of acute and chronic heart failure: The Task Force for the diagnosis and treatment of acute and chronic heart failure of the European Society of Cardiology (ESC). Developed with the special contribution of the Heart Failure Association (HFA) of the ESC. *Eur J Heart Fail* 2016;**18**:891–975.
2 Cleland JG, Tendera M, Adamus J, *et al.* The perindopril in elderly people with chronic heart failure (PEP-CHF) study. *Eur Heart J* 2006;**27**:2338–45.
3 Yusuf S, Pfeffer MA, Swedberg K, *et al.* Effects of candesartan in patients with chronic heart failure and preserved left-ventricular ejection fraction: the CHARM-Preserved Trial. *Lancet* 2003;**362**:777–81.
4 Massie BM, Carson PE, McMurray JJ, *et al.* Irbesartan in patients with heart failure and preserved ejection fraction. *N Engl J Med* 2008;**359**:2456–67.
5 van Veldhuisen DJ, Cohen-Solal A, Bohm M, *et al.* Beta-blockade with nebivolol in elderly heart failure patients with impaired and preserved left ventricular ejection fraction: data From SENIORS (Study of Effects of Nebivolol Intervention on Outcomes and Rehospitalization in Seniors With Heart Failure). *J Am Coll Cardiol* 2009;**53**:2150–8.
6 The Digitalis Investigation Group. The effect of digoxin on mortality and morbidity in patients with heart failure. *N Engl J Med* 1997;**336**:525–33.
7 Pitt B, Pfeffer MA, Assmann SF, *et al.* Spironolactone for heart failure with preserved ejection fraction. *N Engl J Med* 2017;**370**:1383–9.

Heart transplantation

Finn Gustafsson and Kasper Rossing

Introduction

Heart transplantation is the most effective treatment for end-stage HF refractory to medical therapy and pacing. To date, >120,000 heart transplants have been performed worldwide, and >3500 procedures are performed annually (http://www.ishlt.org). Despite this activity, the number of transplantations far from suffice to save the patients in need. The overwhelming reason for this is donor shortage. To this end, mechanical solutions in the form of LVADs are being increasingly used, either as a bridge to transplantation or as final therapy.

Indications for heart transplantations include terminal HF not responding to conventional therapy with an expected 1-year survival of <80%. This is typically estimated by selecting patients with advanced HF symptoms and a peak VO_2 of <12mL/kg/min (<14 in patients intolerant of β-blockers).[1] Contraindications (absolute and relative) include irreversible end-organ dysfunction, recent cancer, obesity (BMI >35kg/m^2), certain chronic infections, fixed pulmonary hypertension, and importantly non-compliance or smoking, substance, or alcohol abuse. Age is not a contraindication, but most patients older than 70 years have comorbidity, leaving heart transplantation an unattractive therapeutic choice.

Median survival after heart transplantation in the registry from the International Society of Heart and Lung Transplantation (ISHLT), including data from the beginning of the registry, is 10.7 years, but >13 years when the analysis is restricted to transplants after 2002, clearly showing that survival is improving because of better patient selection, surgical techniques, and post-transplant medical management. Physical capacity, on average, is lower than that of age-matched controls, but heart transplantation is associated with an enormous improvement in peak VO_2 and quality of life in the majority of patients. Most patients can return to work and lead an active life, including, for instance, travel and sports.

While prognosis after transplantation clearly has improved, multiple medical issues relating to acute or chronic graft rejection, as well as side effects from the necessary immunosuppressive therapy, remain. Leading causes of death late after transplantation include cancer, infection, and allograft vasculopathy (formerly termed chronic rejection). Chronic renal failure affects 20% 10 years after transplantation, and this is independently associated with inferior survival. Other important side effects of immunosuppressive drugs are discussed in ➲ Immunosuppression, p. 174, ➲ Induction therapy, p. 175, and ➲ Maintenance therapy, pp. 176–8.

Transplant immunology and rejection

Rejection of the donor heart results from the recipient's immune system recognizing the transplanted organ as foreign and then mounting an immune response to it, either by antibody- or cellular-mediated mechanisms.

The main target of the recipient's immune response towards the transplanted heart is the major histocompatibility complex (MHC) molecules. MHC molecules are expressed on the surface of a variety of cells and play a key role in the immune system, as they function to display allogeneic peptides to T-cells. In humans, the protein products of the MHC are termed the human leucocyte antigens (HLAs) and are classified into class I (A + B + C) and class II (DR + DQ + DP). HLA class I is present on most nucleated cells and can present alloantigens to a subtype of T-cells termed $CD8^+$ T-cells, which may then trigger an immune response with cell lysis. HLA class II molecules are normally found on antigen-presenting cells (APCs) and display antigens to the $CD4^+$ subtype of T-cells, which facilitate B-cell production of alloantibodies directed against the graft.

Recognition of an alloantigen from the donor by the host T-cells is the primary event which initiates the effector mechanisms of the adaptive immune response, leading to rejection. Donor antigen recognition by the T-cell depends on the binding of the T-cell receptor complex on the surface of the T-cell to an alloantigen/MHC complex on an APC. The APC can be either from the donor (direct pathway) or from the recipient (indirect pathway). In addition, T-cell activation is dependent on a co-stimulatory signal such as binding of the surface molecule CD28 on the T-cell to the surface molecule B7 on the APC. Once activated, T-cells undergo proliferation and differentiation by stimulation of a series of intracellular pathways and autocrine mechanisms, which are important targets of immunosuppressive therapies (see Fig. 3.2.1). Activation of the T-cell by binding to the allogen/MHC complex on the APC, together with the co-stimulatory signal, leads to increased cytoplasmic calcium (Ca^{2+}) concentration, activation of calcineurin, and, in turn, dephosphorylation of the nuclear factor of activated T-cells (NFAT). NFAT then enters the nucleus and promotes transcription of interleukin-2 (IL-2), which leaves the nucleus of the T-cell and binds to the IL-2 receptor on the surface of the T-cell. Binding of IL-2 to the IL-2 receptor (CD27) activates the mammalian target of rapamycin (mTOR), which regulates transition through the cell cycle, leading to T-cell proliferation and differentiation. Based on the timing and underlying mechanisms, rejection is classified into hyperacute, acute, and chronic rejection.

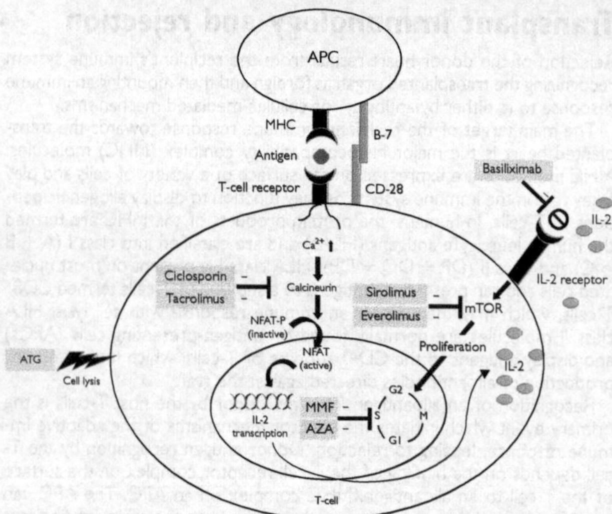

Fig. 3.2.1 Schematic presentation of the initiation of the adaptive immune response triggered by binding of an alloantigen/MHC complex on an antigen-presenting cell to the T-cell receptor on the surface of the T-cell. Mechanisms of action of various immunosuppressants used in heart transplantation are also illustrated. APC, antigen-presenting cell; ATG, anti-thymocyte globulin; AZA, azathioprine; G1, cell cycle gap phase 1; G2, cell cycle gap phase 2; IL-2, interleukin-2; M, cell cycle mitosis phase; MHC, major histocompatibility complex; MMF, mycophenolate mofetil; mTOR, mammalian target of rapamycin; NFAT, dephosphorylated nuclear factor of activated T-cells; NFAT-P, phosphorylated nuclear factor of activated T-cells; S, cell cycle synthesis phase.

Hyperacute rejection

Hyperacute rejection occurs immediately or within hours following transplantation with the reintroduction of blood into the graft. The hyperacute rejection results from preformed antibodies in the recipient to ABO antigens or HLA on the donor endothelium. Binding of preformed antibodies to donor antigens triggers complement and neutrophil activation, leading to extensive destruction of the donor endothelium, microvascular thrombosis, myocardial necrosis, and immediate graft failure. Risk for preformed HLA antibodies increases with pre-transplant blood product transfusions, previous solid organ transplantations, pregnancies, and treatment with durable mechanical ventricular assist systems. Hyperacute rejection is rare and can virtually be eliminated by ABO matching and pre-transplant screening for pre-existing HLA antibodies in the recipient.

Acute rejection

Acute rejection is the commonest form of rejection in heart transplantation and is a potential cause of graft failure and death. The risk of rejection increases with younger recipient age, female gender, re-transplantation, and increased HLA mismatch between donor and recipient. The incidence of acute rejection requiring immediate intensified immunosuppressive treatment has decreased substantially over the last decades, along with improvements in immunosuppressive therapies.[2] Currently, approximately 15% of adult patients will experience an acute rejection requiring treatment during the first year after transplantation, which is associated with increased long-term mortality. The risk of acute rejection is greatest in the first months after transplantation and then declines over the first year. Acute rejection may, however, develop at any time following heart transplantation, and life-long immunosuppression is therefore required.

Acute rejection may be classified as either acute cellular rejection (ACR) or acute antibody-mediated rejection (AMR). ACR is the commonest form of acute rejection. It is mainly caused by T-cells directed against the myocardium of the donor heart, which, if severe, can result in myocyte necrosis and graft failure. ACR is graded based on histologically findings of endomyocardial biopsies, according to the ISHLT criteria, into no rejection (H0R), mild rejection (H1R) with interstitial and/or perivascular infiltrate with up to one focus of myocyte damage, moderate rejection (H2R) with two or more foci of infiltrate with associated myocyte damage, and severe rejection (H3R) with diffuse infiltrate with multifocal myocyte damage ± oedema ± haemorrhage ± vasculitis. The majority of mild rejections will resolve spontaneously on maintenance immunosuppressive therapy, whereas higher-grade rejections require supplemental immunosuppression such as IV methylprednisolone and, in severe cases, anti-thymocyte globulin (ATG).

Acute AMR is less well understood but seems to be predominantly caused by antibodies directed towards the vasculature of the donor heart, leading to complement activation and thereby damage of the vessels and consequently graft dysfunction. AMR can occur in isolation but often coincides with ACR. The grading of AMR, according to the ISHLT criteria, is based on both histopathologic and immunopathologic findings from endomyocardial biopsies. Although not part of the diagnostic criteria for AMR, the recipient may be screened post-transplantation for the formation of *de novo* donor-specific antibodies. The presence of strong and complement-binding donor-specific antigens may indicate the need for treatment, depending on graft function and the clinical situation.

Surveillance of acute rejection

Acute rejection may, if severe, lead to HF and arrhythmias with overt symptoms, but most often patients with mild to moderate rejections have no or only vague symptoms. Therefore, protocol-driven testing is standard practice, with endomyocardial biopsy as the gold standard for detection of rejection and guidance of immunosuppressive therapy. The timing of surveillance biopsies is centre-specific, but in general, biopsies are performed frequently (weekly) early after transplantation where the risk of rejection is greatest and less frequently over time as the risk of rejection declines, typically with the last planned biopsy 1–2 years after transplantation. Additional biopsies are performed when symptoms or cardiac imaging indicate otherwise unexplained graft dysfunction, after previous episodes of rejection, or following major reductions in the immunosuppressive medication such as weaning off corticosteroids or changing to a non-calcineurin inhibitor (CNI)-based immunosuppressive treatment.

Chronic rejection—cardiac allograft vasculopathy

Chronic rejection, now termed cardiac allograft vasculopathy (CAV), is a major cause of late graft failure and mortality after heart transplantation. CAV is a specific form of CAD, characterized by diffuse concentric intimal hyperplasia, which starts in distal small vessels and eventually involves the entire intramyocardial and proximal epicardial arteries. This contrasts with common atherosclerotic lesions which are usually located proximally and are focal and non-circumferential. The prevalence of CAV varies considerably, depending on how vasculopathy is defined and which method is used to detect it. When assessed by coronary angiography, the prevalence of CAV has been reported to be approximately 10% and 30% in survivors at 1 and 5 years after heart transplantation.[3] As patients rarely experience angina due to cardiac denervation, surveillance is applied in most centres. Although angiography remains the most widely used method to assess CAV, this technique shows only the luminal diameters and therefore often misses the intimal thickening associated with early CAV. Using more sensitive techniques, such as intravascular ultrasound (IVUS) of the coronary arteries which provides a cross-sectional image of the wall structure, has demonstrated that CAV develops early after heart transplantation and is present in 50% of patients already 1 year after transplantation.[3]

Whereas multiple factors contribute to the development of CAV, immunologic mechanisms seem to play a predominant role, as both alloimmune and autoimmune responses are causal factors. In addition, many non-immune donor and recipient factors also affect the development of CAV, including hyperlipidaemia, hypertension, diabetes, cytomegalovirus (CMV) infection, and donor-derived CAD (ISHLT's Thirty-First Official Adult Heart Transplant Report—2014). The net result of CAV is chronic graft failure, presenting either as systolic HF or as a restrictive cardiomyopathy with elevated filling pressures despite preserved ejection fraction. Another common presentation of CAV is sudden death.

Prevention of cardiac allograft vasculopathy

Studies have shown that the risk of CAV development depends on the immunosuppressive regimen used, with the lowest rates seen with proliferation signal inhibitors (PSIs). With respect to presumed non-immunologic factors, pravastatin and simvastatin given at the time of transplantation, irrespective of cholesterol levels, have been shown to reduce the risk of CAV in randomized trials. Hence, statins are used in all patients who tolerate them after transplantation. There are no studies documenting the effect on outcome for other cholesterol-lowering drugs. Target levels of blood cholesterol levels have never been established in this setting. Early data suggested that diltiazem was beneficial to prevent CAV, but studies performed in patients treated with statins could not confirm such an effect and diltiazem (which has a significant interaction with several immunosuppressants) are no longer routinely used after transplantation. It is unclear if ACEIs are efficient in preventing CAV. A recent randomized study did not show an effect on plaque burden but indicated that microvascular function might be improved with ramipril.[4] Further studies to confirm this are needed. While there is no evidence that aspirin improves outcome after heart transplantation, it is customary to use it in patients diagnosed with CAV.

Treatment of cardiac allograft vasculopathy

Occasionally, proximal coronary lesions in patients with CAV may be treatable with PCI, and rarely, coronary artery bypass surgery is used. There are no randomized studies to inform about the utility of these strategies. The only definite treatment for severe CAV is cardiac re-transplantation. CAV is the commonest indication for re-transplantation, which accounts for 2–3% of all transplantations performed worldwide. Survival after re-transplantation is significantly lower than after a primary transplant.

Immunosuppression

Development of immunosuppressive therapies over the years has greatly improved survival in heart transplant patients by reducing the incidence of graft failure due to rejection. However, immunosuppression is associated with frequent and serious side effects, including renal failure, malignancies, diabetes, infections, hypertension, dyslipidaemia, neuropathy, and osteoporosis. Overall morbidity and mortality in transplanted patients are, to a large extent, driven by such side effects. The challenge of immunosuppressive therapy is therefore to balance between effects and side effects in the individual patient by continuous adjustment of the immunosuppression, according to the frequency and severity of rejection and the side effects caused by the therapy.

In general, immunosuppressive therapy in heart transplantation consists of a combination of immunosuppressive agents that differ by mechanism of action, thereby minimizing the side effects associated with each class of agent, while maximizing overall effectiveness. The different types of immunosuppression can be divided into induction therapy, which is given for a short period at the time of transplantation, and maintenance therapy, which is given lifelong after transplantation

Induction therapy

Induction therapy mainly consists of polyclonal or monoclonal antibodies against T-lymphocytes. The aim of T-cell-specific antibody induction is to deplete or inhibit the proliferation of the circulating T-lymphocytes in the first days after transplantation, before the full effect of maintenance immunosuppressive treatment is reached, and thus to reduce the frequency and severity of early acute rejection. It has also been suggested that induction therapy may promote acceptance of the graft and allow for long-term reduction of maintenance immunosuppressive treatment. In addition, it may reduce the incidence of chronic allograft vasculopathy and ischaemia–reperfusion injury in the transplanted heart. However, T-cell-specific antibody induction causes profound immunosuppression and may increase the risk of infections, post-transplant lymphoproliferative disorder, and other malignancies. Although approximately 50% of centres use an initial antibody induction therapy, the advantage over an immunosuppressive protocol without induction is not clear and an overall survival benefit of induction therapy has not been demonstrated.

Polyclonal antibodies

Polyclonal antibodies include rabbit and equine ATG. ATG is characterized by its polyclonal nature with a wide range of target molecules, constituting nearly 45 epitopes, ranging from antigens involved in immunity to adhesion and cell signalling molecules and cell surface antigens (Ruan Transplantation Proceedings, 2016). ATG given for induction therapy leads to rapid depletion of B- and T-cells. It is currently being used in approximately 20% of all adult heart transplantations (ISHLT registry slides 2016). Short-term side effects of these agents include thrombocytopenia, leucopenia, cytokine release, and serum sickness. To reduce the side effects induced by cytokine release, it is recommended to give IV corticosteroids and antihistamine before administration of ATG. In addition to its use in induction therapy, ATG is also used together with high-dose glucocorticoids to treat severe acute rejections.

Induction therapy by monoclonal antibodies

Currently, the most widely used monoclonal antibody for induction therapy in heart transplantation is the IL-2 receptor antagonist basiliximab, which is currently used in approximately 30% of adult heart transplants. This antibody does not deplete T-cells but reduces the risk of rejection by preventing clonal proliferation and differentiation of activated T-cells by blocking the IL-2 receptor. This class of compound was developed to increase the specificity of induction therapy, thereby avoiding the toxicity associated with the more diffuse effect of ATG. However, a more favourable outcome of IL-2 receptor antagonist, as compared to ATG, has not been demonstrated.

Several T-cell-depleting monoclonal antibodies have previously been available but have been withdrawn due to infrequent use. These included muromonab–CD3 specific for the CD3 receptor, and daclizumab and alemtuzumab targeting the CD52 surface protein.

Maintenance therapy

Maintenance therapy is given lifelong after transplantation and generally consists of a combination of immunosuppressive agents that differ by mechanism. Such regimens may vary by patient and transplant centre but generally consist of a combination of three different agents, including a CNI (tacrolimus or ciclosporin), an antiproliferative agent [mycophenolate mofetil (MFA) or, less frequently, azathioprine (AZA)], and prednisolone. A more recent class of drugs, known as mTOR inhibitors or signal proliferation inhibitors, includes sirolimus and everolimus. These agents have been used in combination with an antiproliferative agent to allow for CNI dose reduction or withdrawal, as an alternative to an antiproliferative agent in combination with a CNI, or as a fourth agent in patients with ongoing rejection on conventional immunosuppressive therapy with a CNI, an antiproliferative agent, and prednisolone.

Calcineurin inhibitors

CNIs, including ciclosporin and tacrolimus, have remained the cornerstone of most maintenance immunosuppressive regiments in solid organ transplantation, including the heart. These compounds prevent T-cell proliferation and differentiation by inhibiting the enzyme calcineurin which, under normal circumstances, is responsible for activating the transcription of IL-2 leading to T-cell proliferation (see Fig. 3.2.1). The net result is blunting of T-lymphocyte activation and proliferation in response to alloantigens.

Ciclosporin was discovered in 1973 and was the first CNI approved for prevention and treatment of organ rejection by the FDA in 1983. It dramatically improved prognosis after organ transplantation by reducing graft failure due to rejection and substantially prolonged overall survival. To overcome the wide intra- and inter-individual differences in bioavailability of the original oil-based oral formulation of ciclosporin, a microemulsion formula of ciclosporin was introduced in the 1990s. Tacrolimus was discovered in the early 1980s and, from 1989, has been used for the prevention of liver transplant rejection. Since then, its use expanded rapidly into the transplantation of other organs.

Dosing of both oral ciclosporin and tacrolimus is typically titrated based on 12-h trough blood levels, with targets depending on the time since transplantation. In general, the levels are kept highest in the first month post-transplantation (e.g. 200–350ng/mL for ciclosporin and 10–15ng/mL for tacrolimus) and lowered in subsequent periods (e.g. 100–200ng/mL for ciclosporin and 5–10ng/mL for tacrolimus). However, target drug levels should be individualized to balance the risk of rejection with drug toxicities. Both ciclosporin and tacrolimus are available for IV administration where dosing should be reduced to about one-third of the oral dose for both drugs.

Both ciclosporin and tacrolimus have a wide range of side effects, including hypertension, infections, dyslipidaemia, neurotoxicity, diabetes, renal failure, and malignancy. When comparing ciclosporin with tacrolimus, tacrolimus seems to be associated with a lower risk of hypertension, hyperlipidaemia, gingival hyperplasia, and hirsutism. In addition, tacrolimus seems to be superior to microemulsion ciclosporin in heart transplant patients, with regard to survival and prevention of severe rejections.[5] Due to this favourable profile of tacrolimus, it has now largely replaced the use of ciclosporin.[2]

Antimetabolites

Antimetabolites or antiproliferative agents interfere with the synthesis of nucleic acids and exert their immunosuppressive effects by inhibiting the cell cycle of both T- and B-lymphocytes. Antimetabolites include MMF, mycophenolate sodium, and AZA.

AZA was the earlier agent used in this class and served as the mainstay of immunosuppression, even prior to the routine use of ciclosporin. AZA is a prodrug that is first rapidly hydrolysed in the blood to its active form 6-mercaptopurine and subsequently converted to a purine analogue thioinosine monophosphate. This antimetabolite is incorporated into deoxyribonucleic acid (DNA) and inhibits further nucleotide synthesis, thereby preventing mitosis and proliferation of rapidly dividing cells such as activated T- and B-lymphocytes. Major side effects include dose-dependent myelosuppression, particularly leucopenia. Other potentially serious side effects include hepatotoxicity and pancreatitis.

MMF is also a prodrug, which is rapidly hydrolysed to its active form mycophenolic acid, which is a reversible inhibitor of inosine monophosphate dehydrogenase, a critical enzyme for the *de novo* synthesis of guanine nucleotides. Lymphocytes lack a key enzyme in the guanine salvage pathway and are dependent upon the *de novo* pathway to produce purines necessary for ribonucleic acid (RNA) and DNA synthesis. Therefore, both T- and B-lymphocyte proliferation is selectively inhibited. By selectively targeting lymphocyte proliferation, MMF is less likely to produce neutropenia and anaemia than AZA, which affects the proliferation of all dividing cells. MMF is typically administered at a starting dose of 1000–1500mg bd, which is subsequently decreased in response to side effects, which mainly include dose-related leucopenia and GI toxicities such as nausea, gastritis, and diarrhoea. Drug monitoring is not routinely performed. Due to the superiority in survival and rejection with MMF versus AZA, MMF has now replaced AZA as the first-line antiproliferative drug. Also, MMF has been shown to reduce the risk of CAV, compared with AZA.[6]

Mycophenolate sodium is an enteric-coated, delayed-release salt of mycophenolic acid, developed to improve the upper GI tolerability of mycophenolate. It has shown similar effects to MMF, in terms of prevention of rejection, graft loss, and death, with better tolerability.[7] Therefore, a switch from MMF to mycophenolate sodium may be attempted in patients with unacceptable GI side effects to MMF. A dose of 720mg of mycophenolate sodium corresponds to a dose of 1000mg of MMF.

Proliferation signal inhibitors

PSIs or mTOR inhibitors represent the most recent class of drugs used as maintenance therapy in solid organ transplantation. PSIs include sirolimus and everolimus, which have similar mechanisms of action. They inhibit mTOR, which is a protein kinase in the cytoplasm involved in the transduction of signals from the IL-2 receptor to the nucleus, causing cell cycle arrest at the G1 to S phase (see Fig. 3.2.1). The consequence of mTOR inhibition is a reduction of both T- and B-cell proliferation and a differentiation in response to IL-2. They are also known to inhibit the proliferation of endothelial cells and fibroblasts and may have a protective role against malignancies and CMV infections. While everolimus and sirolimus, when used as primary immunosuppressants together with CNIs, have proven efficacy in reducing rejection, compared with AZA, they have not yet been proven superior to MMF. The major advantages of mTOR inhibitors seem to be protection against chronic allograft vasculopathy, as assessed by IVUS of the coronary arteries, which has been documented in several randomized trials comparing PSIs to AZA, MMF, and CNIs.[8,9] In addition, mTOR inhibitors may allow for reduced dosing, or even early withdrawal, of CNIs, leading to significant improvements in renal function by sparing the kidneys from the nephrotoxic effects of CNIs.

Side effects of PSIs include poor wound healing, stomatitis and oral ulcerations, dyslipidaemia, oedema, proteinuria, and non-infectious interstitial pneumonitis. To minimize side effects, regular monitoring of drug serum trough levels is recommended, targeting 5–10ng/mL for sirolimus and 3–8ng/mL for everolimus. Since PSIs potentiate the nephrotoxic effects of CNIs, it is important to reduce the dosing of CNIs if used in combination with a PSI.

Glucocorticoids

Glucocorticoids are non-specific anti-inflammatory agents, with complex effects in the immune system that interrupt multiple steps, including antigen presentation, cytokine production, and proliferation of lymphocytes. Several dosing strategies exist for corticosteroid use, including high doses of IV methylprednisolone at the time of transplantation before tapering of oral prednisone to low maintenance doses begins. High-dose IV methylprednisolone is also used for treatment of episodes of moderate and severe acute rejections. Glucocorticoids have numerous side effects, including glucose intolerance, dyslipidaemia, increased appetite and obesity, osteoporosis, fluid retention, and a predisposition to opportunistic infections. Due to the many side effects associated with long-term use of glucocorticoids, a trial of steroid weaning is recommended in patients with a benign rejection history.[10]

Treatment of acute rejection

Treatment of acute cellular rejection depends on several factors, including the severity, timing, and degree of side effects to the immunosuppressive medication. In general, if there is no rejection, one should consider if the immunosuppressive medication can be reduced to minimize side effects. A mild rejection most often does not require specific treatment, but it may be needed to increase maintenance therapy if drug levels are below targets. A moderate rejection (H2R) and severe rejection (H3R) are generally treated with high-dose glucocorticoid (e.g. 1000mg/day IV for 3 days). In severe rejection, cytolytic therapy with ATG should be considered if haemodynamic compromise is present. In addition, appropriate adjustments of maintenance immunosuppressive therapy should be made to decrease the risk of recurrent rejection. The optimal treatment of antibody-mediated acute rejection is less established but may, if associated with graft dysfunction, include plasmapheresis, IV immunoglobulin, and rituximab.

Drug interactions with immunosuppressive agents

CNIs and PSIs have a wide range of interactions with other medications, mainly through the P450 3A4 pathway. These interactions can create serious consequences in the absence of dose adjustments. Some of the drugs which increase the level of CNIs and PSIs include non-dihydropyridine CCBs, antifungals, and some antibiotics, including all macrolides and ciprofloxacin. Some of the common interactions which lead to reduced levels of CNIs include anti-seizure medications (phenytoin, carbamazepine, and phenobarbital) and rifampicin. These drugs can be used in combination with immunosuppressive therapy but require appropriate monitoring and dose adjustment. CNIs increase drug concentrations of statins, which should be started at low dosing, with slow uptitration. NSAIDs and aminoglycosides potentiate the nephrotoxic effects of CNIs and should be avoided. Allopurinol inhibits the metabolism of AZA, leading to a high risk of severe bone marrow suppression, and the combination should therefore be avoided.

Infections

Heart transplant patients receiving immunosuppressive medication are susceptible to infections. In the first month, patients are most susceptible to infection from donor-transmitted pathogens, as well as nosocomial bacterial and fungal infections. During months 1–6 post-transplant, opportunistic infections, such as *Pneumocystis jiroveci*, may develop, and the sustained level of maximal immune suppression increases the risk for infection from donor-transmitted, or reactivation of, viruses such as CMV and Epstein–Barr virus. Later, infections are dominated by community-acquired infections. Prophylactic treatment against infections may vary between centres but generally include antifungal prophylaxis such as oral nystatin treatment in the first weeks, CMV prophylaxis with oral ganciclovir or valganciclovir for the first 3 months, and anti-protozoal prophylaxis with trimethoprim/sulfamethoxazole usually at least 1 year post-transplant. General antibiotic prophylaxis for infectious endocarditis before dental procedures in cardiac transplant recipients is not recommended by the ESC Task Force. Inactivated vaccines are considered safe in heart transplant patients, and routine seasonal administration of inactivated influenza vaccine is recommended. Live virus vaccines are generally avoided following solid organ transplantation, given the potential for active infection.

Hypertension

Hypertension is common in heart transplant patients. Since antihypertensive treatment in heart transplant recipients has benefits similar to those in the general population, hypertension should be treated to achieve the same goals recommended for the general population. CCBs and ACEIs/ARBs are most commonly used. The non-dihydropyridine CCBs are generally well tolerated and do not require dose reduction of CNIs. In contrast, verapamil and diltiazem increase CNI levels and have negative inotropic effects and are nowadays rarely used for BP control in heart transplant recipients. β-blockers can also be used to treat hypertension but may be associated with decreased exercise capacity.

References

1 Ponikowski P, Voors AA, Anker SD, *et al*. 2016 ESC Guidelines for the diagnosis and treatment of acute and chronic heart failure: The Task Force for the diagnosis and treatment of acute and chronic heart failure of the European Society of Cardiology (ESC). Developed with the special contribution of the Heart Failure Association (HFA) of the ESC. *Eur J Heart Fail* 2016;**18**:891–975.

2 Lund LH, Edwards LB, Dipchand AI, *et al*. The Registry of the International Society for Heart and Lung Transplantation: Thirty-third Adult Heart Transplantation Report—2016; Focus Theme: Primary Diagnostic Indications for Transplant. *J Heart Lung Transplant* 2016;**35**:1158–69.

3 Kobashigawa JA, Tobis JM, Starling RC, *et al*. Multicenter intravascular ultrasound validation study among heart transplant recipients: outcomes after five years. *J Am Coll Cardiol* 2005;**45**:1532–7.

4 Fearon WF, Okada K, Kobashigawa JA, *et al*. Angiotensin-converting enzyme inhibition early after heart transplantation. *J Am Coll Cardiol* 2017;**69**:2832–41.

5 Penninga L, Møller CH, Gustafsson F, *et al*. Tacrolimus versus cyclosporine as primary immunosuppression after heart transplantation: systematic review with meta-analyses and trial sequential analyses of randomised trials. *Eur J Clin Pharmacol* 2010;**66**:1177–87.

6 Eisen HJ, Kobashigawa J, Keogh A, *et al*. Three-year results of a randomized, double-blind, controlled trial of mycophenolate mofetil versus azathioprine in cardiac transplant recipients. *J Heart Lung Transplant* 2005;**24**:517–25.

7 Kobashigawa JA, Renlund DG, Gerosa G, *et al*. Similar efficacy and safety of enteric-coated mycophenolate sodium (EC-MPS, Myfortic) compared with mycophenolate mofetil (MMF) in *de novo* heart transplant recipients: results of a 12-month, single-blind, randomized, parallel-group, multicenter study. *J Heart Lung Transplant* 2006;**25**:935–41.

8 Andreassen AK, Andersson B, Gustafsson F, *et al*. Everolimus initiation with early calcineurin inhibitor withdrawal in *de novo* heart transplant recipients: three-year results from the Randomized SCHEDULE Study. *Am J Transplant* 2016;**16**:1238–47.

9 Gustafsson F, Ross HJ. Proliferation signal inhibitors in cardiac transplantation. *Curr Opin Cardiol* 2007;**22**:111–16.

10 Baraldo M, Gregoraci G, Livi U. Steroid-free and steroid withdrawal protocols in heart transplantation: the review of literature. *Transpl Int* 2014;**27**:515–29.

Hypertension

Hypertension is common in heart transplant patients. Since antihypertensive treatment in heart transplant recipients is broadly similar to that in the general population, hypertension should be treated to achieve the same goals recommended for the general population. CCBs and ACEi/ARBs are most commonly used. The dihydropyridine CCBs are generally well tolerated and do not require dose reduction of CNIs. In contrast, verapamil and diltiazem increase CNI levels and have negative inotropic effects and are therefore rarely used for BP control in heart transplant patients. β-blockers can also be used to treat hypertension but may be associated with decreased exercise capacity.

References

[illegible]

Section 4

Arrhythmias

Section editors

Dan Atar
Antoni Martinez-Rubio

ESC Guidelines advisor

Peter J. Schwartz

Chapter 4.1

Atrial fibrillation

Gheorghe-Andrei Dan and Jan Steffel

Atrial fibrillation

Background

AF is the commonest hospitalized cardiac arrhythmia, with an increasing incidence with age. There are 33 million people with AF around the world, and 18 million people are expected in Europe in the next decade. AF is a risk marker and a risk factor for increased global mortality, stroke, HF, MI, CKD, and dementia. The stroke risk attributable to AF increases with age, more than expected from the increased incidence. There are five classical patterns of AF: first diagnosed AF episode, paroxysmal AF (duration of <7 days, usually <48h, and self-terminating), persistent AF [lasting >7 days and convertible with drugs or by direct current cardioversion (DCCV)], long-standing persistent AF (lasting for >1 year, but still convertible), and permanent AF (not converted and/or accepted). A special form is represented by immediate-relapse AF (IRAF), in which AF recurs within seconds or minutes after electrical or pharmacological conversion. Although catheter-ablative therapies are increasingly being employed in cases where patients are highly symptomatic and refractory to pharmacotherapy, drug therapy remains the mainstay of treatment for the majority of patients with AF and important also in conjunction with ablative therapy.

Electrophysiological basis of atrial fibrillation

AF represents a common electrical phenotype of several mechanisms and risk factors. Different risk factors contribute to modify the atrial substrate. This implies structural and ionic channel remodelling. In the presence of triggers (e.g. ectopic impulses from pulmonary veins), micro-re-entry is finally initiated. The resultant AF is able to self-perpetuate through intrinsic remodelling of the substrate (AF begets AF). Atrial fibrosis and inflammation, representing the result of atrial cardiomyopathy and/or the consequence of AF itself, play a pivotal role in initiating and maintaining AF. Some of rapid atrial impulses are conducted to the ventricles; some only penetrate the atrioventricular node (AVN), increasing its refractoriness; the ventricular rate and irregularity are the result of this concealed conduction of the atrial impulses. During increased sympathetic tone, the AVN refractoriness decreases steeply, leading to a disproportionate increase in heart rate.

Considerations for drug therapy

Drug therapy in AF addresses several main targets:

- Decrease in mortality, mainly due to CV diseases.
- Decrease in stroke rate.
- Decrease in ventricular deterioration and HF.
- Decrease in cognitive impairment and dementia.
- Increase in quality of life.

Clinicians should clearly bear in mind a logistic approach adapted for every patient. Management of AF risk factors, stroke prevention, and acute rate and rhythm therapy in a haemodynamically acutely compromised patient are intended to increase life expectancy. Pharmacological rhythm or rate strategy intended for stable patients or AF ablation and surgery are currently addressing only quality of life and social functioning. In this regard, as it results from many randomized trials, rhythm and rate strategies are considered equivalent and it is mainly to the clinician to choose between one and another strategy for a specific patient or for the moment the patient is evaluated. Obviously, obtaining sinus rhythm is ideal and associated with better outcome, but use of current antiarrhythmic drugs (AADs) is associated with serious adverse effects, including proarrhythmias, and some AADs increase mortality. Therefore, clinicians dealing with AAD therapy should be aware of more than the simple Singh–Vaughan–Williams classification; they need to have knowledge about the pharmacokinetics of AADs, the specific ion channel targeting, the ECG effect, and the cardiac and extra-cardiac adverse actions. In the broadest sense, the most important decisions for pharmacotherapy in AF are whether anticoagulation is warranted for the prevention of thromboembolic complications and whether a rhythm or rate control strategy is preferred and which agent/agents are the most appropriate.

Screening for, and prevention of, atrial fibrillation

Underdiagnosed AF, because silent episodes are frequent and opportunistic screening for AF is warranted in patients with risk factors or in patients with ischaemic stroke or TIAs, as silent episodes bear the same stroke risk as clinically manifest episodes. In patients without known AF and with implanted devices, detection and appropriate management of atrial high-rate episodes (AHREs) (>180 per min and >5–6min) are important, as AHREs are markers for AF and a risk factor for stroke. Primary prevention of AF means prevention of atrial substrate remodelling. Secondary prevention means avoidance of recurrences through prevention of further substrate remodelling, reverse remodelling, and drug or interventional electrophysiologic interventions. Feasibility of recurrence prevention is still a subject of debate. On the other hand, primary prevention seems to be feasible, and early small clinical studies indicate the benefit of so-called 'upstream' therapy due to the antiarrhythmic effect of non-AADs. These drugs include inhibitors of RAAS and statins. However, large randomized studies failed to confirm this benefit. This is not surprising, as the remodelling process was already in place. Inhibition of RAAS is recommended for new-onset AF prevention in patients with hypertension and LVH and in patients with HF with reduced ejection fraction. Also it is indicated as pre-medication to prevent recurrences in patients receiving antiarrhythmic therapy and undergoing electrical cardioversion. Several conditions are particularly prone to developing AF: HF, MI, COPD, sleep apnoea syndrome, CKD, VHD, thyroid dysfunction, obesity, alcoholism, and smoking. In these patients, strict management of the condition is mandatory both for prevention of new-onset AF and for prevention of recurrences.

New (acute)-onset atrial fibrillation

The symptomatology of a first presentation of AF is varied and ranges from those who are symptom-free (often these patients are discovered incidentally) to those *in extremis* with pulmonary oedema and cardiogenic shock. Acute management is largely dependent on symptoms, and the clinician must decide whether acute treatment is necessary. It should be noted that the presence of palpitations add very little to the timing of the AF episode, because many episodes are silent or become silent shortly after the onset of AF and in the same patient, some episodes are symptomatic and others are not. Also it should be emphasized again that AAD therapy is intended for quality of life, and not for life expectancy; therefore, the clinician has to carefully balance the benefits and risk of such therapy in a particular patient.

Intolerable symptoms or haemodynamic instability

Patients presenting with a highly elevated ventricular rate (>150 per min), signs of circulatory collapse (hypotension or pulmonary oedema), chest pain, dyspnoea, or intolerable palpitations should be treated as an acute medical emergency (see Fig. 4.1.1). It is important to consider secondary causes of AF such as thyrotoxicosis, PE, and sepsis, as AF tends to respond poorly in these situations until the underlying cause is treated (see ➔ Secondary atrial fibrillation, pp. 198–9).

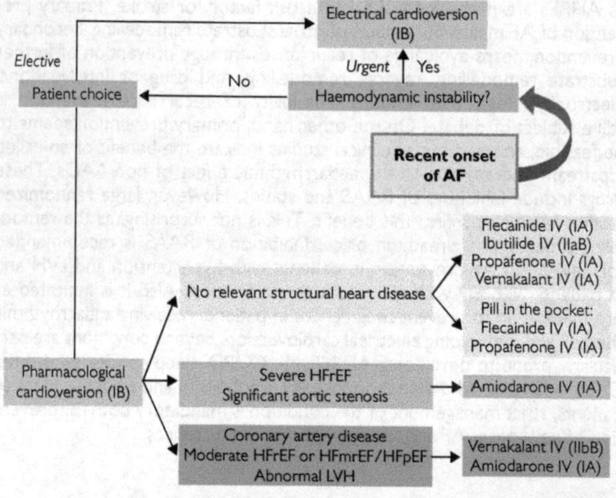

Fig. 4.1.1 Management of an episode of recent-onset AF. Cardioversion could be postponed on an elective basis in such patients. Patients with Wolff–Parkinson–White (WPW) syndrome may present with very high ventricular rates (often >200bpm) and a broad QRS complex (FBI tachycardia: Fast–Broad–Irregular). In this so-called 'pre-excited AF', flecainide is a useful alternative to amiodarone for cardioversion. In contrast, AVN-blocking agents (non-dihydropyridine CCBs, adenosine, and digoxin) should not be used in this situation, as it may lead to increased ventricular rates via uninhibited antegrade accessory pathway conduction.

Patients with circulatory instability should undergo DCCV, independent of the duration of AF. As the efficacy and safety of drug cardioversion is inferior to DCCV, pharmacological cardioversion is not indicated in patients with haemodynamic compromise. In patients with HF, strict control of fluid balance, RAAS inhibition, maintenance of heart rate below 110bpm, and consideration of early rhythm and device strategy are mandatory.

In the absence of haemodynamic instability, cardioversion should not be performed if AF has been present for >48h. In practice, however, there is often no clear history of symptom onset, and indeed patients may be asymptomatic in AF. Moreover, even before 48h, the risk of thromboembolism subsequent to cardioversion increases over time and is higher in those presenting later within the 48-h time window. As such, if in doubt, transoesophageal echocardiography should be performed or, alternatively, anticoagulation initiated in the absence of haemodynamic instability, to increase the safety of cardioversion. This is independent of the mode of cardioversion and applies to electrical, as well as pharmacological, cardioversion. Use of LMWH in this setting is not recommended by guidelines but encountered in practice. The benefit and safety of non-antivitamin K oral anticoagulants (NOACs) in patients were recently evaluated, showing that NOACs are a reasonable alternative to warfarin.

Absent or mild symptoms

These patients generally require no acute drug therapy if the resting ventricular rate is controlled (generally regarded as <110bpm). An assessment of the ambulatory heart rate response, 24-h heart rate profile, structural heart disease (echocardiography), and thromboembolic risk should be made, and the decision to treat and anticoagulate made (see ➔ Anticoagulation, pp. 201–5).

Pharmacotherapy in paroxysmal atrial fibrillation

Pharmacotherapy aims to achieve the following:

- Suppression of AF paroxysms and maintenance of sinus rhythm.
- Control of ventricular rate.
- Prevention of complications such as tachycardia-related cardiomyopathy.
- Prevention of stroke and systemic thromboembolism.

Treatment strategies

Treatment should always be discussed with the patient and tailored to individual needs. In acute, highly symptomatic, or haemodynamically unstable paroxysm, hospital treatment should always be sought and treatment instituted (see ➲ New (acute)-onset atrial fibrillation, pp. 188–9).

Infrequent paroxysms (<1 week)

Simple avoidance of precipitants, such as caffeine and alcohol, may be enough for some. Similarly, lifestyle modification (weight normalization, in particular) has been shown to be highly effective to reduce AF recurrence.

In patients with infrequent bouts, a *pill-in-the-pocket* strategy with a class Ic agent (flecainide 200–300mg single dose or propafenone 450–600mg single dose), in the absence of relevant structural heart disease, may be preferred. This should be combined with low-dose β-blocker therapy to avoid regularization of AF and subsequent rapid conduction to the ventricle. A pill-in-the-pocket strategy can also be used as an add-in for those on low-dose maintenance therapy. For safety reasons, it could be wise to test in hospital for the first time the efficacy of the *pill-in-the-pocket* strategy.

Frequent symptomatic paroxysms

The decision for rhythm versus rate control is an individual one, taking into account the patient's symptoms (at rest/during exercise), age, comorbidities, etc. (see Figs. 4.1.2 and 4.1.3). In addition to pharmacological rhythm control, AF ablation has emerged as a good treatment option for many patients. It is considered a valid choice after a first failure of AAD trial (class IA recommendation) but may also be an option as first-line therapy in selected patients (class IIa recommendation).

It is important to recognize that anticoagulation therapy needs to be continued, based on the CHA_2DS_2-VASc score, independent of the strategy (rate versus rhythm control) or any apparent 'success' of an antiarrhythmic strategy, pharmacological or by AF ablation. Hence, patients who otherwise qualify for anticoagulation need to continue to be anticoagulated also after AF ablation, even if the latter is deemed to have been successful.

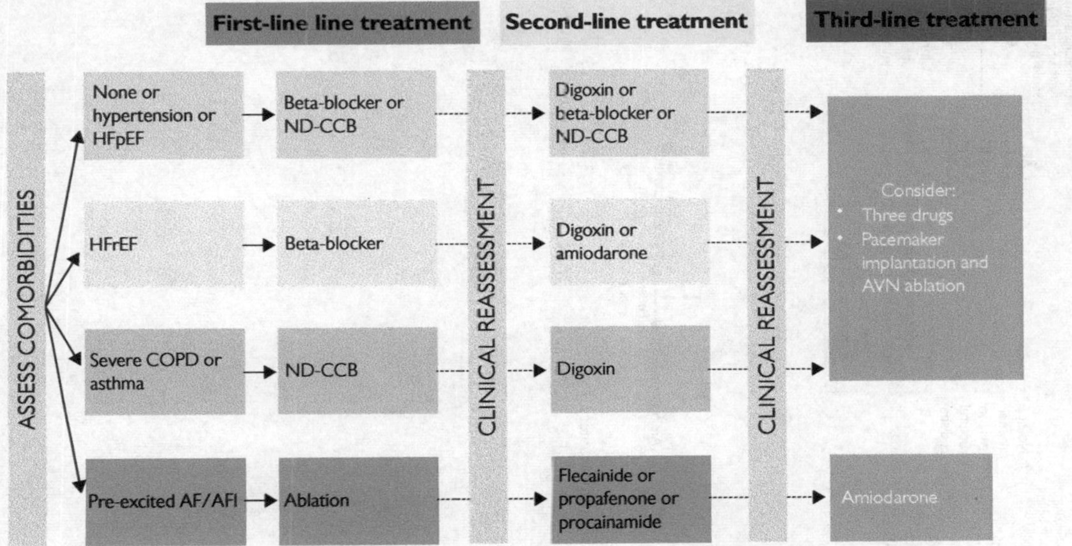

Fig. 4.1.2 Heart rate control. COPD, chronic obstructive pulmonary disease; HFpEF, heart failure with preserved ejection fraction; HFrEF, heart failure with reduced ejection fraction; ND-CCB, non-dihydropyridine calcium channel blocker.

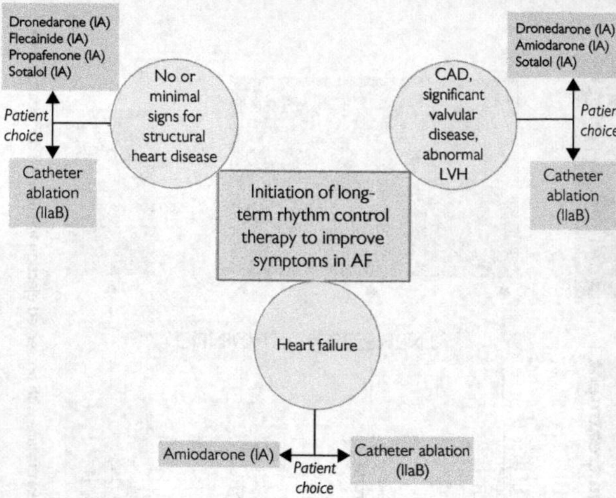

Fig. 4.1.3 Rhythm strategy.

Persistent atrial fibrillation

As with new or paroxysmal AF, treatment should be tailored to the individual and the advantages and disadvantages of a rate or rhythm control strategy discussed with the patient. The major determinant of a treatment strategy is usually the burden of symptoms. It is important to bear in mind the following evidence-based considerations (see Table 4.1.1).

Key points

- Overall there is no significant difference in mortality between rate and rhythm control strategies.
- There is no significant difference in quality of life between rate and pharmacological rhythm control.
- There is no difference in likelihood between strategies of suffering MI or developing congestive cardiac failure, and the 5-year cumulative risk of thromboembolic and haemorrhagic events is similar.
- In patients older than 65 years and in those with CAD or HF [congestive HF (CHF) or ejection fraction <50%], a rhythm control strategy may confer a mortality advantage. In milder HF (up to NYHA class II), there is little difference in mortality outcome between rate and rhythm control. A rhythm control strategy is associated with a greater incidence of hospital admission than rate control. It should be emphasized that rate control is the 'background therapy' for all patients, and the choice of a rhythm control strategy depends both on the patient's condition and the clinician's decision. Some general suggestions are presented in Table 4.1.2.
- Owing to costs associated with DCCV, a greater number of hospital admissions, and generally more expensive medication, the rhythm control strategy is more costly than rate control.
- Appropriate antithrombotic therapy should be offered, based on risk, regardless of the treatment strategy (see ➔ Anticoagulation, pp. 201–5).

Rhythm control agents

As with treatment of acute-onset AF and prophylaxis in paroxysmal AF, agents from Vaughan–Williams classes IC and III are preferred for maintaining sinus rhythm in this group of patients. The choice depends on the presence and degree of cardiac structural substrate alteration. Sotalol, as a drug with combined class II and III electrophysiologic actions, could be valuable if no contraindication to β-blockers or repolarization prolongation drugs (asthma, long QT). A β-blocker should be added to class IC AADs (propafenone or flecainide), in order to prevent rapid ventricular heart rates following transformation into atrial flutter (see Fig. 4.1.3).

Pharmacological cardioversion could be an alternative to DCCV and refers to the use of an IV agent and may be chosen if the patient wishes to be admitted to hospital and does not wish to undergo electrical cardioversion (see Fig. 4.1.1). Several reviews have confirmed a conversion rate of <50%, inferior to electrical conversion; however, during pharmacological cardioversion, there is no need for sedation or fasting. Dofetilide and ibutilide are able to convert recent-onset AF; however, dofetilide is not available in Europe, and ibutilide carries the risk of torsades de pointes (TdP). Vernakalant, a more recently studied drug, is very active in rapidly restoring sinus rhythm in recent-onset AF (but not atrial flutter); it is superior to amiodarone in efficacy and onset of effect. Vernakalant is contraindicated in severe aortic stenosis (AS), hypotension (BP below 100mmHg), severe HF (NYHA class III or IV), and ACS in the last 30 days.

In a less severe acute presentation, or if the patient does not wish to be admitted to hospital, oral treatment should be prescribed, escalation from a standard β-blocker (e.g. metoprolol or atenolol) to sotalol (uptitrated from 80mg bd to 240mg bd) or a class IC agent, in the absence of structural heart disease. In case of treatment failure, another AAD is an acceptable option, the choice depending on the cardiac structural substrate (as in Fig. 4.1.3). Ablation is also an acceptable alternative for these patients and those who failed with amiodarone. For patients who failed ablation, another procedure could improve the results, or hybrid therapy is an alternative (ablation plus AAD). If failure persists, in selected cases and after an MDT evaluation, surgery may be recommended if a rate control strategy is not acceptable.

More detailed information about AAD dosages are found elsewhere.[1]

Rate control strategy for persistent AF patients is discussed in ➲ Permanent atrial fibrillation, pp. 196–7.

When dealing with pharmacological rhythm control strategy, the clinician should be aware of the potential proarrhythmic risk of AADs. Management of proarrhythmias is presented in Fig. 4.1.4.

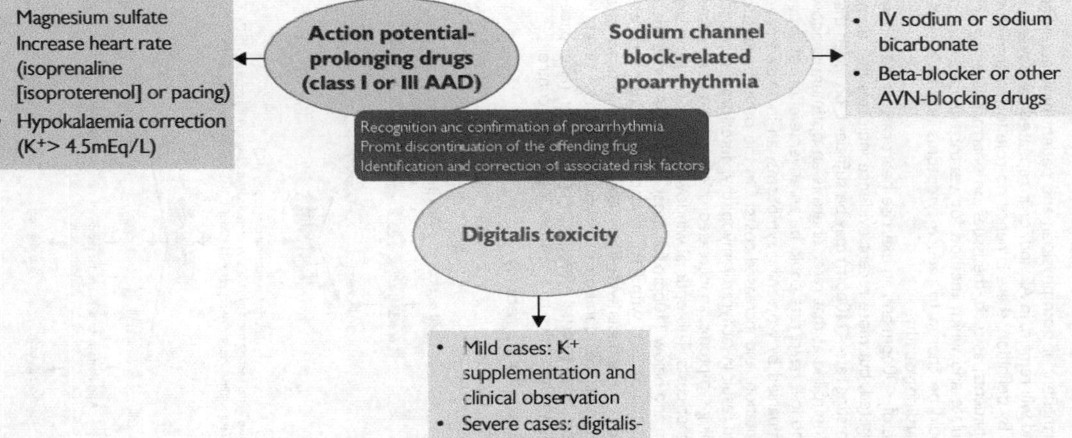

Fig. 4.1.4 Proarrhythmia management.

After Dan GA, *et al.* Antiarrhythmic drugs—clinical use and clinical decision making: a consensus document from the European Heart Rhythm Association (EHRA) and European Society of Cardiology (ESC) Working Group on Cardiovascular Pharmacology, endorsed by the Heart Rhythm Society (HRS), Asia- Pacific Heart Rhythm Society (APHRS) and International Society of Cardiovascular Pharmacotherapy (ISCP). *Europace* 2018;20:731–2.

Permanent atrial fibrillation

AF is considered 'permanent' if both physician and patient have accepted that the patient is, and will remain, in AF and/or if repeated cardioversion attempts have failed. By definition, there is hence no role for rhythm control in this group of patients; as such, the issues on pharmacotherapy are whether to anticoagulate and which method for ventricular rate control strategy (if any) should be chosen to reduce symptoms and to prevent tachycardia-related cardiomyopathy.

A resting heart rate of <90bpm and an exercise heart rate of <180bpm were traditionally targeted, but more recent evidence indicates that more lenient rate control (resting rate <110bpm) may be sufficient, provided that symptoms are well controlled at that rate. There is an optimum window for heart rate, as a too low heart rate could be an adverse effect of drugs controlling HF, accompanied by worsening symptoms, an increased need for pacemaker implantation, and increased costs. On the other hand, too high a heart rate could result in tachycardiomyopathy, deterioration of cardiac function, worsening symptoms, an increased risk for stroke, decreased quality of life, and higher costs. This optimal window includes resting heart rates of above 80bpm and below 110bpm for most patients. A more strict rate control is indicated in patients with CRT in whom a resting heart rate of <80bpm is desired or in patients with significant increase in heart rate during effort (>110bpm at 25% duration of maximum exercise time). In selected cases that have failed to usual measures, AVN ablation (after pacemaker implantation) is an alternative to pharmacological rate control.

Choice of rate-controlling agent(s)

(See Fig. 4.1.5.)

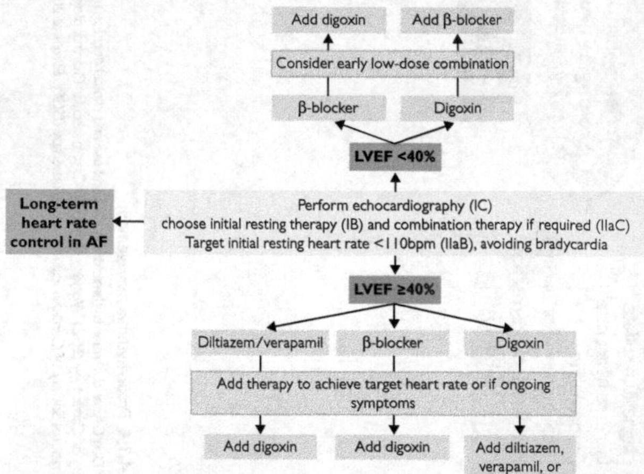

Fig. 4.1.5 Long-term rate-controlling agents in AF.

Key points

- Overall there is no difference in efficacy in ventricular rate control at rest between β-blockers, non-dihydropyridine CCBs (diltiazem or verapamil), and digoxin.
- β-blockers and non-dihydropyridine CCBs improve rhythm irregularity.
- In practice, diltiazem may be preferable to verapamil, owing to a greater negative inotropy with verapamil and its potential for pronounced atrioventricular (AVB) and bradycardia in combination with digoxin.
- Both β-blockers and non-dihydropyridine CCBs are more effective than digoxin at controlling ventricular rates during exercise. Digoxin as monotherapy is therefore only appropriate in those who are sedentary, such as the elderly, and also because it tends to only reduce heart rate at rest, but not during exercise.
- If monotherapy with β-blockers or non-dihydropyridine CCBs fails to control the ventricular rate, there is proven additional benefit from adding digoxin to either a β-blocker (benefit shown only at rest) or CCB (benefit both at rest and during exercise). On this basis, it may be more appropriate to initiate more active people on a non-dihydropyridine CCB for monotherapy, should they require the addition of digoxin at some stage.
- There is increased evidence that digoxin could increase mortality and adverse events in AF patients; however, it still may be a valuable tool in patients with low ejection fraction (in conjunction with β-blocker or not) if a safe drug concentration (in the lower part of the therapeutic range, i.e. 0.5–0.8nmol/L) can be obtained and monitored.

Secondary atrial fibrillation

AF may arise secondarily to structural heart disease, HF, hypertension, surgery, CAD, metabolic disturbances, and toxicity from drugs, including alcohol. It is essential to treat the underlying condition, which may, in itself, terminate or reduce the occurrence of AF prior to any specific AF-directed therapy, unless the patient is haemodynamically compromised. If not mentioned here, these are discussed in the relevant chapters.

Myocardial infarction

In the setting of acute MI, AF is usually transient. It is more likely in the setting of LV dysfunction, LVF, pericarditis, atrial ischaemic damage, and RV infarction. In STEMI, AF carries an increased risk for stroke and higher mortality, and anticoagulation is advised. β-blockers, with well-established benefit post-MI, are important to inhibit the excess sympathetic tone that often predisposes to arrhythmias. Of note, AF itself predisposes to an increased risk for MI.

Thyrotoxicosis

Thyroxine potentiates the effect of the adrenergic system on the heart. One study has demonstrated a 5-fold increased incidence of AF in both overt and subclinical hyperthyroidism [low thyroid-stimulating hormone (TSH) with normal triiodothyronine (T3)/thyroxine (T4)]. The first-line treatment is to establish a euthyroid state, using antithyroid drugs (carbimazole, propylthiouracil, or radioiodine). β-blockade, with either a β1-selective (bisoprolol) or non-selective β-blocker (atenolol, propranolol), has been shown to be beneficial in reducing ventricular rate and HF.

Heart failure

The relation between HF and AF is reciprocal—HF is an important risk factor for AF through atrial substrate remodelling, and AF promotes and worsens HF. The management of AF in patients with HF does not differ from that in patients without HF. Among the specific therapies of AF, only oral anticoagulation for stroke prevention demonstrated outcome benefit in this population. Strict adherence to a specific therapy of HF (RAAS inhibition, β-blockers) is mandatory, as it decreases the AF burden. Pure tachycardiomyopathy and HF as a consequence of AF is rare, but a mixed form is frequent (i.e. worsening of pre-existing HF by high rate and irregularity of AF). In selected patients, catheter ablation can restore LV function and quality of life. Of note, AF is a cause per se for elevation of plasma concentrations of natriuretic peptides, and therefore challenging the diagnostic and prognostic interpretation of natriuretic peptide levels.

Hypertension

Hypertension is a risk factor for AF and a risk factor for stroke and bleeding complications. High BP control is a part of AF management. RAAS inhibition could prevent new-onset AF and AF recurrences in hypertensive patients with LVH (see also ➔ Screening for, and prevention of, atrial fibrillation, p. 187).

Alcohol excess

The Framingham study demonstrated that a high level of alcohol consumption (>36g per day) is associated with a greater risk for developing AF, and the 'holiday heart' syndrome refers to AF triggered by acute alcohol excess. Alcohol is aetiologically important in as many as 63% of cases of new AF in the <65-year age group. Rarely is any treatment, in addition to abstinence, necessary.

Valvular heart disease

VHD, clinically manifest or found exclusively on echocardiographic examination, is present in more than one-third of AF patients. AF worsens the outcome of valvular patients. In terms of stroke prevention in AF, the term of valvular AF is applied only to mitral stenosis (MS) and mechanical valve. Mitral stenosis, a complication of rheumatic heart disease, is now a rare disease in Europe, but still important in developing countries. In patients with MS and AF, the exercise capacity may be increased with AVN-blocking drugs (β-blockers or non-dihydropyridine CCBs). The decision on whether to attempt cardioversion is determined by the clinical pattern of AF, atrial dimensions, stenosis severity, and availability of surgical correction.

Diabetes and obesity

Both diabetes and obesity are risk factors for AF. Diabetes increases the risk of ischaemic stroke. Treatment with metformin decreases the risk for AF in diabetic patients. Obesity is linked to an increased failure rate of AF ablation. Intensive weight loss is associated with fewer AF recurrences if other risk factors are also controlled.

Post-operative atrial fibrillation

AF is common after cardiac surgery, encountered in more than one-third of patients. The presence of post-operative AF is associated with an increased risk of death, stroke, and complications and predicts longer hospitalization. Anticoagulation in mandatory in post-operative AF. The antiarrhythmic decision in post-operative AF is similar to other forms of AF. Preoperative administration of β-blockers or amiodarone decreases the risk of post-operative AF. Other drugs (colchicine, n-3 polyunsaturated fatty acids, magnesium, or corticosteroids) have shown benefit in small trials.

Drugs used in electrical and pharmacological cardioversion

There are several aspects to drug therapy in cardioversion for AF: antithrombotic medication, pre- and post-cardioversion antiarrhythmic therapy, and sedation/anaesthesia during the procedure.

Antithrombotic therapy peri-cardioversion

- If there is no clear history of the time of onset, or symptoms have persisted for >48h, cardioversion should either be deferred and the patient adequately anticoagulated for a minimum of 3 weeks, or transoesophageal echocardiography utilized to exclude left atrial and atrial appendage thrombus prior to DCCV.
- Anticoagulation peri-cardioversion (at least 3 weeks) can be performed either with a NOAC or with warfarin.
- Following cardioversion, whether successful or not, the patient should remain on anticoagulation for a minimum of 4 weeks.
- Patients with a CHA2DS2-VASc score of ≥2 should remain on long-term anticoagulation, unless there is a clear secondary cause of the AF (see ➲ Secondary atrial fibrillation, pp. 198–9). Even then, prudent monitoring may be indicated so not to miss 'true' paroxysmal AF which was erroneously thought to be secondary AF.

Antiarrhythmic therapy for cardioversion

(See Fig. 4.1.1; see ➲ New (acute)-onset atrial fibrillation, pp. 188–9.)

In patients without structural heart disease, class IC antiarrhythmics are effective for restoring sinus rhythm. Ibutilide (class III antiarrhythmic) may be an alternative, if licensed and available, but requires observation for several hours afterwards due to the risk of QTc prolongation and TdP. Vernakalant, an atrial potassium and sodium channel blocker, may be given to patients with mild HF (NYHA class I or II), unless they present with severe AS or hypotension. Vernakalant should not be administered in patients with recent (<30 days) ACS. Finally, amiodarone represents the only drug which can be given also to patients with HF in the absence of other contraindications. Time to cardioversion with amiodarone is longer than with vernakalant or class IC antiarrhythmics. Of note, an important percentage of AF converts spontaneously in <24h; therefore, cardioversion may be deferred for a short interval if AF is asymptomatic or low-symptomatic.

Sedation or anaesthesia peri-cardioversion and facilitated conversion

Drugs used for sedation/anaesthesia in DCCV must provide adequate sedation and analgesia and minimal CV compromise, while enabling rapid recovery. Traditionally, general anaesthetic agents, such as propofol, sevoflurane, and etomidate, have been used safely, with rapid recovery as the main advantage, while dependence of these regimens on input from the anaesthetic department has led others to use IV midazolam, at the expense of prolonged sedation and resedation.

Amiodarone for few weeks before DCCV, sotalol, ibutilide, propafenone, flecainide, or vernakalant, all administered before cardioversion, enhance the success rate of DCCV.

Anticoagulation

Risk stratification

Ischaemic stroke is the most feared complication in patients with AF. So far, anticoagulation is the only therapy that has repeatedly been shown to reduce morbidity (stroke, in particular) and mortality in patients with AF. On the flipside, the fear of causing bleeding, particularly intracranial bleeding, has resulted in marked underutilization of anticoagulants in patients with AF, especially the elderly and patients at risk of falling—even though these patients are at a particularly high risk of stroke.

The most recent 2016 ESC guidelines have reiterated the CHA2DS2-VASc score as the preferred method for risk stratification (see Table 4.1.3).

Anticoagulation is indicated with a class I recommendation in males with a CHA2DS2-VASc score of ≥2 and in females with a CHA2DS2-VASc score of ≥3. Anticoagulation may also be considered (class IIa recommendation) in males with a CHA2DS2-VASc score of 1 and in females with a CHA2DS2-VASc score of 2. In all other patients (males with a CHA2DS2-VASc score of 0 and females with a CHA2DS2-VASc score of 1), no long-term anticoagulation is indicated (see Fig. 4.1.6). However, also these patients require anticoagulation peri-cardioversion (see ➲ Antithrombotic therapy peri-cardioversion, p. 200).

The HAS-BLED score, which was initially introduced to raise awareness of modifiable risk factors, has been 'replaced' for the general risk stratification in the latest guidelines (see Box 4.1.1). Indeed, the HAS-BLED score tracks along very well with the CHA2DS2-VASc, resulting in these patients also having an elevated CHA2DS2-VASc score in most instances. As a result, paradoxically, patients with an elevated HAS-BLED score tend to particularly benefit from anticoagulation. Therefore these patients need to be anticoagulated and carefully monitored. Hence, the primary goal is to look for and—ideally—correct any modifiable risk factors in anticoagulated patients.

Choice of anticoagulant

Until 2009, VKAs were the only class of drugs which had been shown to lead to a reduction in stroke and mortality in AF patients. Since then, four novel anticoagulants (or NOACs), with direct and targeted action on the coagulation cascade (see Fig. 4.1.7), have been studied in four independent large-scale randomized clinical trials in over 70,000 patients.

Overall, these drugs are at least as effective regarding the prevention of stroke and systemic embolism; at the same time, they reduce the most severe forms of bleeding complications (including intracranial haemorrhage) and reduce all-cause mortality, compared with VKAs. As a result, these drugs are today considered standard of care for stroke prevention in AF, especially in patients newly started on anticoagulation (class I A recommendation) (see Fig. 4.1.6).

One important exemption from this are patients with 'valvular AF'. In such patients, VKAs remain the therapy of choice [target international normalized ratio (INR) 2.0–3.0, or 2.5–3.5 in high-risk patients such as those with mechanical mitral prosthesis] and NOACs are contraindicated. Importantly, the term 'valvular AF' specifically refers to patients with at least moderate MS or with a mechanical heart valve. Patients with AF and other valvular disorders [including AS or mitral regurgitation (MR)] can be anticoagulated with NOACs.

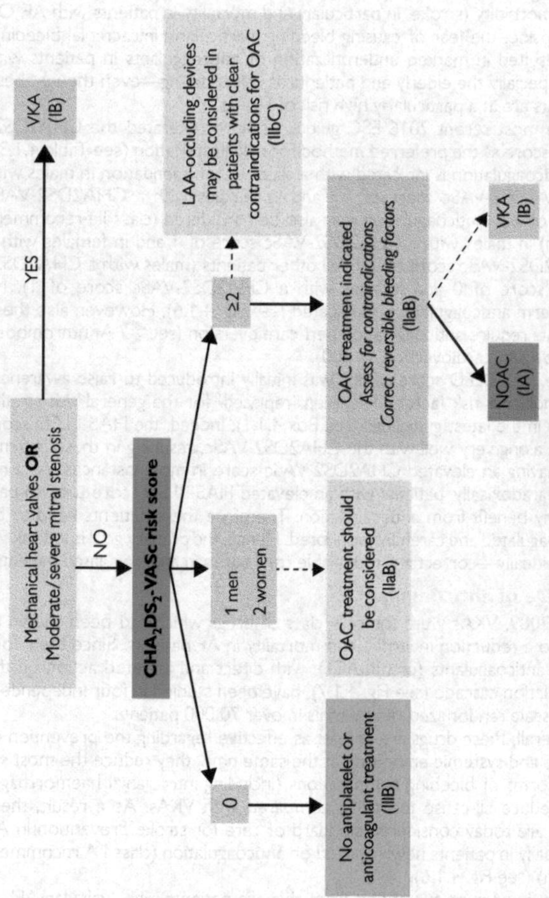

Fig. 4.1.6 Stroke prevention in AF. Summary of the 2016 ESC guidelines.

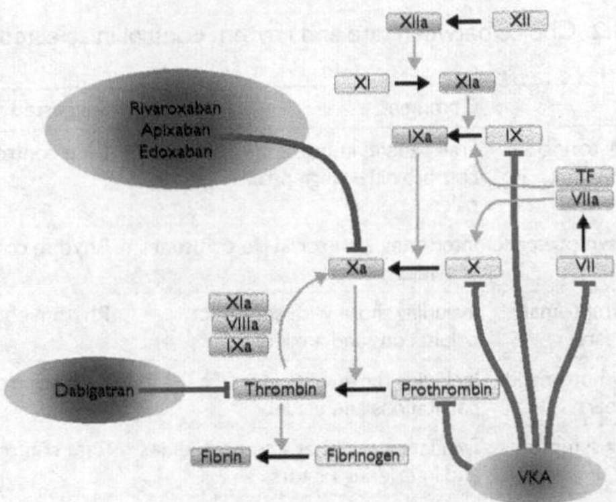

Fig. 4.1.7 Mode of action of NOACs (red) and VKAs (orange).

Modified from: Steffel J, Braunwald E. Novel oral anticoagulants: focus on stroke prevention and treatment of venous thromboembolism. *Eur Heart J* 2011;32(16):1968–76.

Box 4.1.1 Risk factors for bleeding in AF

Modifiable bleeding risk factors:

- Hypertension (especially when SBP is >160mmHg).
- Labile INR or time in therapeutic range <60% in patients on VKAs.
- Medication predisposing to bleeding such as antiplatelet drugs and NSAIDs.
- Excess alcohol (≥8 drinks/week).

Potentially modifiable bleeding risk factors:

- Anaemia.
- Impaired renal function.
- Impaired liver function.
- Reduced platelet count or function.

Table 4.1.1 Available NOACs and criteria for dose reduction

Dabigatran	2 × 150mg/2 × 110mg
Rivaroxaban	1 × 20mg
	(1 × 15mg if CrCl 30–50mL/min)
Apixaban	2 × 5mg
	(2 × 2.5mg if two out of three criteria are met: age >80 years, weight <60kg, creatinine >133micromol/L)
Edoxaban	1 × 60mg
	(1 × 30mg if: CrCl ≤50mL/min, weight ≤60kg, or co-medication with strong P-glycoprotein inhibitor (e.g. verapamil, dronedarone, etc.)

CrCl, creatinine clearance.

Table 4.1.2 Choice between rate and rhythm control in selected patients

Category	Comment	Suggested strategy
Risks of restoring SR outweigh benefits	Frail patient, important comorbidities, high proarrhythmic risk	Rate control
AF highly symptomatic (EHRA III–IV)	Interfering with social life or usual activities	Rhythm control
Minimal symptomatic, age <80 years	Including those with sporadic palpitations and anxiety	Rhythm control
Minimal symptomatic, age >80 years	Including those with sporadic palpitations and anxiety	Rate control
Worsening symptoms	Evaluate and manage comorbidities and interfering factors	Rate control
Deterioration of cardiac function	Evaluate and manage comorbidities and interfering factors	Rhythm control
Failure of rhythm control	After several AAD trials IRAF (?) Ablation failure, not intended or not possible	Rate control
AF accepted	Shared decision-making with the patient	Rate control
Secondary AF	Optimize causal disease Prevent AF (cardiac surgery)	Rhythm control

AAD, antiarrhythmic drug; IRAF, immediate-relapse atrial fibrillation; SR, sinus rhythm.

Table 4.1.3 Stroke risk score CHA2DS2Vasc

Variable	Definition	Value
Congestive heart failure	Sign/symptoms of HF or objective evidence of reduced LVEF	1
Hypertension	Resting BP >140/90mmHg on at least two occasions OR current antihypertensive treatment	1
Age ≥75 years		2
Diabetes mellitus	Fasting glucose >125mg/mL (7mmol/L) OR treatment with hypoglycaemic drugs and/or insulin	1
Stroke, TIA, or thromboembolism		2
Vascular disease	Previous MI, peripheral arterial disease, aortic plaque	1
Age 65–74 years		1
Sex category	Female	1

BP, blood pressure; HF, heart failure; LVEF, left ventricular ejection fraction; MI, myocardial infarction; TIA, transient ischaemic attack.

In contrast, antiplatelet therapy, such as aspirin (ASA), is no longer recommended for stroke prevention in AF. Indeed, while only of limited efficacy, ASA comes with a substantial risk of bleeding. Compared to apixaban (the only NOAC ever compared to ASA in a randomized clinical trial), ASA was substantially less effective at the same rate of major bleeding. As a result, ASA therapy has received a class III recommendation (with an indication of harm) for stroke prevention in AF.

Pharmacokinetic characteristics of NOACs are presented in Table 4.1.4.

A detailed description of anticoagulation in special situations, including renal insufficiency, elderly patients, risk of falling, etc., is beyond the scope of this book. The reader is referred to the relevant literature, including the European Heart Rhythm Association (EHRA) practical guide for the use of NOACs and the most current ESC guidelines.

Table 4.1.4 Absorption and metabolism of NOACs

	Dabigatran	Apixaban	Edoxaban	Rivaroxaban
Bioavailability	3–7%	50%	62%	66% (without food), approximately 100% with food
Prodrug	Yes	No	No	No
Clearance: non renal/renal of absorbed dose if normal renal function	20%/80%	73%/27%	50%/50%	65%/35%
Liver metabolism: CYP3A4	No	Yes (elimination; minor CYP3A4)	Minimal (<4% of elimination)	Yes (elimination)
Absorption with food	No effect	No effect	6–22% more	+39%
Intake with food?	No	No	No	Mandatory
Absorption with H2 blocker/PPI	Plasma level –12 to –30%	No effect	No effect	No effect
Asian ethnicity	Plasma level +25%	No effect	No effect	No effect
GI tolerability	Dyspepsia 5–10%	–	–	–
Elimination half-life	12–17h	12h	9–11h	5–9h (young)/ 11–13h (elderly)

Reproduced from Steffel J, Verhamme P, Potpara TS, et al., Group ESCSD. The 2018 European Heart Rhythm Association Practical Guide on the use of non-vitamin K antagonist oral anticoagulants in patients with atrial fibrillation. *Eur Heart J* 2018; 20 (8):with permission from Oxford University Press.

Atrial flutter

Introduction

Atrial flutter is caused by a macro-re-entrant circuit in the atria. Typical (classical or type I) atrial flutter is the commonest form of atrial flutter, with the macro-re-entrant circuit located in the right atrium in a counterclockwise direction. It is critically dependent upon a region of slow conduction in the isthmus between the tricuspid valve and the inferior vena cava (IVC). Other forms of (atypical) atrial flutter may arise from structural abnormalities and myocardial scarring (e.g. incisional flutter).

It often presents with a ventricular rate of approximately 150bpm, which represents a 2:1 conduction through the AVN, with an atrial rate of around 300bpm. The ventricular rate may be slower in the presence of AVN-blocking drugs or pre-existing AVB.

Conversion to sinus rhythm

The general principles for cardioversion of AF (see ➔ Drugs used in electrical and pharmacological cardioversion, p. 200) also apply to atrial flutter, including—importantly—the indications for anticoagulation pericardioversion. Atrial flutter is converted by low-energy DCCV. AADs were less studied for the pharmacological conversion of atrial flutter, and vernakalant is ineffective in restoring sinus rhythm in atrial flutter.

An important difference to AF is the fact that both pharmacological rhythm-controlling, as well as rate-controlling, therapies may be far less effective for atrial flutter, especially in the long term.

Maintenance of sinus rhythm

In recurrent atrial flutter, isthmus ablation is the treatment of choice, which can be obtained with a high success rate and a low rate of complication.

Alternatively, yet by far less effective, are class IC antiarrhythmics or amiodarone. As in AF, class I agents usually slow the flutter rate, thus increasing the chance that the AVN may not be refractory when flutter waves attempt to conduct to the ventricle. This may result in a 1:1 atrioventricular (AV) conduction, which may be life-threatening. Class I agents should therefore always be co-prescribed with AVN blockers (e.g. β-blockers) in atrial flutter.

Ventricular rate control

Ventricular rate control follows the same principles as for AF but is usually harder to achieve in atrial flutter.

Antithrombotic treatment

No RCTs have been conducted looking specifically at anticoagulation in atrial flutter, and, as such, recommendations are largely extrapolated from AF data. The indication for long-term anticoagulation therefore follows the principles outlined for AF.

AF ablation may cure patients with typical cavo-tricuspid isthmus-dependent atrial flutter. Due to frequent coexistence of atrial flutter and AF, diligently looking for concomitant AF is indispensable in these patients, particularly if the presence of AF would constitute an indication for long-term anticoagulation, according to the CHA2DS2-VASc score.

Reference

1 Dan GA, Martinez-Rubio A, Agewall S, et *al*. Antiarrhythmic drugs—clinical use and clinical decision making: a consensus document from the European Heart Rhythm Association (EHRA) and European Society of Cardiology (ESC) Working Group on Cardiovascular Pharmacology, endorsed by the Heart Rhythm Society (HRS), Asia-Pacific Heart Rhythm Society (APHRS) and International Society of Cardiovascular Pharmacotherapy (ISCP). *Europace* 2018;**20**:731–2an.

Further reading

Boriani G, Proietti M, Laroche C, et *al*.; EORP-AF Long-Term General Registry Investigators. Contemporary stroke prevention strategies in 11 096 European patients with atrial fibrillation: a report from the EURObservational Research Programme on Atrial Fibrillation (EORP-AF) Long-Term General Registry. *Europace* 2018;**20**:747–57.

Dan GA. Changing the paradigm to understand and manage atrial fibrillation. In: Dan GA, Bayés de Luna A, Camm AJ (eds). *Atrial Fibrillation Therapy*. Springer Verlag: London; 2014. pp. 127–65.

Dan GA, Martinez-Rubio A, Agewall S, et *al*. Antiarrhythmic drugs—clinical use and clinical decision making: a consensus document from the European Heart Rhythm Association (EHRA) and European Society of Cardiology (ESC) Working Group on Cardiovascular Pharmacology, endorsed by the Heart Rhythm Society (HRS), Asia-Pacific Heart Rhythm Society (APHRS) and International Society of Cardiovascular Pharmacotherapy (ISCP). *Europace* 2018;**20**:731–2an.

Goette A, Kalman JM, Aguinaga L, et *al*. EHRA/HRS/APHRS/SOLAECE expert consensus on atrial cardiomyopathies: definition, characterization, and clinical implication. *Europace* 2016;**18**:1455–90.

Heidbuchel H, Verhamme P, Alings M, et *al*. Updated European Heart Rhythm Association Practical Guide on the use of non-vitamin K antagonist anticoagulants in patients with non-valvular atrial fibrillation. *Europace* 2015;**17**:euv309.

Kirchhof P, Benussi S, Kotecha D, et *al*. 2016 ESC Guidelines for the management of atrial fibrillation developed in collaboration with EACTS. *Europace* 2016;**18**:1609–78.

Kotecha D, Breithardt G, Camm AJ, et *al*. Integrating new approaches to atrial fibrillation management: the 6th AFNET/EHRA Consensus Conference. *Europace* 2018;**20**:395–407.

Ruff CT, Giugliano RP, Braunwald E, et *al*. Comparison of the efficacy and safety of new oral anticoagulants with warfarin in patients with atrial fibrillation: a meta-analysis of randomised trials. *Lancet* 2014;**383**:955–62.

Savelieva I, Kakouros N, Kourliouros A, Camm AJ. Upstream therapies for management of atrial fibrillation: review of clinical evidence and implications for European Society of Cardiology guidelines. Part I: primary prevention. *Europace* 2011;**13**:308–28.

Steffel J, Verhamme P, Potpara TS, et *al*.; ESC Scientific Document Group. The 2018 European Heart Rhythm Association Practical Guide on the use of non-vitamin K antagonist oral anticoagulants in patients with atrial fibrillation. *Eur Heart J* 2018;**39**(16):1330–93.

Chapter 4.2

Supraventricular (narrow complex) tachycardias

Julio Martí-Almor

Introduction

The term supraventricular tachycardia (SVT) includes an umbrella term used to describe tachycardias (atrial and/or ventricular rates in excess of 100bpm at rest), the mechanism of which involves tissues from the His bundle or above that explains the narrow QRS complex, except for the presence of bundle branch block or antidromic tachycardia in the presence of an accessory pathway. These narrow complex tachycardias (NCTs) can be due to two modalities. The first one, where only atrial tissue is involved, is called atrial tachycardia (AT), including inappropriate sinus tachycardia, focal and multifocal and macro-re-entrant AT (including typical atrial flutter). The second one is AVN-dependent tachycardia, the so-called junctional tachycardia, where the AVN is part of the circuit and blocking it with vagal manoeuvres or adenosine can stop the tachycardia, including AV nodal re-entrant tachycardia (AVNRT) and AV re-entrant tachycardia (in the presence of an accessory pathway) (AVRT).

The epidemiology is not completely known because of incomplete data and failure to discriminate AF, atrial flutter, and other supraventricular arrhythmias. The best available evidence indicates that the prevalence of SVTs in the general population is 2.29 per 1000 persons. SVTs can appear at any age but are especially prevalent in young age and are commoner among females. AF and atrial flutter are treated in ➔ Chapter 4.1. Here we will focus on NCTs.

Diagnosis

AT can originate from the sinoatrial node, the peri-sinoatrial tissue, or any site in the right or the left atria. It may not be easy to determine the nature of a regular NCT on presentation, and often acute treatment is necessary in the absence of an established diagnosis. Nevertheless, some clinical clues can help in the diagnosis, as shown in Table 4.2.1, and some ECG criteria are helpful for the differential diagnosis (see Fig. 4.2.1). In AVNRT, palpitations are generally referred to the neck, and it is difficult to clearly localize the P-wave on the ECG, because it occurs simultaneously with the R-wave. Sometimes, as shown in Fig. 4.2.2, it is possible to see a P-wave mimicking an S-wave in inferior leads or a pseudo-RBBB (RSr') in lead V1. In the case of AVRT via an accessory pathway, the P-wave can be found at 120–140ms after the beginning of the R-wave, as shown in Fig. 4.2.3.

Table 4.2.1 Clinical clues to the differential diagnosis of supraventricular tachycardia

Type of tachyarrhythmia	Typical age at onset of symptoms	Underlying condition	Usual presentation	Findings on baseline ECG
Paroxysmal SVT	All ages	None (normal heart)	Abrupt onset and termination of regular palpitations, diaphoresis	Pre-excitation common in AVRT
AF, atrial flutter, multifocal atrial tachycardia	≥60 years	Heart disease common (hypertension, ischaemic or valvular heart disease)	Abrupt onset of paroxysmal, irregular palpitations; symptoms sometimes persistent and occasionally mild or absent	Signs of LVH; non-specific repolarization abnormalities common
Sinus tachycardia	10–30 years	None (normal heart)	Progressive onset and termination of palpitations	Normal
Ventricular tachycardia	≥50years	Ischaemic heart disease	Abrupt onset and termination of regular palpitations, syncope, or sudden death from cardiac causes	Pathological Q-waves common

AVRT, atrioventricular re-entrant tachycardia through an accessory pathway; AF, atrial fibrillation; LVH, left ventricular hypertrophy; SVT, supraventricular tachycardia.

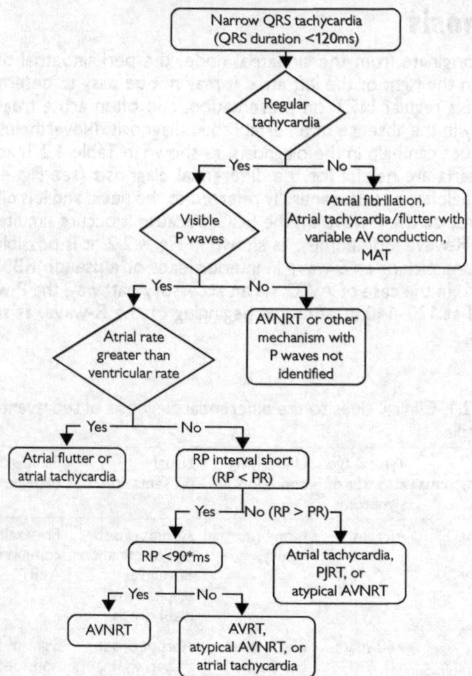

Fig. 4.2.1 Guide to electrocardiographic differential diagnosis of supraventricular tachycardia/regular narrow complex tachycardia. AVNRT, atrioventricular node re-entrant tachycardia; AVRT, atrioventricular re-entrant tachycardia through an accessory pathway; MAT, multifocal atrial tachycardia; PJRT, permanent junctional re-entrant tachycardia.

Vagal manoeuvres (Valsalva manoeuvre, carotid sinus massage, or facial immersion in cold water, rather than eye compression) can be performed, with a reported efficacy of 19–54%. Carotid sinus compression should be performed with caution in older patients, ruling out murmurs by carotid auscultation. Compression should be for 15 and 20s and can be repeated twice. If this fails, adenosine/ATP injection can help to distinguish atrial tachycardia from tachycardia involving the AVN. In addition, the efficacy and safety of etripamil (a short-acting CCB) as nasal spray have recently been reported to terminate paroxysmal SVT induced in the electrophysiological laboratory. It is possible that, in the future, self-administration of such drug would prove useful in patients with tachycardias involving the AVN. Fig. 4.2.4 shows an algorithm indicating the use of IV adenosine for the diagnosis of an underlying rhythm in patients with NCT and how to manage this type of arrhythmia.

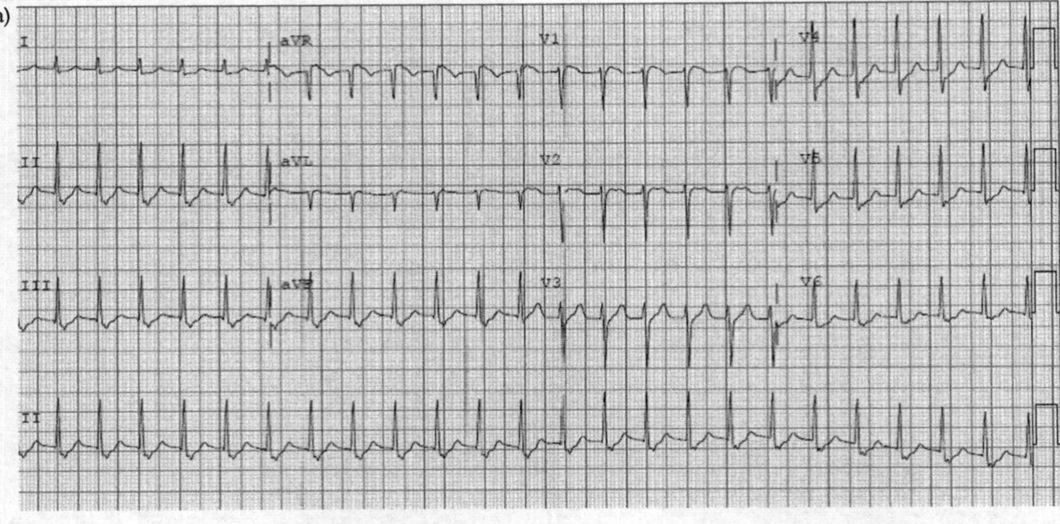

Fig. 4.2.2 (a) An ECG of a female patient with AVNRT, showing the terminal forces in the inferior leads mimicking an S-wave and mimicking a pseudo-RBBB in lead V1. (b) The ECG was recorded when the patient recovered sinus rhythm after adenosine administration.

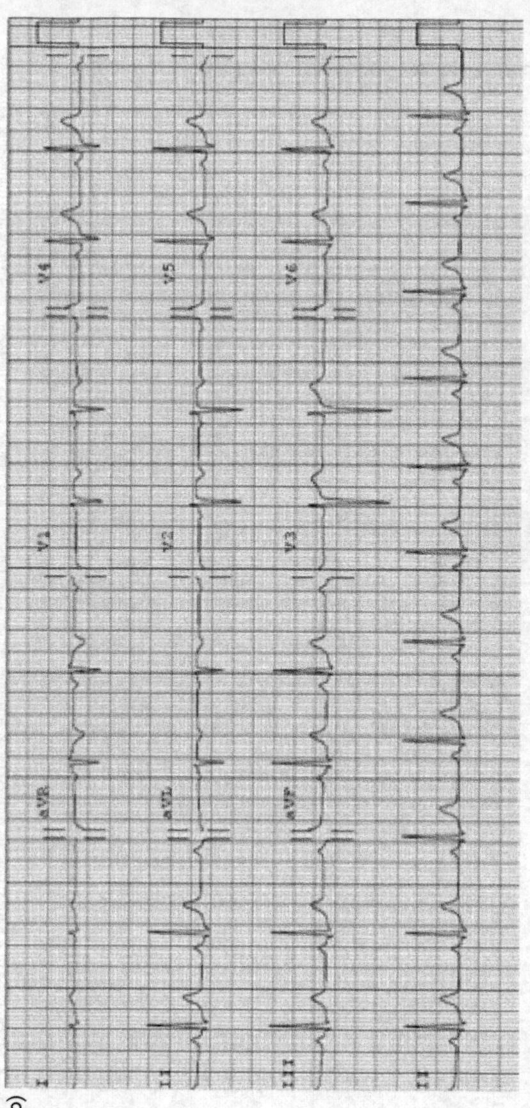

Fig. 4.2.2 (*Contd.*)

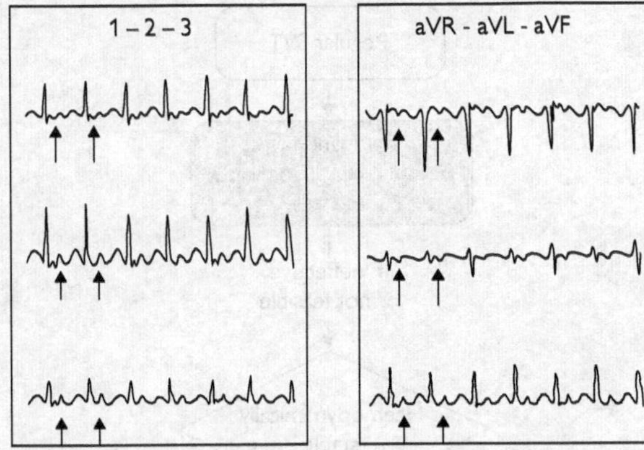

Fig. 4.2.3 AVRT by an accessory pathway. The P-waves can be seen clearly at 140ms after the beginning of the R-wave (as shown by arrows). In this case, the patient was successfully ablated in the mitral annulus using a retro-aortic approach.

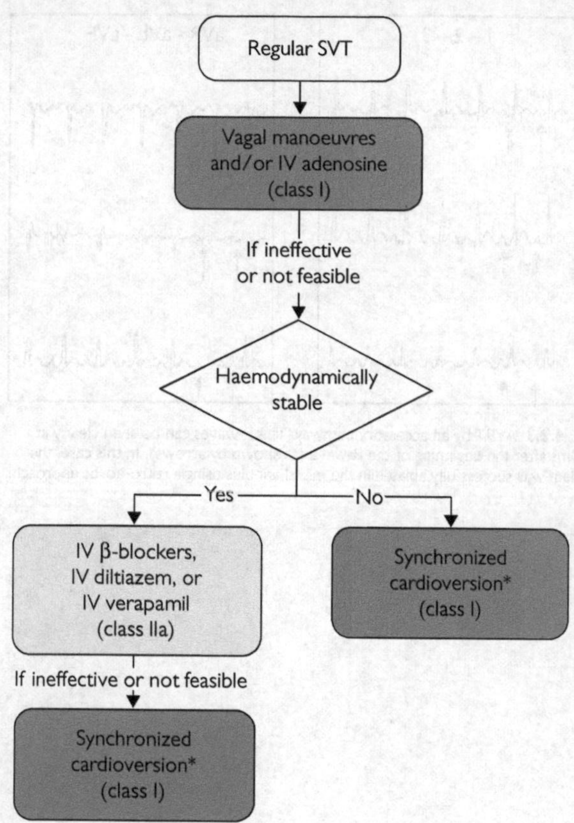

Fig. 4.2.4 Usefulness of vagal manoeuvres or adenosine in the diagnosis of NCT. AVNRT, atrioventricular nodal reciprocating tachycardia; AVRT, atrioventricular reciprocating tachycardia.

Notes:

* Continuous ECG recording should commence on administration.

Adenosine should be given as a push IV injection through the antecubital fossa vein (adenosine is more likely to induce atrial fibrillation if given via a central venous line).

Adenosine is contraindicated in the severely asthmatic, owing to bronchiolar constriction.

Adenosine effects are potentiated by dipyridamole.

Higher rates of atrioventricular block are seen if concomitantly administered with carbamazepine.

Verapamil IV can be used as an alternative atrioventricular-blocking agent for diagnosis/arrhythmia/termination, but it is only recommended to be used by experienced cardiologists.

Treatment

AT originating in, or very close to, the sinoatrial node is mainly treated with pharmacological agents, and ablation is only restricted to some cases of perisinus reciprocating tachycardia not responding to pharmacological therapy.

Ectopic AT originating from any site in the right or left atrium and AVN-dependent tachycardias are usually treated by catheter ablation, which, in recent years, has become the cornerstone treatment for these arrhythmias, reserving pharmacological management for the emergency room scenario. Multifocal AT is difficult to treat pharmacologically. Its presence usually reflects severe chronic lung disease.

Pharmacotherapy

The pharmacological management of supraventricular arrhythmias is summarized in Tables 4.2 2–4.2.4.

Table 4.2.2 Pharmacological options for NCT originating in the sinoatrial node

Type of NCT	Acute treatment	Long-term treatment
Physiological sinus tachycardia	Vagal manoeuvres	β-blockers Non-dihydropyridine CCBs
Inappropriate sinus tachycardia	As above	β-blockers Non-dihydropyridine CCBs Ivabradine (anecdotal evidence, no approved indication) Ablation
Paroxysmal orthostatic tachycardia syndrome (POTS)	As above	β-blockers Fludrocortisone ± bisoprolol SSRIs Other agents; midodrine, clonidine, octreotide, erythropoietin
Sinus node re-entry tachycardia	As above, plus IV amiodarone, non-dihydropyridine CCBs, β-blockers, or digoxin	Little scope for pharmacotherapy—ablation is the mainstay if poorly tolerated or symptoms present

CCB, calcium channel blocker; SSRI, selective serotonin reuptake inhibitor.

Table 4.2.3 Pharmacotherapy for atrial (non-sinus node)-origin NCT

Type of NCT	Acute treatment	Long-term treatment
Focal AT	Reverse digitoxicity/ hypokalaemia Vagal manoeuvres IV adenosine, β-blockers, non-dihydropyridine CCBs, procainamide, flecainide, propafenone, amiodarone, sotalol	β-blockers, non-dihydropyridine CCBs Disopyramide, flecainide, propafenone (in absence of structural/ischaemic heart disease) Sotalol, amiodarone (NB. Class I agents should not be used without AV nodal-blocking agent)
Multifocal AT (irregular rhythm often mistaken for AF)	Correct pulmonary disease or electrolyte disturbances	Non-dihydropyridine CCBs β-blockers often contraindicated due to pulmonary disease No role for antiarrhythmics

AF, atrial fibrillation; AT, atrial tachycardia; AV, atrioventricular; CCB, calcium channel blocker.

Further reading

Blomström-Lundquist C, Sheinman MM, Aliot EM, *et al.* ACC/AHA/ESC Practice Guidelines for the management of patients with supraventricular arrhythmias. *Eur Heart J* 2003;24:1857–97.

Dan GA, Martínez-Rubio A, Agewall S, *et al.* Antiarrhythmic drugs—clinical use and clinical decision making: a consensus document from the European Heart Rhythm Association (EHRA) and European Society of Cardiology (ESC) Working Group on Cardiovascular Pharmacology, endorsed by the Heart Rhythm Society (HRS), Asia Pacific Heart Rhythm Society (APHRS) and International Society of Cardiovascular Pharmacotherapy (ISCP). *Europace* 2018;20:731–2an.

Delacretaz E. Supraventricular tachycardia. *N Engl J Med* 2006;354:1039–51.

Link MS. Evaluation and initial treatment of supraventricular tachycardia. *N Engl J Med* 2012;367:1438–48.

Page RL, Joglar JA, Caldwell MA, *et al.* 2015 ACC/AHA/HRS guideline for the management of adults patients with supraventricular tachycardia. *J Am Coll Cardiol* 2016;67:e27–115.

Wellens HJJ. The value of ECG in the diagnosis of supraventricular tachycardias. *Eur Heart J* 1996;17(Suppl C):10–20.

Table 4.2.4 Pharmacotherapy for junctional/AV nodal rhythms (NB. Ablative therapies have become the mainstay treatment of these rhythms)

Type of NCT	Acute management	Chronic management
AV nodal reciprocating tachycardia (AVNRT)	Vagal manoeuvres IV adenosine IV amiodarone	Non-dihydropyridine CCBs, β-blockers, digoxin Flecainide or propafenone if no ischaemic or structural heart disease 'Pill-in-the-pocket' treatment for infrequent and well-tolerated episodes (further evidence required). Diltiazem 120mg + propranolol 80mg more effective than flecainide
AV reciprocating tachycardia (AVRT)—including WPW syndrome	Vagal manoeuvres IV adenosine (contraindicated in pre-excited AF owing to risk of rapid ventricular response deteriorating into VF)	Non-dihydropyridine CCBs, β-blockers, digoxin (should not be used as monotherapy in those with accessory pathway that may be capable of rapid conduction during AF) Propafenone, flecainide, sotalol, amiodarone. 'Pill-in-the-pocket'—as above
Focal junctional tachycardia	As above IV flecainide	Variable responsiveness to β-blockers, flecainide
Non-paroxysmal junctional tachycardia May be precipitated by: myocardial ischaemia/myocarditis, cardiac surgery, COPD, hypokalaemia, digitoxicity	Correct underlying abnormality, i.e. correct digitoxicity or hypokalaemia	Usually not required, but persisting tachycardia can be suppressed by β-blockers or non-dihydropyridine CCBs

AF, atrial fibrillation; AV, atrioventricular; CCB, calcium channel blocker; COPD, chronic obstructive pulmonary disease; VF, ventricular fibrillation; WPW, Wolff–Parkinson–White.

Chapter 4.3

Ventricular arrhythmias

Martin Borggrefe, Erol Tülümen, and Josep Brugada

Ventricular arrhythmias

Background

Ventricular arrhythmias are abnormal rhythms that originate from below the AVN. They include premature ventricular complexes (PVCs), ventricular tachycardia (VT), and ventricular fibrillation (VF). PVCs are ectopic beats that occur independently of a normal cardiac rhythm. They may be single or repetitive. VTs are classified as non-sustained and sustained VT. By definition, non-sustained ventricular tachycardia (NSVT) lasts ≥3 consecutive beats and <30s, terminates spontaneously, and does not provoke haemodynamic unstability, in which case it would be managed as sustained VT because it is life-threatening. VT can also be classified, according to the morphology of the QRS complexes, as monomorphic and polymorphic VT. VF refers to irregular, uncoordinated ventricular contraction resulting from disorganized electrical activity.

Ventricular arrhythmias may occur in patients with structural heart disease or in patients with a structurally normal heart. Potential underlying causes include:

- Patients with structural heart disease:
  - IHD.
  - Cardiomyopathies: dilated cardiomyopathy (DCM), hypertrophic cardiomyopathy (HCM), arrhythmogenic right ventricular cardiomyopathy (ARVC).
  - VHD, e.g. mitral regurgitation.
- Patients with a structurally normal heart:
  - genetic arrhythmia syndromes: long QT syndrome (LQTS), Brugada syndrome, catecholaminergic polymorphic ventricular tachycardia (CPVT).
  - Idiopathic VT: right ventricular outflow tract VT (RVOT VT), left ventricular outflow tract VT (LVOT VT).

Some causes of ventricular arrhythmias may affect patients with structural heart disease and those with a structurally normal heart:

- Drugs: including antiarrhythmics with pro-arrhythmogenic potential.
- Metabolic abnormalities: electrolyte abnormalities, acidosis, hypoxia.

Symptoms associated with ventricular arrhythmias depend on the frequency, duration, and haemodynamic effects of the arrhythmia. PVCs and non-compromising VT may be asymptomatic or may cause symptoms such as palpitations, shortness of breath, chest discomfort, or dizziness. VT with more profound haemodynamic effects may present with syncope or cardiac arrest. VF rapidly results in collapse and cardiac arrest, due to total ventricular chaos.

Management of ventricular arrhythmias

The focus of this chapter is on the role of antiarrhythmic drugs in the management of ventricular arrhythmias. For practical purposes, the discussion is divided into management of acute ventricular arrhythmias and that of ventricular arrhythmias in the chronic setting. The recommendations for antiarrhythmic drug therapy are based on the ESC 2015 guidelines for the management of patients with ventricular arrhythmias.[1] Where possible, the level of evidence and class of indication for the use of an antiarrhythmic drug for a given situation have been specified.

Table 4.3.1 Acute ventricular arrhythmias—indications for antiarrhythmic drug therapy

Type of arrhythmia	Drug	Comments
Cardiac arrest with shock-resistant VF/VT	Amiodarone (IV) (class III antiarrhythmic)	Amiodarone generally considered first line (class I recommendation/level of evidence C)
	Lidocaine (IV) (class Ib antiarrhythmic)	Lidocaine may be considered as an alternative to amiodarone in ischaemia-driven VF/VT (class IIb recommendation/level of evidence C)
Sustained monomorphic VT	Amiodarone (IV) (class III antiarrhythmic)	Indications for IV amiodarone include: • Haemodynamically unstable sustained VT • Recurrent sustained monomorphic VT despite cardioversion • Recurrent sustained monomorphic VT despite therapy with other antiarrhythmics • In patients with HF, use of amiodarone for acute management of haemodynamically unstable VT and shock-refractory VT is a class I indication (level of evidence B)
	Lidocaine (IV) (class Ib antiarrhythmic)	Lidocaine may be used for treatment of ischaemia-driven stable monomorphic VT
Polymorphic VT with normal QT interval	β-blockers (IV) (class II antiarrhythmic)	IV β-blockers are effective for suppression of polymorphic VT with normal QT interval (class I recommendation/level of evidence B)
	Amiodarone (IV) (class III antiarrhythmic)	IV amiodarone loading is effective for suppression of polymorphic VT with normal QT interval (class I recommendation/level of evidence C)
	Lidocaine (IV) (class Ib antiarrhythmic)	Lidocaine may be effective for management of ischaemia-driven polymorphic VT with normal QT interval
Torsades de pointes	Magnesium sulfate (IV)	IV magnesium sulfate may be considered in patients with LQTS and TdP
	β-blockers (IV) (class II antiarrhythmic)	Patients with bradycardia and TdP may be treated with β-blockers and pacing
	Isoprenaline (IV)	Indicated in recurrent TdP associated with significant pauses in patients who do not have congenital LQTS
	Lidocaine (IV) (class Ib antiarrhythmic)	May be indicated in patients with LQT3 and TdP

The antiarrhythmic drugs listed in Tables 4.3.1–4.3.8 are classified according to their mechanism of action, using the Vaughan–Williams classification. Most of the drugs routinely used for the treatment of ventricular arrhythmias are included in the Vaughan–Williams classification system. One of the limitations of using this system, however, is that some antiarrhythmics do not fit in only one of the categories.

Acute management of ventricular arrhythmias

The management of acute ventricular arrhythmias depends on the haemodynamic effect of the arrhythmia. The following sections outline the guidelines for the management of cardiac arrest and guidelines for the management of stable VT.

Management of cardiac arrest

Cardiac arrest refers to an abrupt loss of CO. Cardiac arrest may arise due to ventricular arrhythmias (VF, pulseless VT), pulseless electrical activity (PEA), or asystole. Patients with cardiac arrest due to ventricular arrhythmia require urgent defibrillation.

AAD therapy is recommended in patients with cardiac arrest and recurrent shock-refractory ventricular arrhythmias (VT/VF). Amiodarone is generally recommended as first line for shock-refractory VT/VF. Lidocaine may be used as an alternative, particularly in patients with evidence of underlying coronary ischaemia. Recommendations for AAD therapy are summarized in Table 4.3.1.

The cardiac arrest algorithm (see Fig. 4.3.1) is based on the 2015 European Resuscitation Council guidelines.[2]

Management of stable ventricular tachycardia

The options for management of stable VT include electrical cardioversion and AAD therapy. It is reasonable to perform electrical cardioversion at any stage in the management of stable VT. Haemodynamically unstable VT requires urgent electrical cardioversion. In patients with monomorphic VT, synchronized shock is recommended.

The choice of AAD therapy for acute ventricular arrhythmias depends on the specific type of ventricular arrhythmia, the haemodynamic effect of the arrhythmia, and the underlying cause of the arrhythmia. The guidelines for AAD therapy for specific arrhythmias are outlined in the next section.

Fig. 4.3.2 shows an algorithm for management of stable VT and is based on the advanced cardiac life support (ACLS) guidelines and ESC guidelines for the management of patients with ventricular arrhythmias.[1]

Antiarrhythmic therapy in patients with acute ventricular arrhythmias

IV preparations of AADs are generally preferred for management of acute ventricular arrhythmias. Therefore, drugs such as sotalol, which are not widely available in an IV preparation, are less commonly used in the acute setting. Table 4.3.1 summarizes ESC (2015) indications for AAD therapy.

Monomorphic ventricular tachycardia

For patients with haemodynamically stable sustained monomorphic VT, the options for AAD therapy include IV amiodarone and lidocaine, and for those who do not present with severe HF or acute MI, they include procainamide and flecainide. Procainamide is often more effective for early termination of stable VT, but it is no longer available in many countries.

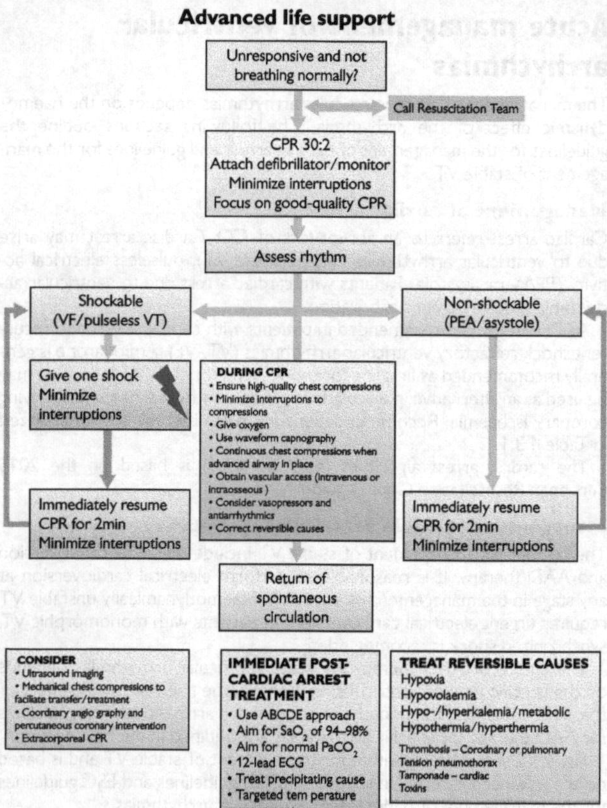

Fig. 4.3.1 Algorithm for the management of cardiac arrest (based on the 2015 European Resuscitation Council guidelines).

Reproduced from Soar J, Nolan JP, Bottiger BW, Perkins GD, Lott C, Carli P, Pellis T, Sandroni C, Skrifvars MB, Smith GB, Sunde K, Deakin CD, Adult advanced life support section C. European Resuscitation Council Guidelines for Resuscitation 2015: Section 3. Adult advanced life support. *Resuscitation* 2015;95:100–47, with permission from Elsevier.

Amiodarone is associated with fewer adverse side effects and may be preferred in HF patients.

Amiodarone is generally considered first line in patients with sustained monomorphic VT with haemodynamic compromise. Lidocaine is an alternative, particularly in patients with underlying coronary ischaemia. Synchronized cardioversion should be considered early in patients with unstable VT.

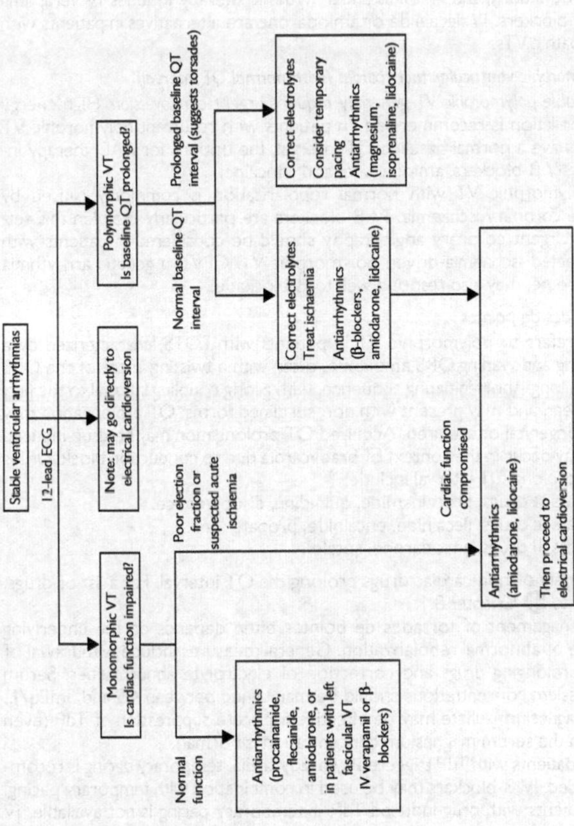

Fig. 4.3.2 Treatment algorithm guide to the management of ventricular tachycardia with pulse.

For patients with recurrent shock, refractory monomorphic VT, either with or without pulse, the first-line AAD is amiodarone. Lidocaine is an alternative in patients with VT in the context of coronary ischaemia. Temporary cardiac pacing and/or sedation/anaesthesia may be considered in certain circumstances for suppression of recurrent VT.

In patients with idiopathic LV fascicular VT (RBBB morphology with left axis deviation), the first-line antiarrhythmic therapy includes IV verapamil or β-blockers. IV flecainide or amiodarone are alternatives in patients with idiopathic VTs.

Polymorphic ventricular tachycardia (with normal QT interval)

Unstable polymorphic VT generally requires urgent cardioversion. High-energy defibrillation is recommended. In patients with recurrent polymorphic VT who have a normal baseline QT interval, the options for AAD therapy include IV β-blockers, amiodarone, and lidocaine.

Polymorphic VT with normal repolarization is commonly caused by acute coronary ischaemia. IV β-blockers are particularly useful in this setting. Urgent coronary angiography should be considered in patients with suspected ischaemia-driven polymorphic VT. CPVT, a genetic arrhythmia syndrome, may also respond well to β-blockade.

Torsades de pointes

TdP refers to polymorphic VT in patients with LQTS, characterized by a waxing and waning QRS amplitude, often with a twisting image of the QRS and a long–short initiating sequence, with a long coupling interval to the first VT beat, and may present with non-sustained forms. QT prolongation may be congenital or acquired. Acquired QT prolongation may be drug-induced or may occur in the context of bradycardia due to conduction block. Drugs that prolong QT interval include:

- Class Ia drugs: procainamide, quinidine, disopyramide.
- Class Ic drugs: flecainide, encainide, propafenone.
- Class III drugs: amiodarone, sotalol.

A variety of non-cardiac drugs prolong the QT interval. For a list of drugs, refer to ➔ Chapter 8.1.

Management of torsades de pointes often depends on the underlying cause of abnormal repolarization. General measures include withdrawal of QT-prolonging drugs and correction of electrolyte abnormalities. Serum potassium concentrations should be maintained between 4.5 and 5mEq/L. IV magnesium sulfate may be effective for acute suppression of TdP (even when the serum magnesium concentration is normal).

In patients with TdP triggered by bradycardia, temporary pacing is recommended. IV β-blockers may be used in combination with temporary pacing. In patients with drug-induced TdP, if temporary pacing is not available, IV isoprenaline may be used as an alternative.

Ventricular arrhythmias secondary to acute coronary ischaemia

PVCs and NSVT are common in patients with ACS. Apart from β-blockers, AAD therapy for suppression of PVCs and NSVT is not indicated. β-blockers are indicated as standard treatment for patients with ACS. In addition to reducing myocardial oxygen demand, β-blockers are effective for suppression of ventricular arrhythmias (see Table 4.3.1).

For patients with sustained ventricular arrhythmias, the choice of AAD depends on LV function. In patients with preserved LV function, options include IV procainamide, amiodarone, flecainide, and lidocaine. Sotalol may also be considered but is not widely available in an IV preparation. In patients with impaired systolic function, amiodarone or lidocaine is recommended. Lidocaine is an effective alternative to amiodarone in patients with underlying coronary ischaemia.

Ventricular arrhythmias are common in the first 48h following acute MI. While sustained ventricular arrhythmias in the peri-infarct period are associated with higher in-hospital mortality, they are not associated with an increased long-term risk. In patients with recurrent ischaemia-driven ventricular arrhythmias, urgent coronary angiography and revascularization should be considered.

Idioventricular rhythms are also common in patients with acute MI, particularly following reperfusion. In the absence of haemodynamic compromise, idioventricular rhythms do not require AAD therapy, apart from β-blockers.

Management of ventricular arrhythmias in the chronic setting

The longer-term treatment goals for patients with ventricular arrhythmias are prevention of sudden cardiac death (SCD) and suppression of symptomatic ventricular arrhythmias. Treatment options include implantation of a cardiac defibrillator (ICD), pharmacological therapy, and radiofrequency ablation. Implantation of an ICD is the main strategy for prevention of SCD, either for primary or secondary prevention. Indications for ICD include:

- Aborted cardiac arrest secondary to VF or VT, with no identifiable cause.
- Spontaneous sustained VT in patients with structural heart disease.
- IHD with impaired LV function (ejection fraction ≤35%), NYHA class II or III HF on optimal medical therapy.
- DCM (non-ischaemic) with severe LV dysfunction (ejection fraction ≤35%) and NYHA class II or III HF on optimal medical therapy, ≥3 months of treatment with optimal pharmacological therapy.
- Inherited conditions associated with life-threatening ventricular arrhythmias, e.g. LQTS, ARVC, HCM, Brugada syndrome.

CRT is recommended to reduce all-cause mortality in patients with an LVEF of ≤35%, LBBB, QRS duration of >120ms, NYHA class III or ambulatory IV HF, and ≥3 months of treatment with optimal pharmacological therapy, who are expected to survive at least 1 year, with good functional status.

CRT should also be considered to reduce all-cause mortality in patients with an LVEF of ≤35%, non-LBBB, QRS duration of >120ms, NYHA class III or ambulatory IV HF, and ≥3 months of treatment with optimal pharmacological therapy, who are expected to survive at least 1 year, with good functional status.

Apart from β-blockers, AADs have not been demonstrated to reduce the incidence of SCD. Chronic AAD therapy is aimed mainly at suppression of ventricular arrhythmias in order to reduce the symptom burden. AADs can be used in isolation or in combination with ICD therapy. In patients with ICDs, AAD therapy may reduce the number of shocks and anti-tachycardia pacing episodes delivered by the device.

In addition to the antiarrhythmic action, a number of drugs have proarrhythmic potential and therefore have to be used with caution. The choice of antiarrhythmic agent often depends on the underlying cause of the ventricular arrhythmia.

An effective alternative treatment for patients with ventricular arrhythmias is radiofrequency ablation. Catheter ablation is particularly useful in patients who are unable to tolerate pharmacological therapy or have arrhythmias that are resistant to AAD therapy. Catheter ablation is also used in patients with ICDs and recurrent arrhythmias that are refractory to drug therapy.

Drug therapy for ventricular arrhythmias in specific patient populations

Patients with impaired left ventricular function due to previous myocardial infarction and patients with symptomatic heart failure

The following section outlines guidelines for chronic management of ventricular arrhythmias in patients with impaired LV function due to previous

MI and in patients with symptomatic HF (irrespective of aetiology). There is significant overlap between the two patient groups, and therefore, not surprisingly, the guidelines for AAD therapy are very similar (see Tables 4.3.2 and 4.3.3). There are, however, some differences relating to the level of evidence and class of indication for some drugs, which are highlighted in Table 4.3.3.

Chronic AAD therapy in these two patient groups is indicated for suppression of symptomatic ventricular arrhythmias, adjunctive therapy in patients with ICD, and alternative therapy in patients who cannot have or refuse ICD therapy. Routine suppression of asymptomatic PVCs and NSVT is not recommended.

Options for chronic AAD therapy include β-blockers, amiodarone, and sotalol. β-blockers should be commenced as standard therapy in patients with impaired LV function, unless specifically contraindicated. In patients with persistent ventricular arrhythmias despite β-blocker therapy, amiodarone may be effective, often in combination with β-blockers. Sotalol may be used as an alternative to amiodarone; however, it is not recommended in patients with severely depressed LV function due to adverse haemodynamic effects.

Class Ia drugs (e.g. procainamide, quinidine, disopyramide) and class Ic drugs (e.g. flecainide, encainide, propafenone) are associated with proarrhythmic effects in patients with IHD and those with impaired ventricular function, and they are therefore contraindicated. CCBs are also particularly contraindicated in patients with severely depressed LV function due to their negative inotropic effects.

In patients with impaired LV function, irrespective of aetiology, optimization of pharmacological HF therapy and, where appropriate, CRT has been demonstrated to reduce the risk of SCD. Guidelines for management of HF are discussed in ➔ Chapter 3.1.

Catheter ablation is recommended in patients presenting with incessant VT, with bundle branch re-entrant tachycardia, electrical storm, or recurrent ICD shocks due to sustained VT, and should be considered in patients with frequent symptomatic PVCs or NSVT as an alternative or as an adjunct to amiodarone.

The indications for ICD therapy, either for primary or secondary prevention of SCD, are listed on ➔ Cardiac resynchronization therapy/implantable cardioverter-defibrillator, p. 157. In patients with underlying IHD, in whom ventricular arrhythmias are precipitated by recurrent coronary ischaemia, coronary revascularization is an important consideration.

Patients with hypertrophic cardiomyopathy

Patients with HCM who have a high risk of SCD require ICD therapy, either for primary or for secondary prevention. ESC guidelines on HCM (2014) recommend the use of a risk calculator (HCM Risk-SCD) that estimates the 5-year risk (http://doc2do.com/hcm/webHCM.html).[3] The predictor variables used in the model are age, maximum LV wall thickness, left atrial size, maximum LVOT gradient, family history of SCD, NSVTs, and unexplained syncope.

In patients with a high risk of SCD (5-year risk of sudden death ≥6%) who cannot have an ICD, amiodarone may be used as an alternative. β-blockers,

Table 4.3.2 Antiarrhythmic drug therapy in patients with impaired LV function due to previous MI

Drug	Indications	Comments
β-blockers (class II antiarrhythmic)	First-line therapy All patients should be commenced routinely on β-blockers, unless specifically contraindicated	Prognostic benefit in patients with impaired LV function due to previous MI May be used as an adjunct to ICD therapy May also be considered as an alternative in patients who refuse or cannot have ICD
Amiodarone (class III antiarrhythmic)	Chronic suppression of symptomatic ventricular arrhythmias unresponsive to β-blockers (class IIa indication/level of evidence C) Patients with an indication for ICD who refuse ICD or cannot have ICD implantation (class IIa indication/level of evidence C) In patients with recurrent ICD shocks due to sustained VT (class I indication/level of evidence B)	Well tolerated in patients with impaired LV function Often used in combination with β-blockers No clear prognostic benefit
Sotalol (class III antiarrhythmic)	Chronic suppression of symptomatic ventricular arrhythmias unresponsive to β-blockers	Greater proarrhythmic potential than amiodarone. Amiodarone therefore generally preferred Not recommended in patients with prolonged QT interval Not recommended in patients with severely depressed LV function No clear prognostic benefit

which are often used as standard therapy in patients with HCM to improve diastolic filling, may have the added benefit of suppressing symptomatic ventricular arrhythmias but are not thought to have the same potential mortality benefit as amiodarone (see Table 4.3.4).

Patients with arrhythmogenic right ventricular cardiomyopathy

ARVC is a condition characterized by fibrofatty infiltration of the RV myocardium and is associated with ventricular arrhythmias and SCD. The impact of ICD therapy or AAD therapy on mortality in patients with ARVC is not established. ICD therapy is indicated in patients with a history of sustained haemodynamically unstable VT or cardiac arrest due to VT/VF. ICD may also be considered for primary prevention in ARVC patients with

Table 4.3.3 Antiarrhythmic therapy in patients with HF

Drug	Indications	Comments
β-blockers (class II antiarrhythmic)	First-line therapy All patients should be commenced routinely on β-blockers, unless specifically contraindicated	Prognostic benefit. β-blockers reduce overall risk of SCD
Amiodarone (class III antiarrhythmic)	Adjunct to ICD therapy—in patients with recurrent appropriate shocks despite optimal device programming (class IIa indication/level of evidence C)	Safe and well tolerated in patients with severely impaired ventricular function Amiodarone is not recommended for the treatment of asymptomatic NSVT (class III indication, level of evidence A)
Sotalol (class III antiarrhythmic)	Adjunct to ICD therapy—in patients with recurrent appropriate shocks, despite optimal device programming, and with contraindication to amiodarone	Greater proarrhythmic potential than amiodarone Amiodarone therefore generally preferred

Table 4.3.4 Antiarrhythmic therapy in patients with HCM

Drug	Indications	Comments
Amiodarone (class III antiarrhythmic)	Chronic therapy for patients with previous sustained VT/VF when ICD is not feasible (class IIa indication/level of evidence C) Chronic therapy for primary prevention in HCM patients with a high risk of SCD when ICD is not feasible (class IIb indication/level of evidence C)	Considered the most effective antiarrhythmic in patients with HCM Useful in prevention of SCD in non-randomized studies
β-blockers (class II antiarrhythmic)	Standard therapy in patients with HCM—improve diastolic filling	No clear evidence for reduction of SCD
β-blockers (class II antiarrhythmic) or disopyramide (class Ia antiarrhythmic)	In patients with obstructive HCM to treat LVOT obstruction	No clear evidence for reduction of SCD

unexplained syncope. In patients with a high risk of SCD who are not candidates for ICD or who have well-tolerated VT, AAD therapy with amiodarone and sotalol may be considered (see Table 4.3.5).

Patients with congenital long QT syndrome

β-blockers (in patients with LQTS, either nadolol or propranolol should be preferred) represent the mainstay of chronic AAD therapy in patients with congenital LQTS. In patients who have a high risk of SCD, i.e. patients with a history of cardiac arrest and those with recurrent syncope or sustained VT while receiving β-blockers, ICD therapy is recommended in combination with β-blockers. Sodium channel blockers (mexiletine, flecainide, or ranolazine) may be considered, in addition to β-blockers, to shorten the QT interval in LQTS type 3 (LQTS3) patients with a QTc of >500ms. The use of β-blockers is not recommended in patients who have symptomatic significant bradycardia associated with LQTS (unless used in combination with permanent pacing) (see Table 4.3.6). Left cardiac sympathetic denervation (LCSD) should be considered in patients with symptomatic LQTS when β-blockers are not effective (multiple ICD shocks despite β-blocker therapy), not tolerated (symptomatic, profound bradycardia), or contraindicated (severe asthma), or when implantation of an ICD is contraindicated or refused.

On an individual basis, in high-risk asymptomatic patients (women with LQTS type 2 and QTc of >500ms; patients with QTc of >500ms and signs of electrical instability; patients with high-risk genetic profiles like carriers of two mutations, including Jervell and Lange–Nielsen syndrome or Timothy syndrome), in addition to β-blocker therapy (or LSCD), primary prophylactic implantation of an ICD should be considered.[1]

Patients with Brugada syndrome

Brugada syndrome is a genetic condition associated with a high risk of ventricular arrhythmias and SCD. Diagnosis is based on characteristic ECG features, associated with a history of aborted SCD or a family history of SCD.

Table 4.3.5 Antiarrhythmic drug therapy in patients with ARVC

Drug	Indications	Comments
β-blockers (class II antiarrhythmics)	As first-line therapy to improve symptoms (class I indication/level of evidence C)	Impact on mortality not well established; titrate to the maximally tolerated dose
Amiodarone (class III antiarrhythmic)	Chronic therapy in patients with sustained VF or VT when ICD implantation is not feasible (class IIa indication/ level of evidence C)	Impact on mortality not established
Sotalol (class III antiarrhythmic)	Chronic therapy in patients with sustained VF or VT when ICD implantation is not feasible and amiodarone is contraindicated	Impact on mortality not established Its use in ARVC has been questioned

Table 4.3.6 Antiarrhythmic drug therapy in patients with congenital LQTS

Drug	Indications	Comments
β-blockers (class II antiarrhythmic)	Chronic therapy for suppression of TdP in patients with a clinical diagnosis of LQTS (class I indication/level of evidence B) Chronic therapy for suppression of TdP in patients with a molecular diagnosis of LQTS who have a normal QT interval (class IIa indication/level of evidence B)	Not recommended in LQTS associated with prominent bradycardia (unless used in combination with permanent pacing)
Mexiletine, ranolazine (class Ib antiarrhythmics) or flecainide (class Ic antiarrhythmic)	As an add-on therapy in patients with LQTS3 with QTc >500ms (class IIb indication/level of evidence C)	Not recommended in LQTS associated with severe bradycardia (unless used in combination with permanent pacing)

ECG abnormalities include RBBB and ST-segment elevation in leads V1–V3. The ECG changes may not be evident until unmasked by provocative tests using flecainide, procainamide, or ajmaline. β-blockers may also augment the ECG changes.

No effective chronic AADs are available for treatment of Brugada syndrome. The mainstay of treatment is ICD therapy. Isoprenaline and quinidine can be used acutely in patients with arrhythmia storm (even in the presence of an ICD, class IIa indication/level of evidence C). Quinidine has also been shown to reduce the frequency of ICD shocks in the long term. Also quinidine should be considered as long-term therapy in patients who qualify for an ICD but present a contraindication or refuse it and in those who require treatment for supraventricular arrhythmias (class IIa indication/level of evidence C).[1]

Patients with short QT syndrome

Short QT syndrome (SQTS) (QTc <340ms) is a very rare, sporadic, or autosomal dominant inherited channelopathy, characterized by abnormally short QT intervals on the ECG and associated with atrial or ventricular tachyarrhythmias and SCD.

In patients with SQTS and VT/VF storm, isoprenaline infusion can be effective. There is no effective chronic antiarrhythmic therapy available for SQTS. ICD therapy is recommended in patients with aborted cardiac arrest or with documented spontaneous VT. Quinidine or sotalol may be considered in patients with SQTS who qualify for an ICD but have a contraindication to ICD therapy or refuse it, and also in asymptomatic patients with SQTS and a family history of SCD (class IIb indication/ level of evidence C).

Patients with catecholaminergic polymorphic ventricular tachycardia

CPVT is an inherited disorder characterized by stress-related polymorphic VT. Patients have a structurally normal heart and normal QT intervals.

β-blockers counteract sympathetic stimulation and are highly effective for suppression of ventricular arrhythmias in patients with CPVT (see Table 4.3.7). β-blockers should be commenced and titrated to maximally tolerated doses in all patients with a diagnosis of CPVT and documented stress-induced ventricular arrhythmias. β-blockers may also be used as prophylactic therapy in patients who are diagnosed with CPVT on the basis of genetic testing with no previous documented arrhythmias. β-blockers are used in combination with ICD therapy in patients with CPVT who have had previous cardiac arrest, recurrent syncope, or polymorphic/bidirectional VT.

LCSD may reduce the frequency of recurrent shocks and should be considered in patients with CPVT when β-blockers either are not effective (multiple ICD shocks despite β-blocker therapy) or cannot be titrated to the maximal dose (symptomatic, profound bradycardia) or are contraindicated (severe asthma).

Patients with a structurally normal heart (idiopathic ventricular tachycardia)
Idiopathic VT may arise in the RVOT (RVOT VT) or the LVOT (LVOT VT). RVOT VT is, by far, the commonest type of idiopathic VT. Chronic therapy with β-blockers or non-dihydropyridine CCBs may be effective for suppression of RVOT VT and LVOT VT. Class Ic drugs may also be used for management of RVOT VT (see Table 4.3.8). Catheter ablation is recommended as first-line therapy in symptomatic patients with idiopathic RVOT and idiopathic left VT (class I indication/level of evidence B) and should be considered in symptomatic drug-refractory VT or in those patients who do not want long-term AAD therapy (class I indication/level of evidence C).

Table 4.3.7 Antiarrhythmic drug therapy in patients with CPVT

Drug	Indications	Comments
β-blockers (class II antiarrhythmic)	CPVT with documented stress-induced ventricular arrhythmias (class I indication/level of evidence C) Prophylactic therapy in patients with a diagnosis of CPVT based on genetic analysis, with no previous episodes of ventricular arrhythmia (class IIa indication/level of evidence C)	May be used in combination with ICD in patients with a high risk of SCD
Flecainide (class Ic antiarrhythmic)	In patients who experience recurrent syncope or polymorphic/bidirectional VT while on β-blockers (class IIa indication/level of evidence C) Prophylactic therapy in patients with a diagnosis of CPVT and carriers of ICD to reduce appropriate ICD shocks (class IIa indication/level of evidence C)	Flecainide should be considered, in addition to β-blockers, in patients with CPVT

Table 4.3.8 Antiarrhythmic drug therapy in patients with idiopathic VT

Drug	Indications	Comments
β-blockers (class II antiarrhythmic)	RVOT VT (class I recommendation/ level of evidence C) LVOT VT	May be used for acute termination or chronic suppression of idiopathic VT
CCBs (class IV antiarrhythmic)	RVOT VT (class I recommendation/ level of evidence C) LVOT VT	May be used for acute termination or chronic suppression of idiopathic VT
Flecainide, encainide, propafenone (class Ic drugs)	RVOT VT (class I recommendation/ level of evidence C)	β-blockers and CCBs usually preferred for RVOT VT
Adenosine	For acute termination of RVOT VT	RVOT VT is typically adenosine-sensitive

Landmark trials for ventricular arrhythmias

Beta-blockers

MUSTT (Multicenter UnSustained Tachycardia Trial)

- Prospective RCT.[4]
- Demonstrated that in patients with CAD, ejection fraction of ≤40%, and asymptomatic NSVT, β-blockers have beneficial effects on survival (5-year mortality of 50% with β-blockers versus 66% without β-blockers; adjusted $p = 0.0001$).
- There was no significant effect of β-blocker therapy on the rate of arrhythmic death or cardiac arrest (adjusted $p = 0.2344$).

Note: multiple studies have demonstrated beneficial effects of β-blockers in patients with CAD (see ➔ Chapter 2.1) and HF (see ➔ Chapter 3.1).

Amiodarone

EMIAT (European Myocardial Infarction Amiodarone Trial)

- Randomized placebo-controlled trial.[5]
- Demonstrated that in high-risk patients post-MI, there was no significant reduction in overall mortality in patients treated with amiodarone, compared with placebo.
- Post hoc analysis demonstrated that a combination of amiodarone and a β-blocker had a significant mortality benefit (unadjusted all-cause mortality reduction of 30%).

CAMIAT (Canadian Amiodarone Myocardial Infarction Arrhythmia Trial)

- Randomized placebo-controlled trial.[6]
- Demonstrated that in high-risk patients post-MI, there was no significant reduction in the incidence of arrhythmic death in patients treated with amiodarone, compared with placebo.
- Post hoc analysis demonstrated that a combination of amiodarone and a β-blocker had a significant mortality benefit (unadjusted all-cause mortality reduction of 60–72%).

SCD-HeFT (Sudden Cardiac Death in Heart Failure Trial)

- Randomized placebo-controlled trial.[7]
- Demonstrated that in patients with NYHA class II or III HF and LVEF of ≤35% on optimal medical therapy, while ICD therapy reduced all-cause mortality, amiodarone had no favourable effect.

Sotalol

SWORD (Survival With Oral D-Sotalol)

- Randomized placebo-controlled trial.[8]
- Demonstrated that in patients with LVEF of ≤40% and either a recent MI or symptomatic HF with a remote MI, sotalol was associated with an increased mortality, presumed secondary to arrhythmias (5.0% mortality in the sotalol group, compared with 3.1% in the placebo group).

Class I antiarrhythmics

CAST I (Cardiac Arrhythmia Suppression Trial I)

- Randomized placebo-controlled trial.[9]
- Demonstrated that in post-MI patients with ventricular premature depolarizations, encainide and flecainide were associated with increased mortality and non-fatal cardiac arrests, compared to placebo (encainide and flecainide-treated patients had a 3.6-fold excessive risk of arrhythmic death, compared with placebo-treated patients).

References

1 Priori SG, Blomström-Lundqvist C. 2015 European Society of Cardiology Guidelines for the management of patients with ventricular arrhythmias and the prevention of sudden cardiac death summarized by co-chairs. *Eur Heart J* 2015;**36**:2757–9.

2 Soar J, Nolan JP, Böttiger BW, *et al.*; Adult advanced life support section Collaborators. European Resuscitation Council Guidelines for Resuscitation 2015: Section 3. Adult advanced life support. *Resuscitation* 2015;**95**:100–47.

3 Authors/Task Force members, Elliott PM, Anastasakis A, Borger MA, *et al.* 2014 ESC Guidelines on diagnosis and management of hypertrophic cardiomyopathy: the Task Force for the Diagnosis and Management of Hypertrophic Cardiomyopathy of the European Society of Cardiology (ESC). *Eur Heart J* 2014;**35**:2733–79.

4 Ellison KE, Hafley GE, Hickey K, et *al.*; Multicenter UnSustained Tachycardia Trial I. Effect of beta-blocking therapy on outcome in the Multicenter UnSustained Tachycardia Trial (MUSTT). *Circulation* 2002;**106**:2694–9.

5 Julian DG, Camm AJ, Frangin G, et *al.* Randomised trial of effect of amiodarone on mortality in patients with left-ventricular dysfunction after recent myocardial infarction: EMIAT. European Myocardial Infarct Amiodarone Trial Investigators. *Lancet* 1997;**349**:667–74.

6 Cairns JA, Connolly SJ, Roberts R, Gent M. Randomised trial of outcome after myocardial infarction in patients with frequent or repetitive ventricular premature depolarisations: CAMIAT. Canadian Amiodarone Myocardial Infarction Arrhythmia Trial Investigators. *Lancet* 1997;**349**:675–82.

7 Bardy GH, Lee KL, Mark DB, *et al.*; Sudden Cardiac Death in Heart Failure Trial I. Amiodarone or an implantable cardioverter-defibrillator for congestive heart failure. *N Engl J Med* 2005;**352**:225–37.

8 Waldo AL, Camm AJ, deRuyter H, *et al.* Effect of d-sotalol on mortality in patients with left ventricular dysfunction after recent and remote myocardial infarction. The SWORD Investigators. Survival With Oral d-Sotalol. *Lancet* 1996;**348**:7–12.

9 Cardiac Arrhythmia Suppression Trial (CAST) Investigators. Preliminary report: effect of encainide and flecainide on mortality in a randomized trial of arrhythmia suppression after myocardial infarction. *N Engl J Med* 1989;**321**:406–12.

Key trials/landmark studies

CAST (Cardiac Arrhythmia Suppression Trial)

- Randomized placebo-controlled trial.
- Demonstrated that in post-MI patients with ventricular premature depolarizations, encainide and flecainide were associated with increased mortality and nonfatal cardiac arrest compared to placebo (encainide and flecainide treated patients had 2.5-fold excess in rate of arrhythmic death compared with placebo-treated patients).

References

[illegible]

Chapter 4.4

Bradyarrhythmias

Haran Burri

Background

Bradycardia is defined as a heart rate of <60bpm. However, patients do not usually develop symptoms until the heart rate falls to <50bpm. Bradycardias can be divided broadly into sinus bradycardia and bradycardia due to AV conduction block.

Sinus bradycardia

Sinus bradycardia may be physiological or pathological. Examples of physiological sinus bradycardia include nocturnal sinus bradycardia and bradycardia in trained athletes. Pathological sinus bradycardia may arise due to extrinsic causes (e.g. drugs, metabolic disorders) or intrinsic sinus node dysfunction, i.e. sick sinus syndrome. Sick sinus syndrome is characterized by failure to generate or transmit impulses at the sinus node. Most patients with sinus bradycardia who have normal sinus node function are asymptomatic. Symptoms, e.g. dizziness, syncope, and dyspnoea, are commoner in patients with sinus node dysfunction.

Bradycardia due to atrioventricular conduction block

AV conduction block can be classified into first-degree, second-degree, or third-degree heart block, according to the part of the conduction system affected and the appearance on the surface ECG as follows.

First-degree heart block

- The majority of cases are due to conduction delay at the level of the AVN.
- The ECG is characterized by a prolonged PR interval (>200ms).

Second-degree heart block

- Mobitz I (or Wenckebach):
  - The great majority of cases are due to conduction delay at the level of the AVN.
  - The ECG is characterized by progressive prolongation of the PR interval, followed by failure to conduct a beat.
- Mobitz II:
  - All cases are due to dysfunction of the conduction system distal to the AVN (His–Purkinje system).
  - ECG: constant PR interval, with intermittent failure to conduct beats.

Third-degree heart block

- May be due to dysfunction of the conduction system at the level of, or distal to, the AVN (His–Purkinje system).
- ECG: complete AV dissociation.

First-degree and Mobitz I second-degree heart block are generally considered to be benign conditions and may be physiological (e.g. in patients with high vagal tone) or pathological. Mobitz II second-degree AVB and third-degree AVB are almost always pathological and may arise due to degeneration of, or injury to, conduction tissue. Mobitz II second-degree AVB is associated with a higher risk of developing symptomatic bradycardias and progressing to third-degree AVB. In patients with third-degree AVB, atrial impulses are not conducted to the ventricles and an escape rhythm is generated from an accessory pacemaker distal to the AVN. The escape rhythm may originate from the bundle of His or the distal ventricular conduction system. Patients with more distal ventricular pacemakers have a broad complex escape rhythm on the surface ECG.

In patients with partial AVB, i.e. bundle branch block and fascicular block, AV conduction is maintained and therefore, bradycardia is rare. There is, however, a risk of progression to complete heart block, and hence symptomatic bradycardia. In isolated bundle branch or fascicular block, progression to complete heart block is rare. In patients with bifascicular and trifascicular block, the risk of development of complete heart block is higher; however, the overall incidence is still low.

In patients with AVB, symptoms are commoner with higher degrees of block. Most patients with first-degree and Mobitz I second-degree AVB are asymptomatic. However, very prolonged PR intervals may result in AV dyssynchrony ('P on T'), with simultaneous atrial and ventricular contraction, leading to symptoms such as dyspnoea and exercise intolerance. Patients with higher degrees of AVB may present with symptoms such as dizziness, syncope, shortness of breath, fatigue, and chest pain. Patients with complete heart block, especially those with a broad complex escape rhythm, are at risk of developing haemodynamic compromise due to severe bradycardia or asystolic cardiac arrest. Those with QT prolongation are also at risk of TdP.

Management of bradycardias

The following section is divided into management of acute bradycardias and management of bradycardias in the chronic setting. The role of pharmacological agents is restricted to the management of acute bradycardia, which is the main focus of this chapter.

Acute management of bradycardias

The management of acute bradycardia depends on the severity, haemodynamic effect, and underlying cause of the bradycardia. Principles of management of symptomatic bradycardias in the acute setting include correction of reversible underlying causes and, where appropriate, use of drugs to increase the heart rate or temporary cardiac pacing.

The algorithm in Fig. 4.4.1 outlines the 2015 European Resuscitation Council guidelines for the management of acute bradycardia. The next section contains a discussion on the role of drugs for the management of acute bradycardia and guidelines for the specific management of drug-induced bradycardia.

Drugs for acute management of bradycardias

Atropine is considered the first-line pharmacological agent for acute management of severe or haemodynamically compromising bradycardia. In patients who do not respond to initial treatment with atropine, alternatively, second-line drugs such as isoprenaline, adrenaline, and dopamine may be used. Pharmacological therapy and transcutaneous pacing are often used as temporizing measures until transvenous pacing is initiated. Table 4.4.1 outlines drugs used in acute management of bradycardia.

Management of drug-induced bradycardias

In the majority of patients with drug-induced bradycardia, the only treatment required is withdrawal of the offending drug. Common cardiac drugs that may cause bradycardia include β-blockers, CCBs, digoxin, and class I and III antiarrhythmics. Non-cardiac drugs that may induce bradycardia are covered in ➔ Chapter 9.1.

In patients with bradycardia due to toxic levels of rate-slowing drugs, in addition to the drugs listed in Table 4.4.2, specific antidotes may be used in certain circumstances. Such measures are often reserved for patients with profound bradycardia with evidence of end-organ hypoperfusion or a high likelihood of clinical deterioration.

Cardiac pacemakers

The management of patients with bradycardias in the chronic setting depends on the presence of symptoms, the correlation of symptoms to the bradycardia, the mechanism of bradycardia (e.g. sinus dysfunction, nodal versus infra-nodal block), and the underlying cause of the bradycardia. Patients with physiological bradycardia are usually asymptomatic and do not require specific treatment. The management of symptomatic bradycardias due to extrinsic causes involves correction of potential underlying causes, e.g. withdrawal of rate-limiting drugs. Pacemaker implantation represents the mainstay of treatment of patients with sinus dysfunction and intrinsic conduction disease who have symptomatic bradycardia. Pacemaker

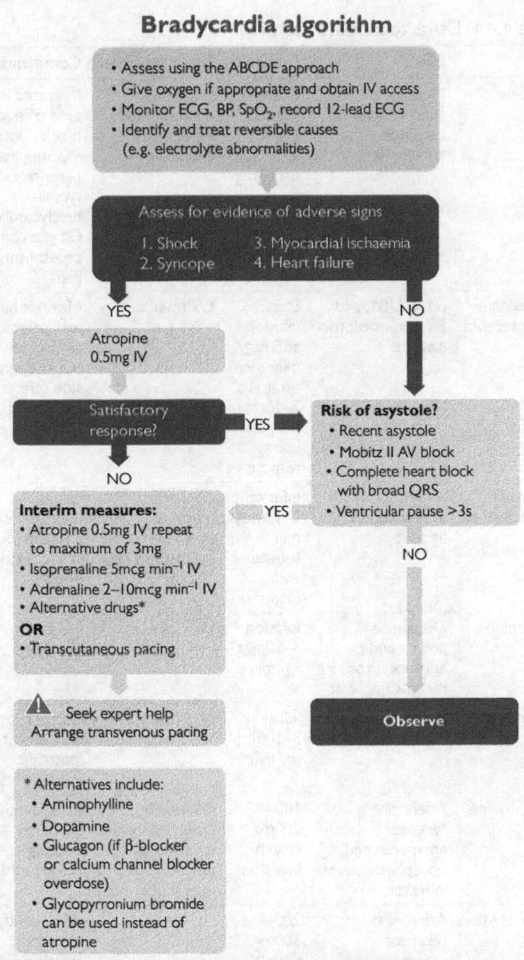

Fig. 4.4.1 Acute management of bradycardia according to the 2015 European Resuscitation Council guidelines. ABCDE, Airway, Breathing Circulation, Disability, Exposure; AV, atrioventricular; BP, blood pressure; ECG, electrocardiogram; IV, intravenous; SpO_2, oxygen saturation measured by pulse oximetry.

Reproduced from Soar J, Nolan JP, Bottiger BW, Perkins GD, Lott C, Carli P, Pellis T, Sandroni C, Skrifvars MB, Smith GB, Sunde K, Deakin CD, Adult advanced life support section C. European Resuscitation Council Guidelines for Resuscitation 2015: Section 3. Adult advanced life support. *Resuscitation* 2015;95:100–47, with permission from Elsevier.

Table 4.4.1 Drugs to increase heart rate

Drug	Effect	Dosage	Pharmacokinetics	Comments
Atropine	Muscarinic acetylcholine receptor antagonist	0.5mg IV (repeat every 3–5min to max 3mg)	t½ 3–4h; approximately 50% renal excretion	Indicated in case of nodal block. Doses <0.5mg may paradoxically worsen bradycardia. CI: glaucoma, prostatism, ileus
Isoprenaline/ isoproterenol	α1, α2, β1, and β2-adrenoceptor agonist	Start infusion at 5mcg/ min, then titrate to 2–10mcg/ min, based upon response	t½ 1min	May not be well tolerated over many hours due to side effects (trembling, headache, etc.)
Adrenaline (epinephrine)	α- and β-adrenoceptor agonist	Infusion 2–10mcg/ min (titrate with response)	t½ 3min, followed by slower elimination (t½ 10min)	Useful if hypotension is an issue (due to vasoconstricting effect)
Dopamine	Dopamine and α- and β-adrenoceptor receptor agonist	Infusion 4–10mcg/ kg/min	t½ 2min	No bolus injections
Dobutamine	β1-adrenoceptor receptor agonist	Infusion 3–10mcg/ kg/min	t½ 2min	Useful if concurrent inotropic insufficiency
Theophylline	Adenosine receptor antagonist and phosphodiesterase inhibitor	100–200mg, slow IV injection	t½ 4–24h (affected by age, smoking, hepatic function, drug interaction, etc.)	Infrequently used for treating bradycardia
Aminophylline	Adenosine receptor antagonist and phosphodiesterase inhibitor	200–300mg, slow IV injection		Infrequently used for treating bradycardia

All drugs should be used with caution in cases of cardiac ischaemia.

CI, contraindication; t½, half-life.

implantation is also indicated in asymptomatic patients with infra-nodal AVB or severe conduction disease who are deemed to have a high risk for developing high-degree AVB (e.g. alternating bundle branch block).

Pacemakers may be single-chamber (ventricular or, exceptionally, atrial), dual-chamber (AV), or biventricular (indicated in case of LV systolic dysfunction or for treating HF by CRT). An international code is used to designate the: (1) pacing chamber (A = atrium, V = ventricle, D = dual, O = none); (2) sensing chamber (A, V, D, O); (3) function (I = inhibited, T= triggered, D = both, O = none); (4) rate response (R = with rate response); and (5) multichamber pacing (A = bi-atrial, V = biventricular). Thus, a single-chamber rate-responsive pacemaker would be programmed in a VVIR mode, and a DDD mode would be programmed in a patient with a dual-chamber pacemaker with isolated AVB.

Tables 4.4.3, 4.4.4 and 4.4.5 summarize the ESC/EHRA 2013 guideline indications for permanent cardiac pacing.

Effect of drugs on cardiac pacing

A number of AADs can interfere with pacemaker function by increasing pacing thresholds (with loss of capture, potentially leading to bradycardia/asystole). These are listed in Box 4.4.1.

Box 4.4.1 Effect of drugs on pacing thresholds

Increased pacing threshold

1. Flecainide.
2. Propafenone.
3. Sotalol.
4. Mineralocorticoids.

Possibly increased pacing threshold

1. β-adrenergic blockers.
2. Ibutilide.
3. Lidocaine.
4. Procainamide.
5. Quinidine.

Decreased pacing threshold

1. Atropine.
2. Adrenaline.
3. Isoprenaline.
4. Glucocorticoids.

Table 4.4.2 Specific treatment options for bradycardia due to drug toxicity

Drug causing bradycardia	Treatment	Comments
β-blocker	Glucagon	First-line antidote Inotropic effect not mediated by β-receptors; therefore, more effective for β-blocker toxicity 2–10mg bolus, followed by 2–5mg/h infusion
	Inotropes: adrenaline, dobutamine, isoprenaline	Competitive β-receptor agonists High doses often required to overcome the effect of β-blockade
	Phosphodiesterase inhibitors: amrinone, milrinone	Inotropic; however, causes peripheral vasodilatation which exacerbates hypotension—therefore, not commonly used Can be used in combination with vasoconstricting inotropes
	High-dose insulin	Evidence restricted to case reports Infusion in combination with dextrose—monitor glucose and potassium levels
CCBs	IV calcium	First-line antidote Partially overcomes calcium blockade Calcium chloride or calcium gluconate can be given as boluses or infusion—monitor levels
	Glucagon	Can be used as bolus or infusion: 2–10mg bolus, followed by 2–5mg/h infusion
	High-dose insulin	As with β-blocker, toxicity evidence restricted to case reports
Digoxin	Digoxin-specific antibodies	First-line antidote Digoxin-specific antibodies (Fab fragments)

Table 4.4.3 Indications for permanent pacing in patients with persistent bradycardia

Recommendations	Class	Level
1. Sinus node disease: pacing is indicated when symptoms can be clearly attributed to bradycardia	I	B
2. Sinus node disease: pacing may be indicated when symptoms are likely to be due to bradycardia, even if the evidence is not conclusive	IIb	C
3. Sinus node disease: pacing is not indicated in patients with SB which is asymptomatic or due to reversible causes	III	C
4. Acquired AV block: pacing is indicated in patients with third- or second-degree type 2 AV block, irrespective of symptoms	I	C
5. Acquired AV block: pacing should be considered in patients with second-degree type 1 AV block which causes symptoms or is found to be located at intra- or infra-His levels at EPS	IIa	C
6. Acquired AV block: pacing is not indicated in patients with AV block which is due to reversible causes	III	C

AV, atrioventricular; EPS, electrophysiological study; SB, sinus bradycardia.
Reproduced from Brignole M, Auricchio A, Baron-Esquivias G, Bordachar P, Boriani G, Breithardt OA *et al*. 2013 ESC guidelines on cardiac pacing and cardiac resynchronization therapy: the task force on cardiac pacing and resynchronization therapy of the European Society of Cardiology (ESC). Developed in collaboration with the European Heart Rhythm Association (EHRA). *Europace* 2013;**15**:1070–1118 with permission from Oxford University Press.

Table 4.4.4 Indication for pacing in documented intermittent bradycardia

Recommendations	Class	Level
1. Sinus node disease (including brady-tachy form): pacing is indicated in patients affected by sinus node disease who have the documentation of symptomatic bradycardia due to sinus arrest or sinus-atrial block	I	B
2. Intermittent/paroxysmal AV block (including AF with slow ventricular conduction): pacing is indicated in patients with intermittent/paroxysmal intrinsic third- or second-degree AV block	I	C
3. Reflex asystolic syncope: pacing should be considered in patients ≤40 years with recurrent, unpredictable reflex syncopes and documented symptomatic pause/s due to sinus arrest or AV block or a combination of the two	IIa	B
4. Asymptomatic pauses (sinus arrest or AV block): pacing should be considered in patients with a history of syncope and documentation of asymptomatic pauses of >6s due to sinus arrest, sinus-atrial block, or AV block	IIa	C
5. Pacing is not indicated in reversible causes of bradycardia	III	C

AV, atrioventricular.
Reproduced from Brignole M, Auricchio A, Baron-Esquivias G, Bordachar P, Boriani G, Breithardt OA *et al*. 2013 ESC guidelines on cardiac pacing and cardiac resynchronization therapy: the task force on cardiac pacing and resynchronization therapy of the European Society of Cardiology (ESC). Developed in collaboration with the European Heart Rhythm Association (EHRA). *Europace* 2013;**15**:1070–1118 with permission from Oxford University Press.

Table 4.4.5 Indications for pacing in bundle branch block

Recommendations	Class	Level
1. BBB, unexplained,syncope and abnormal EPS: pacing is indicated in patients with syncope, BBB and positive EPS defined as HV interval of ≤70ms, or second- or third-degree His–Purkinje block demonstrated during incremental atrial pacing or with pharmacological challenge	I	B
2. Alternating BBB: pacing is indicated in patients with alternating BBB with or without symptoms	I	C
3. BBB, unexplained syncope with non-diagnostic investigations: pacing may be considered in selected patients with unexplained syncope and BBB	IIb	B
4. Asymptomatic BBB: pacing is not indicated for BBB in asymptomatic patients	III	B

BBB, bundle branch block; EPS, electrophysiological study.

Reproduced from Brignole M, Auricchio A, Baron-Esquivias G, Bordachar P, Boriani G, Breithardt OA *et al.* 2013 ESC guidelines on cardiac pacing and cardiac resynchronization therapy: the task force on cardiac pacing and resynchronization therapy of the European Society of Cardiology (ESC). Developed in collaboration with the European Heart Rhythm Association (EHRA). *Europace* 2013;15:1070–1118 with permission from Oxford University Press.

Further reading

Brignole M, Auricchio A, Baron-Esquivias G, *et al.* 2013 ESC guidelines on cardiac pacing and cardiac resynchronization therapy: the task force on cardiac pacing and resynchronization therapy of the European Society of Cardiology (ESC). Developed in collaboration with the European Heart Rhythm Association (EHRA). *Europace* 2013;15:1070–118.

Burri H. Pacemaker programming and troubleshooting. In: Ellenbogen KA, Wilkoff BL, Kay N, Lau CP, Auricchio A (eds). *Clinical Cardiac Pacing, Defibrillation, and Resynchronization Therapy*, 5th ed. Elsevier: Philadelphia, PA; 2016. pp. 1037–62.

Soar J, Nolan JP, Bottiger BW, *et al.* European Resuscitation Council Guidelines for Resuscitation 2015: Section 3. Adult advanced life support. *Resuscitation* 2015;**95**:100–47.

Chapter 4.5

Syncope

Ricardo Ruiz-Granell

Background

Syncope is a transient loss of consciousness of short duration, with rapid, total, and spontaneous recovery, resulting from transient global cerebral hypoperfusion.

The classification of syncope can be based on pathophysiology, as follows:[1,2]

- *Neurally mediated, reflex, neurocardiogenic, or vasovagal syncope*. It is the commonest type of syncope in the general population. Different triggering events induce a reflex response, like the Bezold–Jarisch reflex, that gives rise to vasodilatation and/or bradycardia, leading to cerebral hypoperfusion. There are episodes in which vasodepression predominates, episodes in which bradycardia or asystole are the principal components, and mixed forms, even in the same individual. Also the triggering events might vary considerably in individual patients. The classical vasovagal syncope is mediated by emotional or orthostatic stress. Reflex syncope in specific scenarios (micturition, defecation, coughing) is known as situational syncope. Carotid sinus syncope occurs with mechanical pressure over the carotid sinuses. However, the clinical presentation can be atypical, without clear triggering events or without premonitory symptoms. Detailed clinical history is crucial to the diagnosis. Tilt test and prolonged ECG monitoring, even with implantable devices, are the most useful tests in difficult cases.
- *Orthostatic hypotension* refers to syncope in which the upright position (most often movement from sitting or lying to an upright position) causes arterial hypotension. Volume depletion and inability of the autonomic nervous system to respond to the challenges imposed by an upright position are the two major causes. Clinical history, orthostatic tests, and neurologic evaluation are the main components for diagnosis.
- *Cardiac arrhythmias*. Brady- and tachyarrhythmias can provoke a decrease in CO, causing syncope. Cardiac evaluation and documentation of the arrhythmia (spontaneous episodes and/or induced in the electrophysiological study) usually lead to diagnosis.
- *Structural heart disease* can lead to syncope when circulatory demands outweigh the impaired ability of the heart to increase its output. Diagnosis is based on cardiac evaluation.
- *Steal syndromes* can cause syncope when a blood vessel has to supply both part of the brain and an arm. History taken and neurologic and imaging tests are the main diagnostic elements.

When a patient with syncope is first seen in an emergency department or in cardiology clinic, there is an evaluation pathway that should be followed. Firstly, the presence of a true transient loss of consciousness has to be established. Hence, falls without unconsciousness, coma, TIAs, seizures, psychogenic episodes, and other forms of non-syncopal episodes of altered consciousness have to be excluded. Secondly, some forms of syncope can be diagnosed in the initial evaluation (the diagnostic criteria can be found in the ESC Guidelines). When initial evaluation does not reveal the cause of syncope, risk stratification has to be performed. Severe structural heart disease, IHD, clinical or ECG features suggesting arrhythmic syncope, and important comorbidities, such as severe anaemia or electrolyte disturbances, are markers of risk for major CV events or SCD. Patients with a high-risk profile should be hospitalized for early evaluation and treatment. In these patients, if a cardiac or an arrhythmic cause of syncope is demonstrated, appropriate treatment can be established. If the evaluation is negative, a long-term ECG monitoring strategy with implanted devices is usually adopted, given the patients' high risk and the tests do not have 100% diagnostic sensitivity, although neurally mediated syncope is the commonest diagnosis obtained. Low-risk patients usually do not need hospitalization, except in special cases of comorbidities or body injury. Low-risk patients with single or rare episodes do not need further evaluation. Neurally mediated syncope is the most probable cause of their syncope, so advice on general measures (see ➔ Management of neurally mediated syncope, pp. 254–5) can be useful for these patients. When syncopal episodes are frequent causing severe impairment to the quality of life or occur in patients with particular occupational risks, tests including the tilt table test or long-term ECG monitoring can help to confirm the benign underlying causes of the syncope.

Treatment of arrhythmias, structural heart disease, and steal syndromes are reviewed elsewhere. In this chapter, we will review the pharmacological management of neurally mediated and orthostatic hypotension syncope.

Management of neurally mediated syncope

The aims of treatment of reflex syncope are to reduce the number of recurrences, to avoid body injury, and to improve the quality of life. Given the benign nature of the condition, treatment should always begin with lifestyle measures. Pharmacological and non-pharmacological invasive treatment, including cardiac ganglia plexi ablation and dual-chamber pacemakers, should be reserved for difficult cases.

General measures

Non-pharmacological measures are probably the mainstay of treatment, and the following should be considered:

- Reassurance of the benign nature of this kind of syncope.
- Education about recognition and possible avoidance of triggers (warm environment, prolonged standing, volume depletion, etc.). Direct treatment of known triggers (cough, psychological assistance to cope with triggering situations such as in medical or dental settings, etc.).
- Education about early recognition of prodromal symptoms is essential to recognize impending symptoms and apply preventative manoeuvres.
- Education about preventative manoeuvres when prodromal symptoms are recognized. Adopting a supine position may avoid progression to syncope. Physical counter-pressure manoeuvres, like leg crossing, arm tensing, or handgrip, have been shown to be effective in reducing syncope burden.
- Avoidance of unnecessary hypotensive drugs or substances (e.g. alcohol).
- Increasing water and salt intake, if not contraindicated, has been a current recommendation in patients with reflex syncope, although there is a lack of evidence of its effects and in the long-term balance of risks and benefits.
- In patients with syncope triggered by an upright position, tilt training or orthostatic training can be conducted, although some randomized trials have failed to demonstrate their benefit in reducing syncope burden.

Pharmacological treatment

Multiple drugs have been tested for the treatment of vasovagal syncope, but the evidence supporting their use is scarce. In most cases, randomized trials have not been conducted or have not demonstrated their benefit over placebo. The most studied drugs include the following.

- α-agonists: their benefit results from vasoconstriction (preventing vasodepression) and venoconstriction (preventing venous pooling). Etilefrine was studied in a randomized trial and showed no significant effect. Midodrine was studied in a few small randomized trials in children and adults, with inconsistent results. A meta-analysis showed midodrine to be associated with a reduction in syncope burden. Midodrine should be avoided in patients with a history of hypertension, HF, or urinary retention.

- Fludrocortisone: this mineralocorticoid is widely used in patients with neurally mediated syncope; it induces water and sodium retention, as well as potassium excretion. In the Prevention of Syncope Trial 2 (POST 2), there was a marginal reduction in syncope burden in patients treated with fludrocortisone, following a period of dose stabilization. This effect has not been demonstrated in children.
- β-blockers: these are widely used for the treatment of vasovagal syncope, despite the fact that various randomized studies failed to show their significant effects. Recently, an analysis of Prevention of Syncope Trial 1 (POST 1) showed an age-related effect, being significant in patients aged over 42 years.
- Selective serotonin reuptake inhibitors (SSRIs): since administration of serotonin during the tilt table test can induce syncope due to its central effects on heart rate and BP, SSRIs, such as paroxetine and fluoxetine, have been tested for the prevention of reflex syncope, with inconsistent results. Thus, there is no evidence to support their systematic use.
- Other: other drugs used to prevent neurocardiogenic syncope include disopyramide, hyoscine, clonidine, theophylline, and ephedrine. However, there is no consistent evidence supporting their use.

Non-pharmacological treatment

- Cardiac ganglionated plexus ablation is a recent approach to treat selected patients with neurocardiogenic syncope, but data are still scarce and there are no large trials studying this technique.
- Dual-chamber pacemakers. Cardiac pacing can prevent the cardioinhibitory response during neurocardiogenic syncope but has no effect on the vasodepressor response. Thus, its efficacy in preventing syncope would probably depend on a precise selection of patients. Several studies failed to demonstrate a significant effect, while others showed that a marginal effect could be attributed to a placebo effect of the pacemaker. More recently, it was demonstrated that in patients older than 40 years, with multiple recurrences and with asystole documented during a spontaneous syncopal episode, implantation of a dual-chamber pacemaker with algorithms to detect reductions in the heart rate can significantly reduce the syncopal burden. This effect is particularly significant if it is proven that the patient does not have a vasodepressor response in the tilt table test.

Management of orthostatic hypotension

Aetiology and diagnosis

The transition from lying or sitting to an upright position triggers some reflexes that maintain the BP. Failure of some of these mechanisms can provoke an abnormal fall in the BP during orthostatism, so-called orthostatic hypotension, that can result in neurological manifestations, including syncope.

Orthostatic hypotension is a frequent cause of syncope, especially in the elderly. There are non-neurological and neurological causes of orthostatic hypotension. The most important non-neurological causes include: failure of regulation (somatic alteration), e.g. old age, anorexia, post-gastrectomy; failure of vascular reactivity (after intense exercise, physical deconditioning, fever, heat exposure, arteriovenous fistula, cardiac shunt); hypovolaemia (haemorrhage, severe burns, dehydration); reduced venous tone (varicose veins, compression by tumours, pregnancy); circulating vasodilators (carcinoid syndrome, mastocytosis, hyperbradykininism); and endocrine disorders (Addison's disease, hyperaldosteronism, phaeochromocytoma). The main neurological causes are either primary or secondary. Primary autonomic failure can be acute or subacute, as in acute autonomic neuropathy, or chronic, as in pure autonomic failure (Bradbury–Eggleston syndrome), multisystem atrophy (Shy–Drager syndrome), and autonomic failure with Parkinson's disease. There is a great number of diseases that can result in secondary autonomic failure, e.g. diabetic, alcoholic, or amyloid neuropathies, human immunodeficiency virus (HIV) infection, Guillain–Barré syndrome, transverse myelitis, Chagas' disease, paraneoplastic syndromes, spinal cord trauma, dopamine β-hydroxylase deficiency, neural growth factor deficiency, etc.

The diagnosis of orthostatic hypotension is based on the clinical history and active orthostatic tests. The tilt test and Valsalva and handgrip manoeuvres can help in the diagnosis. The nature and extent of autonomic involvement require specialized assessment.

General measures

Education of patients with orthostatic hypotension is the mainstay of treatment and is essential to the success of any therapeutic strategy. It is based on the following measures:

- To avoid activities and habits that precipitate hypotension. Patients have to learn to 'break down' their transition from lying to standing into two or three phases; they have to avoid inactivity, as well as strenuous exercise, standing for long periods of time, copious meals, and alcohol consumption.
- To normalize the circulating volume and to avoid day–night imbalance. Acute fluid intake has been shown to be useful in patients with neurogenic orthostatic hypotension for occasional, temporary relief. Abundant water and liberal salt intake should be promoted, unless contraindicated. Nocturnal hypertension and excessive nocturnal diuresis can worsen early diurnal hypotension. Elevating the head of the bed by 5–20° can avoid excessive interstitial liquid reabsorption during the night, nocturnal diuresis, and hypertension.

- To use compression garments to improve venous return in an upright posture.
- To avoid, if possible, offending medications such as antihypertensives, diuretics, vasodilators, antidepressants, nasal sprays with vasoconstrictors, β-agonists drugs, etc.
- To practise manoeuvres that increase BP such as leg crossing, arm tensing, handgripping, squatting, etc. It is important to teach the patient to recognize symptoms of an impending syncope and to execute those manoeuvres immediately. Slow deep breathing before and during a change of position has been demonstrated to increase BP and also can be useful.

Pharmacological treatment

Numerous drugs have been used for orthostatic hypotension. Unfortunately, there is no drug that can avoid a fall in BP during orthostatism without producing side effects or hypertension during clinostatism.

Fludrocortisone is possibly the most commonly used drug, with inconsistent results. It increases the plasma volume through water and salt retention and also increases the sensitivity of vascular catecholamine receptors. Hypertension in the decubitus position, weight increase, oedema, and hypokalaemia are the commonest side effects.

Drugs with α-agonist effects (ephedrine, phenylephedrine, phenylpropanolamine) also have been widely used, and the best results have been obtained with midodrine. In a recent randomized trial, midodrine was found to be superior to a combination of midodrine and pyridostigmine or pyridostigmine alone.

Subcutaneous octreotide has been used for postprandial hypotension because of its effect on the mesenteric vasculature. Desmopressin can be useful in cases of excessive nocturnal diuresis. Subcutaneous erythropoietin has also been tested.

Droxidopa seems to reduce orthostatic hypotension in Parkinson's disease. Clonidine has been shown to have a paradoxical effect in patients with autonomic failure, but only in those with severe post-ganglionic impairment. Atomoxetine is being studied in autonomic failure.

References

1 Moya A, Sutton R, Ammirati F, *et al*. Task Force for the Diagnosis and Management of Syncope; European Society of Cardiology (ESC); European Heart Rhythm Association (EHRA); Heart Failure Association (HFA); Heart Rhythm Society (HRS). Guidelines for the diagnosis and management of syncope (version 2009). *Eur Heart J* 2009;**30**:2631–71.

2 Brignole M, Moya A, de Lange FJ, *et al*.; ESC Scientific Document Group. 2018 ESC Guidelines for the diagnosis and management of syncope. *Eur Heart J* 2018;**39**:1883–948.

Further reading

Moya A. Therapy for syncope. *Cardiol Clin* 2015;**33**:473–81.

Shen WK, Sheldon RS, Benditt DG, *et al*. 2017 ACC/AHA/HRS Guideline for the Evaluation and Management of Patients With Syncope: Executive Summary: A Report of the American College of Cardiology/American Heart Association Task Force on Clinical Practice Guidelines and the Heart Rhythm Society. *Circulation* 2017;**136**:e25–59.

Pharmacological therapy in OH

Section 5

Structural heart disease

Section editors

Claudio Ceconi
Francesca Mantovani

ESC Guidelines advisor

Erland Erdmann

Chapter 5.1

Valvular heart disease

Francesca Mantovani

Introduction

The commonest causes of structural defects in the heart are valvular heart disease (VHD), heart muscle disease (cardiomyopathy), and congenital structural heart diseases. Less commonly, heart damage may be caused by infection.

Any of the four valves of the heart can be affected, although left-sided valvular disease is far commoner than right-sided disease. VHD is frequent and often requires intervention. The aims of the evaluation of patients with VHD are to diagnose, quantify, and assess the mechanism of VHD, as well as its consequences. Decision-making should ideally be made through a collaborative approach between cardiologists, cardiac surgeons, imaging specialists, anaesthetists, and, if needed, general practitioners, geriatricians, or intensive care specialists—called a 'Heart Team' approach.

Mitral regurgitation

In Europe, mitral regurgitation (MR) is the second most frequent valve disease requiring surgery. According to the mechanism of MR, it can be divided into primary (due to valve leaflet abnormality) or secondary (also termed as functional, resulting from geometrical distortion of the subvalvular apparatus secondary to LV remodelling). Moreover, according to the presentation, MR can be acute or chronic. Acute MR is usually caused by papillary muscle rupture following acute MI or by ruptured chordae in degenerative mitral valve disease. Acute MR should be suspected in patients presenting with acute pulmonary oedema or shock, whereas chronic MR can be asymptomatic for a long time.

Primary mitral regurgitation

The commonest aetiology of primary MR in developed countries is degenerative MR, including mitral valve prolapse disease. Endocarditis is also one of the causes of primary MR.

Echocardiography is the principal investigation to establish the diagnosis, mechanism, severity, reparability, and consequences of MR. Valve repair, when feasible, is the optimal surgical treatment in patients with severe MR who have symptoms.

In asymptomatic patients with signs of LV dysfunction, surgery may be indicated. If LV function is preserved, surgery should be considered in patients with new-onset AF or pulmonary hypertension. Early surgery may be considered in patients at low operative risk where there is a high likelihood of durable valve repair on the basis of the valve lesion and the surgeon's experience.

Among the transcatheter procedures, currently, only edge-to-edge mitral repair is widely adopted. Percutaneous edge-to-edge repair may be considered in patients with symptomatic severe primary MR who fulfil the echocardiographic criteria of eligibility and are judged inoperable or to be at high surgical risk by the Heart Team, avoiding futility.

Medical management

There is no evidence supporting the use of vasodilators (including ACEIs) in MR without HF. However, when HF has developed, ACEIs are beneficial and should be considered. β-blockers and spironolactone should also be considered in the setting of LV dysfunction.

Anticoagulation is required in the presence of AF (either permanent or paroxysmal) or when there is a history of thromboembolism or left atrial thrombus and for 3 months after mitral valve repair.

Secondary mitral regurgitation

Secondary or functional MR results from geometrical distortion of the left ventricle due to idiopathic cardiomyopathy or CAD. In the latter, MR is also called ischaemic MR. Secondary MR is a dynamic condition, and its severity may change according to the loading condition: hypertension, medical therapy, exercise. Echocardiography is useful to establish the diagnosis and to differentiate secondary from primary MR in patients with CAD or HF. Severe secondary MR should be corrected at the time of coronary artery bypass surgery. The indications for isolated mitral valve surgery in symptomatic patients with severe secondary MR and severely depressed systolic LV function, who cannot be revascularized or who present with cardiomyopathy, are questionable.

Among the transcatheter procedures, currently, only edge-to-edge mitral repair is widely adopted. Percutaneous edge-to-edge repair may be considered in patients with symptomatic severe primary MR who fulfil the echocardiographic criteria of eligibility and are judged inoperable or to be at high surgical risk by the Heart Team, avoiding futility.

Medical management

In severe secondary MR, such as in ischaemic cardiomyopathy, optimal medical therapy should be the first step, in line with guidelines on the management of HF.

ACEIs and β-blockers, with the addition of an aldosterone antagonist, in the presence of symptoms of HF, may reduce MR by progressive inverse remodelling of the left ventricle. Diuretics are required in the presence of fluid overload. Nitrates, diuretics, and sodium nitroprusside reduce filling pressures, and hence the regurgitant fraction; therefore, they may be useful for treating acute dyspnoea. Inotropic agents and IABPs can be added in cases of hypotension. MR in this setting may be exacerbated by dyssynchrony of the ventricles, and resynchronization therapy may be beneficial, in accordance with related guidelines.

Mitral stenosis

Rheumatic fever is the predominant aetiology of mitral stenosis (MS) and has greatly decreased in developed countries, although MS still results in significant morbidity and mortality worldwide. Conversely, in recent years, an increase in the degenerative aetiology of MS has emerged.

Echocardiography is the main method used to assess the severity and consequences of MS, as well as the extent of anatomic lesions.

Symptoms may not develop for years and then present with a gradual decrease in functional capacity with exertional dyspnoea. Intervention is indicated in symptomatic patients with significant MS (mitral valve area ≤1.5cm^2) by percutaneous commissurotomy if the anatomy is suitable, or alternatively by open surgery, including valve replacement.

Medical management

Dyspnoea can be transiently ameliorated by diuretics or long-acting nitrates. β-blockers or non-dihydropyridine CCBs can improve exercise tolerance by prolonging diastole and increasing LV filling time, hence improving CO. Patients with either permanent or paroxysmal AF require anticoagulation, with the INR in the range of 2.5–3. In patients in sinus rhythm, anticoagulation is recommended with a history of thromboembolism or in the presence of left atrial thrombus. It should also be considered when dense spontaneous echo contrast is seen on transoesophageal echocardiography or in cases of enlarged left atrial volumes of >60mL/m^2. Aspirin and other antiplatelet agents are not valid alternatives.

Aortic stenosis

Aortic stenosis (AS) is the commonest type of VHD in Europe and North America. AS primarily presents as calcific AS in adults of advanced age. The second commonest aetiology develops due to turbulent flow across a congenitally abnormal aortic valve (most frequently bicuspid aortic valve), typically at a younger age. Rheumatic AS has become rare.

While AS progresses, there are usually no symptoms until the aortic orifice is reduced to about 1cm^2. At this stage, the usual triad of possible symptoms consists of angina, syncope, and dyspnoea, progressing to HF.

Echocardiography reveals the valve morphology, diagnosis of AS, the severity, the consequences on the left ventricle, and coexisting ascending aortic dilatation (up to 60% of cases associated with bicuspid aortic valve), when present.

Aortic valve replacement (AVR) should be recommended in all symptomatic patients with severe AS. Transcatheter aortic valve implantation (TAVI) is indicated in patients with severe symptomatic AS who are not suitable for AVR (due to high-risk profile or technical contraindications), as assessed by a 'heart team', and who are likely to gain improvement in their quality of life and to have a life expectancy of >1 year, after consideration of their comorbidities. In the asymptomatic patient, the wide variability in the rate of progression of AS heightens the need for patients to be carefully educated about the importance of follow-up and reporting symptoms as soon as they develop.

Medical management

Symptomatic patients require early intervention, because no medical therapy for AS is able to improve outcome, compared to the natural history. However, patients not suitable for surgery or TAVI, or those awaiting these procedures, may be treated with digoxin and diuretics if they experience HF symptoms. Importantly, coexisting hypertension should be treated. Therapy should be carefully titrated to avoid hypotension, and patients should be re-evaluated frequently. Treatment of atrial arrhythmia is beneficial, as its presence leads to loss of the atrial contribution to ventricular filling.

Although several retrospective reports have shown beneficial effects of statins and ACEIs, randomized trials have consistently shown that statins do not affect the progression of AS.

Statin therapy should therefore not be used in AS patients where their only purpose is to slow progression.

Aortic regurgitation

Aortic regurgitation (AR) may be caused primarily by disease of the aortic valve leaflets and/or abnormalities of the aortic root. Congenital diseases, mainly bicuspid aortic valve, is a common finding. AR can be associated with abnormalities of the aortic root, especially in patients with connective tissue diseases, including Marfan's syndrome. AR presentation can be acute or chronic, where acute severe AR represents an emergency condition, most frequently caused by infective endocarditis and aortic dissection, with a poor prognosis without intervention, due to haemodynamic instability. Chronic severe AR may be asymptomatic for a long time because the left ventricle gradually enlarges. Symptoms—dyspnoea, palpitations, and angina—occur late, developing once LV failure has occurred.

Analysis of the mechanism of AR influences patient management, particularly when valve repair is considered. Echocardiography and other imaging modalities, mainly angio-computed tomography (CT) and angio-magnetic resonance (MR), are essential in the diagnosis and follow-up of AR, as well as in monitoring aortic root dilatation and potential complications.

In patients with severe AR, symptom onset is an indication for surgery. Surgery is indicated in asymptomatic patients with severe AR and impaired LV function.

Also, surgery is recommended, irrespective of the severity of AR, when the pathology of the aortic root is above certain thresholds, especially in patients with Marfan's syndrome or those with bicuspid valves.

Medical management

Inotropic agents and vasodilators may be used for short-term therapy to improve conditions in patients with severe HF before surgery. In patients with chronic severe AR and HF, vasodilators (ACEIs or ARBs) may be useful in the presence of arterial hypertension, if surgery is contraindicated, or post-operatively in cases of persistent LV dysfunction. Their benefit in asymptomatic patients without hypertension, in order to delay surgery, is unproven.

In the setting of patients with Marfan's syndrome, β-blockers should always be considered since they have been shown to slow aortic root dilatation and reduce the risk of aortic complications. Preliminary findings suggest that ARBs have an intrinsic effect on the aortic wall by preserving elastin fibres, but their clinical benefit remains to be proven by ongoing trials.

Recommendations to avoid strenuous physical exercise and competitive and isometric sport should be given to patients with Marfan's syndrome and others with borderline aortic root dilatation approaching the threshold for intervention. Screening the proband's first-degree relatives with appropriate imaging studies is indicated in Marfan's patients and those with bicuspid aortic valve disease.

Tricuspid regurgitation

Trivial tricuspid regurgitation (TR) is a frequent finding in normal subjects. Pathological TR is more often secondary, rather than due to primary valve damage. TR can be secondary to annular dilatation and leaflet tethering related to RV volume and/or pressure overload.

The commonest cause is pressure overload caused by pulmonary hypertension, resulting from left-sided heart disease (i.e. mitral valve disease).

Predominant symptoms are those of associated valve disease, and even severe TR may be well tolerated for long time. Echocardiography is the ideal technique to evaluate TR, to distinguish between primary and secondary forms, to measure the degree of annular dilatation, and to evaluate the pulmonary systolic pressure and RV dimensions and function.

If technically possible, valve repair with ring annuloplasty is preferable to valve replacement, and surgery should be performed early enough to avoid irreversible RV dysfunction.

The need for correction of TR is usually considered at the time of surgical correction of left-sided valve lesions. Surgery is indicated in patients with severe TR. Surgery should be considered in patients with moderate primary TR, as well as in patients with mild or moderate secondary TR if the tricuspid annulus is dilated.

Medical management

Patients with TR respond well to diuretic therapy, but specific therapy of the underlying disease is warranted in order to avoid irreversible RV damage, organ failure, and poor results of late surgical intervention.

Tricuspid stenosis

Tricuspid stenosis (TS) is mostly of rheumatic origin and therefore is now rare in the Western world. Frequently, TS is associated with left-sided valve lesions, especially MS, that dominate the clinical presentation. Therefore, its detection requires careful evaluation.

TS evaluation is particularly difficult by echocardiography, since no generally accepted grading of TS severity exists, but only a transvalvular gradient cut-off is considered indicative of clinically significant TS. The presence of commissural fusion, the anatomy of the valve, and the subvalvular apparatus are the most important determinants of reparability and the degree of concomitant TR.

Surgery is indicated in symptomatic patients with severe isolated TS or in those with severe TS undergoing left-sided valve intervention. The lack of pliable leaflet tissue is the main limitation for valve repair. Even though this is still a matter of debate, biological prostheses for valve replacement are usually preferred over mechanical ones because of the higher risk of thrombosis carried by the latter and the satisfactory long-term durability of the former in the tricuspid position. Percutaneous balloon valvuloplasty can be attempted as a first approach if TS is isolated or if percutaneous commissurotomy can be performed on the mitral valve.

Medical management

Diuretic therapy is useful in the presence of HF to eliminate fluid overload and its associated symptoms, as well as improve hepatic function, but is of limited efficacy.

Combined and multiple valve diseases

Significant stenosis and regurgitation can be found on the same valve; also, disease of multiple valves may be encountered in several conditions (rheumatic heart disease and degenerative valve disease). In these cases, valve diseases influence each other, and assessment of severities and management could be particularly tricky. Also, there is a lack of data on mixed and multiple valve diseases, and this does not allow for evidence-based recommendations.

As a general principle, it is important to establish the predominant VHD and treat it according to the relative guideline indications.

Antithrombotic management in valvular heart disease

Thromboembolism and anticoagulant-related bleeding represent the majority of complications in patients with prosthetic valves. Antithrombotic management should address effective control of modifiable risk factors for thromboembolism, in addition to the prescription of antithrombotic drugs.

Oral anticoagulation using a VKA is recommended lifelong for all patients with a mechanical prosthesis, as well in those with surgical or transcatheter-implanted bioprostheses with other indications for anticoagulation (AF, VTE, hypercoagulable state, or, with a lesser degree of evidence, severely impaired LV dysfunction with an ejection fraction of <35%). The addition of low-dose aspirin to VKAs in patients with mechanical prostheses should be considered after thromboembolism despite an adequate INR and may be considered in the case of concomitant atherosclerotic disease.

When choosing an optimal target INR, patient risk factors and the thrombogenicity of the prosthesis, as determined by reported valve thrombosis rates for that prosthesis in relation to specific INR levels, should be considered (see Table 5.1.1). INR recommendations in individual patients may need to be revised downwards if recurrent bleeding occurs, or upwards in the case of embolism, despite an acceptable INR level.

The substitution of VKAs by direct oral inhibitors of factor IIa or Xa is contraindicated in patients with mechanical prostheses.

The use of low-dose aspirin should be considered for the first 3 months after surgical implantation of an aortic bioprosthesis. Oral anticoagulation using a VKA should still be considered for the first 3 months after surgical implantation of a mitral or tricuspid bioprosthesis or after mitral or tricuspid valve repair.

Table 5.1.1 INR recommendations

Prosthesis thrombogenicity*	Patient-related risk factors§	
	No risk factor	Risk factor ≥1
Low	2.5	3.0
Medium	3.0	3.5
High	3.5	4.0

* Prosthesis thrombogenicity: low = Carbomedics, Medtronic Hall, ATS, Medtronic Open-Pivot, St Jude Medical, On-X, Sorin Bicarbon; medium = other bileaflet valves with insufficient data; high = Lillehei-Kaster, Omniscience, Starr–Edwards (ball-cage), Bjork–Shiley, and other tilting-disc valves.

§ Patient-related risk factors: mitral or tricuspid valve replacement, previous thromboembolism, AF, mitral stenosis of any degree, LV ejection fraction <35%.

The first post-operative month is a high-risk period for thrombo-embolism. The addition of aspirin to anticoagulant therapy decreases the post-operative thromboembolic risk but increases the bleeding risk and cannot be recommended routinely.

DAPT should be considered for the first 3–6 months after TAVI, followed by lifelong single antiplatelet therapy in patients who do not need oral anticoagulation for other reasons, while single antiplatelet therapy may be considered after TAVI in the case of high bleeding risk.

Interruption of anticoagulant therapy

Anticoagulation during non-cardiac surgery requires very careful management, based on risk assessment. It is recommended not to interrupt oral anticoagulation for most minor surgical procedures (including dental extraction and cataract removal) and those procedures where bleeding is easily controlled. Appropriate techniques of haemostasis should be used, and the INR should be measured on the day of the procedure. Major surgical procedures require an INR not exceeding 1.5. In patients with a mechanical prosthesis, oral anticoagulant therapy should be stopped before surgery and bridged with heparin. UFH remains the only approved heparin treatment in patients with mechanical prostheses. SC LMWH is often used as an alternative to UFH for bridging; however, LMWH is not approved in patients with mechanical prostheses, due to the lack of controlled comparative studies with UFH. When LMWH is used, it should be administered twice a day using therapeutic doses, adapted to body weight and renal function, and, if possible, with monitoring of anti-Xa activity with a target of 0.5–1.0U/mL.

Management of overdose of vitamin K antagonists and bleeding

The risk of major bleeding increases considerably when the INR exceeds 4.5 and increases exponentially above an INR of 6.0. An INR of ≥6.0 therefore requires rapid reversal of anticoagulation.

In the absence of bleeding, management depends on the target INR, the actual INR, and the half-life of the VKA used. Possible strategies are to stop oral anticoagulation and to allow the INR to fall gradually or to give oral vitamin K in increments of 1 or 2mg. If the INR is >10, high doses of oral vitamin K (5mg) should be considered. The oral route carries a lower risk of anaphylaxis; therefore, it should be favoured over the IV route. Immediate reversal of anticoagulation is required only for severe bleeding—defined as not amenable to local control, threatening life or important organ function (e.g. intracranial bleeding), causing haemodynamic instability, or requiring an emergency surgical procedure or transfusion. IV prothrombin complex concentrate has a short half-life and, if used, should therefore be combined with oral vitamin K, whatever the INR. When available, use of IV prothrombin complex concentrate is preferred over fresh frozen plasma. The optimal time to restart anticoagulant therapy should be discussed in relation to the location of the bleeding event, its evolution, and interventions performed to stop bleeding and/or to treat the underlying cause. Bleeding while in the therapeutic INR range is often related to an underlying pathological cause, and it is important that it is identified and managed.

Prosthetic valve thrombosis

Obstructive prosthetic valve thrombosis

Obstructive prosthetic valve thrombosis should be suspected promptly in any patient with any type of prosthetic valve, who presents with a recent onset of dyspnoea or an embolic event. Suspicion should be higher in cases of recent inadequate anticoagulation or in cases of an increased coagulability status (e.g. dehydration, infection, etc.). The diagnosis should be confirmed by echocardiography (transthoracic and/or transoesophageal echocardiography) or cinefluoroscopy or CT.

The management of prosthetic thrombosis is challenging, whatever the option taken. Re-do high-risk surgery is most often performed under emergency conditions. On the other hand, fibrinolysis carries risks of bleeding, systemic embolism, and recurrent thrombosis.

Urgent or emergency valve replacement is recommended for obstructive thrombosis in critically ill patients without contraindications to surgery. If thrombogenicity of the prosthesis is an important factor, it should be replaced with a less thrombogenic prosthesis.

Fibrinolysis should be considered when surgery is not available or is very high risk or for thrombosis of right-sided prostheses.

In cases of haemodynamic instability, a short protocol is recommended, using either IV recombinant tissue plasminogen activator (alteplase, rTPA) 10mg bolus + 90mg in 90min with UFH, or streptokinase 1,500,000U in 60min without UFH. Longer durations of infusions can be used in stable patients.

Fibrinolysis is less likely to be successful in mitral prostheses, in chronic thrombosis, or in the presence of a pannus, which can be difficult to distinguish from a thrombus.

Non-obstructive prosthetic valve thrombosis

Non-obstructive prosthetic thrombosis is diagnosed using transoesophageal echocardiography. It can be diagnosed in routine exams following mitral valve replacement or during a workup after an embolic event. Management depends mainly on the occurrence of a thromboembolic event and the size of the thrombus. Close monitoring by echocardiography is mandatory. The prognosis is favourable with medical therapy in most cases of a small thrombus (<10mm). A good response with gradual resolution of the thrombus obviates the need for surgery. Conversely, surgery should be considered for large (≥10mm) non-obstructive prosthetic thrombus complicated by embolism or which persists despite optimal anticoagulation. Fibrinolysis may be considered if surgery is at high risk but carries a risk of bleeding and thromboembolism. Valve thrombosis occurs mainly in mechanical prostheses. However, cases of thrombosis of bioprostheses have been reported after surgery or transcatheter valve implantation. Anticoagulation using a VKA and/or UFH is the first-line treatment of bioprosthetic valve thrombosis.

Management of thromboembolism

Thromboembolism after valve surgery is multifactorial in origin. Although thromboembolic events frequently originate from the prosthesis, many others arise from other sources and are part of the background incidence of strokes and TIAs in the general population.

Thorough investigation of each episode of thromboembolism is therefore essential, rather than simply increasing the target INR or adding an antiplatelet agent. Prevention of further thromboembolic events involves:

- Treatment or reversal of risk factors such as AF, hypertension, hypercholesterolaemia, diabetes, smoking, infection, and prothrombotic blood test abnormalities.
- Optimization of anticoagulation control, if possible with patient self-management, on the basis that better control is more effective than simply increasing the target INR. This should be discussed with the neurologist in cases of a recent stroke.
- Low-dose aspirin (≥100mg daily) may be added, if it was not previously prescribed, after careful analysis of the risk–benefit ratio, avoiding excessive anticoagulation.

Marfan's syndrome

Marfan's syndrome is the commonest heritable connective tissue disorder. Transmitted as an autosomal dominant disease, Marfan's syndrome is essentially associated with mutations in the gene that encodes fibrillin-1, a glycoprotein in the extracellular matrix. A deficiency of fibrillin may lead to weakening of the supportive tissues and dysregulation of transforming growth factor beta (TGF-β). Prognosis is mainly determined by progressive dilatation of the aorta, at any level, but most frequently at the aortic root level, leading to aortic dissection or rupture, which are the major causes of death.

Diagnosis

Marfan's syndrome diagnosis requires an MDT. According to the revised Marfan's nosology, a definite diagnosis requires occurrence of at least two of the following: aortic root aneurysm, ectopia lentis, a family history of Marfan's syndrome, and documented fibrillin-1 mutation. Diagnosis can be made also in the presence of an aortic aneurysm and a systemic score of ≥7 points (made up of specific skeleton anomalies/deformities, pneumothorax, dural ectasia, skin striae, myopia, and mitral valve prolapse). Marfan's syndrome can be confused with other heritable connective tissue disorders that closely mimic Marfan's symptoms, such as Loeys–Dietz syndrome, familial aortic aneurysm, bicuspid aortic valve with aortic dilatation, familial ectopia lentis, MASS phenotype, and Ehlers–Danlos syndrome, because of the considerable clinical overlap between the various syndromes.

Assessment of the aortic root and distal ascending aortic levels is made by echocardiography, which also provides evaluation of the LV function, the aortic valve and AR, or mitral valve prolapse and regurgitation. CMR or CT should be performed in every patient, providing imaging of the entire aorta, including aortic dimensions beyond the root.

Early identification and establishment of the diagnosis are critical, since prophylactic surgery can prevent aortic dissection and rupture. Replacement of the aortic valve and ascending aorta has become a low-risk and very durable operation in experienced hands. Marfan's syndrome has, however, been associated with a considerably higher risk of re-dissection and recurrent aneurysm than other aetiologies of aortic disease.

In patients with anatomically normal aortic valves, valve-sparing operations with root replacement by a vascular prosthesis and with reimplantation of the coronary arteries into the prosthesis or remodelling of the aortic root have now become the preferred surgical procedures. If necessary, all parts of the aorta can be replaced with a prosthesis.

Stent grafting in patients with Marfan's syndrome is currently not recommended, unless the risk of conventional open surgical repair is deemed prohibitive. Even after repair of the ascending aorta, Marfan's syndrome patients remain at risk for dissection of the residual aorta.

Patients should be advised to avoid exertion at maximal capacity and competitive and isometric sports. Women with an aortic diameter of >45mm are strongly discouraged from becoming pregnant without prior repair, because of the high risk for dissection. An aortic diameter of <40mm rarely presents a problem, although a completely safe diameter does not exist.

With an aortic diameter of between 40 and 45mm, previous aortic growth and a family history are important for advising on pregnancy with or without aortic repair.

Medical therapy

Rigorous antihypertensive medical treatment, aiming at an SBP of <120mmHg and 110mmHg in patients with aortic dissection, is important. β-blockers might reduce the rate of aortic dilatation and might improve survival. Losartan is potentially useful because it leads to TGF-β antagonism and can be effective in reducing the rate of dilatation of the aortic root. Clinical trials are presently ongoing to evaluate its beneficial effect.

Further reading

Baumgartner H, Bonhoeffer P, De Groot NM, *et al.*; Task Force on the Management of Grown-up Congenital Heart Disease of the European Society of Cardiology (ESC); Association for European Paediatric Cardiology (AEPC); ESC Committee for Practice Guidelines (CPG). ESC Guidelines for the management of grown-up congenital heart disease (new version 2010). *Eur Heart J* 2010;**31**:2915–57.

Baumgartner H, Falk V, Bax JJ, *et al.*; ESC Scientific Document Group. 2017 ESC/EACTS Guidelines for the management of valvular heart disease. *Eur Heart J* 2017;**38**:2739–91.

Erbel R, Aboyans V, Boileau C, *et al.*; ESC Committee for Practice Guidelines. 2014 ESC Guidelines on the diagnosis and treatment of aortic diseases: Document covering acute and chronic aortic diseases of the thoracic and abdominal aorta of the adult. The Task Force for the Diagnosis and Treatment of Aortic Diseases of the European Society of Cardiology (ESC). *Eur Heart J* 2014;**35**:2873–926.

Loeys BL, Dietz HC, Braverman AC, *et al*. The revised Ghent nosology for the Marfan syndrome. *J Med Genet* 2010;**47**:476–85.

Chapter 5.2

Myocarditis and pericardial syndromes

Giovanni Boffa and Claudio Ceconi

Myocarditis

Myocarditis is defined as inflammatory disease of the myocardium, diagnosed by established histological, immunological, and immunohistochemical criteria.[1] The clinical presentations of myocarditis[1] can be very different: mild symptoms (chest pain and palpitations), pseudo-ACS, new onset or chronic HF, cardiogenic shock, ventricular arrhythmia, and SCD.

Causes of myocarditis

- Infectious:
  - Viral, bacterial, spirochaetal, fungal, protozoal, parasitic, rickettsial.
- Immune-mediated:
  - Allergens, alloantigens, autoantigens.
- Toxic:
  - Drugs, heavy metals, hormones, physical agents.
- Idiopathic.

The clinical course is variable. Acute myocarditis resolves in about half of cases in a few weeks; about 25% of patients will develop DCM, and 12–25% may acutely deteriorate and either die or need heart transplantation or ventricular mechanical assistance. Arrhythmias are commonly associated with severe myocarditis and may be the cause of SCD.

Management of myocarditis

Aetiology-targeted therapy is indicated when supported by evidence. However, in the vast majority of patients with myocarditis, the most important targets of treatment are HF and arrhythmias.

Management of systolic LV dysfunction should follow the recommendations of current ESC guidelines on HF. The proposed flow chart suggests diuretics and the combination of ACEIs (or ARBs) and β-blockers as first-line pharmacological treatment. In patients who remain symptomatic despite optimal management, additional treatment with aldosterone antagonists should be considered. No data are yet available about the effectiveness of sacubitril/valsartan complex and ivabradine in patients with myocarditis and LV dysfunction. Immunosuppression is indicated only in giant cell myocarditis and can be taken in consideration in proven autoimmune forms of myocarditis, including cardiac sarcoid myocarditis occurring in extra-cardiac immune disease.

In patients with severe LV dysfunction, inotropic support may be necessary, and ventricular assist devices may represent a bridge to recovery or to heart transplantation.

There are no specific treatments of arrhythmias in myocarditis, and so management should follow the recommendations of the current ESC guidelines. Cardioverter–defibrillator implantation must be deferred in the acute phase because myocarditis may heal. In patients with myocarditis and severe ventricular arrhythmia, a wearable cardioverter–defibrillator can represent a bridge to recovery, ICD implantation, or heart transplantation.

Pericardial syndromes

Pericardial diseases are relatively common in clinical practice, and new diagnostic strategies have been proposed for the triage of patients with pericarditis and pericardial effusion and allow accurate diagnosis.

Pericardial syndromes include different clinical presentations of pericardial diseases with distinctive signs and symptoms that can be grouped as specific 'syndromes'. The classical pericardial syndromes include pericarditis, pericardial effusion, cardiac tamponade, and constrictive pericarditis.

A simple aetiological classification is to consider infectious and non-infectious causes of pericardial diseases (see Box 5.2.1).

Pericarditis is the commonest disease of the pericardium encountered in clinical practice; it is defined as an inflammation of the pericardium. In the majority of cases, pericarditis is an acute, self-limiting condition.

In a proportion of cases, no cause is found, i.e. idiopathic pericarditis. The majority of cases of pericarditis are either idiopathic or due to viral infection.

Chest pain is the commonest symptom associated with pericarditis. The pain is typically exacerbated by lying flat and by deep inspiration. Physical examination may reveal low-grade pyrexia and a pericardial friction rub. The presence of a significant pericardial effusion causing tamponade may be associated with hypotension, tachycardia, and pulsus paradoxus. A comprehensive summary of the pericardial syndromes is summarized in Table 5.2.1.

Elevation of markers of inflammation, i.e. C-reactive protein (CRP) and erythrocyte sedimentation rate (ESR), as well as elevation of the white blood cell count, is a common and supportive finding in patients with acute pericarditis and may be helpful for monitoring the activity of the disease and the efficacy of therapy.

Management of pericarditis

Management of pericarditis depends on the pattern of disease, the underlying cause, and the presence or absence of complications. The following section outlines the ESC guidelines[2] for treatment of pericarditis.

Most cases of pericarditis, particularly idiopathic and viral pericarditis, are uncomplicated and are associated with self-limiting symptoms. The only treatment required in such cases is anti-inflammatory therapy (see Table 5.2.2).

The choice of drug should be based on the history of the patient, the presence of concomitant diseases, and physician expertise. Colchicine is recommended at low, weight-adjusted doses to improve the response to medical therapy and prevent recurrences. Corticosteroids should be considered as a second option in patients with contraindications and failure of aspirin or NSAIDs because of the risk of favouring the chronic evolution of the disease.

Approximately 15–30% of patients with idiopathic acute pericarditis who are not treated with colchicine will develop either recurrent or incessant disease, while colchicine may halve the recurrence rate.[2,3]

Incessant pericarditis (i.e. cases with persistent symptoms without clear-cut remission after the acute episode) and *chronic* pericarditis (disease processes lasting >3 months) (see Table 5.2.2), by definition, need a more prolonged treatment period.

Box 5.2.1 Aetiology of pericardial diseases

Infectious causes

- *Viral*: enteroviruses (Coxsackie viruses, echoviruses), herpesviruses (Epstein–Barr virus, cytomegalovirus, human herpesvirus 6), adenoviruses, parvovirus B19 (possible overlap with aetiologic viral agents of myocarditis).
- *Bacterial: Mycobacterium tuberculosis, Coxiella burnetii, Borrelia burgdorferi*; rarely *Pneumococcus* species (spp.), *Meningococcus* spp., *Gonococcus* spp., *Streptococcus* spp., *Staphylococcus* spp., *Haemophilus* spp., *Chlamydia* spp., *Mycoplasma* spp., *Legionella* spp., *Leptospira* spp., *Listeria* spp., *Providencia stuartii*.
- *Fungal* (rare): *Histoplasma* spp. (more likely in immunocompetent patients), *Aspergillus* spp., *Blastomyces* spp., *Candida* spp. (more likely in immunocompromised host).
- *Parasitic* (rare): *Echinococcus* spp., *Toxoplasma* spp.

Non-infectious causes

- *Autoimmune:*
  - Systemic autoimmune and auto-inflammatory diseases (systemic lupus erythematosus (SLE), Sjögren's syndrome, rheumatoid arthritis (RA), scleroderma, systemic vasculitides (i.e. eosinophilic granulomatosis with polyangiitis or allergic granulomatosis, previously named Churg–Strauss syndrome, Horton disease, Takayasu disease, Behçet's syndrome), sarcoidosis, familial Mediterranean fever, inflammatory bowel disease, Still disease.
- *Neoplastic*:
  - Primary tumours (rare, above all pericardial mesothelioma).
  - Secondary metastatic tumours (common, above all lung and breast cancers, lymphoma).
- *Metabolic*:
  - Uraemia, myxoedema, anorexia nervosa, other rare.
- *Traumatic and iatrogenic*:
  - *Early onset—direct injury* (penetrating thoracic injury, oesophageal perforation).
  - *Indirect injury* (non-penetrating thoracic injury, radiation injury).
  - *Delayed onset—pericardial injury syndromes* (post-MI syndrome, post-pericardiotomy syndrome, post-traumatic, including forms after iatrogenic trauma (e.g. PCI, pacemaker lead insertion, and radiofrequency ablation).
  - *Drug-related*: lupus-like syndrome (procainamide, hydralazine, methyldopa, isoniazid, phenytoin); antineoplastic drugs (often associated with cardiomyopathy, may cause pericardiopathy): doxorubicin and daunorubicin, cytosine arabinoside, fluorouracil, cyclophosphamide; penicillins as hypersensitivity pericarditis with eosinophilia; amiodarone, methysergide, mesalazine, clozapine, minoxidil, dantrolene, practolol, phenylbutazone, thiazides, streptomycin, thiouracils, streptokinase, *p*-aminosalicylic acid, sulfa-drugs, ciclosporin, bromocriptine, several vaccines, granulocyte-macrophage colony-stimulating factor (GM-CSF), anti-tumour necrosis factor (TNF) agents.
- *Other*: amyloidosis.

Recurrent pericarditis is diagnosed with a documented first episode of acute pericarditis, a symptom-free interval of 4–6 weeks or longer, and evidence of subsequent recurrence of pericarditis (see Table 5.2.2). Aspirin or NSAIDs remain the mainstay of therapy. Colchicine is recommended on top of standard anti-inflammatory therapy, without a loading dose and using weight-adjusted doses (i.e. 0.5mg od if the body weight

Table 5.2.1 Definitions and diagnostic criteria for pericarditis

Pericarditis	Definition and diagnostic criteria
Acute	Inflammatory pericardial syndrome to be diagnosed with at least two of the four following criteria: 1. Pericarditic chest pain 2. Pericardial rubs 3. New widespread ST-elevation or PR-depression on ECG 4. Pericardial effusion Additional supporting findings: • Elevation of markers of inflammation (i.e. CRP, ESR, and white blood cell count) • Evidence of pericardial inflammation by an imaging technique (CT, CMR)
Incessant	Pericarditis lasting for >4 to 6 weeks, but <3 months
Recurrent	Recurrence of pericarditis after a documented first episode of acute pericarditis and a symptom-free interval of 4–6 weeks or longer
Chronic	Pericarditis lasting for >3 months

Reproduced from Adler Y. *et al.* (2015) ESC Guidelines for the diagnosis and management of pericardial diseases: The Task Force for the Diagnosis and Management of Pericardial Diseases of the European Society of Cardiology (ESC). *Eur Heart J*. 2015 Nov 7;36(42):2921–64 with permission from Oxford University Press.

Table 5.2.2 Commonly prescribed anti-inflammatory therapy for acute pericarditis

Drug	Dosing	Treatment duration	Tapering
Aspirin	750–1000mg every 8h	1–2 weeks	Decrease doses by 250–500mg every 1–2 weeks
Ibuprofen	600mg every 8h	1–2 weeks	Decrease doses by 200–400mg every 1–2 weeks
Colchicine	0.5mg od (<70kg) or 0.5mg bd (≥70kg)	3 months	Not mandatory, alternatively 0.5mg every other day (<70kg) or 0.5mg once (≥70kg) in the last weeks

Reproduced from Adler Y. *et al.* (2015) ESC Guidelines for the diagnosis and management of pericardial diseases: The Task Force for the Diagnosis and Management of Pericardial Diseases of the European Society of Cardiology (ESC). *Eur Heart J*. 2015 Nov 7;36(42):2921–64 with permission from Oxford University Press.

is <70kg or 0.5mg bd if it is ≥70kg, for ≥6 months), in order to improve the response to medical therapy, improve remission rates, and prevent recurrences.[2,3]

In cases of incomplete response to aspirin/NSAIDs and colchicine, corticosteroids may be used, but they should be added at low to moderate doses to aspirin/NSAIDs and colchicine as triple therapy, and not to replace these drugs, in order to achieve better control of symptoms. Although corticosteroids provide rapid control of symptoms, they favour chronicity, more recurrences, and side effects.[2,4,5] If corticosteroids are used, their tapering should be particularly slow, and in cases of recurrence, every effort should be made not to increase the dose or to reinstate corticosteroids. In selected infection-negative cases, AZA, IV immunoglobulin (IVIG) (immunomodulatory, but also antiviral), and anakinra, a recombinant IL-1b receptor antagonist, have been used, but strong evidence-based data are lacking.[2]

Treatment of the underlying cause of pericarditis

Treatment directed at the underlying cause of pericarditis is indicated in the following situations:

- Pericarditis due to bacterial infection:
  - Without appropriate antibiotic therapy, purulent bacterial pericarditis is usually fatal.
  - Empirical antibiotic therapy may be commenced, pending culture results. The choice of antibiotic is then tailored, based on the sensitivity of the causative organism.
  - Pericardial drainage is necessary for purulent pericarditis.
  - Intrapericardial thrombolysis should be considered to reduce the risk of constriction (level of evidence C, class IIa recommendation).
- Tuberculous pericarditis:
  - In the absence of antituberculous chemotherapy, tuberculous pericarditis is associated with high mortality.
  - Steroids may be considered as an adjunct to antituberculous therapy (level of evidence C, class IIb recommendation).
- Uraemic pericarditis:
  - Most patients with uraemic pericarditis respond to renal replacement therapy.
  - NSAIDs and corticosteroids (systemic or intrapericardial) may be considered when intensive dialysis is ineffective.
- Pericarditis due to autoimmune inflammatory conditions:
  - Treatment of the underlying disease and inflammatory condition may be effective.

Management of complications associated with pericarditis

- In patients with a significant pericardial effusion complicated by pericardial tamponade, urgent pericardiocentesis is essential. Patients with recurrent pericardial effusions may require a subxiphoid pericardiotomy.
- Patients with constrictive pericarditis may require a pericardiectomy.

References

1 Caforio AL, Pankuweit S, Arbustini E, *et al.*; European Society of Cardiology Working Group on Myocardial and Pericardial Diseases. Current state of knowledge on aetiology, diagnosis, management, and therapy of myocarditis: a position statement of the European Society of Cardiology Working Group on Myocardial and Pericardial Diseases. *Eur Heart J* 2013;**34**:2636–48.

2 Adler Y, Charron P, Imazio M, *et al.*; ESC Scientific Document Group. 2015 ESC Guidelines for the diagnosis and management of pericardial diseases: The Task Force for the Diagnosis and Management of Pericardial Diseases of the European Society of Cardiology (ESC). *Eur Heart J* 2015;**36**:2921–64.

3 Imazio M, Brucato A, Belli R, *et al.* Colchicine for the prevention of pericarditis: what we know and what we do not know in 2014—systematic review and meta-analysis. *J Cardiovasc Med* 2014;**15**:840–6.

4 Lotrionte M, Biondi-Zoccai G, Imazio M, et al. International collaborative systematic review of controlled clinical trials on pharmacologic treatments for acute pericarditis and its recurrences. *Am Heart J* 2010;**160**:662–70.

5 Brucato A, Brambilla G, Moreo A, *et al.* Long-term outcomes in difficult-to-treat patients with recurrent pericarditis. *Am J Cardiol* 2006;**98**:267–71.

Further reading

Alabed S, Cabello JB, Irving GJ, Qintar M, Burls A. Colchicine for pericarditis. *Cochrane Database Syst Rev* 2014;**8**:CD010652.

Chapter 5.3

Cardiomyopathy

Giovanni Boffa

Cardiomyopathy

Disease of the heart muscle is referred to as cardiomyopathy. Broadly, there are three main types of functional impairment in cardiomyopathy, although often there is some overlap:

- Hypertrophic cardiomyopathy (HCM).
- Dilated cardiomyopathy (DCM).
- Restrictive cardiomyopathy.

Hypertrophic cardiomyopathy

HCM is characterized by the presence of increased LV wall thickness that is not explained by loading conditions.[1] The prevalence of HCM in different adult populations is reported in the range of 0.02–0.23%. In 40–60% of cases, HCM is an autosomal dominant trait caused by mutations in cardiac sarcomere protein genes; in 5–10% of cases, HCM is caused by other genetic disorders, and in 25–30% of cases, it is sporadic. The LV diastolic function is impaired to various degrees in the majority of patients, and about two-thirds of patients have resting or provocable LVOTO. HCM can be asymptomatic or cause a wide range of clinical manifestations: symptoms and signs of HF (secondary to diastolic dysfunction), angina (due to increased myocardial oxygen demand and microvascular dysfunction), arrhythmias, syncope, and SCD.

Management

Management of HCM is directed towards minimizing symptoms and reducing complications. Use of prophylactic drug therapy in asymptomatic or minimally symptomatic patients to prevent or delay disease progression remains unfounded.

- β-*blockers*: reduce myocardial oxygen demand and improve LV filling via their negative chronotropic and inotropic effects. As a consequence, they may alleviate angina, as well as dyspnoea, and decrease LVOTO. Patients with symptomatic LVOTO should be treated initially with non-vasodilating β-blockers titrated to the maximum tolerated dose. Evidence-based data on the relative efficacy of individual β-blockers are not available.

There are no data to support the use of antiarrhythmics for the prevention of SCD in HCM. Use of β-blockers (and/or amiodarone) is today recommended only in patients with an ICD, who continue to have symptomatic ventricular arrhythmias or recurrent shocks despite optimal treatment. Use of β-blockers is recommended for controlling the ventricular rate in patients with paroxysmal, persistent, or permanent AF. Moreover, β-blockers are indicated, in addition to an ACEI, for the treatment of HF in patients with HF due to systolic compromise of LV function.

- *CCBs: verapamil* or *diltiazem* can be used when β-blockers are contraindicated or ineffective. The benefit of CCBs is thought to derive from their ability to address the hypercontractile systolic function, while improving diastolic relaxation and filling of the LV. Caution is needed when administering these drugs, especially in those with high LV filling pressure, as their vasodilating property may exaggerate the LV outflow gradient. *Dihydropyridine CCBs* are not recommended for the treatment of LVOTO.

CCBs can be successfully used to treat angina and reduce the ventricular rate in AF.

- *Disopyramide*: if β-blockers or CCBs alone are not sufficiently effective in reducing the outflow tract gradient, this class IA AAD may be added (titrated up to a maximum tolerated dose of usually 400–600mg/day). Disopyramide can abolish basal LV outflow pressure gradients and improve exercise tolerance.
- *Diuretics*: can improve dyspnoea in patients with increased pulmonary capillary pressure due to severely compromised LV diastolic function, and their use is mandatory if signs of fluid retention are present.
- Infective endocarditis prophylaxis is no longer recommended, even in patients with an outflow gradient.

The role of non-pharmacological treatment is of paramount importance in specific groups of patients. Septal reduction therapy (surgical myectomy or alcoholic ablation) is recommended in very symptomatic patients with an LV outflow gradient of 50mmHg, despite maximum tolerated medical therapy. ICD implantation is indicated in patients who have survived a cardiac arrest due to VT or VF, or who have spontaneous sustained VT causing syncope or haemodynamic compromise.

Cardiac transplantation may be indicated for end-stage patients who meet standard eligibility criteria. Ventricular assist devices can be used as a bridge to heart transplantation or destination therapy in selected patients.

Dilated cardiomyopathy

According to the position statement of the ESC Working Group on Myocardial and Pericardial Disease, DCM is defined by the presence of LV or biventricular dilatation and systolic dysfunction in the absence of abnormal loading conditions or CAD sufficient to cause global systolic impairment. The causes of DCM can be classified as genetic or non-genetic (drugs and toxins, myocarditis, peripartum DCM). Treatment of symptomatic patients should follow the therapeutic algorithm proposed by the 2016 ESC guidelines. The first-line treatment includes diuretics, ACE inhibition (or angiotensin receptor blockade), β-blockade, and aldosterone antagonism. The complex neprilysin inhibitor sacubitril/valsartan is recommended to replace ACEIs in patients who remain symptomatic despite optimal treatment. The I_f channel inhibitor ivabradine should be considered for patients in sinus rhythm and with a resting heart rate of >70bpm.

In symptomatic patients despite optimal medical treatment and with LVEF of <35%, implantation of ICD is recommended, with cardiac resynchronization function if the QRS duration is ≥150ms and in the presence of an LBBB QRS morphology.

LVAD implantation and heart transplantation can be the only solution in advanced HF patients.

Reference

1 Authors/Task Force members, Elliott PM, Anastasakis A, Borger MA, et al. 2014 ESC Guidelines on diagnosis and management of hypertrophic cardiomyopathy. The Task Force for the Diagnosis and Management of Hypertrophic Cardiomyopathy of the European Society of Cardiology (ESC). *Eur Heart J* 2014;35:2733–79.

Further reading

Pinto YM, Elliott PM, Arbustini E, *et al*. Proposal for a revised definition of dilated cardiomyopathy, hypokinetic non-dilated cardiomyopathy, and its implications for clinical practice: a position statement of the ESC working group on myocardial and pericardial diseases. *Eur Heart J* 2016;37:1850–8.

Chapter 5.4

Pulmonary hypertension

James Tonkin, Kate Ryan, and Brendan Madden

Introduction

Pulmonary hypertension describes an elevation in PAP as a consequence of one or more disease processes. Diagnosis is made during right heart catheterization with a mean pulmonary artery pressure (mPAP) of >25mmHg at rest.[1]

Pulmonary hypertension is divided into groups 1 to 5. Group 1 is characterized by plexogenic pulmonary arteriopathy on histology. In this group of patients, often described as having pulmonary arterial hypertension (PAH), the left atrial filling pressure is normal. This is measured at right heart catheterization as the pulmonary capillary wedge pressure (PCWP) and should be <15mmHg. PAH is also associated with an elevated pulmonary vascular resistance of >3 Wood units.

Group 2 is typically characterized by a PCWP of >15mmHg and is associated with left heart disease. This is the commonest cause of pulmonary hypertension, accounting for 68% of cases. Group 1 disorders only account for 2.7% of all cases.

Aetiology

(See Table 5.4.1.)[2]

Table 5.4.1 Aetiology of pulmonary hypertension

1 Primary causes 1' Pulmonary veno-occlusive disease and pulmonary capillary haemangiomatosis	1.1 Idiopathic 1.2 Heritable (BMPR2 and others) 1.3 Drug- and toxin-induced 1.4 Associated with: 1.4.1 Connective tissue disease 1.4.2 HIV infection 1.4.3 Portal hypertension 1.4.4 Congenital heart disease 1.4.5 Schistosomiasis 1'.1 Idiopathic 1'.2 Heritable (EIF2AK4) 1'.3 Drug- and toxin-induced 1'.4 Connective tissue disease (1'.4.1) or HIV infection (1'4.2)
2 Left heart disease	2.1 Left ventricular systolic dysfunction 2.2 Left ventricular diastolic dysfunction 2.3 Valvular disease 2.4 Congenital/acquired left heart inflow/outflow tract obstruction and congenital cardiomyopathies 2.5 Congenital/acquired pulmonary vein stenosis
3 Chronic lung disease	3.1 Chronic obstructive pulmonary disease 3.2 Interstitial lung disease 3.3 Mixed restrictive and obstructive pattern 3.4 Sleep-disordered breathing 3.5 Hypoventilation disorders 3.6 Chronic exposure to high altitude 3.7 Developmental lung diseases
4 Chronic thromboembolic pulmonary hypertension	4.1 Chronic thromboembolic pulmonary hypertension 4.2 Other pulmonary artery obstructions
5 Miscellaneous	5.1 Haematological disorders 5.2 Systemic disorders 5.3 Metabolic disorders 5.4 Others: thrombotic microangiopathy, fibrosing mediastinitis, chronic renal failure, segmental pulmonary hypertension

Pathophysiology

The pulmonary circulation is a low-pressure system. Typical systolic pulmonary arterial pressures are 15–30mmHg, associated with an mPAP of 9–20mmHg.

The pressure in the right ventricle is significantly lower than that in the left ventricle. It is thin-walled and suited to deliver large volumes of deoxygenated blood at low pressures to the lungs. Increases in PAP lead to increased strain on the right ventricle. This can lead to RV dilatation and impaired contractility. Furthermore, RV strain can lead to occlusion of the right coronary artery.

RV dilatation can cause septal flattening, restricting LV filling. This reduction in LV output impairs RV filling, eventually causing RV failure and circulatory collapse. RV failure is the commonest cause of death in patients.

Pathophysiology of group 1 disorders

In group 1 disorders, pulmonary vascular resistance is increased through structural changes to the pulmonary vascular bed. It occurs via three mechanisms:

1. Pulmonary artery vasoconstriction.
2. Vessel wall hyperplasia and proliferation.
3. In-vessel thrombosis.

These changes are influenced by genetic factors, systemic disorders, and environmental triggers. They occur predominantly via three pathways.

The nitric oxide pathway

Reduced activation of endothelial nitric oxide synthase (eNOS) occurs in pulmonary hypertension. eNOS stimulates the production of NO (see Fig. 5.4.1), which induces the guanylate cyclase enzyme. Guanylate cyclase converts guanosine triphosphate (GTP) to cyclic guanosine monophosphate (cGMP). cGMP inhibits the proliferation, and causes the relaxation, of pulmonary artery smooth muscle.

cGMP activates myosin light chain phosphatase to reduce the phosphorylation of myosin and reduces vascular tone. In addition, it prevents the influx of calcium, leading to less hypertrophy and hyperplasia. NO also reduces platelet aggregation and adhesion.

cGMP is broken down by PDE5. This is the mechanism through which PDE5 inhibitors, such as sildenafil, work.

The endothelin pathway

Pro-endothelin is converted into endothelin-1 (ET1) by the endothelin-converting enzyme (present in endothelial cells). ET1 is a potent

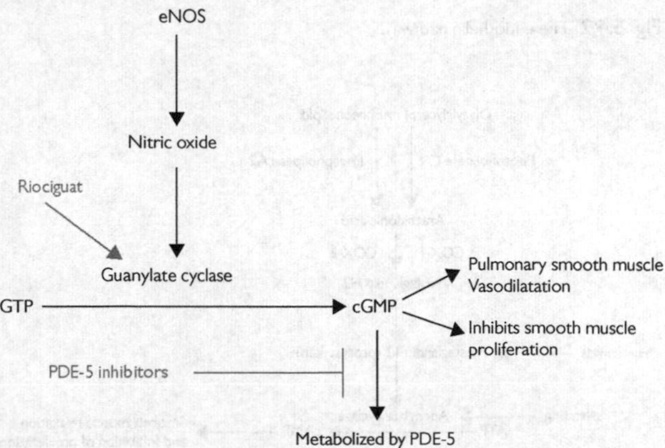

Fig. 5.4.1 The nitric oxide pathway.

vasoconstrictor. It acts as an agonist to ETa receptors (present in smooth muscle cells) and ETb receptors (present in smooth muscle cells and on endothelial cells). Activation of ETa receptors leads to pulmonary artery smooth muscle contraction, proliferation, and hypertrophy. However, ETb receptors on endothelial cells lead to the production of prostacyclin (PGI2) and NO. Endothelin receptor antagonists (ERAs) can block ETa and ETb receptors or ETa receptors alone (see Fig. 5.4.2).

The prostacyclin pathway

PGI2 is produced through the arachidonic acid pathway (see Fig. 5.4.3). Diacylglycerol or phospholipids are converted by phospholipase C and phospholipase A2 to arachidonic acid. This is then converted by COXs into prostaglandin H2. Prostaglandin H2 is converted by prostacyclin synthase into PGI2.

Prostacyclin stimulates adenylate cyclase, converting ATP into cyclic adenosine monophosphate (cAMP), which acts on pulmonary artery smooth muscle cells to cause smooth muscle relaxation and inhibit proliferation.

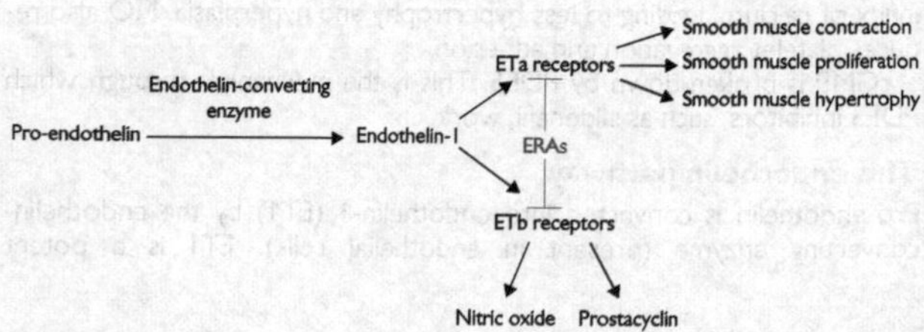

Fig. 5.4.2 The endothelin pathway.

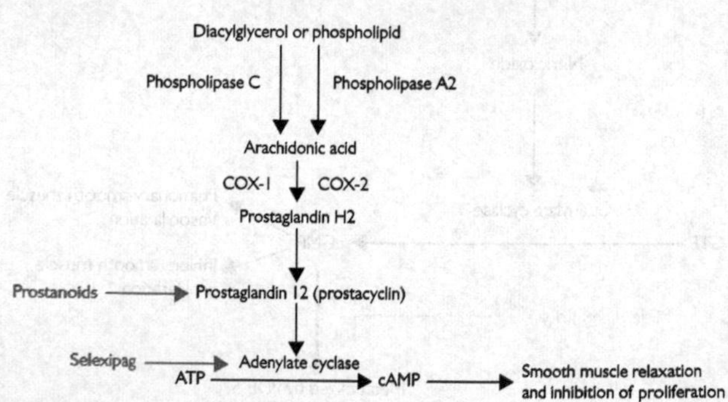

Fig. 5.4.3 The prostacyclin pathway.

Genetics

Genetic mutations have been identified in the bone morphogenetic type 2 receptor (BMPR2), a TGF-β ligand. The protein prevents smooth muscle proliferation and endothelial dysfunction; mutations in this receptor can lead to plexogenic pulmonary arteriopathy. Seventy-five per cent of hereditary PAH and 25% of sporadic PAH have heterozygous *BMPR2* mutations. Mutations in eukaryotic translation initiation factor 2 α kinase 4 (EIF2AK4) have been found in familial and sporadic cases of pulmonary veno-occlusive disease (PVOD).

Histopathology

Pulmonary arteries are usually thin-walled with a wide lumen to reduce pulmonary vascular resistance. However, in PAH, vascular abnormalities, known as plexogenic pulmonary arteriopathy, occur.[3]

1. Medial hypertrophy of pulmonary smooth muscle cells extending to the arterioles—this process is reversible upon treatment.
2. Cellular intimal proliferation occurring in arteries and arterioles—this can lead to blockage of the vessels; this process is also reversible.
3. Intimal fibrosis—deposition of collagen in the intima in a concentric pattern; once this occurs, it is irreversible.
4. Plexiform lesions—dilated segments of pulmonary arteries occur beyond branching points. Fibrinoid necrosis can occur within the cavity wall, and beyond this, the vessel becomes thin-walled and tortuous. This is an irreversible process and suggests severe disease.
5. Dilatation lesions—thin-walled, tortuous arteries without intraluminal plexuses.
6. Fibrinoid arteritis—fibrinoid necrosis of the arterial wall, with intimal proliferation.

Pathophysiology of group 1' diseases

Group 1' diseases comprise PVOD and pulmonary capillary haemangiomatosis (PCH). These are uncommon conditions with pathological changes in pulmonary veins and pulmonary capillaries. In PVOD, there is fibrous intimal thickening of pulmonary venules and veins, leading to occlusion. This leads to raised pulmonary venous resistance. In PCH, there is cellular proliferation of pulmonary capillaries, leading to increased pulmonary vascular resistance. Although these patients develop pulmonary hypertension, pulmonary vasodilators can cause decompensation due to reduced left atrial filling in the presence of increased venous resistance.

Pathophysiology of groups 2–5 diseases

Group 2 diseases

Pulmonary hypertension due to left heart disease can be caused by restrictive disease, cardiomyopathy, or VHD. It occurs in 60% of patients with HFrEF and in up to 70% of those with HFpEF. Restriction of forward blood flow leads to pulmonary venous hypertension and subsequent PAH. Left atrial pressure is elevated due this restriction of anterograde flow; this is measured as a raised PCWP.[4]

Initially, the pulmonary vascular resistance may be normal. Pulmonary arteries respond to compensate for raised pulmonary venous pressure. However, vascular remodelling occurs through the release of thromboxane A2 and serotonin (5-HT) and activation of the RAS. This leads to raised pulmonary vascular resistance, initially at exercise and then at rest.

Group 3 diseases

Pulmonary hypertension secondary to chronic lung disease can be secondary to obstructive lung disease, restrictive lung disease, or sleep-disordered breathing. Hypoxic pulmonary vasoconstriction is a mechanism whereby the pulmonary circulation redistributes blood to areas well ventilated, to improve ventilation/perfusion (V/Q) matching.[5] In addition to this, cigarette smoke causes inflammation through TNF-α and IL-6 pathways, leading to pulmonary vasoconstriction. It impairs vasodilatation by antagonizing NO and causes smooth muscle proliferation through endothelin and vascular endothelial growth factor (VEGF).

Group 4 diseases

Pulmonary hypertension secondary to chronic thromboembolic disease is characterized by previous or recurrent PE; 0.5–2% of patients with acute PE will go on to develop chronic thromboembolic pulmonary hypertension (CTEPH). Fibrous obstruction due to previous PEs cause obstruction to the pulmonary circulation, leading to elevated pulmonary vascular resistance. Platelets also release serotonin, causing pulmonary vasoconstriction.

Distal thromboembolic disease may show similarities with group 1 diseases with vascular remodelling and plexogenic changes. There are higher levels of asymmetric dimethylarginine, which is an inhibitor of NO and inhibits vasodilatation and promotes vascular smooth muscle proliferation.

Clinical features

History

The commonest symptom is exertional breathlessness. However, patients also report fatigue, light-headedness, chest pain, and cough. Orthopnoea and paroxysmal nocturnal dyspnoea can also occur. These symptoms usually suggest RV dysfunction. Syncope suggests severe RV failure. Abdominal distension and oedema also occur. Severe mechanical obstruction by large pulmonary arteries can lead to haemoptysis, wheeze, and myocardial ischaemia.

Clinical examination

Features of pulmonary hypertension include:

- Parasternal heave.
- Loud P2 and S4.
- Pansystolic murmur of TR and *v* waves in the JVP.
- Raised JVP, S3, and ascites, suggesting RV failure.

  Other clinical features to suggest the aetiology include:
- Cyanosis/clubbing associated with Eisenmenger's and congenital heart disease.
- Sclerodactyly and Raynaud's phenomenon in systemic sclerosis.
- Caput medusae and splenomegaly seen in portal hypertension.

World Health Organization functional class

The World Health Organization (WHO) functional classification in pulmonary hypertension is a predictor of survival and disease progression.

1. Patients with pulmonary hypertension but are not limited by ordinary physical activity.
2. Patients are comfortable at rest, but ordinary activity leads to symptoms such as shortness of breath or fatigue.
3. Patients with marked limitation of physical activity but are comfortable at rest.
4. Patients unable to carry out any activity without symptoms.

Investigations

ECG

While often normal, there may be features of pulmonary hypertension such as right axis deviation, P-pulmonale, and incomplete or complete RBBB.

Patients can also develop AF, atrial flutter, or multifocal atrial tachycardias.

Chest radiograph

Chest X-ray may show prominent central pulmonary arteries, with absence of pulmonary vessels peripherally. Underlying chronic lung diseases or features of pulmonary oedema in patients with left heart disease can be seen. Pulmonary artery calcification can be seen in left-to-right shunts.

Echocardiography

Echocardiography is the initial screening test for pulmonary hypertension (see Fig. 5.4.4). The TR jet is used as an estimate for the RV systolic pressure. However, this can be an overestimate or an underestimate.

A TR velocity of <2.8m/s, without other signs of pulmonary hypertension, represents a low risk for pulmonary hypertension.

A TR velocity of 2.8–3.4m/s represents an intermediate risk for pulmonary hypertension.

A TR velocity of >3.4m/s represents a high risk for pulmonary hypertension.

An echocardiogram may show other features such as TR, RV dilatation, and impaired RV systolic function. Pericardial effusions and severe TR are

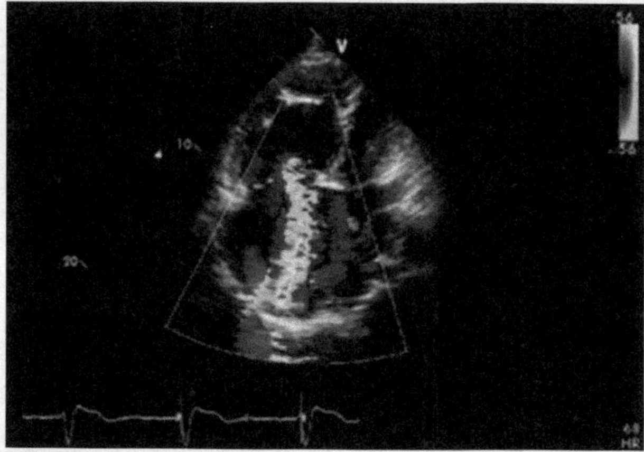

Fig. 5.4.4 An echocardiogram showing a tricuspid regurgitant jet which is used to estimate the pulmonary artery systolic pressure.

Reproduced from Madden BP. Pulmonary Hypertension and pregnancy. *Int J Obstet Anesth* 2009;**18**;156–164 with permission from Elsevier.

indicators of poor prognosis. RV size and TR velocity can be used to determine the response to treatment. Tricuspid annular plane systolic excursion (TAPSE) measures shortening of the right ventricle. A TAPSE of <15mm is associated with higher mortality.

The echocardiogram may also suggest left heart disease aetiology such as impaired LVEF, diastolic dysfunction, or VHD. An atrial septal defect (ASD) or VSD can also be seen.

Pulmonary function tests

Pulmonary function tests can indicate whether chronic lung disease is contributing to pulmonary hypertension. However, pulmonary function tests can be abnormal in PAH as well. Most PAH patients have a low transfer factor [diffusion of carbon monoxide (DLCO)]. Patients with interstitial lung disease, PVOD, and scleroderma may have a very low DLCO.

V/Q or computed tomography pulmonary angiography

V/Q scanning assesses pulmonary blood flow and ventilation to look for mismatch. In PE or CTEPH, there may be one or multiple areas of mismatched ventilation and perfusion defects. During CT pulmonary angiography (CTPA) (see Fig. 5.4.5), contrast is given to visualize the pulmonary arterial circulation. In pulmonary hypertension, the pulmonary artery is often larger than the aorta. There may also be enlargement of the segmental pulmonary arteries, with small arterioles. Reflux of contrast into the inferior vena cava (IVC) and hepatic veins suggests TR. In CTEPH, filling defects may be laminated or crescentic, adherent to the wall, or web-like. The distribution determines whether the thrombus is surgically accessible.

Overnight pulse oximetry or polysomnography

Overnight pulse oximetry as a screening test or polysomnography can help diagnose obstructive sleep apnoea or obesity hypoventilation syndrome.

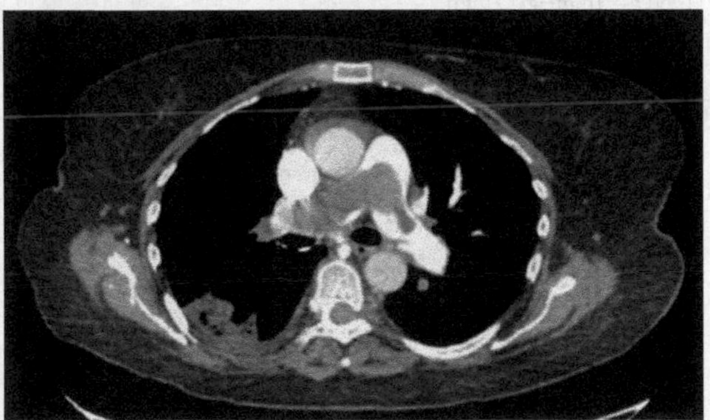

Fig. 5.4.5 CT pulmonary angiogram showing a large central thrombus in the main pulmonary artery.

Blood tests

BNPs are released in response to ventricular stretch and their levels are elevated in pulmonary hypertension.[6]

High D-dimer values, although not specific for pulmonary hypertension, are seen in those with more severe haemodynamics.

Full blood count, urea and electrolytes, and thyroid function tests should be checked in all patients. LFTs may indicate liver disease and hepatic congestion and should be monitored for patients on ERA therapy. Serology testing for HIV and hepatitis and an autoimmune panel should be performed in those with unexplained causes. Those with CTEPH should have thrombophilia screening with antiphospholipid antibodies and lupus anticoagulant.

The 6-minute walk test

The 6-minute walk test (6MWT) is a measure of functional capacity as a surrogate of oxygen consumption. However, motivation and musculoskeletal limitations can affect the result.

Right heart catheter study

The right heart catheter study remains the gold standard in the diagnosis of pulmonary hypertension, to assess haemodynamics and perform vasoreactivity testing. This procedure, performed under local anaesthesia, is used to measure right-sided pressures. Using a sheath in either the basilic, internal jugular, subclavian, or femoral vein, a pulmonary artery catheter is inserted. ECG monitoring occurs throughout to detect arrhythmias.

Mean, systolic, and diastolic pressures are measured for the right atrium, right ventricle, and pulmonary artery, as well as PCWP. Blood gases are taken for SvO_2 and can be taken at the pulmonary artery, RV, and right atrial levels to look for evidence of shunts.

Thermodilution or the Fick method is used to measure CO, and pulmonary vascular resistance can be calculated in Wood units (1 WU = 1mmHg/L/min).

$$PVR = (mPAP - PCWP)/CO$$

Vasodilator testing

In patients with idiopathic or drug-induced PAH, vasodilator testing can be used to determine the suitability for CCBs. IV esoprostenol, IV adenosine, inhaled NO, or inhaled iloprost is given at the time of the right heart catheter study.

A positive result is a >10mmHg drop in mPAP to <40mmHg, with an increased or unchanged CO. Vasodilator testing should be avoided in patients with an elevated PCWP or low CO.

Management (general measures)

The aim of treatment is to maintain good functional status and preserve RV function. This involves specific pulmonary hypertension therapies and treatment of underlying causes.

Treatment goals

- To improve functional class (class I or II).
- 6MWT of >380m.
- Normal size and function of the right ventricle on echocardiography.
- Normal BNP levels.
- Right atrial pressure of <8mmHg, cardiac index of >2.5mL/kg/min.

General management of group 1 diseases

Despite advances in therapy, maternal mortality remains high during pregnancy and puerperium. Patients should be counselled regarding birth control, and the progesterone-only pill is preferred. If women decide to proceed to delivery, they should be managed in a specialist centre with an MDT approach.[7]

Pneumococcal and influenza vaccinations are recommended, as pneumonia is a common cause of death. Physical activity is encouraged within their symptom limits.

Oxygen is also used for patients with PaO_2 of <8, and ambulatory oxygen for patients who get symptomatic benefit. Patients with WHO functional classes 3 and 4 and those with arterial blood oxygen pressure of below 8kPa should be considered for in-flight oxygen.[2]

Psychosocial support is essential, as anxiety and depression are common. Patients should be signposted to local support groups and psychological services. Charities such as the Pulmonary Hypertension Association are invaluable for providing education for patients, family, and carers.

Thrombosis is known to be a pathological contributor to PAH. There is a survival benefit in patients with idiopathic PAH taking anticoagulants. However, in scleroderma-associated pulmonary hypertension, anticoagulation is avoided.[8]

Iron deficiency anaemia is common and, if detected, should be investigated. Often absorption is impaired and patients often require IV replacement. Diuretics are used to control oedema and ascites. All patients should be managed in designated (or shared-care) centres with expertise in pulmonary hypertension.

Calcium channel blockers

Only 5–10% of patients have a haemodynamic response to acute vasodilators. Patients with idiopathic or anorexigen-induced pulmonary hypertension, with a vasodilator response, have improved survival with CCBs. Other group 1 pulmonary hypertension patients (even if they have a positive vasodilator response) do not have a survival benefit with CCBs.

High-dose CCBs are used: nifedipine (120–140mg daily), diltiazem (240–720mg), or amlodipine (20mg). Common side effects include headache, lower limb oedema, and hypotension. After 3–4 months, these patients are reassessed for response.

If CCBs do not improve functional status or show haemodynamic improvement, advanced vasodilator therapy is started.

Advanced vasodilator therapy

There are five groups of advanced vasodilator therapy:

- PDE-5 inhibitors.
- ERAs.
- Prostacyclin analogues (prostanoids).
- Selective prostacyclin receptor agonists.
- Guanylate cyclase stimulators.

Phosphodiesterase type 5 inhibitors

PDE-5 inhibitors prevent the breakdown of cGMP. cGMP causes smooth muscle relaxation and inhibits proliferation. Side effects include headaches, hearing loss, dyspepsia, myalgia, flushing, epistaxis, hypotension, and visual disturbances.

Sildenafil

- Oral and IV formulations; dosed at 25–50mg tds.
- Sildenafil was shown in the double-blind RCT Sildenafil Use in Pulmonary Arterial Hypertension (SUPER) to improve exercise capacity, functional class, and mPAP. These results have been replicated in other trials and persist over the longer term. Improvements in quality of life have also been shown.

Tadalafil

- 40mg od; orally active.
- In the Pulmonary Arterial Hypertension and Response to Tadalafil (PHIRST) study: 40mg was found to improve 6MWT, time to clinical deterioration, and health-related quality of life. However, statistically significant improvements in functional class were not seen.

Vardenafil

- 5mg bd; orally active
- RCTs have shown improvements in exercise capacity and right heart catheterization measurements, when compared to placebo.

Endothelin receptor antagonists

ERAs can block either ETa or both ETa and ETb receptors. This prevents smooth muscle proliferation and the vasoconstricting effects of endothelin. ETb receptors cause vasodilatation; however, selective ETa antagonists have not been shown to be more effective. All agents can cause hepatic transaminitis and so require frequent liver function testing. Sitaxentan is no longer used due to hepatotoxicity. Other side effects include oligospermia and anaemia, and all are teratogenic.

Bosentan

- Bosentan blocks ETa and ETb receptors.
- 125mg bd.
- Licensed for WHO functional class II–IV disease.
- The Bosentan Randomized Trial of Endothelin Antagonist Therapy-1 (BREATHE-1) and Endothelin Antagonist tRial in miLdlY symptomatic PAH patients (EARLY) RCTs showed improved 6MWT, WHO functional status, and Borg score for breathlessness, as well as haemodynamics, at right heart catheterization.

Ambrisentan

- Ambrisentan is a selective ETa receptor antagonist. It is licensed in WHO functional class II and III disease.
- 5–10mg od.
- The Pulmonary Arterial Hypertension, Randomized, Double-Blind, Placebo-Controlled, Multicenter, Efficacy Study 1 and 2 (ARIES 1 and 2), both RCTs against placebo, showed improvements in 6MWT, WHO functional class, time to clinical worsening, and BNP levels.

Macitentan

- Macitentan: ETa and ETb receptor antagonist, but with a 50-fold higher affinity for ETa receptors. It is licensed for WHO functional class II and III disease.
- 10mg od.
- In the Study with an Endothelin Receptor Antagonist in Pulmonary arterial Hypertension to Improve cliNical outcome (SERAPHIN) trial, 10mg macitentan showed a statistical improvement in time to admission, functional class, and 6MWT. There was also a non-statistical trend towards improved mortality.

Prostanoids

Prostanoids replenish prostacyclin, usually produced by endothelial cells. They stimulate adenylate cyclase to convert ATP to cAMP. This leads to smooth muscle relaxation and inhibits proliferation of smooth muscle cells, as well as platelet aggregation. Due to oral agents lacking efficacy in trials, these are typically given via a central venous catheter (CVC), SC, or as an aerosol.

Epoprostenol

Epoprostenol is licensed for WHO functional class III and IV disease. It is given as a continuous IV infusion through a tunnelled CVC due to its short half-life. Side effects include flushing, headache, diarrhoea, jaw, and leg pain. Administration can precipitate high-output HF, and infection and thrombosis of the CVC can occur.

When added to conventional therapy, epoprostenol improves 6MWT and haemodynamics at right heart catheterization. It also improves functional class and overall mortality.

Treprostinil

Treprostinil is an analogue of epoprostenol, which can be given SC, inhaled, or via a CVC. It is licensed for WHO functional class II–IV disease.

The subcutaneous form improves exercise capacity and haemodynamics. However, infusion site pain frequently occurs, and a subcutaneous catheter is required. A randomized trial compared inhaled treprostinil to placebo in patients already on sildenafil or bosentan. Improvements were seen in 6MWT, quality of life, and BNP levels, but not breathlessness or functional class. Unfortunately, an oral form has not been shown to be effective. The FREEDOM-C study showed no improvements in exercise capacity or functional class.

Iloprost

Iloprost can be given as an aerosol or via a CVC. The main side effects include flushing and jaw pain. Inhaled iloprost added to conventional therapy has been shown to improve NYHA class, 6MWT, breathlessness, and quality of life in patients with functional class III or IV.

Beraprost

Beraprost is an oral prostacyclin. Side effects include headache, flushing, jaw pain, and diarrhoea. Used as monotherapy in patients with functional class III or IV, it improves 6MWT, but not haemodynamics at right heart catheterization. However, the effect seems to be short-lived, with no benefit seen at 12 months.

Selexipag

Selexipag is an oral prostacyclin receptor agonist. The main side effects include headaches, diarrhoea, nausea, and jaw pain. The Prostacyclin (PGI2) Receptor Agonist In Pulmonary Arterial Hypertension (GRIPHON) trial randomized patients to selexipag or placebo, including treatment-naïve, and on PDE-5 inhibitors, ERAs, or both.[9] There was no statistically significant mortality benefit. However, there was a statistically significant improvement in the composite endpoint of death or complication of pulmonary hypertension. Selexipag also improves exercise capacity and pulmonary vascular resistance at right heart catheterization.

Riociguat

Riociguat is a soluble guanylate cyclase stimulator. It enhances cGMP production; however, it cannot be used with PDE-5 inhibitors due to a risk for hypotension. The Riociguat clinical Effects Studied in Patients with Insufficient Treatment response to PDE-5 inhibitors (RESPITE) study looked at patients with PAH who had an insufficient response to sildenafil and switched them to riociguat after a washout period. The riociguat group had improved functional class, 6MWT, and haemodynamics at right heart catheterization. The main adverse effect is syncope.

Combination treatment

Combination treatments are used in pulmonary hypertension to target different pathways. Treatment usually starts with monotherapy and progressing to dual/triple therapy to achieve treatment targets. However, in those with severe disease, combination therapy is sometimes started upfront. When deciding on combination therapy, drug interactions need to be taken into account.

Sildenafil and bosentan are often used together. However, in COMPASS-2, there was no improvement in mortality or functional status, but a modest improvement in exercise capacity. Bosentan is noted to reduce the plasma concentration of sildenafil by inducing CYP3A4.

Ambrisentan and tadalafil do not interact in the same way. The Ambrisentan and Tadalafil in Patients with Pulmonary Arterial Hypertension (AMBITION) study compared combined ambrisentan and tadalafil to monotherapy. While it did not improve mortality, admissions were reduced and exercise capacity increased.

The Bosentan Randomized Trial of Endothelin Antagonist Therapy-2 (BREATHE-2) looked at the addition of bosentan to esoprostenol. There was a trend towards improvements in exercise capacity and functional class; however, this was not statistically significant.

There is more evidence for the combination of prostanoids and PDE-5 inhibitors. A double-blind, placebo-controlled trial compared sildenafil to placebo in patients on IV epoprostenol. This showed improvement in exercise capacity, haemodynamics, time to clinical worsening, and health-related quality of life.

Sildenafil and riociguat together are contraindicated. The PATENT-PLUS study was terminated early due to unfavourable outcomes.[10]

Treatment algorithm

1. Vasoreactivity test: responders—stepwise increase to high-dose CCBs.
2. If negative: group into low, medium, or high risk.
   - Low risk: oral monotherapy or oral combination therapy.
   - High risk: initial combination therapy with IV epoprostenol.
3. If inadequate response—proceed to double or triple sequential therapy.
4. If inadequate response—consider referral for transplantation.

Management of group 2 diseases

Pulmonary hypertension is common in patients with left heart disease and is often seen as a marker of the severity of the disease. Optimization of the underlying disease is the priority, and this includes valve repair/replacement and treatment of HF and modifying risk factors for CV disease. Other causes such as coexisting respiratory disease or thromboembolic disease should be treated. Advanced vasodilator therapies do not improve exercise capacity or symptoms and can precipitate acute LV failure.

Management of group 3 diseases

This group is categorized into moderate disease (mPAP >25) and severe disease (mPAP >35 or >25 with low CO).

Treatment is directed at the underlying condition and treating the concurrent heart disease or CTEPH. Long-term oxygen therapy has been shown to reduce progression in COPD, and diuretics help optimize fluid balance. Vasodilators are not used, as they reverse hypoxic vasoconstriction and impair gas exchange by reversing mechanisms that improve V/Q matching. Trials of PDE-5 inhibitors and ERAs have not shown a benefit and, in some cases, worsened exercise capacity in COPD and pulmonary fibrosis.

Management of chronic thromboembolic pulmonary hypertension

All patients who are diagnosed with CTEPH require lifelong anticoagulation.

Pulmonary thromboendarterectomy

Pulmonary endarterectomy is the treatment of choice. This involves removal of fibrous obstructive tissue from the pulmonary tree.

V/Q, CT, and MRI are used to determine operability. Twenty to 40% of cases of CTEPH are inoperable.

A median sternotomy is performed, and the patient is placed on extracorporeal circulation. Two incisions are made in the proximal pulmonary artery, and the fibrous occlusion is removed. There is a 5% mortality associated with the procedure, and 5–10% have pulmonary hypertension afterwards.

Percutaneous balloon angioplasty remains an evolving technique for patients unsuitable for pulmonary endarterectomy. Reperfusion injury and pulmonary artery perforation remain as significant complications.

Medical therapy

Diuretics and oxygen are often needed. Vasodilator therapy is off licence for use in CTEPH to treat microvascular disease. These are often used as a bridge to surgery for patients with significant pulmonary hypertension.

Sildenafil has been shown to improve pulmonary vascular resistance, exercise capacity, and functional status in patients with inoperable CTEPH. Bosentan has been used in patients with inoperable disease. In the Bosentan Effects in iNopErable Forms of chronIc Thromboembolic pulmonary hypertension (BENEFiT) trial, there were statistically significant improvements in pulmonary vascular resistance, but not in 6MWT. Inhaled prostanoids have also been shown to improve haemodynamics preoperatively.

Riociguat has shown promising effects in CTEPH. The Chronic Thromboembolic Pulmonary Hypertension Soluble Guanylate Cyclase–Stimulator Trial 1 (CHEST-1) and CHEST-2 showed improvements in exercise capacity and WHO functional class in patients with inoperable or persistent CTEPH. This is currently used for patients with inoperable CTEPH.

Other surgical treatments

Atrial septostomy

Atrial septostomy is occasionally used in Eisenmenger's syndrome and group 1 diseases. It is only used in patients on maximal medical therapy and with WHO functional class IV with refractory right HF.

Either through a surgical incision or balloon dilatation via a right heart catheter, a right-to-left shunt is formed through the atrial septum. This decompresses the right ventricle, increases LV preload, and improves CO. It is typically used as a palliative procedure or as a bridge to lung transplantation. The mortality rate has been quoted as 15%.

Lung transplantation

Lung transplantation is occasionally used as treatment for patients with advanced pulmonary hypertension, who have not responded to conventional medical therapy. It is most commonly used for idiopathic pulmonary hypertension, usually involving bilateral lung transplantation. Referral is advised for patients with WHO functional class III or IV or those with progressive disease.

Post-operatively, there is immediate improvement in afterload; however, RV function does not improve immediately. NO, inotropes, and vasopressors are required in the immediate post-operative period. RV assist devices are sometimes required. Graft dysfunction is a concern in the post-operative period, secondary to ischaemia–reperfusion injury, haemorrhage, infection, or acute rejection.

The procedure has a 5-year survival of approximately 75%. Outcomes are better for bilateral lung transplantation for idiopathic PAH. However, in Eisenmenger's syndrome, the outcomes are best for combined heart–lung transplantation.

Management of specific diseases

HIV

The pathogenesis of how HIV infection leads to pulmonary hypertension is unclear. The prevalence is estimated at 0.46%. Although uncommon, it is associated with higher mortality. Anticoagulation should be avoided due to bleeding risk and drug reactions. Pulmonary hypertension is sometimes reversible with antiviral therapy. The algorithm should follow that for group 1 diseases. However, drug interactions need to be considered.

Portal hypertension

Pulmonary hypertension can occur in up to 5% of patients with portal hypertension. However, this does not correlate with the severity of portal hypertension estimated by the Model for End-stage Liver Disease (MELD) score. Treatment is similar to patients with idiopathic pulmonary arterial hypertension. However, anticoagulation is avoided due to bleeding risk. Propranolol (used for prophylaxis of variceal bleeds) is usually stopped due to its negatively inotropic effects.

PDE-5 inhibitors, ERAs, prostanoids, and riociguat have been used. Bosentan is avoided due to hepatotoxicity and hepatic clearance, and ambrisentan and macitentan are often used instead.

All patients considered for liver transplantation should be screened for pulmonary hypertension, as this is a risk factor for poor outcome after transplantation. Patients should be treated for pulmonary hypertension, and MDT discussion regarding transplantation is needed.

Pulmonary veno-occlusive disease and pulmonary capillary haemangiomatosis

In addition to CT imaging, bronchoalveolar lavage is necessary to look for alveolar haemorrhage for diagnosis. This may show a higher percentage of haemosiderin-laden macrophages. At right heart catheterization, the PCWP is often normal. Vasodilator testing can lead to acute pulmonary oedema. In hereditary cases, patients should be tested for the *EIF2AK4* mutation. Occasionally, patients need to proceed to surgical lung biopsy to make the diagnosis.

All patients should be referred for transplantation on diagnosis. Oxygen and diuretics can be used, and occasionally, slow IV doses of epoprostenol as a bridge to transplantation. However, vasodilators can precipitate pulmonary oedema.

Congenital heart disease and Eisenmenger's syndrome

Systemic-to-pulmonary shunts lead to high pressure in the pulmonary circulation and pulmonary arteriopathy. When pulmonary vascular resistance is greater than systemic vascular resistance, a right-to-left shunt occurs (Eisenmenger's syndrome). However, pulmonary hypertension can also occur in patients with congenital heart disease without shunts, due to an elevated left atrial pressure.

PDE-5 inhibitors, ERAs, and prostanoids are used in Eisenmenger's syndrome. However, CCBs are not. Sildenafil has been shown to improve functional class and haemodynamics. Bosentan improves exercise capacity and mPAP.

If pulmonary thromboembolism or features of congestive cardiac failure are present, patients should be anticoagulated. If there are symptoms of hyperviscosity and the haematocrit exceeds 65%, venesection should be considered.

Heart–lung transplantation is performed in specific cases.

Connective tissue disease and systemic sclerosis

PAH is associated with systemic sclerosis, SLE, mixed connective tissue diseases, Sjögren's syndrome, RA, and dermatomyositis.

In systemic sclerosis, pulmonary hypertension can occur as PAH or as a consequence of interstitial lung disease or left heart disease. All patients should undergo annual echocardiography, lung function testing including transfer factor, and blood tests including BNP levels, anti-centromere antibodies, and serum urate levels. The DETECT study has identified an algorithm to determine who should proceed to right heart catheterization.

In patients with SLE and connective tissue disease, immunosuppression can lead to improvement in 6MWT. Patients typically do not respond to CCBs. Also, in systemic sclerosis, there is a higher risk for bleeding, and so the risks and benefits need to be considered before starting anticoagulation. Advanced vasodilator therapy, particularly epoprostenol, is used in connective tissue disease and scleroderma-associated pulmonary hypertension.

Pulmonary hypertension and general anaesthesia

In pulmonary hypertension, the right ventricle is sensitive to changes in preload and afterload. Anaesthetic agents typically lower systemic vascular resistance, reducing the venous return and RV filling. Further to this, hypoxia, hypercarbia, hypothermia, acidaemia, pain, and high PEEP can increase pulmonary vascular resistance. Arterial lines are often used to detect drops in systemic vascular resistance. Pulmonary artery catheters can also be used to detect PAPs and monitor CO. Anaesthetic agents that do not increase PAPs, such as isoflurane, and those that do not cause myocardial depression, such as fentanyl, are often used. Planning around general anaesthesia should involve an MDT, including surgeons, anaesthetists, intensivists, and pulmonary hypertension specialists.[11]

Pulmonary hypertension emergencies

Advanced right ventricular failure

There is high mortality in patients with PAH admitted to the ICU with RV failure. Triggers, such as infection, anaemia, and arrhythmias, should be identified and treated early. Infection and anaemia can increase cardiac demand, while arrhythmias and thromboembolism increase afterload. Patients are closely monitored with an arterial line, a pulmonary artery catheter, and serial echocardiography.

Fluid balance should be optimized with IV diuretics. IV prostacyclin and PDE-5 inhibitors reduce afterload but can lead to hypotension. Inhaled NO and iloprost can be used, particularly in intubated patients post-cardiac surgery. Inotropes (such as dobutamine, milrinone, and levosimendan) support the right ventricle, while vasopressin and noradrenaline are used as vasopressors.

High-flow oxygen and NIV are used for respiratory support. Intubation should be avoided, as it frequently leads to haemodynamic collapse due to non-selective vasodilatation.

Veno-arterial extracorporeal membrane oxygenation

If patients are considered for heart–lung transplantation and have not responded to medical therapy, veno-arterial extracorporeal life support can be considered as a bridge to transplantation. This can be done without the need for intubation.

Arrhythmias

Atrial arrhythmias are common in pulmonary hypertension and can precipitate RV failure, as CO is reduced with reduced ventricular filling. The commonest arrhythmias are AF and atrial flutter.

Reverting to sinus rhythm and maintenance of sinus rhythm is key to survival. A study showed that those who remain in sinus rhythm had a 2-year mortality of 6%, compared to 82% in those with persistent AF. Electrical cardioversion and radiofrequency ablation are used to restore sinus rhythm. Digoxin and amiodarone are used to maintain sinus rhythm, as these are not negatively inotropic.

Haemoptysis

Haemoptysis in PAH is usually as a result of abnormal pulmonary vessels eroding into bronchi. Once haemoptysis occurs, anticoagulation should be stopped. Bronchoscopic intervention is often not effective at controlling bleeding, and bronchial artery embolization is required. Patients should also be considered for lung transplantation. Occasionally, repeated embolization is needed as a bridge to transplantation.

Mechanical complications

Dilatation of the pulmonary artery, dissections, and aneurysms can lead to mechanical obstruction of bronchi, pulmonary veins, coronary arteries, or recurrent laryngeal nerves. Patients can present with breathlessness, anginal chest pain, or vocal changes. Abnormal dilatation of the pulmonary arteries can be diagnosed on CT with contrast. If left main stem occlusion occurs, angiography with stenting can be done. All patients with mechanical complications should be considered for transplantation.

References

1 Hoeper MM, Bogaard HJ, Condliffe R, *et al*. Definitions and diagnosis of pulmonary hypertension. *J Am Coll Cardiol* 2013;**62**(Suppl):D42–50.

2 Galiè N, Humbert M, Vachiery JL, *et al*.; ESC Scientific Document Group. 2015 ESC/ERS Guidelines for the diagnosis and treatment of pulmonary hypertension. The Joint Task Force for the European Society of Cardiology (ESC) and the European Respiratory Society (ERS). *Eur Heart J* 2015;**37**:67–119.

3 Lourenco AP, Fontoura D, Henriques-Coelho T, Leite-Moreira AF. Current pathophysiological concepts and management of pulmonary hypertension. *Int J Cardiol* 2012;**155**:350–61.

4 Moraes DL, Colucci WS, Givertz MM. Secondary pulmonary hypertension in chronic heart failure: the role of the endothelium in pathophysiology and management. *Circulation* 2000;**102**:1718–23.

5 Wright JL, Levy RD, Churg A. Pulmonary hypertension in chronic obstructive pulmonary disease: current theories of pathogenesis and their implications for treatment. *Thorax* 2005;**60**:605–9.

6 Wilkins MR, Paul GA, Strange GW, *et al*. Sildenafil versus endothelial receptor antagonist for pulmonary hypertension (SERAPH) study. *Am J Respir Crit Care Med* 2005;**171**:1292–7.

7 Madden BP. Pulmonary hypertension and pregnancy. *Int J Obstet Anesth* 2009;**18**:156–64.

8 Olsson KM, Delcroix M, Gohfrani HA, *et al*. Anticoagulation and survival in pulmonary arterial hypertension: results from the Comparative, Prospective Registry of Newly Initiated Therapies for Pulmonary Hypertension (COMPERA). *Circulation* 2014;**129**:57–65.

9 Sitbon O, Channick R, Chin KM, *et al*.; GRIPHON Investigators. Selexipag for the treatment of pulmonary arterial hypertension. *N Engl J Med* 2015;**373**:2522–33.

10 Galiè N, Müller K, Scalise AV, Grünig E. PATENT-PLUS: a blinded, randomised and extension study of riociguat plus sildenafil in pulmonary arterial hypertension. *Eur Respir J* 2015;**45**:1314–22.

11 Madden BP (ed). *Treatment of pulmonary hypertension. Current Cardiovascular Therapy*. Springer International Publishing: Cham, Switzerland; 2015.

angiography with [illegible] can be done; all patients who [illegible] ications should be considered for transplantation.

References

1. [illegible]
2. [illegible] N, Humbert M, Vachiery JL, et al. 2015 ESC/ERS Guidelines for the diagnosis and treatment of pulmonary hypertension [illegible] (ERS). *Eur Heart J* 2016;37:67–119.
3. [illegible] pulmonary hypertension [illegible]
4. [illegible] pulmonary hypertension [illegible]
5. [illegible]
6. [illegible]
7. [illegible]
8. [illegible] pulmonary hypertension [illegible]
9. [illegible]
10. [illegible]
11. [illegible]

Section 6

Management of cardiovascular disease in pregnancy and lactation and in the presence of comorbidities

Section editors

Debasish Banerjee
David Goldsmith

ESC Guidelines advisor

Xavier Garcia-Moll

Chapter 6.1

Kidney disease

Debasish Banerjee, Robin Ramphul, and David Goldsmith

Introduction

CV events are commoner in CKD patients, and prognosis is poor; the pathophysiology in these patients is different from that in patients without CKD and is poorly understood. There are few robust clinical guidelines in this area, due to the fact that patients with CKD are systematically excluded from many major trials and nephrologists have not been able to conduct many appropriate interventional studies (and those that have been conducted frequently do not show positive findings). The rate of CV events increases and prognosis worsens in patients with reduced kidney function, which is worst in dialysis, with partial improvement with kidney transplantation. In clinical practice, pharmacotherapy is suboptimal, and despite appropriate treatment, patient prognosis remains poor. Hence, a better understanding of CV drugs among nephrologists, cardiologists, internists, and non-nephrologists is necessary for improved and timely care of these patients.

CKD patients are classified according to the eGFR and the level of proteinuria, as shown in Fig. 6.1.1. The Modification of Diet in Renal Disease Study (MDRD) and the Chronic Kidney Disease Epidemiology Collaboration (CKD-EPI) equations are used to determine the stages of CKD; yet most studies use the Cockcroft–Gault equation to determine safe drug dosing in CKD patients. The differences between these different derived GFR values, while often clinically trivial, can sometimes be substantial. Patients on dialysis and those post-kidney transplantation are often referred to as CKD-D and CKD-T, respectively.

Renal elimination of drugs

Many drugs are filtered and excreted unchanged through the kidney. Other drugs are metabolized prior to excretion. Drug elimination through the kidney is determined by the following factors.

- Drug filtration across the glomerulus: drug molecules of <20kDa and that are not protein-bound are filtered freely. When partially protein-bound, only free drug molecules are filtered through the glomerulus. The elimination of small free drug molecules decreases with progressive CKD.
- Tubular secretion of drugs: this involves two types of transporters:
  - Organic anion transporters—these can transport across a concentration gradient and hence are very effective, e.g. glucuronides, sulfates, furosemide, bendroflumethiazide, probenecid, and penicillins. The secretion of transporter-dependent drugs decreases with decreasing kidney function.
  - Organic cation transporters, e.g. for morphine, pethidine, triamterene.
- Diffusion across the tubular membrane: this is easier for lipid-soluble drugs and depends on the concentration gradient. The tubular fluid pH is very important for excretion of polar, non-lipid-soluble drugs, such as furosemide, digoxin, gentamicin, methotrexate, atenolol, penicillins, etc. For example, ionization is pH-dependent, and hence, alkaline urine favours the loss of phenobarbital.

Altered protein binding may affect drug elimination in the kidney, as described above. **Inhibition of tubular excretion** by certain drugs may affect the excretion of others, e.g. probenecid and penicillin/zidovudine; verapamil, amiodarone, quinidine, and digoxin; and aspirin, NSAIDs, and methotrexate. Some drugs can alter **urine flow and urine pH**, thereby affecting the elimination of other drugs, e.g. diuretics and lithium; and sodium bicarbonate and phenobarbital.

			Presistent albuminuria categories Description and range		
			A1	A2	A3
			<30 mg/g <3 mmol/mg	30–300 mg/g 3–30 mg/mmol	>300 mg/g >30 mg/mmol
eGFR categories Description and range	G1	>90 ml/min/1.73m²			
	G2	60–89 ml/min/1.73m²			
	G3a	45–59 ml/min/1.73m²			
	G3b	30–44 ml/min/1.73m²			
	G4	15–29 ml/min/1.73m²			
	G5	<15 ml/min/1.73m²			

Fig. 6.1.1 CKD categories by eGFR and albuminuria and associated risk (KDIGO classification). Green = low risk (if no other markers of CKD: no CKD); yellow = moderate risk; orange = high risk; red = very high risk.

Management of acute coronary syndrome (STEMI/unstable angina/ NSTEMI)

ACS is common in patients with CKD and those on dialysis. The incidence of NSTEMI is higher in CKD patients, although STEMI is also common, compared to the general population.[1] Prognosis of CKD patients after MI is poor, and presentation can be atypical, with less obvious chest pain and more prominent HF. Often these patients do not receive optimal care, due to a lack of knowledge about the safety and efficacy of appropriate medicines which are routinely used in non-CKD patients. This section provides guidance, based on available evidence on the management of CKD (including dialysis and kidney transplant) patients with ACS. In mild CKD and an eGFR of >60mL/min/1.73m^2, there is very little difference in management. However, knowledge about drug safety and efficacy is important for CKD stages 4 and 5 (see Table 6.1.1).[2,3]

Prehospital management

Transport time from the onset of chest pain to a hospital should be kept to a minimum. There is no direct evidence to support this statement in CKD patients, but kidney failure patients suffer sudden death due arrhythmias much more commonly than non-CKD cohorts. Hence, the time to reach hospital may be even more relevant to prevent out-of-hospital deaths.

Management in the emergency department

CKD patients presenting with chest pain are high risk, and if the initial ECG is non-diagnostic, then multiple ECGs are necessary, along with estimation of blood biomarkers such as serial troponin assays. Bedside echocardiography looking for RWMAs can be useful. Baseline troponin values are often elevated in predialysis CKD and dialysis patients, and so a rising troponin is necessary to establish a diagnosis of ACS.

Aspirin

Aspirin 150–375mg should be given to chew, as there is some trial and observational study evidence that aspirin therapy is associated with lower mortality, without a significant increase in the risk for bleeding in CKD patients. Observational data show benefit in both predialysis CKD and dialysis patients.

Clopidogrel

Clopidogrel reduces further events in mild to moderate CKD, without a marked increased risk for bleeding, as demonstrated in further analyses of RCTs (loading dose of 300mg, maintenance dose of 75mg od) in ACS patients. Prasugrel (loading dose of 60mg and maintenance dose of 10mg od) and ticagrelor (loading dose of 180mg and maintenance dose of 90mg bd) have both been shown to be better than clopidogrel in patients with mild CKD, similar to those without CKD, without an increased risk for bleeding, although none has been tested in ESRD patients. All antiplatelet agents should be used with caution due to an increased risk for bleeding.

Morphine

Morphine can be administered for pain at 4mg IV, followed by 2–8mg every 15min (caution: the metabolites accumulate and can cause toxicity). It may

Table 6.1.1 Pharmacotherapy of acute coronary syndrome in predialysis CKD and dialysis patients

	Recommendation for use	Dose modification
Aspirin	Should be used in all CKD patients	Not necessary
Oral P2Y12 receptor antagonist	Should be considered in mild to moderate CKD patients only	No dose reduction necessary
β-blockers	Should be used in all CKD patients	Carvedilol and metoprolol require no dose modification. Dose reduction necessary for atenolol
ACEIs	Should be used in all patients	Dose reduction may be necessary, but kidney function and potassium levels should be monitored
Statins	Should be used in all patients	No dose reduction necessary
Fibrinolysis	Should be considered in all patients when PPCI is not available. PPCI is the therapy of choice	No dose reduction necessary
Glycoprotein IIb/IIIa antagonist	May be considered but increases the risk of bleeding	Dose reduction necessary
UFH	Should be considered in all patients	No dose reduction necessary
Other anticoagulants	Enoxaparin may be used, but with an increased risk of bleeding Fondaparinux and bivalirudin may be considered, as they are associated with less bleeding in CKD stages 3–4	Enoxaparin requires dose reduction

Source data from Ibanez, B., *et al*, ESC Scientific Document Group. 2017 ESC Guidelines for the management of acute myocardial infarction in patients presenting with ST-segment elevation: The Task Force for the management of acute myocardial infarction in patients presenting with ST-segment elevation of the European Society of Cardiology (ESC). *Eur Heart J* 2018;39:119–177 and Roffi, M., *et al*, Management of Acute Coronary Syndromes in Patients Presenting without Persistent ST-Segment Elevation of the European Society of Cardiology. 2015 ESC Guidelines for the management of acute coronary syndromes in patients presenting without persistent ST-segment elevation: Task Force for the Management of Acute Coronary Syndromes in Patients Presenting without Persistent ST-Segment Elevation of the European Society of Cardiology (ESC). *Eur Heart J* 2016;37:267–315.

also impact antiplatelet action, e.g. delaying the onset of, and decreasing exposure to, ticagrelor.

Nitrates

Nitrates may be used for pain control, provided the SBP is >90mmHg, in all CKD patients.

Oxygen

Oxygen, if indicated in the presence of hypoxaemia on pulse oximetry, can be administered in all CKD patients.

Beta-adrenergic blocking agents

These agents are proven to improve outcome post-MI. Short-acting drugs are preferred. Long-acting drugs require careful monitoring of heart rate. Carvedilol, metoprolol, and bisoprolol (10mg daily if eGFR is <20mL/min/1.73m^2) are all safe to use. Atenolol tends to accumulate, due to its renal clearance, and hence a dose reduction may be necessary for safety (maximum dose of 50mg daily if the eGFR is 15–30mL/min/1.73m^2; maximum dose of 25mg daily if the eGFR is <15mL/min/1.73m^2). Large observational studies support the use of β-blockers in both predialysis and dialysis patients, with a 30-day mortality reduction of 30% and 22%, respectively.

Angiotensin-converting enzyme inhibitors

Use of ACEIs is associated with improved outcome in post-MI patients with LV dysfunction. However, they may be associated with hyperkalaemia and worsening kidney function in predialysis patients. So if judged necessary, they should be used with careful monitoring of creatinine and potassium levels. The new oral potassium binders may help with the management of hyperkalaemia in CKD patients on ACEIs if the potassium level is >5.5mEq/L. However, they have not been tested in ACS patients.

Mineralocorticoid receptor blockers

Although aldosterone blockers have been recommended for post-MI patients with LV systolic dysfunction, their use is restricted in patients with significant CKD and high potassium levels because of the risk for hyperkalaemia.[4]

Fibrinolysis

Data on fibrinolysis are limited to a pooled analysis of RCTs and observational cohorts. There is some evidence of an increased risk for intracranial haemorrhage in patients with severe CKD, from 0.6% in patients with normal eGFR of >90mL/min/1.73m^2 to 3% in those with severe CKD (eGFR <30mL/min/1.73m^2). However, large observational studies indicate no difference in in-hospital mortality with fibrinolysis in moderate CKD and higher mortality with severe dysfunction. Angiographic flow after fibrinolysis was similar in patients with severe CKD. Hence, fibrinolysis can be an option in patients with all stages of CKD when PCI is not available.

Primary percutaneous coronary intervention

There is high-grade evidence of benefits of PPCI for the management of patients with STEMI in the general population. Data from large observational studies suggest a decrease in mortality with PPCI in CKD patients with eGFR of 30–59mL/min/1.73m^2. However, contrast-induced acute kidney injury (AKI) in patients undergoing PPCI is commoner in patients with significant CKD (21% risk with creatinine level of >133micromol/L versus 6% in those with creatinine levels <133micromol/L), which, in turn, is associated with an increased risk of death and dialysis. Hence, use of low-volume and iso-osmolar contrast, with adequate rehydration, is necessary, with use of normal saline and, in selected cases, *N*-acetylcysteine and sodium bicarbonate, particularly in patients with CKD stages 3b and 4 and stage 3a with other risk factors, including diabetes.[5] However, a recent study of CKD stage 3 did not show benefits of hydration.[6] The benefits of PPCI outweigh the risk associated with contrast-induced AKI, and hence, it should be offered to patients with CKD and post-kidney transplantation, with adequate hydration and a minimum possible volume of contrast.[2] Patients on haemodialysis or peritoneal dialysis may be offered PPCI. However, the benefits are not clear, despite a very high mortality, up to 73% at 2 years.

Statins

Post-MI statin treatment is associated with improved 1-year mortality in patients with CKD stages 2–4 in a retrospective analysis. An RCT of simvastatin treatment in primary prevention reduced atherosclerosis events by 17% in both CKD and haemodialysis patients.[7] There are several observational studies which have demonstrated improved outcomes in post-ACS patients. Thus, there is evidence for use of statins in both primary and secondary prevention of atherosclerotic artery disease.

Glycoprotein IIb/IIIa antagonist therapy

Glycoprotein IIa/IIIb therapy in CKD patients is associated with some reduction in ischaemic events, but an overall increase in bleeding events. If used, doses should be reduced for eptifibatide (50% reduction for eGFR <50mL/min/1.73m^2; after ACS: 180mcg/kg bolus, followed by an infusion of 1mcg/kg/min for up to 72h) and tirofiban (25mcg/kg IV over 3min, followed by an infusion of 0.075mcg/kg/min for up to 18h post-PCI; if eGFR <30mL/min/1.73m^2).

Anticoagulation

UFH remains the recommended anticoagulation agent by major guidelines for ACS, both STEMI and NSTEMI. It is mainly cleared by the reticuloendothelial system and very minimally by the kidney.

Enoxaparin in patients with moderate CKD provides an added benefit but has an increased risk for bleeding, even with a dose adjustment of 1mg/kg/day. Fondaparinux, compared to enoxaparin, was associated with better outcome in moderate CKD with unstable angina and NSTEMI (GFR <58mL/min) but has not been tested in patients with severe kidney failure, and it is excreted through the kidneys. Bivalirudin is similar in efficacy, compared to UFH, but may be expected to have less major bleeding complications in moderate CKD; it has not been tested in severe CKD (reduce the rate to <1.4mg/kg/h if eGFR is 30–60mL/min/1.73m^2). Thus, the newer agents have not been tested in patients with severe CKD and are not associated with significantly improved outcome.

Management of heart failure in chronic kidney disease

Kidney disease in patients with HF is common, is associated with poor prognosis, and is often difficult to manage due to associated biochemical abnormalities.

CKD, present normally in around one-third of chronic HF patients, and worsening renal function in patients during admissions for acute HF, which occurs in one-tenth of patients, are both associated with high mortality.

HFpEF in patients with CKD is probably as common as HFrEF but is difficult to diagnose, as fluid overload due to CKD has the same symptoms and signs as does congestion due to HF. HF in patients on dialysis is associated with very high mortality, and even a diagnosis of 'fluid overload' (which is often clinically conflated with HF) is equally serious.

Patients with CKD stages 1–3 have often been included in clinical trials of HF by chance, but those with CKD stages 4–5 and dialysis patients have been routinely excluded.[8] Thus, there is some evidence to support the use of most guideline-recommended life-prolonging therapy in CKD stages 1–3, but such evidence in CKD stages 4–5 and in dialysis and post-kidney transplantation patients is worryingly lacking.

Management of HF involves symptom control and use of drugs to improve survival. Management of chronic HF patients with CKD requires careful use of ACEIs/ARBs, β-blockers, and mineralocorticoid inhibitors to improve prognosis, while monitoring serum creatinine and potassium levels. Management of acute decompensated HF may require large doses of diuretics and cautious use of ACEIs/ARBs or MRAs, again with regular monitoring of serum creatinine levels and electrolytes (see Table 6.1.2).

ACE inhibitors in patients with heart failure and chronic kidney disease

Subgroup analysis of several RCTs of ACEIs in HF patients with CKD have shown benefits, with a reduction in mortality and hospitalizations with enalapril and lisinopril in CKD patients with an eGFR of <60mL/min/1.73m^2 and <45mL/min/1.73m^2, respectively. Angiotensin receptor blockers can be used in patients intolerant of ACEI.

Use of ACEIs and ARBs together is associated with adverse outcomes, such as hyperkalaemia and AKI, even in non-CKD patients, and hence, dual blockade in CKD patients is not recommended.

Beta-blockers in patients with heart failure and chronic kidney disease

Data from trials with metoprolol and carvedilol have suggested improvement in all-cause mortality in CKD patients with an eGFR of <60mL/min/1.73m^2. Carvedilol has been shown to be beneficial in a small RCT of dialysis patients.[9] β-blockers should be used in all HFrEF patients. Evidence suggests nebivolol may be useful in elderly HFpEF and HFmEF patients.[8]

Table 6.1.2 Pharmacotherapy in patients with CKD and heart failure

Agents	CKD stages 1, 2, and 3	CKD stages 4 and 5
ACEIs	Should be used in all patients with HFrEF, with monitoring of creatinine and potassium levels	May be used in HFrEF patients, with monitoring of creatinine and potassium levels. Dose modification may be necessary
β-blockers	Should be used in all HFrEF patients	May be used in HFrEF patients
Mineralocorticoid receptor antagonists	Should be used in HFrEF, with careful monitoring of potassium levels	May be used in HFrEF patients, with caution and monitoring of potassium levels
ARBs	Should be used in all HFrEF patients with caution	May be used in HFrEF patients, with monitoring of creatinine and potassium levels
Ivabradine	May be used in HFrEF patients in sinus rhythm and already on ACEIs and β-blockers	Unknown effects
Hydralazine and isosorbide dinitrate	Should be considered in HFrEF patients intolerant to ACEIs/ARBs	May be considered in HFrEF patients intolerant to ACEIs/ARBs

Source data from Ponikowski P, *et al*, Authors/Task Force Members, Document Reviewers. 2016 ESC Guidelines for the diagnosis and treatment of acute and chronic heart failure: The Task Force for the diagnosis and treatment of acute and chronic heart failure of the European Society of Cardiology (ESC). Developed with the special contribution of the Heart Failure Association (HFA) of the ESC. *Eur J Heart Fail* 2016;18:891–975.

Mineralocorticoid receptor antagonists in heart failure and chronic kidney disease

These agents are proven to be beneficial in patients with HFrEF who remain symptomatic after adequate treatment with ACEIs and β-blockers, and after an MI. Close to half of the patients in a large RCT of spironolactone and one-third of those in a trial of eplerenone had an eGFR of <60mL/min/1.73m^2 at baseline and benefited from therapy. Hence, these drugs should be used in CKD patients with HFrEF.

Hyperkalaemia is common in patients with HF and CKD, particularly in those on ACEIs and MRAs. Potassium levels of >5.5mmol/L may be present in one-third of patients with CKD stages 4 and 5, which may require careful management to maximize the use of ACEIs and MRAs, including use of loop diuretics, correction of metabolic acidosis, advice on low-potassium diet, and, in the future, on use of novel potassium binders.

Ivabradine

Trials of ivabradine included patients with an eGFR of <60mL/min/1.73m^2. However, no trial has included patients with CKD stages 4 and 5. Benefits may exist in CKD stage 3, but further evidence is needed.

Diuretic therapy

Diuretics are key in treating and preventing fluid overload in patients with HF and CKD. Patients with chronic HF and CKD stages 1–3 may benefit from thiazide diuretics. However, patients with CKD stages 4–5 may need loop diuretics, as thiazide diuretics are less effective with an eGFR of <30mL/min/1.73m^2. Use of loop diuretics can be challenging, due to changes in creatinine and electrolytes, although helpful in tempering RAAS-induced hyperkalaemia. In acute decompensated HF, both continuous and bolus IV loop diuretics are equally effective in achieving symptom control. Adequate diuretic therapy combining different agents remains the mainstay in relieving congestion in acute decompensated HF, even compared to ultrafiltration. A combination of a loop diuretic and a potassium-sparing diuretic may help prevent hypokalaemia, although this is unusual in advanced CKD. Hyponatraemia is common with diuretics particularly thiazides, which is managed by diuretic dose reduction, fluid restriction, and in future may be with vasopressin receptor antagonists. In HF patients on dialysis, who may have very low urine output, fluid removal during dialysis is often associated with symptomatic intradialytic hypotension and may require daily isolated ultrafiltration.

Neprilysin and angiotensin receptor blocker

The role of the sacubitril/valsartan combination is established in non-CKD patients but is yet to become widely used. An RCT showing benefit in HF patients excluded patients with an eGFR of 30mL/min/1.73m^2 or less and further excluded patients with rising creatinine levels of >2.5mg/dL during the run-in phase. It may be used in stable CKD stages 1–3; in CKD 4 up to eGFR 20ml/min/1.73m^2.

Management of arrhythmias in chronic kidney disease

Supraventricular tachyarrhythmias are usually associated with narrow QRS complexes. They can be sustained or paroxysmal, originating from the atria, the AVN, or AV accessory pathways. AF is the commonest of such arrhythmias, and its management is discussed separately in ➲ Management of atrial fibrillation in chronic kidney disease, pp. 330–5. Acute management of paroxysmal supraventricular arrhythmias requires the use of IV adenosine or verapamil/diltiazem. An initial episode of atrial flutter requires cardioversion, but recurrent episodes may require sotalol, dofetilide, disopyramide, amiodarone, or catheter ablation, unless the patient is haemodynamically unstable, needing urgent cardioversion (see Table 6.1.3).

Ventricular arrhythmias are associated with wide QRS. They originate from the ventricular myocardium or the His–Purkinje system and include premature ventricular beats, sustained and non-sustained ventricular arrhythmias, and VF. They are common in all CKD patients and particularly those on dialysis, and they are the most frequent cause of death. Several drug classes are recommended in ventricular arrhythmias, including β-blockers, CCBs (diltiazem, verapamil), sodium channel-blocking agents (mexiletine, disopyramide, flecainide, propafenone), potassium channel-blocking agents (sotalol, dofetilide), and amiodarone. Despite the fact that ICDs are the most effective agents in the prevention of SCD due to ventricular arrhythmias, and bearing in mind that there is a 6.5% rate of SCD in patients on haemodialysis, most patients on haemodialysis are not eligible for ICD therapy, according to current guidelines. A retrospective analysis of ICD use in dialysis patients has failed to demonstrate benefits and has shown high rates of associated infections. A prospective trial using a wearable defibrillator is ongoing.

Table 6.1.3 Antiarrythmia agents, route of elimination, half-life, and dose adjustments in CKD

Drug	Elimination	Half-life (h)	Renal dose adjustment
Atenolol	Renal	6–9	eGFR 15–35mL/min/1.73m^2: max 50mg od eGFR <15mL/min/1.73m^2: max 25mg od
Acebutolol	Renal/hepatic	6–7	eGFR 25–50mL/min/1.73m^2: half dose eGFR <25mL/min/1.73m^2: quarter dose
Metoprolol	Hepatic	3–8	None
Nadolol	Renal	10–24	eGFR <50mL/min/1.73m^2: increase dose interval
Sotalol	Renal	12	eGFR 30–60mL/min/1.73m^2: half dose eGFR 10–30mL/min/1.73m^2: quarter dose eGFR <10mL/min/1.73m^2: avoid
Verapamil	Hepatic/renal	4.5–12	None
Diltiazem	Hepatic	3–4.5	Lower starting dose
Flecainide	Hepatic 75%/renal	7–22	eGFR <35mL/min/1.73m^2: reduce dose, max 100mg od
Mexiletine	Hepatic	10–14	
Disopyramide	Renal 50%/hepatic	4–10	Reduce dose
Quinidine	Hepatic 75%/renal	6–8	Caution
Propafenone	Hepatic	2–8	None
Dofetilide	Renal	10	Avoid
Amiodarone	Hepatic	40–55	None
Dronedarone	Hepatic	13–19	eGFR <30mL/min/1.73m^2: avoid
Digoxin	Renal	38–48	Reduce dose, monitor plasma level

Management of atrial fibrillation in chronic kidney disease

AF is a common arrhythmia in patients with CKD, with a prevalence estimated to be 20% in the non-dialysis-dependent CKD population and between 13% and 27% in the chronic dialysis-dependent CKD population. There is an elevated risk of thromboembolism, particularly stroke, and bleeding, when compared to the general population without CKD. The most effective way to reduce the risk of thromboembolism in the general population is through anticoagulation, but the higher bleeding risk, especially in those on dialysis, complicates management, often resulting in underuse of anticoagulation in this high-risk group. The large trials supporting the use of anticoagulation to reduce the risk of stroke in non-valvular AF (NVAF) have largely excluded patients with moderate to severe renal impairment (eGFR <30mL/min/1.73m^2), and data in the CKD and dialysis populations are limited to observational studies only and often have conflicting messages (see Table 6.1.4). Thus, it is unclear whether anticoagulation is safe and effective at reducing the risk of stroke in the CKD population. Catheter ablation for AF in CKD patients is relatively safe in expert hands but is less effective than non-CKD patients.

Stroke and systemic thromboembolism prevention

Aspirin

There is no evidence to suggest aspirin is effective at reducing the risk of stroke in patients with AF and CKD or those on dialysis, although there is an increased risk of bleeding. Therefore, in patients at an increased risk of stroke, aspirin monotherapy should not be used in the place of anticoagulation.

Aspirin and warfarin

Combination therapy with aspirin and warfarin did not reduce the risk of stroke in one study, but the risk of significant bleeding was increased. Therefore, this combination should be avoided.

Warfarin

There are no RCTs investigating the effect of warfarin on stroke risk reduction in the CKD population with AF. Observational data have been conflicting, with some studies reporting a reduced incidence of stroke, while others reported no significant difference and even an increased risk of stroke.[10] Similarly, the risk of significant bleeding with warfarin was increased.

In a meta-analysis consisting of 11 studies, in a total of >48,500 patients including >11,600 warfarin users, warfarin was associated with a significant reduction in the risk of stroke and no effect on major bleeding in the CKD population. Contrary to this, however, warfarin had no effect on the risk of stroke but significantly increased the risk of bleeding in the dialysis population. Hence, warfarin may reduce the risk of ischaemic stroke in the CKD population without a significant increase in the risk of haemorrhage, but in the dialysis population, warfarin may not reduce the risk of ischaemic stroke but increase the risk of occurrence of major bleeding. Warfarin is given at

Table 6.1.4 Anticoagulation for atrial fibrillation in CKD

	Recommendation for use	Dose modification
Aspirin	No evidence of benefit	Not necessary
Warfarin	Should be considered for prevention of stroke and systemic thromboembolism in CKD stages 1–5. May reduce stroke risk in CKD, but not in dialysis, patients. Bleeding risk appears to be elevated in dialysis patients	No dose reduction necessary, but more frequent monitoring of INR/prothrombin time may be required to maintain within target range
Apixaban	Should be considered for prevention of stroke and systemic thromboembolism in CKD stages 1–3. May be considered for use in CKD stages 4–5 and dialysis	5mg bd if eGFR >30mL/min/1.73m^2 (or 2.5mg bd if age >80 or weight <60kg). Reduce to 2.5mg bd if eGFR <30mL/min/1.73m^2 and use with caution, particularly in CKD stage 5 on dialysis (FDA approval only)
Dabigatran	Should be considered for prevention of stroke and systemic thromboembolism in CKD stages 1–3. May be considered for use in CKD stage 4	110–150mg bd if eGFR ≥30mL/min/1.73m^2 (avoid if eGFR <30)
Edoxaban	Should be considered for prevention of stroke and systemic thromboembolism in CKD stages 1–3. May be considered in CKD stage 4	60mg od if eGFR ≥50mL/min/1.73m^2. Reduce to 30mg od if eGFR 15–49mL/min/1.73m^2. Use with caution if eGFR <30mL/min/1.73m^2. Contraindicated if eGFR <15mL/min/1.73m^2
Rivaroxaban	Should be considered for prevention of stroke and systemic thromboembolism in CKD stages 1–3. May be considered in CKD stage 4	20mg od if eGFR ≥50mL/min/1.73m^2; 15mg od if eGFR 15–49mL/min/1.73m^2. Use with caution if eGFR <30mL/min/1.73m^2. Avoid if eGFR <15mL/min/1.73m^2

Source data from Kirchhof P, *et al*, 2016 ESC Guidelines for the management of atrial fibrillation developed in collaboration with EACTS. *Eur Heart J* 2016;37:2893–2962.

variable doses, adjusted to a target INR of 2.5. Close monitoring of the INR to ensure it remains within the specified range of 2–3 may help to reduce the risk of stroke, while minimizing the risk of significant haemorrhage. However, recent data suggest that the time within the therapeutic range in CKD and dialysis patients is significantly lower than in non-CKD cohorts, despite best efforts.

Direct oral anticoagulants

Unlike warfarin, DOACs have predictable pharmacokinetics and do not require frequent monitoring and have fewer diet and drug interactions.[11] They all undergo renal excretion, albeit to varying degrees, and therefore, the risk of bleeding increases with the severity of renal impairment. As a result, dose modification is recommended.

Apixaban

Apixaban is an oral, irreversible direct factor Xa inhibitor, given at 5mg bd or 2.5mg bd if any two of the following three conditions are present: age ≥80 years, body weight ≥60kg, or serum creatinine ≥133micromol/L. The Apixaban for Reduction in Stroke and Other Thromboembolic Events in Atrial Fibrillation (ARISTOTLE) trial demonstrated that apixaban, when compared to warfarin, was associated with a reduced risk of stroke, thromboembolism, major bleeding, and all-cause mortality in patients with moderate CKD (eGFR <50mL/min/1.73m^2). However, patients with moderate to severe renal dysfunction (i.e. eGFR <25mL/min/1.73m^2) were excluded from the study. There have been no studies investigating the efficacy and safety of apixaban in patients with severe renal dysfunction (eGFR <25mL/min/1.73m^2). Although the US FDA has approved apixaban for use in severe renal impairment, including in patients on dialysis, this recommendation was based on pharmacokinetic data obtained from two open-label, parallel-group, single-dose studies, which included seven patients with an eGFR of <30mL/min/1.73m^2 and not on dialysis and eight patients with ESRD on haemodialysis.[12] Until further more robust evidence is obtained, apixaban should be used with considerable caution in patients with moderate to severe renal impairment (eGFR <25mL/min/1.73m^2) and particularly in dialysis patients. Any such patient offered apixaban should be informed of the data limitations, and alternative anticoagulation such as warfarin considered.

Dabigatran

Dabigatran is an oral, reversible direct thrombin inhibitor. The Randomized Evaluation of Long-Term Anticoagulation Therapy (RE-LY) trial showed that, at a dose of 150mg bd, dabigatran, when compared to warfarin, resulted in lower rates of stroke and systemic thromboembolism and no significant difference in the rate of major bleeding across the range of renal function groups. A lower dose of dabigatran 110mg bd resulted in few major bleeds, when compared to warfarin, but similar stroke risk reduction across the renal function groups. Patients with an eGFR of <30mL/min/1.73m^2 were excluded from the RE-LY study. However, using pharmacokinetic modelling, the US FDA has approved dabigatran at a reduced dose of 75mg bd for NVAF in patients with an eGFR of 15–30mL/min/1.73m^2. There are very few data to support the use of dabigatran in this severe renal impairment population, and until more robust studies have investigated the efficacy and safety of dabigatran in this patient population, it should be used with extreme caution, with consideration given to alternative anticoagulants such as warfarin, and patients should be clearly informed of the data limitations. Dabigatran is contraindicated in patients on dialysis and with an eGFR <15mL/min/1.73m^2.

Edoxaban

Edoxaban is an oral, reversible direct factor Xa inhibitor, given at 60mg od for patients with an eGFR of >50mL/min/1.73m^2 and 30mg od for those with an eGFR of 15–50mL/min/1.73m^2. The Effective Anticoagulation with Factor Xa Next Generation in Atrial Fibrillation–Thrombolysis in Myocardial Infarction 48 (ENGAGE AF-TIMI 48) trial was a large multicentre RCT comparing two dose regimens of edoxaban with warfarin (60mg and 30mg od) and included patients with an eGFR of up to 30mL/min/1.73m^2. When compared to warfarin, both doses of edoxaban were similar in terms of efficacy in preventing stroke and systemic embolism and were associated with significantly lower rates of bleeding and death from CV causes. Pharmacokinetic data were used to support edoxaban at a reduced dose of 30mg od for severe renal impairment (eGFR 15–30mL/min/1.73m^2), and it should be used with caution in the absence of robust clinical studies in this subgroup. Consideration should be given to alternative anticoagulants, such as warfarin, in this scenario, and patients should be clearly informed of the data limitations. Edoxaban is contraindicated in patients on dialysis and with an eGFR of <15mL/min/1.73m^2.

Rivaroxaban

Rivaroxaban is an oral direct factor Xa inhibitor. The Rivaroxaban Once Daily Oral Direct Factor Xa Inhibition Compared with Vitamin K Antagonism for Prevention of Stroke and Embolism Trial in Atrial Fibrillation (ROCKET-AF) trial was a large multicentre RCT comparing rivaroxaban to warfarin. The trial demonstrated a trend, albeit not statistically significant, towards a lower risk of stroke, systemic embolism, and fatal bleeding in the moderate renal impairment subgroup (eGFR 30–49mL/min/1.73m^2), compared to warfarin. The recommended dose is 20mg od for eGFR of >50mL/min/1.73m^2 and 15mg od for eGFR of 15–49mL/min/1.73m^2, although there is little clinical evidence to support the use of rivaroxaban in patients with an eGFR of <30mL/min/1.73m^2, and it should be used with caution in this patient population. There are no clinical data for eGFR of <15mL/min/1.73m^2, and therefore, rivaroxaban is not recommended in this population.

Rhythm control in atrial fibrillation

Pharmacological cardioversion therapies

Flecainide

Flecainide is a sodium channel blocker with antiarrhythmic class 1c properties. It has been shown to prevent paroxysmal AF, compared to placebo, in the general population, and in selected patients, it has been shown to be feasible and safe when it is self-administered out-of-hospital (pill-in-pocket approach). Thirty-five per cent is excreted unchanged in the urine. A dose reduction is recommended in renal impairment (eGFR <35mL/min/1.73m^2).

Propafenone

Propafenone is a sodium channel blocker and a class Ic antiarrhythmic agent. It is used in the treatment of paroxysmal AF and cardioversion of AF to sinus rhythm. In selected patients, it has been shown to be feasible and safe when it is self-administered out-of-hospital (pill-in-pocket approach). It undergoes extensive first-pass metabolism in the liver, producing metabolites with antiarrhythmic activity similar to propafenone. Less than 1% of propafenone and 38% of its metabolites are excreted unchanged in the urine. It should be used with caution and initiated under hospital conditions, with ECG and BP monitoring.

Amiodarone

Amiodarone is a class III antiarrhythmic agent but has other mechanisms of action, exhibiting class I, II, and IV activity also. It is used in the treatment of acute symptomatic AF for both rate control and cardioversion to sinus rhythm; paroxysmal and persistent AF to maintain sinus rhythm; and permanent AF for rate control when other interventions have failed or are not tolerated. Amiodarone has been shown to increase the success rate of electrical cardioversion if given up to 4 weeks beforehand, but because of the potential for side effects, this is not routinely recommended. It may be appropriate in cases where electrical cardioversion is unlikely to be successful or if a previous attempt has failed. Amiodarone is metabolized in the liver and excreted through hepatic and biliary routes, with almost no elimination via the kidneys. No dose adjustment is needed in mild renal impairment, but it is best avoided in severe renal failure. Thyroid dysfunction and pulmonary toxicity remain concerns with long-term use.

Sotalol

Sotalol is a non-selective β1-adrenergic receptor antagonist that has class II and III antiarrhythmic activity. It is indicated in the treatment of paroxysmal and persistent AF to maintain sinus rhythm and has been shown to increase the success rate of electrical cardioversion if given up to 4 weeks beforehand, but because of the potential for side effects, this is not routinely recommended. It may be appropriate in cases where electrical cardioversion is unlikely to be successful or if a previous attempt has failed. Sotalol is not metabolized, and 70% is excreted unchanged via the kidneys. Doses should be reduced by 50% in moderate renal impairment (CrCl 30–60mL/min/1.73m^2) and by 75% in severe renal impairment (CrCl 10–30mL/min/1.73m^2). Sotalol should be used with caution in renal impairment, hypokalaemia, and hypomagnesaemia and in the elderly because of its proarrhythmic effects.

Dronedarone

Dronedarone is an antiarrhythmic drug, similar to amiodarone in structure and which exhibits class I, II, III, and IV antiarrhythmic activity. There is less risk for thyroid dysfunction and lung toxicity, compared to amiodarone. It is used in non-permanent AF to maintain sinus rhythm and to control the ventricular rate. Serum creatinine levels are increased as a result of partial inhibition of the tubular organic cationic transporter system, rather than causing renal dysfunction. It undergoes extensive first-pass metabolism and, along with its metabolites, is excreted predominantly in faeces (84%), with

6% undergoing renal excretion mainly as active and inactive metabolites. No pharmacokinetic difference was observed in patients with mild to severe renal impairment, and no dose adjustment needs to be made for renal impairment. It is contraindicated in moderate to severe HF (NYHA classes III and IV), as it has been shown to be associated with increased mortality in these patient populations.

Ibutilide

Ibutilide is an IV antiarrhythmic agent used for cardioversion of resistant AF to sinus rhythm. It is well tolerated in renal impairment, but caution should be exercised in hypokalaemic and hypomagnesaemic states, as it may increase the risk for arrhythmias (TdP). It is unavailable in Europe.

Dofetilide

Dofetilide is renally excreted and needs dose adjustment in renal impairment, as there is an increased risk for ventricular arrhythmias. However, it is not available in Europe and Australia.

Management of hypertension in chronic kidney disease

Hypertension (see Table 6.1.5) is both a cause and a consequence of CKD. High BP levels are associated with a higher CV risk in CKD patients. However, the relationship of BP with CV events is often not clear in dialysis patients where low BP levels are also associated with poor outcomes and may represent severe cardiomyopathy. Management of high BP in patients with CKD is aimed at reducing CV events and the progression of renal impairment, and the strategy employed is determined by the presence of coexisting comorbidities, especially diabetes and other CV diseases, albuminuria, age, risk of progression of CKD, the presence of retinopathy in diabetics, and tolerance to treatment.

The pathophysiology of high BP in dialysis patients is complex, involving several issues unique to dialysis patients. This includes chronic fluid retention, advanced vascular disease, autonomic dysfunction, and fluctuations in BP with ultrafiltration and dialysis treatment, among others. The backbone of management focuses on achieving a normal extracellular fluid volume using ultrafiltration on dialysis and salt and fluid dietary restriction. This is rarely achieved consistently, and often pharmacological therapy for hypertension is required nonetheless. There is no compelling evidence to recommend one class of antihypertensive agent over another, and, as such, any established use of these drugs in the general population or CKD patients should be applied to dialysis patients until better evidence emerges. There is no evidence for a definition, or a target therapeutic threshold, for any particular BP level in dialysis patients.

Lifestyle modification

Lifestyle modification is a simple and inexpensive method to lower BP and should be considered in every patient with hypertension. In addition, it may offer benefits other than improving BP control, e.g. reducing weight and lowering cholesterol with diet modification.

Lifestyle modification recommendations, as suggested by Kidney Disease: Improving Global Outcomes (KDIGO) guidelines on the management of hypertension in patients with CKD, are as follows:

- Maintaining a healthy weight (BMI 20–25).
- Lowering salt intake to 2g (90mmol) of sodium or 5g of sodium chloride per day.
- Undertaking regular exercise, as tolerated, aiming for at least 30min five times a week.
- Limiting alcohol intake to no more than two standard drinks for men and one standard drink for women per day.

Pharmacotherapy to lower blood pressure

With the exception of ACEIs and ARBs, which can help to lower albuminuria, there is no strong evidence to support the preferential use of any particular antihypertensive agent in patients with CKD. The choice of antihypertensive therapy tends to be tailored to the individual, taking into consideration issues such as the presence of albuminuria, comorbidities,

Table 6.1.5 Pharmacotherapy of hypertension in CKD

	Recommendation for use	Dose modification
ACEIs	May be used in all CKD patients, particularly those with albuminuria, diabetes, HF, MI, stroke, and high CV risk	No dose reduction is necessary, but the starting dose may need to be modified and kidney function and potassium levels should be monitored
Aldosterone antagonists	May be used in resistant hypertension and oedema	No dose reduction necessary, but kidney function and potassium levels should be monitored. Avoid in severe renal impairment
Direct renin inhibitors (aliskiren)	May be considered in mild to moderate CKD, in addition to conventional therapy	Avoid if eGFR <30mL/min/1.73m^2. Contraindicated in diabetics or if eGFR <60mL/min/1.73m^2 when used in combination with ACEI or ARB
Thiazides and thiazide-like diuretics	May be used in all CKD patients, although they are less effective in when eGFR falls below 30–50mL/min/1.73m^2	No dose reduction necessary
Loop diuretics	May be used in all CKD patients, although they are less effective in severe renal impairment	No dose reduction necessary (higher doses required, as GFR declines)
Potassium-sparing diuretics	May be used in mild renal impairment	Avoid in moderate to severe renal impairment
β-blockers	May be used in all CKD patients	Carvedilol and metoprolol require no dose modification. Dose reduction necessary in severe renal impairment for atenolol Dose reduction necessary for bisoprolol if eGFR <20mL/min/1.73m^2 (max 10mg daily)
Calcium channel antagonists	May be used in all CKD patients	No dose reduction necessary, except for nicardipine and nimodipine. Start diltiazem at lower dose
Centrally acting α-agonists	May be considered in all patients with resistant hypertension	No dose reduction necessary for methyldopa and clonidine. Maximum single dose of 0.2mg and maximum daily dose of 0.4mg if eGFR 30–60mL/min/1.73m^2, and avoid moxonidine if eGFR <30mL/min/1.73m^2
α-blockers	May be considered in all CKD patients	No dose reduction necessary
Direct vasodilators	May be considered in patients with resistant hypertension	Dose reduction recommended if eGFR <30mL/min/1.73m^2 for hydralazine. Use minoxidil with caution in severe renal impairment

compliance, adverse effects, and drug interactions, among others. Often, patients will require two or three agents to achieve a desired BP target.

Renin–angiotensin–aldosterone system blockers

This class of antihypertensive agents typically includes ACEIs, ARBs, aldosterone antagonists, and direct renin inhibitors (DRIs).

ACEIs and ARBs are indicated as first-line therapy in CKD patients with albuminuria, as they have a favourable impact on renal and CV outcomes. They are also recommended for use in hypertensive, diabetic patients with albuminuria. An initial acute decline in the GFR, thought to be due to a haemodynamic effect, may be seen, the magnitude of which is inversely proportional to the long-term rate of change in GFR. An acute fall in the GFR of up to 30% (or a rise in creatinine levels of 30%) is often accepted as the physiological effect of ACEI or ARB initiation, whereas larger declines in the GFR may occur as a result of volume depletion, clinically significant renal artery stenosis, or co-administration with other medications that affect GFR such as NSAIDs.[13] This acute decline in the GFR is typically reversible upon cessation of therapy.

ACEIs and ARBs should be initiated and used with caution in patients with intravascular volume depletion, renal artery stenosis, sepsis, and concurrent use of NSAIDs and diuretics, as they may lead to rapid and large declines in the GFR, producing AKI, and rarely requiring emergency dialysis, with attendant clinical risk. Patients already on ACEI or ARB therapy should have their therapy withheld or stopped in these cases. Likewise, patients who develop intercurrent illness that may result in dehydration, such as diarrhoea, vomiting, and fever, who are already on ACEIs or ARBs should have their treatment withheld until the acute illness has resolved (but few patients and doctors appear to know and use this important information).

In the general population, ACEIs and ARBs have been recommended for use in patients with diabetes and hypertension, HF, MI, stroke, and high CV risk, and they may be considered for use in these patients with CKD.

Monitoring for hyperkalaemia is an important safety intervention in patients starting on, or continuing with, RAAS-blocking agents, particularly in patients with moderate to severe CKD or when used in combination with potassium-sparing diuretics, NSAIDs, COX-2 inhibitors. ACEIs and ARBs used in combination increase the risk for hyperkalaemia, hypotension, and decline in kidney function, and their combined use is no longer recommended.

Aldosterone antagonists, such as spironolactone and eplerenone, are recommended for use in non-CKD patients with HF. It is unclear whether they have the same prognostic benefit in patients with CKD. The risk of side effects, such as hyperkalaemia, is elevated, particularly in patients with advanced CKD. They have proven anti-albuminuric effects when used in combination with ACEIs or ARBs, although not in patients with an eGFR of <70mL/min/1.73m^2. In CKD patients, they are often used in the treatment of resistant hypertension and/or oedema and may be considered for use in CKD patients with HF or as an additional therapy to ACEIs and ARBs to reduce albuminuria. However, the risk of side effects, such as hyperkalaemia, particularly in patients with moderate to severe CKD, are elevated. Concomitant use of other diuretics may help to mitigate the risk of hyperkalaemia but does not negate it. Aldosterone antagonists should be used with caution and closely monitored.

The DRI aliskiren has been approved for the treatment of hypertension. Limited data are available in patients with CKD, although one RCT investigating the combination of aliskiren and losartan was encouraging, suggesting significant reductions in albuminuria in patients with CKD, with no difference in the rates of adverse events. However, the Aliskiren Trial in Type 2 Diabetes Using Cardiorenal Endpoints (ALTITUDE) trial, a larger RCT investigating aliskiren in addition to conventional treatment, was terminated early due to increased risks of adverse events (renal impairment, hypotension, and hyperkalaemia). It is therefore contraindicated in combination with an ACEI or ARB in patients with diabetes or in patients with an eGFR of <60mL/min/1.73m^2. In all other patients, the combination of a DRI and an ACEI or ARB is not recommended.

Thiazides and thiazide-like diuretics

These diuretics exert their effect by promoting the excretion of salt and water but may also have a vasodilatory effect. Their diuretic effect diminishes, as the eGFR falls below 30mL/min/1.73m^2, although their antihypertensive effect may be preserved. For this reason, loop diuretics are often preferred in patients with CKD stages 4 and 5. Thiazide and thiazide-like diuretics have been extensively studied and are thought to be similar in effect, clinical outcomes, and cost. Although they are renally excreted, no dose adjustment is required in patients with CKD. They potentiate the effect of other antihypertensive agents, particularly ACEIs and ARBs, and help to prevent hyperkalaemia. Their side effects, particularly hyperglycaemia, hyperuricaemia, and altered plasma lipid concentrations, should be considered in patients at risk of metabolic syndrome.

Loop diuretics

Loop diuretics, such as furosemide, are commonly used in the management of hypertension with oedema, particularly in patients with advanced CKD. They are effective in the short term but may not be as effective as thiazides in the long term. Concomitant use of a loop diuretic and a thiazide may potentiate the diuretic and antihypertensive effects. They may help to reduce the risk of hyperkalaemia by promoting the excretion of potassium. Larger doses are required to achieve the desired effect, as the GFR falls. They are often discontinued once haemodialysis is started, as their efficacy is debatable and ultrafiltration is far more effective in dealing with inappropriate volume expansion. In peritoneal dialysis, where continued preservation of residual renal function for as long as possible is desirable, they are often continued until the urine output becomes negligible.

Potassium-sparing diuretics

Examples of these include amiloride and spironolactone. They are usually avoided in CKD, especially in severe renal impairment, due to their potential to cause hyperkalaemia and because they are not as effective in reducing oedema as thiazides or loop diuretics. In salt-wasting nephropathy, amiloride helps to reduce the risk for hyponatraemia. Aldosterone antagonists have been discussed previously.

Beta-blockers

β-blockers are a large class of CV drugs that are effective in the treatment of hypertension. In addition to their antihypertensive effect, β-blockers are recommended for use in HF, AF, and CAD in the general population. In CKD patients, β-blockers reduce mortality in patients with HF. Since the pharmacology of each β-blocker varies, the choice of the most appropriate one will depend on the risk of accumulation, as this may lead to concentration-dependent side effects such as bradycardic arrhythmias. Renally excreted β-blockers, such as atenolol, are more likely to accumulate, and therefore, dose adjustments need to be made in severe renal impairment. Metoprolol, carvedilol, and propranolol undergo hepatic metabolism and are less likely to accumulate in renal impairment (although manufacturers of propranolol advise caution in renal impairment). Bisoprolol undergoes both renal excretion and hepatic metabolism and may accumulate in severe renal impairment. Using β-blockers in combination with other bradycardia-inducing drugs, such as non-dihydropyridine CCBs, is not recommended, as this increases the risk of bradycardic arrhythmias. Lipid-soluble β-blockers may cross the blood–brain barrier and, if used with other centrally acting agents, may result in drowsiness and confusion.

Calcium channel antagonists

Calcium channel antagonists are valuable agents in the treatment of hypertension in patients with CKD and, with the exception of nicardipine and nimodipine, do not need dose adjustment in renal impairment. Two major subclasses exist: dihydropyridines (DCAs) such as amlodipine and nifedipine, and non-dihydropyridines (NDCAs) such as diltiazem and verapamil. DCAs are more selective for vascular smooth muscle, leading to vasodilatation, a side effect of which can be fluid retention. NDCAs act directly on the myocardium, including the sinoatrial and atrioventricular nodes, resulting in a reduction in myocardial contractility and heart rate.

DCAs tend to exert their effect predominantly on the afferent arteriole at the glomerulus, resulting in an increase in albuminuria, whereas NDCAs typically do not exhibit this effect.

NDCAs and β-blockers, used together, should be avoided, particularly in advanced CKD, as this combination may lead to bradycardia, complete heart block, or asystole. NDCAs can increase CNI (ciclosporin and tacrolimus) and mTOR (sirolimus, everolimus) concentrations. Thus, some physicians have used them to increase these immunosuppressant blood concentrations (in order to reduce cost).

Centrally acting alpha-adrenergic agonists

Centrally acting α-adrenergic agonists (CAAAAs) inhibit sympathetic activity within the brain and are a valuable adjunct to hypertensive therapy in patients with CKD and resistant hypertension. They reduce heart rate and promote vasodilatation. As a result, fluid retention and oedema are common side effects, and therefore, they are often used in combination with a diuretic. Other side effects include sedation, hypotension, GI symptoms, and dry mouth. Clonidine can suppress sinoatrial node and AVN function, leading to significant bradycardia, particularly in patients with CKD or sinoatrial node dysfunction. Rebound hypertension may also occur if clonidine at high doses is suddenly discontinued. No dose reductions are required for clonidine and methyldopa in renal impairment, although they should be started at small doses and increased gradually. Moxonidine is extensively renally cleared, and therefore, a dose reduction is recommended in patients with moderate renal impairment (eGFR 30–60mL/min/1.73m^2) and should be avoided if the eGFR is <30mL/min/1.73m^2. In addition, moxonidine should be avoided in patients with HF.

These drugs have the advantage of not interacting with other antihypertensive drugs or immunosuppressants, although caution is advised when using drugs with similar side effects [such as central nervous system (CNS) depression].

Alpha-blockers

α-blockers, such as doxazosin and prazosin, exert their effect by causing peripheral vasodilatation. They are often used in patients with CKD as adjuncts to antihypertensive therapy after ACEIs, ARBs, β-blockers, and calcium channel antagonists have been considered. α-blockers are often considered in men with benign prostatic hypertrophy, as they reduce the symptoms associated with this. α-blockers are metabolized by the liver; hence, no dose reduction is required in patients with CKD. A common side effect is hypotension, and therefore, they are often started at low doses and gradually increased.

Direct vasodilators

Hydralazine and minoxidil cause vascular smooth muscle relaxation, and therefore vasodilatation. They are potent antihypertensive agents used as an adjunct to existing therapy in cases of resistant hypertension. They can cause significant fluid retention (including pericardial effusion) and tachycardia, and for this reason, they should be used in combination with a β-blocker and loop diuretic. Minoxidil has the additional unwanted side effect of hypertrichosis, while hydralazine can cause an SLE-like syndrome. A dose reduction is necessary for hydralazine if the eGFR is <30mL/min/1.73m^2, and minoxidil should be used with caution in severe renal impairment.

References

1 Szummer K, Lundman P, Jacobson SH, *et al.*; SWEDEHEART. Relation between renal function, presentation, use of therapies and in-hospital complications in acute coronary syndrome: data from the SWEDEHEART register. *J Intern Med* 2010;**268**:40–9.

2 Ibanez B, James S, Agewall S, *et al.*; ESC Scientific Document Group. 2017 ESC Guidelines for the management of acute myocardial infarction in patients presenting with ST-segment elevation: The Task Force for the management of acute myocardial infarction in patients presenting with ST-segment elevation of the European Society of Cardiology (ESC). *Eur Heart J* 2018;**39**:119–77.

3 Roffi M, Patrono C, Collet JP, *et al.*; ESC Scientific Document Group. 2015 ESC Guidelines for the management of acute coronary syndromes in patients presenting without persistent ST-segment elevation: Task Force for the Management of Acute Coronary Syndromes in Patients Presenting without Persistent ST-Segment Elevation of the European Society of Cardiology (ESC). *Eur Heart J* 2016;**37**:267–315.

4 Rossignol P, Cleland JG, Bhandari S, *et al.* Determinants and consequences of renal function variations with aldosterone blocker therapy in heart failure patients after myocardial infarction: insights from the Eplerenone Post-Acute Myocardial Infarction Heart Failure Efficacy and Survival Study. *Circulation* 2012;**125**:271–9.

5 Weisbord SD, Gallagher M, Jneid H, *et al.*; PRESERVE Trial Group. Outcomes after angiography with sodium bicarbonate and acetylcysteine. *N Engl J Med* 2018;**378**:603–14.

6 Nijssen EC, Rennenberg RJ, Nelemans PJ, *et al*. Prophylactic hydration to protect renal function from intravascular iodinated contrast material in patients at high risk of contrast-induced nephropathy (AMACING): a prospective, randomised, phase 3, controlled, open-label, non-inferiority trial. *Lancet* 2017;**389**:1312–22.
7 Baigent C, Landray MJ, Reith C, *et al*.; SHARP Investigators. The effects of lowering LDL cholesterol with simvastatin plus ezetimibe in patients with chronic kidney disease (Study of Heart and Renal Protection): a randomised placebo-controlled trial. *Lancet* 2011;**377**:2181–92.
8 Ponikowski P, Voors AA, Anker SD, *et al*.; Authors/Task Force Members, Document Reviewers. 2016 ESC Guidelines for the diagnosis and treatment of acute and chronic heart failure: The Task Force for the diagnosis and treatment of acute and chronic heart failure of the European Society of Cardiology (ESC). Developed with the special contribution of the Heart Failure Association (HFA) of the ESC. *Eur J Heart Fail* 2016;**18**:891–975.
9 Cice G, Ferrara L, D'Andrea A, *et al*. Carvedilol increases two-year survival in dialysis patients with dilated cardiomyopathy: a prospective, placebo-controlled trial. *J Am Coll Cardiol* 2003;**41**:1438–44.
10 Kumar S, de Lusignan S, McGovern A, *et al*. Ischaemic stroke, haemorrhage, and mortality in older patients with chronic kidney disease newly started on anticoagulation for atrial fibrillation: a population based study from UK primary care. *BMJ* 2018;**360**:k342.
11 Kirchhof P, Benussi S, Kotecha D, *et al*. 2016 ESC Guidelines for the management of atrial fibrillation developed in collaboration with EACTS. *Eur Heart J* 2016;**37**:2893–962.
12 Wang X, Tirucherai G, Marbury TC, *et al*. Pharmacokinetics, pharmacodynamics, and safety of apixaban in subjects with end-stage renal disease on hemodialysis. *J Clin Pharmacol* 2016;**56**:628–36.
13 Holtkamp FA, de Zeeuw D, Thomas MC, *et al*. An acute fall in estimated glomerular filtration rate during treatment with losartan predicts a slower decrease in long-term renal function. *Kidney Int* 2011;**80**:282–7.

Chapter 6.2

Pregnancy and lactation

Anita Banerjee, Debasish Banerjee, and Vivekanand Jha

Cardiac disease in pregnancy

CV diseases complicate the course of 0.2–4% of all pregnancies.[1] Cardiac disease remains a significant cause of maternal death at around 1%. The conditions most frequently encountered during pregnancy are congenital heart disease in developed nations and rheumatic heart disease in the developing world. With more pregnancies at an advanced maternal age and an increasing prevalence of traditional CV risk factors among women, the incidence and spectrum of CV diseases during pregnancy are shifting, with a rising prevalence of atherosclerotic CV disease and HF.[2]

Women with pre-existing cardiac disease may exhibit decompensation of cardiac function during pregnancy, leading to maternal, as well as fetal, mortality and morbidity. Maternal morbidity is primarily due to pulmonary oedema, a cerebrovascular accident (CVA), or arrhythmias. Obstetric complications include preterm delivery, premature rupture of membranes, and postpartum haemorrhage. Fetal and neonate morbidity manifests as small-for-gestational age babies and prematurity complicated by respiratory distress syndrome and intracerebral haemorrhage.

This chapter will provide an approach to the management of cardiac disease in pregnancy, with updates from the ESC's Registry of Pregnancy and Cardiac Disease (ROPAC). Optimum care should be provided ideally within the setting of a joint obstetric cardiac clinic and with multidisciplinary team (MDT) input, involving the cardiologist, high-risk obstetrician, obstetric anaesthetist, and obstetric physician.

Risk stratification of cardiac disease can help a woman of reproductive age in making an informed choice on whether to embark on a pregnancy, inform about the risks of continuing a pregnancy, and help with management. Several classification schemes have been developed to estimate maternal cardiac risk; the CARPREG (CARdiac disease in PREGnancy) classification considers both congenital and acquired cardiac diseases, and the ZAHARA (Zwangerschap bij vrouwen met een Aangeboren HARtAfwijking) classification considers congenital heart disease only. The modified WHO classification, summarized in Table 6.2.1, however, appears to be the most reliable in predicting maternal risks, since it takes into consideration any underlying heart disease.

Table 6.2.1 Modified WHO classification of maternal risk in women with cardiac disease*

WHO class	I	II	III	IV
Risk of maternal mortality	Minimal	Small increase	Significant increase	Pregnancy contraindicated
Risk of maternal morbidity	Mild	Moderate	Severe	Severe (termination should be considered)
	Uncomplicated/mild: Pulmonary stenosis Patent ductus arteriosus Mitral valve prolapse Successfully repaired simple lesions Isolated ventricular or atrial ectopic beats	Repaired tetralogy of Fallot Unoperated atrial/ventricular septal defect Majority of arrhythmias	Mechanical valve Systemic right ventricle Fontan circulation Cyanotic heart disease (unrepaired) Other complex congenital heart disease Aortic dilatation 40–45mm in Marfan's syndrome Aortic dilatation of 45–50mm in aortic disease associated with bicuspid aortic valve	Severe systemic ventricular dysfunction (LVEF <30%, NYHA classes III–IV) PAH of any cause Native severe coarctation Aortic dilatation of >50mm in aortic disease associated with bicuspid aortic valve Marfan's syndrome with aortic dilatation of >45mm
		Individualized risk II or III to be determined Mild left ventricular impairment Hypertrophic cardiomyopathy		

* Source data from Regitz-Zagrosek V, Roos-Hesselink JW, Bauersachs J, *et al.*; ESC Scientific Document Group. 2018 ESC Guidelines for the management of cardiovascular diseases during pregnancy. *Eur Heart J* 2018;39:3165–241 and Thorne S, MacGregor A, Nelson-Piercy C. Risks of contraception and pregnancy in heart disease. *Heart* 2006 Oct;92(10):1520–1525.

Physiological changes in pregnancy

CV adaptations to pregnancy start in the first trimester. The first change is an increase in plasma volume as a result of salt and water retention by the kidneys, seen as early as 4 weeks' gestation. This, in combination with a fall in the SVR, leads to rise in CO and a drop in BP from the fifth week of gestation. The drop in SVR reaches its nadir at 20–32 weeks' gestation and then rises to pre-pregnancy level before term. The heart rate increases by approximately 10bpm in the second half of pregnancy. The CO increases further during the intrapartum period and immediately after delivery. The CV changes and ECG findings are summarized in Box 6.2.1 and Table 6.2.2.

Changes in respiratory physiology include a 40–50% rise in minute ventilation due to an increased tidal volume at the expense of the functional residual capacity. The forced expiratory volume remains stable. About 60–70% of women experience a sensation of dyspnoea during normal pregnancy. However, the respiratory rate does not increase; hence, any rise may be associated with significant pathology.

Other significant adaptive changes include an increase in the renal blood flow and GFR by 50%. Altered renal haemodynamics, along with endocrine changes, lead to significant water and sodium retention by the renal tubules, and mildly reduced serum sodium levels and serum osmolality. Changes in the haematological system include a lowered haemoglobin concentration, contributed partly by an increased blood volume, and a state of hypercoagulability secondary to pregnancy-induced changes in coagulation factor concentrations.

Box 6.2.1 Common ECG abnormalities in a normal pregnancy

- Atrial and ventricular ectopics are common
- Small Q-wave and inverted T-wave in lead III
- ST-depression and T-wave inversion in inferior lateral leads
- Left-axis shift of QRS complex

Table 6.2.2 Common cardiovascular changes throughout pregnancy

	First trimester	Second trimester	Third trimester	Intrapartum	Early post-delivery	Late changes (>2 weeks)
SVR	↓	↓	↑ beginning to rise by term	↓	↑	↑
Blood pressure	↓	↓	↑ to pre-pregnancy	↔	↑	↔
Cardiac output	↑	↑	↔	↑	↑	↓
Stroke volume	↑	↑	↑	↑	↑	↓

Drug metabolism in pregnancy

GI absorption and bioavailability of drugs are affected by delayed gastric emptying, increased gastric pH, and reduced intestinal motility. This may lead to delayed absorption of high-permeability drugs. Haemodynamic changes, such as renal blood flow and GFR, affect drug distribution and elimination, as do alterations in hepatic metabolism. The increased plasma volume, particularly in early pregnancy, may cause a reduction in drug concentration. Lowered serum albumin levels, however, may increase the non-protein-bound fraction of other drugs, as the pregnancy progresses.

Drug safety in pregnancy

There are sparse drug safety data on many of the cardiac drugs prescribed in pregnancy. Drugs causing teratogenicity and embryopathy, such as warfarin, ACEIs, and ARBs, should be used with caution in women of childbearing age. Counselling women regarding the potential side effects and advising on appropriate contraception are imperative. The type of anticoagulation to be used for mechanical heart valves, the risks versus benefits of switching medication, or the continuation of warfarin in the pregnancy should be carefully considered. In the ROPAC registry, two-thirds of all cardiac medications used were β-blockers.[4] There has been controversy regarding the effects of β-blockers during pregnancy, but recent data suggest it is the underlying disease, rather than β-blockers, that is associated with low birthweight.

Recognizing the increased prevalence of women with pre-existing medical conditions requiring medication during pregnancy and the detrimental effects of withholding medication, the US FDA has amended the *Pregnancy and Lactation Labeling Final Rule*. The new rules remove the pregnancy letter categories A, B, C, D, and X and require the label to be updated when needed. The final rule requires that the labelling includes relevant information about pregnancy testing, contraception, and infertility and creates a consistent format for providing information.

Management of hypertension in pregnancy

Hypertensive disorders affect up to 10% of all pregnant women. Hypertension is a risk factor for kidney injury, stroke, HF, placental abruption, intrauterine growth retardation (IUGR), and prematurity. Appropriate management of BP improves maternal and fetal outcome. Severe systolic hypertension is an independent risk factor for stroke in pregnancy. Distinguishing between the different hypertensive disorders is important for appropriate management. The definitions of hypertensive disorders in pregnancy and the stages of hypertension are summarized in Tables 6.2.3 and 6.2.4.

The BP targets continue to be debated. A large international study found that there was no detriment to maintaining the DBP at 80–85mmHg, i.e. less tight control.[5] They found no significant differences in perinatal or maternal adverse outcomes. Evidence of end-organ damage, CKD, diabetes mellitus, or cardiac disease should prompt a lower target (SBP <130mmHg).

Among hypertensive women of childbearing age, the antihypertensive medication should be reviewed as part of pre-pregnancy planning (see Table 6.2.5). Target BP and preventative measures should be discussed, including smoking cessation, optimal weight management, and lifestyle modifications. An evaluation of end-organ damage and exclusion of

Table 6.2.3 Definitions of hypertensive disorders in pregnancy

Chronic hypertension Incidence 1–5%	BP ≥140/90mmHg Precedes pregnancy Occurs before 20 weeks' gestation Persistent 3 months post-delivery	25% will have PET
Gestational hypertension Incidence 6–7%	Occurs after 20 weeks' gestation BP ≥140/90mmHg No proteinuria or abnormal blood tests	Future risk A marker for risk of future chronic hypertension
Pre-eclampsia (PET) Incidence 5–7%	New-onset protein: creatinine ratio >0.3 BP ≥140/90 mmHg	Future risks 2-fold ↑ IHD 4-fold ↑ hypertension Reoccurrence rate of PET in future pregnancies 25–60%

Table 6.2.4 Stages of hypertension in pregnancy

Mild	Moderate	Severe
140–149/90–99mmHg	150–59/100–109mmHg	>160/110mmHg

Table 6.2.5 Antihypertensive use in pregnancy and safety profile

Class of drug	Teratogenic	Side effects Contraindications (CI)	Crosses placenta	Transfer to breast milk	Breastfeeding
Calcium channel blockers: Amlodipine Nifedipine	No	Leg oedema Flushing Palpitations CI: aortic stenosis	Yes	Yes	Limited data No adverse effects from amlodipine Compatible Nifedipine concentrations in breast milk are similar to those in maternal plasma
β-blockers: Bisoprolol Metoprolol	No	Bronchospasm Bradycardia CI: asthma	Yes	Yes	Limited data Compatible Propranolol concentrations in breast milk are similar to those in maternal plasma
α/β-blockers: Labetalol	No	Bronchospasm Bradycardia CI: asthma	Yes	Yes	Compatible
Central α-adrenergic: Methyldopa	No	Sedation 5% hepatitis Depression	Yes	Yes	Compatible
α-adrenergic blockers: Doxazosin Prazosin	No	Postural hypotension	Yes	Yes	Prazosin preferred postpartum

(Continued)

Table 6.2.5 *(Contd.)*

Class of drug	Teratogenic	Side effects Contraindications (CI)	Crosses placenta	Transfer to breast milk	Breastfeeding
Vasodilator: Hydralazine	No	Headaches Flushing Tachycardia Palpitations CI: heart rate >120bpm	Yes	Yes	Compatible
ACEIs	Yes Fetal anomalies in all three trimesters 8% Lowest incidence of birth defects with exposure in the first trimester	CI: during pregnancy	Yes	Yes	Introduce postpartum with captopril and enalapril
Diltiazem	Yes Skeletal anomalies		Yes	Yes	Limited data

potential secondary causes of hypertension should be considered, e.g. phaeochromocytoma, Cushing's disease, or Conn's syndrome. A systematic review and meta-analysis found adverse outcomes of pregnancy were common in women with chronic hypertension. Counselling regarding the risk of superimposed pre-eclampsia (PET) and the risk of preterm delivery and maternal and fetal complications should be discussed.

Preventative measures for PET include the administration of 75–150mg nocte of aspirin from 12 weeks' gestation for high-risk groups, including all hypertensives. A systematic review and meta-analysis found that low-dose aspirin before 16 weeks' gestation reduced the incidence of PET and IUGR. There is growing evidence of a dose-dependent effect of aspirin. A recent study found that when 150mg aspirin was administered from 11–14 weeks' gestation until 36 weeks' gestation to women, who in their first-trimester screening were deemed high risk for preterm PET (before 34 weeks' gestation), there was a reduced incidence of preterm PET.[6] Calcium supplementation of ≥1g a day reduces the risk of PET, particularly in women with a low-calcium diet.

During hypertensive emergencies, the aim is to normalize the maternal physiological parameters and protect the organs, the goal being to lower the BP to <160/110mmHg. BP lowering should occur over several hours and can be achieved orally or parenterally. One systematic review suggested that a single oral agent can be as effective in reducing BP as parenteral agents. Parenteral magnesium sulfate may be needed for seizure prophylaxis, to control BP and reduce the risk of eclampsia. This has been supported by evidence from the Use the Collaborative Eclampsia Trial. A loading dose of 4g should be given IV over 5min, followed by an infusion of 1g/h maintained for 24h. Recurrent seizures should be treated with a further dose of 2–4g given over 5min.

Postpartum hypertension peaks on days 3–5 postpartum, likely due to volume expansion and fluid shifts. NSAIDs should be avoided in women with PET and AKI. In gestational hypertension, the BP falls to normal pre-pregnancy levels within a few weeks. Therefore, a review of the medication prior to discharge and planning for follow-up are necessary to titrate or cease medication.

Management of heart failure in pregnancy

Maternal mortality remains high for women with cardiomyopathy and HF in pregnancy. In addition, cardiomyopathy increases the risk for HF and ventricular arrhythmias. Diagnosis may be missed, as symptoms like tiredness, shortness of breath, and palpitations may be attributed to pregnancy. In the large worldwide ROPAC registry, 13.1% of the 1321 enrolled women developed HF.[7] Cardiomyopathy also increases the risk for preterm delivery and admission to an intensive care setting. Acute HF develops more frequently in the third trimester, intrapartum, and immediately postpartum. Women with cardiac disease and superimposed PET had a 30% risk of developing HF in the pregnancy. For causes of heart failure in pregnancy, see Box 6.2.2.

The goals of treatment remain the same as for non-pregnant women with HF, including control of heart rate, reduction in cardiac afterload, and increase in cardiac contractility (see Table 6.2.6).[2] Hydralazine and nitrates should be used to offload, instead of ACEIs and ARBs. If inotropic agents are required, dopamine and levosimendan can be used. Early delivery may be needed if LV function worsens and symptomatic HF develops despite medical management.

Box 6.2.2 Causes of heart failure in pregnancy

- Pre-existing structural heart disease—congenital or acquired
- Coronary artery disease
- Hypertensive disorders
- Cardiomyopathy—dilated/hypertrophic/restrictive
- Peripartum cardiomyopathy
- Arrhythmias

Table 6.2.6 Drugs used in heart failure during pregnancy

	Teratogenic	Side effects Contraindications	Crosses placenta	Transfer to breast milk	Breastfeeding
Reduce preload					
Diuretics: Furosemide	No	Risk of intravascular depletion	Yes	No	↓ Milk production
Calcium channel blockers: Nifedipine Amlodipine	No	Leg oedema Flushing Palpitations	Yes	Yes	Compatible Nifedipine concentrations in breast milk are similar to those in maternal plasma
β-blockers: Bisoprolol Metoprolol	No	Bronchospasm Bradycardia	Yes	Yes	Limited data Compatible
Reduce after load					
Hydralazine	No	Headaches Flushing Tachycardia Palpitations	Yes	Yes	Compatible

(*Continued*)

Table 6.2.6 (*Contd.*)

	Teratogenic	Side effects Contraindications	Crosses placenta	Transfer to breast milk	Breastfeeding
Nitrates	No		Unknown	Unknown	Compatible
Increase contractility of the heart					
Digoxin	No		Yes	Yes	Compatible
Levosimendan	No		Yes	Yes	Compatible
Dopamine	No		Yes	Yes	Compatible
Spironalactone Eplerenone	Risk of anti-androgen effect Not associated with adverse effects Can be used when other medications ineffective		Yes	Yes	Compatible

Peripartum cardiomyopathy

Peripartum cardiomyopathy (PPCM) is characterized by reduced ejection fraction (<45%), presenting towards the end of pregnancy or within 5 months of delivery, in a woman without known pre-existing structural heart disease. The incidence is 1 in 300–3000. Risk factors include advanced age, multiparity, multiple pregnancies, PET, and African heritage. Treatment includes standard HF management and anticoagulation to prevent intracardiac mural thrombus. If maximal medical management fails, women may require additional support by a ventricular assist device or extracorporeal membrane oxygenation to bridge them until recovery or cardiac transplantation. The risk of relapse in a future pregnancy is greater in women with persistent LV dysfunction, compared to those who show complete recovery (50% versus 20%). Novel approaches to management are being evaluated. A recent RCT has shown bromocriptine may be beneficial in the management of PPCM.[8] The cathepsin D-cleaved 16kDa form of prolactin has been considered to mediate PPCM.

Management of valvular heart disease in pregnancy

All women with VHD planning to become pregnant should be carefully assessed prior to conception. The increased CO, tachycardia, and fall in the peripheral vascular resistance increase transvalvular gradients, compromising the valve function. A general, as well as lesion-specific, cardiac risk assessment is required. Where possible, correction prior to pregnancy can improve outcomes. Stenotic lesions can be more problematic than regurgitant lesions (see Table 6.2.7).

Mitral stenosis

Pre-existing mitral stenosis is commonly due to rheumatic heart disease. Severe mitral stenosis (valve areas of <1.5 cm^2) increases the risk for cardiac failure and arrhythmias. AF may occur due to the dilated atrium, requiring therapeutic anticoagulation (see ➔ Management of arrhythmias in pregnancy, p. 361). Standard failure management includes use of β-blockers, diuretics, and digoxin. Where indicated, mitral balloon valvuloplasty should be performed prior to pregnancy.

Aortic stenosis

This is most likely to be a bicuspid valve, which may also be associated with aortic coarctation. β-blockers or a non-dihydropyridine CCB may be of benefit, but vasodilators are to be avoided. Aortic balloon valvuloplasty should be considered prior to pregnancy. Pregnancy need not be discouraged in asymptomatic women, even those with severe aortic stenosis, when the LV size and function, as well as the exercise test, are normal and severe LVH (posterior wall ≥15mm) has been excluded.

Table 6.2.7 Adverse effects and treatment options for stenotic valvular heart disease in pregnancy

Valve	Maternal adverse effects	Fetal adverse effects	Treatment options
Aortic stenosis	HF 10% Arrhythmias 3–25%	IUGR Prematurity Small-for-gestational age All risks up to 25%	β-blockers
Mitral stenosis	Moderate to severe mitral stenosis Valve area <1.5cm^2 Risk of AF 15% and HF Mortality 3%	IUGR 20–30% Prematurity 5–20% Stillbirth 1–3%	β-blockers, digoxin

Source data from Sliwa K, Johnson MR, Zilla P, Roos-Hesselink JW. Management of valvular disease in pregnancy: a global perspective. *Eur Heart J* 2015 May 7;36(18):1078–1089.

Management of congenital heart disease in pregnancy

With appropriate pre-conceptual counselling and the development of specialized adult congenital services, the outcome of pregnancy in women with congenital heart disease has improved substantially, among those who have undergone prior corrective surgery and those with favourable NYHA class baselines and little use of medication pre-pregnancy. Simple lesions give a normal life expectancy; however, complex conditions, such as a single ventricle, a systemic RV, cyanotic heart disease, PAH, and Fontan circulation, are associated with significant morbidity, including HF, postpartum haemorrhage, arrhythmias, and decline in ventricular function. Women with congenital heart disease should have a fetal echocardiogram at 18–22 weeks' gestation for a detailed screen. The risk of congenital fetal cardiac anomalies is estimated to be 3–5% in the offspring of women with congenital heart disease. In cyanotic congenital heart disease, the degree of maternal hypoxaemia is an important predictor of fetal outcome. When the resting maternal oxygen saturation is >90%, the live birth rate is 92%, whereas it declines to 12% when the maternal oxygen saturation is <85%.[4] Maternal complications include VTE, SVT, and infective endocarditis.[5]

Management of prosthetic heart valves during pregnancy

All women with a prosthetic valve should receive counselling prior to pregnancy. Balancing the risk of valve thrombosis and haemorrhage and the risk to the fetus requires a multidisciplinary approach to care. ROPAC more recently undertook a review from the worldwide registry of 212 metallic heart valves (MHVs) and 134 tissue heart valves (THVs) (see Table 6.2.8).[10] The majority of MHVs were for acquired conditions, whereas the congenital group had THVs. The probability of an adverse-free event was higher in the THV group than the MHV group (79.1% versus 58.1%, respectively). HF events and maternal and fetal outcomes were comparable in developed versus emerging countries.

Due to the risk of infective endocarditis all women with prosthetic valves are recommended to have prophylactic antibiotics for all surgical procedures. It is common practice to give prophylactic antibiotics at the time of a Caesarean section or if there is confirmation of β-haemolytic streptococcal colonization.

There are different strategies proposed as therapeutic options for anticoagulation in pregnancy (see Table 6.2.9). Currently, no specific management plan has been found to be supreme. Current guidelines suggest continuing VKAs despite an increased risk for pregnancy loss. VKAs are associated with a lower risk for valve thrombosis in the second and third trimesters, compared to UFH and LMWH (see Table 6.2.10). However, regimens that include VKAs had lower live birth rates. The risk for miscarriages and late fetal death was increased in women on VKAs in the first trimester, and this continued throughout pregnancy. A dose-dependent increase in fetal complications with warfarin has been described. A daily warfarin dose of <5mg appears to have a better outcome. To minimize the risk for fetal intracerebral haemorrhage, VKAs should be replaced with LMWH 10–14 days before delivery. One single-centre study with enoxaparin alone found 14.9% had a thrombotic event and a third had antepartum or postpartum haemorrhage. Women with adverse events were more likely to be non-compliant and had subtherapeutic factor Xa levels.

Table 6.2.8 Overall risk of all valvular heart diseases in pregnancy from ROPAC registry

Overall serious complication	>40%
Maternal mortality	1.4%
Pregnancy loss	18.4%
Valve thrombosis	4.7% associated with a 20% mortality
Haemorrhage	23.1%

Source data from van Hagen IM, Roos-Hesselink JW, Ruys TP, Merz WM, Goland S, Gabriel H, *et al.* Pregnancy in Women With a Mechanical Heart Valve: Data of the European Society of Cardiology Registry of Pregnancy and Cardiac Disease (ROPAC). *Circulation* 2015 Jul 14;132(2):132–142.

Table 6.2.9 Options for antithrombotic strategy for valvular heart disease in pregnancy

Warfarin >5mg or warfarin at any dose	Warfarin <5mg
Discontinue 6–12 weeks, replace by LMWH or UFH	Continue oral anticoagulant throughout pregnancy until 36th week
Twice-daily SC LMWH Dose adjustment for anti-Xa level of 0.8–1.2U/mL 4–6h post-dose Task Force advises weekly control of peak anti-Xa levels	To minimize the risk of fetal intracerebral haemorrhage, oral anticoagulants are to be discontinued 10–14 days before delivery, to allow clearance of the drug, and switched to LMWH

Table 6.2.10 Antithrombotic drugs used in pregnancy

	Teratogenicity	Side effects Contraindications	Transfer across placenta	Transfer to breast milk	Breastfeeding
Warfarin	Yes Chondrodysplasia punctata, nasal hypoplasia, short proximal limbs 5% risk	Dose-dependent risk of intracerebral haemorrhage, miscarriage, and stillbirth Bleeding	Yes	Yes, minimal	Compatible
LMWH	No	Bleeding	No	No	Compatible
UFH	No	Bleeding	No	No	Compatible

The indications for anticoagulation during pregnancy include AF, prosthetic valve thrombosis, and VTE. If warranted, thrombolysis is not contraindicated for a massive PE in pregnancy. There is increasing evidence for the use of thrombolytic agents in pregnancy, including in cases of thrombosis of prosthetic valves, stroke, and PE. Thrombosis of prosthetic valves is a life-threatening event. Management warrants fibrinolysis if immediate surgical removal is not possible. A low-dose infusion of tissue plasminogen activator from a single-centre prospective study found a 100% thrombolysis rate and a fetal mortality rate of 20%. Some recommend the addition of aspirin 75mg throughout pregnancy to reduce the risk of a thrombotic event.

The new-generation oral anticoagulants, including dabigatran and rivaroxaban, in animal studies have been shown to have adverse effects on the fetus and are not recommended in pregnancy.

Management of pulmonary hypertension in pregnancy

A mPAP of >25mmHg at rest is indicative of PAH. Maternal morbidity and mortality are high in women with PAH, especially in the third trimester and in the first few weeks postpartum, because of VTE, refractory right HF, and pulmonary hypertensive crisis. Therapeutic options include inhaled iloprost or IV prostaglandin. Endothelin-1 receptor antagonists are not usually recommended for use in pregnancy. Early referral to a specialist centre and an MDT approach are paramount. Maternal mortality has improved to 17–33%, and neonatal survival rate to 87–89%, with the introduction of newer agents for the management of PAH.

Management of aortopathies in pregnancy

The risk of dissection occurs in the last trimester (50%) or early postpartum (38%). Risk factors include hypertension and increasing maternal age. Certain conditions leave patients more susceptible, including women with bicuspid aortic valve and inherited diseases (Marfan's, Ehlers–Danlos type IV, and Loey–Dietz). The risk of dissection in Marfan's syndrome is 1% with a non-dilated aorta. The risk increases with dilatation of >4.5cm. Treatment with β-blockers is thought to be beneficial as a preventative measure.

Takayasu's arteritis is a chronic, inflammatory, progressive, idiopathic arteriopathy, afflicting young women of reproductive age, causing narrowing, occlusion, and aneurysms of the aorta and its branches. This condition is seen in India, East Asia, and Latin America. During pregnancy, such patients warrant special attention. Possible presentation can be with hypertension, organ dysfunction, and stenosis, hindering uterine blood flow. Pregnancy does not interfere with disease progression, but Takayasu's arteritis has several adverse implications in pregnancy, including miscarriage, PET, IUGR, intrauterine death (IUD), and placental abruption. The aims of treatment are control of inflammation, prevention, and treatment of complications such as hypertension. The possibility of revascularization by percutaneous angioplasty, use of endoprosthesis, or surgical correction for occlusive and stenotic lesions should be explored.

Management of arrhythmias in pregnancy

Most palpitations in pregnancy are benign. Premature extra beats and sustained tachyarrhythmias are common. SVT is exacerbated in 20–44% of cases. AF and atrial flutter are rare.

Acute conversion of SVT includes a trial of vagal manoeuvres, followed by IV adenosine. Second-line agents include verapamil and metoprolol (see Table 6.2.11). For long-term management, β-blockers are preferred, with flecainide and sotalol as second-line agents. Synchronized direct current (DC) conversion is indicated in the case of CV compromise. For persistent CV compromise, general anaesthesia and intubation are advised, with a rapid sequence induction anaesthetic procedure after 20 weeks' gestation to reduce the risk of aspiration. Manual displacement of the uterus is also recommended to reduce vena caval compression after 20 weeks' gestation.

Approximately 1.4% of pregnant women develop ventricular tachyarrhythmias, more commonly in the third trimester. Risk factors include NYHA class >1 and cardiomyopathy. The management is similar to that for the non-pregnant state and is to add β-blockers and procainamide. Haemodynamic compromise requires immediate DC cardioversion.

Pregnancy outcomes for women with ICDs are good. The ICD is switched off during a Caesarean section, to prevent inappropriate discharge from electrical interference by diathermy, which may be misinterpreted and deliver inappropriate shocks. Women should be delivered in specialized centres.

Table 6.2.11 Drugs used to manage arrhythmias in pregnancy

	Teratogenicity	Transfer across placenta	Transfer to breast milk	Breastfeeding
Adenosine	No	No	No	Compatible
Metoprolol	No	Yes	Yes	Compatible
Sotalol	No	Yes	Yes	Compatible
Flecainide	No	Yes	Yes	Compatible
Verapamil	No	Yes	Yes	Compatible
Procainamide	No	Yes	Yes	Compatible
Propafenone	No	Yes	Yes	Compatible
Amiodarone	17% transient neonatal hypothyroidism	Yes	Yes	No

Management of acute coronary syndrome in pregnancy

There is a 3-fold increase in ACS during pregnancy than in the non-pregnant population. More women now conceive with pre-existing IHD. Hormone-derived vasculopathy increases the risk for coronary artery dissection in pregnancy, most commonly at the time of delivery and in the early postpartum period. The initial management is the same as that for the non-pregnant state.[2] For percutaneous angiography and intervention, access should be gained by the radial artery, with a lead shield used to protect the fetus and a pelvic tilt to reduce the effects of aorto-venocaval compression. BMS are preferred for revascularization to minimize the requirement for long-term DAPT. Current guidelines suggest refraining from use of the glycoprotein IIb/IIIa drugs bivalirudin, prasugrel, and ticagrelor. No lipid-lowering agent should be administered during pregnancy and lactation. Delivery should be postponed for 2 weeks after the cardiac event, if possible. Women with pre-existing IHD are at an increased risk of maternal cardiac events in pregnancy. A retrospective study found women had more obstetric and fetal complications. Hormone-derived vasculopathy increases the risk for coronary artery dissection in pregnancy, most commonly at the time of delivery and in the early postpartum period. For drugs used for ACS in pregnancy, see Table 6.2.12.

Table 6.2.12 Drugs used for acute coronary syndrome in pregnancy

	Teratogenicity	Transfer across placenta	Transfer to breast milk	Breastfeeding
Aspirin (low dose)	No	Yes	Yes	Compatible
Clopidogrel	No	Yes	Yes	Compatible
Prasugrel		No data	No data	No
Ticagrelor		No data	No data	No
Statins	Little data	Data lacking	Data lacking	No

Cardiac arrest in pregnancy

One in 12,000 hospital admissions are complicated by a cardiac arrest in pregnancy in the United States. The commonest causes include amniotic fluid embolism, HF, haemorrhage, MI, and sepsis. Manual uterine displacement is advised in women at >20 weeks' gestation to improve maternal cardiopulmonary resuscitation. A perimortem Caesarean section should be considered within the first couple of minutes into a cardiac arrest situation in women at >20 weeks' gestation to improve maternal cardiopulmonary resuscitation. All standard cardiac arrest medications can be administered.

Obstetric management for women with cardiac disease

Seamlessly coordinated care should be the goal in the management of pregnancy in women with cardiac disease. Women stratified as high risk should be managed and delivered at a specialist centre, with input from the MDT. It is important to draw up a delivery plan prior to delivery with MDT input, considering factors including current cardiac status and obstetric history. Where possible, vaginal delivery can be considered, unless there are obstetric reasons/indications or concerns for further deterioration of cardiac function during delivery. In asymptomatic women, spontaneous delivery at term can be considered. A planned induction is advised when further monitoring is required, including telemetry and an arterial line. Standard guidelines do not exist, due to a lack of prospective data and the influence of individual characteristics of the women. Management therefore should be individualized.

Intrapartum management

Assisted second stage of labour may be helpful to minimize maternal effort. Women with cardiac disease are most at risk of pulmonary oedema during the second stage and immediately postpartum. Following delivery, there is an immediate rise in CO due to relief of the IVC and contraction of the uterus, leading to an autotransfusion. During the first 12–24h post-delivery, monitoring of volume status and fluid balance is important. Fluid overload can occur for several reasons: iatrogenic fluid infusions, oxytocin infusions, β-agonists for tocolysis, or high-dose steroids for fetal lung maturation. Obstetric medication may be indicated for the prevention of postpartum haemorrhage and induction of labour (see Table 6.2.13).

Table 6.2.13 Common obstetric drugs administered

Usage	Drug	Risks	Suitability
PPH	Carboprost PG2α agonist	Vasospasm Bronchospasm	Avoid in PAH, shunt lesions, and single ventricle
PPH	Ergometrine	Severe hypertension Coronary vasospasm Pulmonary oedema	Avoid in ACS, aortopathies, PAH, and hypertension/PET
Prevention of PPH and augmentation of labour	Oxytocin	Bolus injection can cause sudden vasodilatation and severe hypotension	*Alternatively, administer as a slow infusion*
PPH, IOL, medical termination	Misoprostol PGE1 agonist		Well tolerated No contraindication for cardiac conditions
IOL	Dinoprostone PGE2 agonist	It has been suggested dinoprostone has a more profound effect on BP than PGE1 agonists	Well tolerated No absolute contraindication for cardiac conditions

ACS, acute coronary syndrome; BP, blood pressure; IOL, induction of labour; PAH, pulmonary arterial hypertension, PET, pre-eclampsia; PG, prostaglandin; PPH, postpartum haemorrhage.

Follow-up of women with cardiac disease

Long-term follow-up of all women with cardiac disease is important. Haemodynamic changes take several weeks to return to pre-pregnancy state. Early cardiac reassessment is required in women with impaired ventricular function or VHD that may have deteriorated further. Now, a review of the medication and contraception should be discussed, taking into consideration the woman's preferences and the risks versus benefits. Below is a table of the contraceptive options for the women (see Table 6.2.14).

Table 6.2.14 Contraception options with risks versus benefits for women with cardiac disease[11,12]

Class of drugs	Risks	Benefits	Suitability
Combined oestrogen and progesterone pill	High-dose oestrogen combinations carry an increased risk of: • Thrombosis • Hypertension • Dose-related increase in MI		Not suitable for many cardiac conditions
Progesterone-only pill		No significant change in BP, lipid profile, or thrombotic risk	Suitable for women on long-term anticoagulation
Intrauterine device Intrauterine system Copper IUD Levonorgestrel—Mirena®	Avoid if history of previous infective endocarditis PAH women to be inserted in a hospital setting, risk of bradycardia in response to cervical instrumentation	Good lipid profile: • ↑ HDL with Mirena® levonorgestrel releasing coil	
Injectable contraception Depot injection Depo-Provera® Subdermal implant Nexplanon®	Risk of haematoma if on anticoagulation	No cardiac contraindication	

BP, blood pressure; HDL, high-density lipoprotein; IUD, intrauterine device; MI, myocardial infarction; PAH, pulmonary arterial hypertension.

Source data from Mohan AR, Nelson-Piercy C. Drugs and therapeutics, including contraception, for women with heart disease. *Best Pract Res Clin Obstet Gynaecol* 2014 May;28(4):471–482 and Roos-Hesselink JW, Cornette J, Sliwa K, Pieper PG, Veldtman GR, Johnson MR. Contraception and cardiovascular disease. *Eur Heart J* 2015 Jul 14;36(27):1728–34, 1734a–1734b.

References

1 Roos-Hesselink JW, Ruys TP, Stein JI, *et al.* Outcome of pregnancy in patients with structural or ischaemic heart disease: results of a registry of the European Society of Cardiology. *Eur Heart J* 2013;**34**:657–65.
2 Regitz-Zagrosek V, Roos-Hesselink JW, Bauersachs J, *et al.*; ESC Scientific Document Group. 2018 ESC Guidelines for the management of cardiovascular diseases during pregnancy. *Eur Heart J* 2018;**39**:3165–241.
3 Thorne S, MacGregor A, Nelson-Piercy C. Risks of contraception and pregnancy in heart disease. *Heart* 2006;**92**:1520–5.
4 Ruys TP, Maggioni A, Johnson MR, *et al.* Cardiac medication during pregnancy, data from the ROPAC. *Int J Cardiol* 2014;**177**:124–8.
5 Magee LA, von Dadelszen P, Rey E, *et al.* Less-tight versus tight control of hypertension in pregnancy. *N Engl J Med* 2015;**372**:407–17.
6 Poon LC, Wright D, Rolnik DL, *et al.* Aspirin for Evidence-Based Preeclampsia Prevention trial: effect of aspirin in prevention of preterm preeclampsia in subgroups of women according to their characteristics and medical and obstetrical history. *Am J Obstet Gynecol* 2017;**217**:585.e1–5.
7 Ruys TP, Roos-Hesselink JW, Hall R, *et al.* Heart failure in pregnant women with cardiac disease: data from the ROPAC. *Heart* 2014;**100**:231–8.
8 Hilfiker-Kleiner D, Haghikia A, Berliner D, *et al.* Bromocriptine for the treatment of peripartum cardiomyopathy: a multicentre randomized study. *Eur Heart J* 2017;**38**:2671–9.
9 Sliwa K, Johnson MR, Zilla P, Roos-Hesselink JW. Management of valvular disease in pregnancy: a global perspective. *Eur Heart J* 2015;**36**:1078–89.
10 van Hagen IM, Roos-Hesselink JW, Ruys TP, *et al.* Pregnancy in women with a mechanical heart valve: data of the European Society of Cardiology Registry of Pregnancy and Cardiac Disease (ROPAC). *Circulation* 2015;**132**:132–42.
11 Mohan AR, Nelson-Piercy C. Drugs and therapeutics, including contraception, for women with heart disease. *Best Pract Res Clin Obstet Gynaecol* 2014;**28**:471–82.
12 Roos-Hesselink JW, Cornette J, Sliwa K, Pieper PG, Veldtman GR, Johnson MR. Contraception and cardiovascular disease. *Eur Heart J* 2015;**36**:1728–34, 1734a–b.

Chapter 6.3

Liver disease

Nina Hojs, Aftab Ala, and Debasish Banerjee

Introduction

Liver injury can be related to a variety of pathophysiological mechanisms, with the common causes being chronic infections with hepatitis B or C and alcoholic and non-alcoholic fatty liver disease (NAFLD).[1] With liver dysfunction, drug pharmacokinetics and pharmacodynamics may be altered via different mechanisms. Drug pharmacokinetics are altered as a result of blood shunting beyond the liver (both porto-systemic and intra-hepatic), impaired hepatocellular function, impaired biliary excretion, and decreased protein binding, and ascites or oedema which increases the volume of distribution for hydrophilic drugs.[1,2] Cytochrome P450 (CYP450) activity, which includes the major liver enzymes involved in drug metabolism, is variably reduced in patients with cirrhosis.[3]

There is no simple endogenous marker to predict hepatic function with respect to the elimination capacity of specific drugs.[3] Although not developed for this purpose, the Child–Pugh classification (see Table 6.3.1) is the most widely used assessment of hepatic dysfunction. Impairment of drug elimination only occurs late in the evolution of chronic liver disease, and thus, modification of the drug regimen should be needed only in the

Table 6.3.1 The Child–Pugh score and classification

Criteria		Number of points
Total bilirubin (micromol/L)	<34.2	1
	34.2–51.3	2
	>51.3	3
Albumin (g/L)	>35	1
	28–35	2
	<28	3
INR	<1.7	1
	1.7–2.2	2
	>2.2	3
Ascites	Absent	1
	Slight	2
	Moderate	3
Encephalopathy	Absent	1
	Grade 1–2	2
	Grade 3–4	3
Number of points together	**Class**	
5–6	A	
7–9	B	
10–15	C	

presence of significant hepatic dysfunction (Child–Pugh classes B and C).[3] The MELD score, which depends on kidney function, bilirubin, INR, and sodium values, can also be used for this purpose. Acute liver disease often affects drug elimination to a lesser extent than does cirrhosis.[3]

In order to predict the kinetic behaviour of drugs in cirrhotic patients, agents can be grouped according to their extent of hepatic extraction.[1] For drugs with a high hepatic extraction (β-blockers, calcium channel antagonists, morphine, certain statins, etc.), bioavailability increases as hepatic clearance decreases in cirrhotic patients.[1,2] If such drugs are administered orally to cirrhotic patients, their initial dose has to be reduced according to the hepatic extraction. Furthermore, their maintenance dose has to be adapted, irrespective of the route of administration. For drugs with a low hepatic extraction, their bioavailability after administration is not affected by liver disease, but hepatic clearance may be affected. For such drugs, only the maintenance dose has to be reduced, according to the estimated decrease in hepatic drug metabolism. For drugs with an intermediate hepatic extraction (amiodarone, certain statins), initial oral doses should be chosen in the low range of normal for cirrhotic patients and maintenance doses should be reduced as for high-extraction drugs.[1,2]

It must also be taken into account that many patients with liver disease have concurrent kidney failure, which may also affect drug metabolism.

The common CV conditions and their therapy which may affect patients with liver disease, such as hypertension, IHD, HF, and AF, are discussed in ➔ Arterial hypertension, pp. 370–2; ➔ Coronary artery disease, pp. 375–7; ➔ Heart failure, p. 382; and ➔ Arrhythmias, p. 378, respectively.

Arterial hypertension

Arterial hypertension (see Table 6.3.2) is seldom found in patients with liver disease, with the exception of NAFLD. Subjects with arterial hypertension may become normotensive during the development of chronic liver disease, and arterial hypertension is rarely manifested in patients with cirrhosis. The prevalence of essential hypertension in patients with cirrhosis is <15%.

Table 6.3.2 Antihypertensives in liver disease[2,4,5]

Drug	Recommendation of use
ACEIs	
Ramipril	Usual dose with frequent monitoring
Enalapril	Usual dose with frequent monitoring
Lisinopril	Usual dose with frequent monitoring
Fosinopril	Usual dose with frequent monitoring
ARBs	
Losartan	Initiate with lower dose, 25mg od
Candesartan	Initiate with lower dose, 4mg od
Calcium channel antagonists	
Nifedipine	Dose reduction may be necessary
Diltiazem	Dose reduction may be necessary
Amlodipine	Initiate with lower dose
Diuretics	
Spironolactone	Usual dose with frequent monitoring
Bendroflumethiazide	No dose reduction; monitor electrolytes
Hydrochlorothiazide	No dose reduction; monitor electrolytes
Furosemide	No dose reduction; monitor electrolytes
β-blockers	
Metoprolol	Dose reduction may be necessary
Atenolol	Usual dose with frequent monitoring
Bisoprolol	Dose reduction may be necessary
Others	
Doxazosin	Usual dose with frequent monitoring
Methyldopa	Precaution; initiate with lower dose
Clonidine	Initiate with lowest possible dose
Isosorbide mononitrate	Caution in severe hepatic impairment
Minoxidil	Usual dose with frequent monitoring; maybe a lower dosage interval

For treating arterial hypertension in liver disease, the same drugs are used as in subjects without liver disease. However, certain drugs may be preferred to others and caution is required with some of them.

Angiotensin-converting enzyme inhibitors and angiotensin receptor blockers

ACEIs and ARBs may be preferred in treating hypertension, since they may reduce the progression of liver fibrosis and portal hypertension. The majority of ACEIs (except fosinopril) are excreted by the kidneys; hence, drug toxicity is not a major concern in patients with liver dysfunction. However, some ACEIs (e.g. enalapril, ramipril) are prodrugs, which require transformation by the liver into active metabolites. With liver dysfunction, a reduction in prodrug transformation and inactivation of the active drug may occur.[4] Data are scarce, but changes in prodrug transformation are mostly clinically insignificant.

Calcium channel antagonists

Most calcium channel antagonists are mainly metabolized by the liver and undergo extensive first-pass metabolism.[4] In liver cirrhosis, clearance decreases, the half-life is prolonged, bioavailability doubles, and the volume of distribution increases. Amlodipine is unique because it has greater bioavailability and lower liver clearance than other calcium channel antagonists; it may accumulate with chronic oral dosing.[4] Verapamil and diltiazem are also transformed into active metabolites by the liver. The dose of a calcium channel antagonist needs to be reduced in liver dysfunction, i.e. a low starting dose with continued monitoring for side effects.

Diuretics

Diuretic therapy is commonly used to treat decompensated cirrhosis with ascites.[2] Spironolactone is the first-line diuretic recommended in this case. In cases of an inadequate response to spironolactone, thiazide diuretics are added to the regimen. Thiazides are terminated if the patient does not respond after 3 days and are replaced with a loop diuretic. Loop diuretics are mostly metabolized by the liver and excreted by the kidney.[4] Furosemide and torasemide have altered pharmacokinetic and pharmacodynamic profiles in cirrhosis, and the natriuretic potency of both is markedly reduced in liver cirrhosis.[2] No dose adjustments of loop diuretics are necessary if renal function is normal in cirrhosis.[4]

Beta-blockers

β-blockers are given as prophylaxis for variceal bleeding, resulting in vasoconstriction in the splanchnic compartment, which increases preload and improves diastolic function. β-blocker therapy may also prevent bleeding from portal hypertensive gastropathy and the development of spontaneous bacterial peritonitis. In general, hydrophilic β-blockers are excreted unchanged by the kidneys, and lipophilic β-blockers are largely metabolized by the liver. No dose adjustments are necessary for atenolol, nadolol, esmolol, and acebutolol.[4] When using metoprolol or bisoprolol, dose reductions may be necessary. Propranolol should be administered cautiously. Reduction of the initial dosage of carvedilol has been suggested in patients with liver cirrhosis.[4] The drug's manufacturer, however, recommends that carvedilol should not be administered in patients with clinically manifest hepatic impairment.

Alpha-blockers

Prazosin is subjected to high first-pass metabolism.[4] Moderate to severe hepatic impairment may increase its bioavailability and reduce its clearance. Dose reduction is necessary, and adjustments should be based on clinical response and patient tolerance.

Terazosin is extensively metabolized by the liver but does not undergo significant first-pass metabolism.[4] It has a significantly longer half-life than prazosin, allowing once-daily dosing. Its bioavailability is 90%. Hepatic impairment may prolong the duration of its effect because of impaired metabolism. The dose should be reduced, and the drug should be used with caution.

The liver extensively metabolizes doxazosin. However, no dose adjustments are necessary in mild to moderate hepatic impairment.

Centrally acting antihypertensives

Methyldopa is metabolized extensively in the liver. Biotransformation is reduced with hepatic impairment. A rare fatal hepatic necrosis has been reported after use of this drug. It is contraindicated in patients with active hepatic disease such as acute hepatitis and active cirrhosis. The drug should be used with caution in patients with a history of previous liver disease or dysfunction, and the dose should be reduced and adjusted based on patient response.[4]

Clonidine metabolism is reduced with hepatic impairment; therefore, its bioavailability increases.[4] The lowest possible dose is recommended in patients with moderate to severe liver dysfunction.

Direct vasodilators

Hydralazine undergoes extensive hepatic metabolism and significant first-pass effect; its bioavailability is 50% in slow acetylators and 30% in fast acetylators. Its half-life is increased in hepatic impairment, and a reduction in dose or prolonged dosage intervals may be indicated.[4]

No extensive pharmacodynamic studies of minoxidil use in patients with hepatic impairment exist. One pharmacokinetic analysis suggests a longer dosage interval may be appropriate.

Isosorbide mononitrate (ISMN) should be used with caution in severe hepatic impairment.

Glyceryl trinitrate is described in ➔ Coronary artery disease, pp. 375–7.

Dyslipidaemia

The liver plays an essential role in lipid metabolism. With liver dysfunction, lipoprotein synthesis is reduced; therefore, plasma cholesterol and TG levels are lower. Serum cholesterol might have an independent prognostic value in patients with liver cirrhosis.

In NAFLD, an atherogenic lipid profile, consisting of high TG, low HDL-C, increased LDL particles, increased very low-density lipoprotein (VLDL) cholesterol, and elevated apolipoprotein B100 levels, is present. This type of atherogenic dyslipidaemia is strongly linked to adverse CV outcomes.

Hypercholesterolaemia is also a common feature of primary biliary cholangitis (PBC) and other forms of cholestatic liver disease. However, till now, data have suggested that these patients are not at an increased risk of atherosclerosis. For patients without other known risk factors for CAD, dietary modification and exercise are suggested. For those with risk factors for CAD, a treatment approach similar to that for patients without PBC is suggested.

Statins

The potential hepatotoxic risk of statins in patients with an underlying liver disease has been examined in a number of studies; their conclusion is that statins can be used safely in patients with liver disease.[6] Whether one statin is safer than another in cirrhosis has not been formally studied—although pravastatin and pitavastatin, in contrast to the others, do not undergo metabolism by CYP450, which may be impaired in severe hepatic disease.[2] Because of the absence of evidence, the best statin therapeutic algorithm is unknown and a cautious attitude should be adopted. Several authors recommend to start with a low dose (because of a possible greater incidence of liver enzyme elevations with higher doses) and to check the liver enzymes after 2 weeks.[7] They also propose that liver biochemistry monitoring should be performed every month for the first 3–4 months and 4 times a year thereafter. If the levels of transaminases increase to >3 times the baseline values, discontinuation of the drug should be considered. Clinical correlation with worsening of the underlying disease, as well as exclusion of alcohol abuse and drug interactions, should be done before attempting permanent discontinuation of the drug. After an episode of elevation of liver enzymes and once levels return to baseline, rechallenge may be considered.

Other lipid-lowering agents

Among other lipid-lowering agents, nicotinic acid (niacin) should be used cautiously in patients who are alcoholic or have a history of liver disease or unexplained elevation in hepatic enzymes.[6] Liver enzymes should be monitored every 6–12 weeks during the first year of nicotinic acid use or even more frequently.[6] Resin-binding agents, including fenofibrate and clofibrate, can lead to an increased risk of developing gallstones, which can affect hepatic enzymes, and they should be monitored according to their labelling.[6] Use of fenofibrate in liver disease has not been studied and is currently contraindicated. Ezetimibe can be used without dose adjustment in patients with Child–Pugh A cirrhosis; its use is not recommended in patients with more severe hepatic impairment. Bile acid resins have not been implicated in causing hepatic injury; in fact, colestyramine is often considered hepatoprotective.[6] Overall, there are very limited data to suggest that other lipid-lowering agents should not be used in chronic liver disease (see Table 6.3.3).[6]

Table 6.3.3 Lipid-lowering agents in liver disease[4,5]

Drug	Recommendation of use
Simvastatin	Start at lowest dose and titrate cautiously; regularly check liver enzymes
Atorvastatin	Start at lowest dose and titrate cautiously; regularly check liver enzymes
Rosuvastatin	Start at lowest dose and titrate cautiously; regularly check liver enzymes
Ezetimibe	Use with caution in patients with mild hepatic impairment; use is not recommended in patients with moderate or severe hepatic impairment
Fenofibrate	Contraindicated

Coronary artery disease

It was originally believed that the incidence of CAD in liver diseases (see Table 6.3.4) is low.[8] The more recent literature reports a prevalence of CAD varying between 2.5% and 27% in patients who have cirrhosis being considered for liver transplantation.[8] One of the latest and largest studies found that the prevalence of obstructive CAD among cirrhotic patients without symptoms or a history of heart attack did not differ significantly from that among a propensity score-matched non-hepatic control group.[8] However, patients with liver cirrhosis were at a higher risk for non-obstructive lesions, which have a more favourable course.[8]

Patients with NAFLD have been consistently shown to have an increased risk for CAD, which is the leading cause of death in this group.[9] There is growing evidence that NAFLD is an independent CV disease risk factor, and there are plausible biological mechanisms by which NAFLD could contribute to CV disease, including: (1) poor nutrition (e.g. high fat, high carbohydrate, high fructose intake), genetic factors—*PNPLA3* genotype; (2) visceral ectopic fat, adipose tissue inflammation, and T2DM promoting long-chain fatty acids, hyperinsulinaemia, and adipocytokines; and (3) intestine dysbiosis attenuating the primary and secondary bile acid pool. These factors contribute to hepatic stellate cell and Kupffer cell activation, lipotoxicity oxidative stress, and collagen matrix deposition. Since NAFLD is the commonest liver disorder in Western countries, and as the number of patients with NAFLD is increasing, it is likely that the number of patients with synchronous liver and CV disease will increase as well.

Chronic hepatitis C virus (HCV) infection is a multisystem disease that leads to increased risks of cirrhosis and its complications, as well as extrahepatic disturbances, including cryoglobulinaemia and CV and metabolic alterations (also T2DM). Recent accumulating evidence suggests that HCV infection can increase CV risk and that viral eradication can improve CV outcomes in the clinical setting.

Table 6.3.4 Coronary artery disease drugs in liver disease[2,4,5,9]

Drug	Recommendation of use
Aspirin	Use depends on the bleeding risk; usual dose with frequent monitoring; avoid in Child–Pugh C cirrhosis
Clopidogrel	Usual dose with frequent monitoring; avoid in Child–Pugh C cirrhosis
Ticagrelor	Avoid in Child–Pugh C cirrhosis
Prasugrel	Precaution
Bivalirudin	Usual dose
Glyceryl trinitrate	Dose reduction may be necessary; avoid in severe hepatic impairment
Morphine	Reduce dose and frequency by half

Aspirin

Cirrhosis has been listed as an absolute contraindication for aspirin use due to GI bleeding risk.[9] However, aspirin prophylaxis for primary or secondary prevention of arterial events should not be withheld from all patients with cirrhosis. Although data are largely lacking, the bleeding risk of primary and secondary prophylaxis are likely increased in patients with liver disease, compared to that in the general population, in particular in patients with varices. In patients with varices, aspirin is likely contraindicated for primary, and perhaps also for secondary, prevention.[9] In high-risk patients, such as patients with non-alcoholic steatohepatitis-related cirrhosis, the use of aspirin likely justifies the bleeding risk.[9]

P2Y12 receptor inhibitors

Inhibitors of the P2Y12 receptor, which block ADP-induced platelet aggregation, are an integral part of treatment of CAD.[9] A major disadvantage of the irreversible P2Y12 inhibitors is that they require metabolic activation by the liver, which may result in unpredictable pharmacokinetics in patients with cirrhosis.

The pharmacokinetics and pharmacodynamics of clopidogrel are unaltered in patients with Child–Pugh A or B cirrhosis; yet significant liver impairment or cholestatic jaundice is stated as contraindications in the Summary of Product Characteristics (SPC).[9] No pharmacokinetic differences in patients with Child–Pugh B cirrhosis were demonstrated for prasugrel, and chronic liver disease is not a contraindication, according to the package insert, although caution is advised.[9] Ticagrelor does not require metabolic activation but is cleared by the liver.[9] Severe chronic liver disease is a contraindication for ticagrelor use, according to the package insert. Since most of the P2Y12 inhibitors state (severe) liver disease as a contraindication, the role of these drugs in patients with cirrhosis is unclear. Use of P2Y12 inhibitors for the prevention of arterial events in cirrhosis may be limited to those patients without varices, since the rate of variceal bleeding in patients receiving antiplatelet agents following stent placement was substantial (12.5%).[9]

Glycoprotein IIb/IIIa receptor antagonists

Glycoprotein IIb/IIIa receptor antagonists are sometimes used in the setting of ACS prior to, or during, PCI. One of their significant side effects is thrombocytopenia. Their use should be carefully considered in patients with known liver dysfunction, since data on complications and bleeding risks in these patients are limited.

Direct thrombin inhibitors

The safety and efficacy of bivalirudin have not been specifically studied in patients with hepatic impairment, since it is minimally metabolized by the liver. No dose adjustment is necessary in hepatic impairment.

Nitrates

Glyceryl trinitrate undergoes very rapid and near-complete hepatic metabolism. Lower doses of oral preparations (50%) are advised in hepatic impairment because bioavailability may increase.[4] Also lower doses of ISDN are recommended in these patients. ISDN and ISMN should be avoided in severe hepatic impairment.[4]

Opioids

Opioids should be used cautiously since they can cause sedation, constipation, and sudden encephalopathy. Their administration should be observed. The clearance of opioids in patients with hepatic insufficiency is decreased. Therefore, the initial dose must be decreased and the intervals between doses should be increased.

Inhibitors of late sodium current

Ranolazine undergoes extensive hepatic metabolism. Because of its potential to prolong the corrected QT interval, it should be used with caution in moderate hepatic impairment and is contraindicated in cirrhotic patients.

Metabolic agents

No dose adjustments are necessary when using trimetazidine in patients with liver disease.

The use of lipid-lowering agents, ACEIs, β-blockers, calcium channel antagonists, anticoagulation therapy, thrombolytics, and ivabradine in liver disease is described in ➔ Dyslipidaemia, pp. 373–4; ➔ Arterial hypertension, pp. 370–2; ➔ Anticoagulation therapy, pp. 379–80; ➔ Thrombolytic therapy, p. 381; and ➔ Heart failure, p. 382, respectively.

Arrhythmias

The risk for arrhythmias in liver cirrhosis is influenced by factors such as cirrhotic cardiomyopathy (CCM), cardiac ion channel remodelling, electrolyte imbalances, impaired autonomic function, hepatorenal syndrome, metabolic abnormalities, advanced age, inflammatory syndrome, stressful events, impaired drug metabolism, and comorbidities. Close monitoring of cirrhotic patients is needed for arrhythmias, particularly when QT interval-prolonging drugs are given or if electrolyte imbalances or hepatorenal syndrome appear (see Table 6.3.5).

AF and atrial flutter are arrhythmias that are more frequently diagnosed in cirrhotic patients and are significantly associated with arteriosclerosis, hypercholesterolaemia, and diabetes mellitus.

Antiarrhythmics agents

Amiodarone has low bioavailability because of poor absorption. It undergoes extensive hepatic metabolism to the active metabolite desethylamiodarone. No dosage reduction is required in hepatic impairment.[4]

Lidocaine is a highly extracted flow-dependent drug, which is eliminated almost exclusively by the liver. The systemic clearance is reduced by approximately 40% in cirrhosis, and the volume of distribution is increased.[4] The half-life in the longer phase of metabolism is increased almost 3-fold. The dose should be reduced by 40–50% in cirrhosis, and serum levels should be monitored.

Quinidine is extensively metabolized by the liver and has a narrow therapeutic index. Its half-life in cirrhotics can be significantly prolonged, and therefore, less frequent dosing or a smaller dose may be required.[4] Its clearance does not seem to be significantly altered.

Propafenone needs to be reduced (by a factor of 2–3) in patients with moderate to severe liver disease.[10]

Sotalol does not need dosage adjustments in patients with hepatic impairment.[10]

Adenosine is a short-acting drug that is not hepatically eliminated. No dosage adjustments are necessary in hepatic failure.[4]

Dronedarone is contraindicated in patients with severe hepatic impairment. Very rarely, it can be the cause of life-threatening hepatic toxicity (1 in 1000–10,000). Elevated enzyme levels occur at rates of between 1 in 10 and 100. The EMA and FDA advise periodic testing during treatment.

β-blockers and calcium channel antagonists are described in ➲ Arterial hypertension, pp. 370–2.

Table 6.3.5 Antiarrhythmics in liver disease[2,4,5,10]

Drug	Recommendation of use
Amiodarone	Usual dose with frequent monitoring
Lidocaine	Reduce dose by a factor of 2–3; avoid in Child–Pugh C cirrhosis
Propafenone	Reduce dose by a factor of 2–3
Sotalol	No reduction
Adenosine	Usual dose with frequent monitoring
Dronedarone	No dose adjustment needed in Child–Pugh A or B cirrhosis

Anticoagulation therapy

Liver disease leads to a form of 'rebalanced' haemostasis, in which diminished hepatic function leads to both procoagulant and anticoagulant effects (see Table 6.3.6). All stages of the haemostatic process may be abnormal, including primary haemostasis (platelet adhesion and activation), coagulation (generation and cross-linking of fibrin), and fibrinolysis (clot dissolution). Patients with severe liver disease and abnormalities of coagulation testing should not be assumed to be 'auto-anticoagulated', because standard coagulation testing does not assess prothrombotic and fibrinolytic changes. Factors that contribute to increased risks of both bleeding and thrombosis include altered blood flow, diminished numbers and function of platelets, and inflammatory alterations in endothelial cells.

As patients with cirrhosis develop indications for anticoagulation therapy (e.g. AF, VTE, portal vein thrombosis), doctors are left to make difficult decisions when selecting therapeutics, with little evidence to rely on. Current practice supports the use of LMWH or VKAs in select patients with cirrhosis requiring anticoagulation. UFH is an alternative in cirrhotic patients for shorter-term use and in cases of severe renal dysfunction and/or haemodynamic instability. Fondaparinux is an option in HIT; however, limited data exist on its use in cirrhotic patients.

LMWH is the most widely studied anticoagulant in cirrhotic patients, demonstrating efficacy in treatment and an acceptable safety profile.[11] Monitoring with anti-Xa level for LMWH dosing adjustment is not recommended, because anti-Xa levels can be lower in cirrhotic patients, compared to normal controls, after administration of a prophylactic or therapeutic dose of LMWH. The anti-Xa assay may underestimate the true degree of anticoagulation.

VKAs have particular limitations in cirrhotic patients, including a low therapeutic index, drug and dietary interactions, and the need for monitoring with

Table 6.3.6 Anticoagulation therapy in liver disease[4,5,11]

Drug	Recommendation of use
LMWH	Precaution; monitoring anti-Xa not recommended
UFH	Dose reduction may be necessary
Warfarin	Initiate at lower dose
Dabigatran	Not specified
Apixaban	Child–Pugh A cirrhosis: no adjustment Child–Pugh B cirrhosis: caution Child–Pugh C cirrhosis: avoid
Rivaroxaban	Child–Pugh A cirrhosis: no adjustment Child–Pugh B cirrhosis: caution Child–Pugh C cirrhosis: avoid
Edoxaban	Child–Pugh A cirrhosis: no adjustment Child–Pugh B and C cirrhosis: avoid

the INR. As the INR was designed for warfarin dosing in non-cirrhotic patients, the actual therapeutic window for an effective anticoagulant effect in patients with hepatic dysfunction is not known. In cirrhotic patients with an innately elevated INR due to hepatic dysfunction, selecting and maintaining a target range of VKAs is empirical and challenging.[11]

DOACs are desirable, as they do not require routine monitoring; they can be taken orally, and they have a quick onset of action and an equivalent or lower risk of bleeding versus VKAs.[11] Unfortunately, patients with chronic liver disease were excluded from clinical trials that demonstrated efficacy and safety, when compared to traditional anticoagulation. Data are now emerging that support the use of DOACs in well-compensated cirrhotic patients; however, further studies are necessary. Dabigatran has no specific recommendations for dosing or use in patients with hepatic impairment in the available approved prescribing guidance. Rivaroxaban is not recommended for use in patients with Child–Pugh B or C cirrhosis or in any patient with a B hepatic disease associated with a coagulopathy. Apixaban requires no dose adjustment in patients with Child–Pugh A cirrhosis. No specific recommendations are made for patients with Child–Pugh B cirrhosis, and the medication is not recommended in patients with Child–Pugh C cirrhosis. Edoxaban should not be used in patients with Child–Pugh B and C cirrhosis; no dosage adjustment is needed in patients with Child–Pugh A cirrhosis.[11]

Cirrhotic patients on anticoagulation therapy should be monitored closely for signs and symptoms of bleeding and thrombosis.

Thrombolytic therapy

Thrombolytic therapy is used for different indications, e.g. acute MI, PE, acute ischaemic stroke, and portal vein thrombosis. Thrombolytic therapy is relatively contraindicated in patients with advanced liver disease.

Alteplase is removed rapidly from the liver, and therefore, liver blood flow is rate-determining for its clearance.[4] Patients with severely impaired blood flow may have excessively high plasma alteplase concentrations and represent a group of patients in whom dosage adjustment may be necessary.

Peripheral artery disease

NAFLD is significantly associated with CV diseases, including PAD. No data exist about PAD in other cases of hepatic impairment. The management of patients with PAD is aimed at lowering the risk of CV disease progression and improving symptoms. Management includes physical activity, smoking cessation, long-term antithrombotic therapy with aspirin or clopidogrel, lipid-lowering therapy, and treatment of hypertension and diabetes. The use of these drugs in patients with liver disease has been described in ➲ Coronary artery disease, pp. 375–7; ➲ Dyslipidaemia, pp. 373–4; and ➲ Arterial hypertension, pp. 370–2, respectively. In patients with claudication, the addition of cilostazol, a PDE inhibitor, may improve symptoms. Cilostazol should be avoided in patients with moderate and severe hepatic impairment. For patients with ischaemic rest pain or ulceration, where the limb is threatened, revascularization is a priority to restore perfusion and limit tissue loss. Some patients with acute thrombosis superimposed on chronic stenosis or occlusion may benefit from thrombolytic therapy.

Cirrhotic cardiomyopathy

Cardiac dysfunction is frequently observed in patients with cirrhosis and has long been linked to the direct toxic effect of alcohol. CCM has recently been identified as an entity, regardless of the aetiology of cirrhosis. Increased CO due to hyperdynamic circulation is a pathophysiological hallmark of the disease. The main clinical features of CCM include attenuated systolic contractility in response to physiologic or pharmacologic strain, diastolic dysfunction, electrical conductance abnormalities, and chronotropic incompetence.

No specific treatment exists for CCM. Given the pivotal role of the cirrhosis itself in the development of circulatory abnormalities, efforts should be made to effectively treat the underlying cirrhotic disease. Liver transplantation is the only established effective treatment for patients with end-stage liver disease and associated cardiac failure. Liver transplantation has been shown to reverse systolic and diastolic dysfunction and the prolonged QT interval after transplantation.

When HF becomes evident, treatment principles should be the same as for non-cirrhotic HF described in ➲ Heart failure, p. 382.

Heart failure

When HF is present in patients with liver disease, treatment should follow the same guidelines as in patients without liver disease. However, in patients with liver disease, cardiac afterload reduction will not be well tolerated in those with advanced cirrhosis who are significantly vasodilated. Therefore, vasodilators, like ACEIs, should be used carefully. Diuretics are indicated in patients with water retention. Aldosterone antagonists may have beneficial effects in the reduction of LV dilatation and wall thickness, and are potentially useful in the improvement of diastolic function. β-blockers reduce the hyperdynamic load, improve the prolonged QT interval, lower portal pressure, and potentially reduce the degree of shunting of cardiotoxins from the splanchnic to the systemic circulation. The use of cardiac glycosides is currently not warranted, since short-acting cardiac glycosides did not improve cardiac contractility in patients with alcoholic cirrhosis and LV dysfunction. No dose adjustment is needed for ivabradine in patients with mild hepatic impairment. Caution is advocated when treating patients with moderate hepatic impairment, and ivabradine is contraindicated in patients with severe hepatic insufficiency (as a substantial increase in systemic exposure is predicted).

Adverse effects of cardiovascular drugs on the liver

CV drugs can cause hepatic injury, which can be either acute or chronic. Acute injury may be mainly cytotoxic, which involves cellular destruction, cholestatic injury that consists of an obstruction of bile flow, or a mixed presentation of both.[4] Cytotoxic hepatic injury may be due to necrosis, steatosis, or both. Chronic hepatic injury may include chronic active hepatitis, chronic steatosis, chronic cholestasis, phospholipidosis, veno-occlusive disease, pseudoalcoholic liver disease, fibrosis and cirrhosis, peliosis hepatis, granulomatous disease, or hepatic neoplasms.[4] A list of CV drugs causing acute hepatic injury is presented in Table 6.3.7.

Table 6.3.7 Cardiovascular drugs causing acute hepatic injury[4]

Cytotoxic and mixed	Cholestatic and mixed
Amiodarone	Captopril
Aspirin	Enalapril
Carvedilol	Lisinopril
Diltiazem	Furosemide
Nifedipine	Thiazides
Methyldopa	Ticlopidine
Nicotinic acid	Verapamil
	Warfarin

References

1 European Medicines Agency. *Guideline on the evaluation of the pharmacokinetics of medicinal products in patients with impaired hepatic function*. European Medicines Agency: London; 2005.

2 Lewis JH, Stine JG. Review article: prescribing medications in patients with cirrhosis—a practical guide. *Aliment Pharmacol Ther* 2013;37:1132–56.

3 Dourakis S. Drug therapy in liver disease. *Ann Gastroenterol* 2008;**21**:215–17.

4 Sokol SI, Cheng A, Frishman WH, Kaza CS. Cardiovascular drug therapy in patients with hepatic diseases and patients with congestive heart failure. *J Clin Pharmacol* 2000;**40**:11–30.

5 Perianez-Parraga L, Martinez-Lopez I, Ventayol-Bosch P, Puigventos-Latorre F, Delgado-Sanchez O. Drug dosage recommendations in patients with chronic liver disease. *Rev Esp Enferm Dig* 2012;**104**:165–84.

6 Gupta NK, Lewis JH. Review article: the use of potentially hepatotoxic drugs in patients with liver disease. *Aliment Pharmacol Ther* 2008;**28**:1021–41.

7 Calderon RM, Cubeddu LX, Goldberg RB, Schiff ER. Statins in the treatment of dyslipidemia in the presence of elevated liver aminotransferase levels: a therapeutic dilemma. *Mayo Clin Proc* 2010;**85**:349–56.

8 An J, Shim JH, Kim SO, *et al*. Prevalence and prediction of coronary artery disease in patients with liver cirrhosis: a registry-based matched case-control study. *Circulation* 2014;**130**:1353–62.

9 Lisman T, Kamphuisen PW, Northup PG, Porte RJ. Established and new-generation antithrombotic drugs in patients with cirrhosis—possibilities and caveats. *J Hepatol* 2013;**59**:358–66.

10 Klotz U. Antiarrhythmics: elimination and dosage considerations in hepatic impairment. *Clin Pharmacokinet* 2007;**46**:985–96.

11 Intagliata NM, Maitland H, Caldwell SH. Direct oral anticoagulants in cirrhosis. *Curr Treat Options Gastroenterol* 2016;**14**:247–56.

Section 7

Major drug interactions

Section editors

Ljubica Vukelic Andersen
Birgitte Klindt Poulsen

Chapter 7.1

Major drug interactions

Maja Hellfritzsch Poulsen
and Marlene Lunddal Krogh

Introduction

A common definition of interactions is when the effects of one drug are changed by the presence of another drug, food, herbal medicine, or other exogenic substances. As a consequence, interactions can cause both an enhanced or a reduced effect of a drug, but also, just as importantly, a decreased or an increased risk of side effects, and thereby an increased risk of toxicity. We most commonly refer to interactions as being unwanted and unsought, but we must also remember that some interactions are used intentionally to obtain a more effective treatment such as combining antihypertensive drugs in order to reach the target BP.

Many drug–drug interactions (DDIs) are mainly theoretical and have never been proved to cause harm to patients, but some are potentially harmful and it is some of the latter that we will focus on in this chapter. The CV drugs that we have chosen to focus on are mainly those with the highest risk of severe side effects and/or with a narrow therapeutic window leaving only little room for changes in plasma concentrations before patients may experience potentially harmful symptoms. Importantly, there is large patient variability concerning whether or not patients develop symptoms due to an interaction, and thereby making the interaction clinically relevant for the individual patient. This makes it difficult to predict what might happen when a patient is given two or more drugs that interact. Avoiding interactions is often not possible, but with some appropriate precautions, co-medication is often possible despite clinically relevant interactions. Much of the information gathered in this chapter has been retrieved from relevant international databases and online tools, including Micromedex and Drugs.com, as well as updated books such as *Stockley's Drug Interactions*, tenth edition for references, along with a few chosen studies and relevant ESC guidelines.

Mechanisms of interactions

Based on the underlying mechanism, DDIs can be categorized into pharmacokinetic (PK) and pharmacodynamic (PD) DDIs. It may be too simple sometimes to blame an interaction on just one specific mechanism, as we know that some clinically important interactions are more complex. Nevertheless, for clarification purposes, most of the DDIs in this chapter will be explained by the most important mechanism.

In PK-related interactions, one drug causes changes in the absorption, distribution, metabolization, and/or excretion of another drug. Many of these interactions can be proven by changes in the plasma concentration of the affected drug. PD-related interactions are based upon the mechanism of action of the drug and the side effects. PK changes are often more predictable, whereas PD changes are often unpredictable, individual, and reflected by an augmented or a reduced effect and/or side effects.

Part of drug metabolism includes oxidation caused by CYP450 enzymes, which are mainly located in the liver and intestine. These enzymes are divided into families and subfamilies and are named with the prefix 'CYP', followed by an Arabic number and a numerical number for the specific enzyme. These enzymes differ according to their substrates and genetic characteristics, but all can be induced and inhibited. When one drug is metabolized by several CYP enzymes, the clinical effect depends on the capacity of all enzymes involved.

P-glycoprotein (P-gp) is one of the most important ATP-binding cassette transporters in humans and is responsible for the transport of some drugs and metabolites in several organs such as the intestine, liver, and kidney, as well as the brain where it serves as a part of the blood–brain barrier. In the intestine, P-gp actively transports drugs that are substrates back to the lumen, thereby inhibiting the absorption of the drug, probably as a protective mechanism against toxic xenobiotics. P-gp has some individual variations and, like CYP450 enzymes, can be inhibited or induced, which can therefore have consequences in terms of developing toxicity or treatment failure.

In addition to the influence of CYP enzymes and P-gp, the metabolism of drugs can be changed in other ways, e.g. by the blood flow in the liver and/or kidneys.

Some clinically important principles of PK interactions are shown in Table 7.1.1, along with some clinical examples. It is important to note that interactions caused by inhibition of CYP450 enzymes start within a few days and cease when the inhibiting drug is no longer present, whereas interactions due to enzyme induction usually develop over several days to weeks and may persist for a long time after the inducing drug has been withdrawn.

Table 7.1.2 shows the most common inhibitors, inducers, and substrates of the most common CYP450 enzymes, as well as of P-gp. This list is not exhaustive but shows some of the relevant potentially interacting drugs. Concerning CYP1A2, in addition to drugs, smoking is also mentioned because tobacco smoke induces this enzyme and smoking cessation, as well as starting smoking just a few cigarettes, may cause important changes in the plasma concentrations of the enzyme substrates. This is important, since smoking cessation is highly warranted in cardiac patients.

Table 7.1.1 Clinically important principles of pharmacokinetic drug interactions and clinically relevant examples

Mechanism	Commonest causes with clinical relevance	Clinical examples
Absorption	Induction and inhibition of drug transporter proteins such as P-gp	Increased absorption of digoxin due to inhibition of P-gp by clarithromycin
	Chelation or complex formation	Activated charcoal inhibits the absorption of dabigatran
Distribution	Protein binding	Often only relevant to the interpretation of therapeutic drug monitoring
Metabolism	Inhibition of CYP450 enzymes	Increased plasma concentration of simvastatin due to inhibition of CYP3A4 by amiodarone, thereby increasing the risk for muscle symptoms
	Induction of CYP450 enzymes	Reduced plasma concentration of ciclosporin by rifampicin, causing an increased risk of transplant rejection
Excretion	Changes in renal tubular excretion	Reduced excretion of digoxin due to spironolactone
	Changes in renal blood flow	NSAIDs cause a rise in the plasma concentration of lithium

NSAID, non-steroidal anti-inflammatory drug; P-gp, P-glycoprotein.

Table 7.1.2 Examples of substrates, inhibitors, and inducers of the commonest CYP450 enzymes and P-gp, as well as genetic differences for some of the enzymes

CYP enzyme or transporter	Substrates	Inhibitors	Inducers	Characteristics
1A2	Clozapine, duloxetine, imipramine, olanzapine	Amiodarone, ciprofloxacin, fluvoxamine	Carbamazepine, efavirenz, rifampicin, smoking	Some genetic variation
2B6	Ketamine, methadone	Clopidogrel, voriconazole	Carbamazepine, phenytoin, rifampicin	
2C9	Celecoxib, diclofenac, irbesartan, losartan, naproxen, valproate, warfarin	Amiodarone, fluconazole, metronidazole, miconazole, voriconazole,	Carbamazepine, dicloxacillin, efavirenz, rifampicin, St John's wort	Approximately 4% are slow metabolizers
2C19	Amitriptyline, citalopram, clopidogrel, labetalol	Esomeprazole, fluoxetine, oral contraceptives	Carbamazepine, efavirenz, rifampicin, St John's wort	Approximately 3% of Caucasians and 20% of Asiatics are slow metabolizers. There are several inactivating mutations in the gene coding for CYP2C19 and genotyping is possible

(Continued)

Table 7.1.2 (*Contd.*)

CYP enzyme or transporter	Substrates	Inhibitors	Inducers	Characteristics
2D6	Aripiprazole, atenolol, carvedilol, codeine, duloxetine, flecainide, fluoxetine, metoprolol, paroxetine, propafenone, risperidone, tramadol, venlafaxine	Amiodarone, celecoxib, citalopram, **duloxetine**, **fluoxetine**, methadone, **paroxetine**, **sertraline**, **terbinafine**		Approximately 7–8% of Caucasians and 1–2% of Afro-Americans and Asiatics are slow metabolizers due to multiple inactivating mutations in the *CYP2D6* gene. Approximately 1% are ultra-fast metabolizers. Genotyping of both fast and slow metabolizers is possible
3A4	Amlodipine, apixaban, atorvastatin, diltiazem, edoxaban, felodipine, rivaroxaban, sildenafil, simvastatin, tamoxifen, verapamil	Amiodarone, **clarithromycin**, **erythromycin**, **grapefruit juice**, **itraconazole**, **ketoconazole**, **verapamil**, **voriconazole**	Carbamazepine, efavirenz, phenobarbital, rifampicin, St John's wort	Expressed in the liver and gut wall
P-gp	Atorvastatin, carvedilol, digoxin, diltiazem, losartan, morphine, simvastatin, verapamil	Amiodarone, clarithromycin, erythromycin, itraconazole, ketoconazole, voriconazole, verapamil	Carbamazepine, phenobarbital, rifampicin, St John's wort	Close relationship with CYP3A4

This table is not exhaustive but shows examples. Drugs in boldface are strong and moderate inhibitors.

Challenges and consequences of polypharmacy

There is no agreed definition of polypharmacy, and suggestions of whether it means receiving three, five, or six different drugs or whether it means receiving the wrong drugs have not been established. What the exact definition might be does not matter that much; what matters is that the more drugs a patient is taking, the more complicated it can be to obtain an overview of all drugs and the potential interactions, especially when adding or removing drugs from the medication list.

These complex medication lists are often the reason for drug dosing errors, harmful interactions, and drug toxicity, which may lead to hospitalizations. Several studies have shown that 5–12% of all hospitalizations are caused by drugs and that just a few groups of drugs cause the majority of hospitalizations, namely anticoagulants, antiplatelets, NSAIDs, opioids, and antihypertensives, because of their side effects.[1] In particular, concerning antithrombotics, the combination of antiplatelets and anticoagulants, or the combination of any of those with NSAIDs, carries a high risk of severe bleeding.

Some of the precautions that can be taken to avoid harmful interactions are the following:

- Identification of high-risk drugs with a narrow therapeutic window and potentially severe side effects, e.g. anticoagulants, antiarrhythmic drugs, digoxin, and many antipsychotics.
- Identification of those patients who are more fragile and susceptible to harmful side effects, including the elderly and also patients with impaired organ function, e.g. renal, liver, or mental impairment.
- Considering closer drug monitoring, e.g. measurements of INR and plasma concentrations, as well as closer monitoring of safety, e.g. ECG and renal function.
- Considering a dose reduction upfront.
- Making regular medication reviews and discontinuing drugs that are no longer needed.
- Remembering to provide the patient with thorough information on which symptoms they should be aware of, and also considering giving information to relatives and caregivers, as well as to your colleagues who are also taking the case of this patient.

Specific drugs with a high risk of clinically important interactions

Interactions affecting antiarrhythmic drugs

AADs are highly heterogenous but are often regarded as being high-risk drugs because of the risk of toxicity leading to severe ventricular arrhythmia. Both PK and PD interactions differ among these drugs. Concerning PD interactions, a major issue is the risk of QT interval prolongation, and thereby a risk of TdP, due to the combination of drugs that have the ability to prolong the QT interval. However, this risk may also arise due to PK interactions or due to side effects of other drugs causing metabolic disturbances. There is some consensus on not to combine drugs with a high risk of causing prolongation of the QT interval and to be cautious when combining drugs with a moderate risk. Some of the most commonly used AADs are discussed in more detail in the following sections.

Beta-adrenoceptor antagonists

At present, β-adrenoceptor antagonists are generally considered as almost ideal AADs because of their broad antiarrhythmic effect and good safety profile. PK interactions vary among these drugs (see Table 7.1.2), with the most lipophilic β-adrenoceptor antagonists primarily metabolized by CYP2D6. Hence, drugs that inhibit this enzyme, e.g. propafenone, the antifungal terbinafine when used systemically, antidepressants such as fluoxetine, paroxetine (strong inhibitors), duloxetine, and sertraline, and cimetidine (moderate inhibitors), increase the plasma concentration of these β-adrenoceptor antagonists. Verapamil inhibits the hepatic breakdown of lipophilic β-adrenoceptor antagonists, increasing their plasma concentration. The most water-soluble β-adrenoceptor antagonists (e.g. atenolol and sotalol) are mainly excreted by the kidneys and are therefore rarely subjected to DDIs. β-adrenoceptor antagonists have a broad therapeutic index, and most patients tolerate a rise in their plasma concentrations, with the exception of HF patients in whom slow and careful titration may be warranted. Concerning PD interactions, there is a risk of additive cardiac depressant effects, such as hypotension and bradycardia, when used in combination with other drugs with similar side effects. β-adrenoceptor antagonists inhibit the competitive binding of catecholamines to β-adrenoceptors, thereby potentially decreasing the effect of these drugs, but with some differences between the drugs. β1-selective drugs (e.g. atenolol and metoprolol) selectively block receptors in cardiac tissue, but at high dosages, they also affect β2 receptors. Non-selective drugs block receptors (β2) in the lung and blood vessels (e.g. propranolol and carvedilol—carvedilol also block α1 receptors).

Calcium channel antagonists

Verapamil and diltiazem are mainly metabolized by CYP3A4. Thus, drugs that inhibit CYP3A4, e.g. erythromycin, clarithromycin, most azole antifungals, and some antiviral agents, increase the plasma concentration of these calcium channel antagonists, and inducers, such as rifampicin, will decrease their plasma concentration (see Table 7.1.2). The main issue concerning interactions with verapamil is its ability to inhibit CYP3A4 and P-gp. Verapamil may nearly double plasma digoxin levels[2] and increase the levels of dabigatran, quinidine, ciclosporin, simvastatin, atorvastatin, and lovastatin. Diltiazem interacts with the same drugs, but to a lesser extent. Verapamil and diltiazem inhibit the AVN, causing PD interactions with other drugs that also inhibit the AVN, e.g. β-adrenoceptor antagonists, digoxin, and amiodarone. Verapamil cause arteriolar dilatation and exerts a direct negative inotropic effect on the heart. The negative inotropic effect of combining verapamil and disopyramide is considerable.

Amiodarone

Amiodarone is also mainly metabolized by CYP3A4. Thus, certain protease inhibitors, ketoconazole, itraconazole, clarithromycin, and verapamil may decrease the metabolism and increase the serum concentrations of amiodarone. Furthermore, amiodarone is also a substrate for P-gp. Grapefruit juice, usually >200mL a day, inhibits P-gp in the intestinal mucosa and can increase the bioavailability of oral amiodarone, resulting in increased plasma levels and a risk of toxicity.[3] Therefore, grapefruit juice should be avoided during treatment with oral amiodarone. Concomitant use of P450 enzyme inducers, e.g. rifampicin, may lead to decreased serum concentrations and loss of efficacy. Amiodarone inhibits several of the P450 enzymes (mainly CYP1A1/2, CYP3A4, CYP2C9, and CYP2D6), as well as P-gp. It thereby has the potential to increase the plasma levels of many of the enzyme substrates, e.g. metoprolol, some antidepressants, and some statins. The use of statins that are P450 substrates in combination with amiodarone has been associated with reports of myopathy/rhabdomyolysis, and this is why a maximum dose of 20mg of simvastatin should be considered when given in combination with amiodarone. In addition, digoxin plasma levels and the anticoagulant effect of warfarin are increased. Thus, the dose of digoxin, as well as that of warfarin, should be reduced, and plasma digoxin levels and INR should be monitored. Also, the effect of dabigatran and the other NOACs are increased. Concerning PD interactions, the main issue concerns the co-administration of amiodarone with drugs known to prolong the QT interval, e.g. some other AADs, some antipsychotics, some antidepressants, some fluoroquinolone and macrolide antibiotics, and some azole antifungals. In addition, concomitant use of drugs with depressant effects on the sinoatrial and atrioventricular nodes can potentiate the electrophysiological and haemodynamic effects of amiodarone, resulting in bradycardia, sinus arrest and AVB, and hypotension. Recently, severe bradycardia has been reported when combining amiodarone with the new direct-acting antiviral drugs used to treat chronic HCV infection—sofosbuvir and daclatasvir. Thus, either another AAD should be used or the heart rate should be monitored, especially during the first 48h. Due to the very long half-life of amiodarone of up to 100 days, in cases of maintenance treatment, the interactions may last several months after stopping amiodarone.

Digoxin

The main DDIs with digoxin are due either to P-gp or to the fact that digoxin is excreted by the kidneys. The clinically relevant PK interactions due to

P-gp[2] are related to concomitant treatment with, for example, amiodarone, clarithromycin, verapamil, and other inhibitors of P-gp (see Table 7.1.2). In addition to P-gp inhibition, the interactions due to reduced renal excretion can also be due to drugs that reduce renal blood flow, e.g. NSAIDs, ACEIs, and spironolactone. Another type of interactions with digoxin is with drugs that, through inducing low levels of potassium, may increase the risk of toxicity. Such drugs include, for example, diuretics and amphotericin. None of these drugs are contraindicated, but attention should be paid to maintaining the potassium levels within the upper part of the normal range and, in cases of PK interactions, to monitor the side effects and, in some cases, serum digoxin levels.

Flecainide and propafenone

Flecainide is mainly metabolized by CYP2D6, and propafenone by several CYP enzymes. See Table 7.1.2 for drugs that inhibit or induce these enzymes. Both drugs may induce AVB, and potential PD interactions are with other drugs with the same profile. Careful observation of the QT and QRS intervals and for proarrhythmias should be considered.

Oral anticoagulants

Oral anticoagulants are widely used in the prophylaxis and treatment of thrombosis. Most anticoagulant users are elderly persons with a high frequency of comorbid conditions and concomitant medications, making them particularly susceptible to DDIs. Due to the potency of oral anticoagulants, DDIs can have serious consequences, potentially leading to thrombosis, bleeding complications, hospitalizations, and death.

The PK DDIs vary between the individual oral anticoagulant drugs, whereas the PD DDIs are similar in all oral anticoagulants.

Warfarin

VKAs are especially prone to clinically significant DDIs due to their extensive liver metabolism and narrow therapeutic index.

The most potent of warfarin's enantiomers (S-enantiomer) is metabolized by CYP2C9, and inhibition of CYP2C9 will result in decreased metabolism of warfarin, leading to an increased anticoagulant effect. Conversely, induction of CYP2C9 will result in increased metabolism and thereby a decreased anticoagulant effect.[4] A list of drugs known to inhibit or induce CYP2C9 can be found in Table 7.1.2.

INR should be monitored closely when initiating, as well as stopping, therapy with drugs serving as inhibitors and inducers of CYP2C9 in warfarin-treated patients, and the warfarin dose may have to be adjusted. If short-term therapy with a strong CYP2C9 inducer or inhibitor is necessary, warfarin therapy should be paused and replaced by LMWH during the treatment course and reinitiated afterwards.

The markedly less potent R-enantiomer is metabolized by CYP3A4. While the metabolism of R-warfarin indeed can be affected by concomitant therapy with inhibitors or inducers of CYP3A4, this will rarely lead to clinically significant changes in the anticoagulant activity of warfarin due to the low potency of R-warfarin.[4]

The list of drugs reported to potentially interact with warfarin is long. While some of the drugs on the list involve an interference with warfarin metabolism through the CYP system, other apparent DDIs more likely reflect an interaction between warfarin and the condition being treated or the side effects to the drug (e.g. dyspepsia leading to a change in food intake). Therefore, INR changes in relation to a change in drug therapy may be unpredictable despite detailed knowledge of the drug's interference with the CYP system. For this reason, monitoring of INR should be considered in the context of any change in drug therapy.

Other vitamin K antagonists

Similar to warfarin, acenocoumarol is primarily metabolized by CYP2C9, and is therefore likely to interact with inhibitors and inducers of CYP2C9 (see Table 7.1.2).

CYP-dependent metabolism is less pronounced for phenprocoumon than for warfarin and acenocoumarol (60% versus 100%), making this pathway less important for the total elimination of phenprocoumon. Thus, the potential for CYP-mediated DDIs is lower for phenprocoumon than for warfarin and acenocoumarol. Further, the predominant CYP enzyme involved in phenprocoumon metabolism is CYP3A4 (the role of CYP2C9 is minor), and DDIs involving phenprocoumon will therefore more likely be caused by concomitant therapy with drugs interfering with the activity of CYP3A4 (see Table 7.1.2) than CYP2C9.

Non-vitamin K antagonist oral anticoagulants

An often mentioned benefit of NOACs, compared to VKAs, is the lower potential for DDIs. With a lower degree of liver metabolism and a wider therapeutic index, NOACs are indeed involved in fewer clinically relevant DDIs. However, while VKA dosing can be titrated 'to fit' the DDI, the options are limited in the context of NOACs due to their fixed dosing regimens. Concomitant treatment with a drug known or expected to interact significantly with NOACs will therefore lead to either a dose reduction or discontinuation of one of the agents (i.e. contraindicated combinations).

Importantly, NOACs are newly marketed drugs, and most of our knowledge concerning NOACs and DDIs is currently based on PK studies using differences in total drug exposure [i.e. area under the curve (AUC)] between NOAC users exposed to and those unexposed to the potentially interacting drug as a proxy for a DDI. The precise correlation between changes in the AUC and the effectiveness and safety of NOACs remains to be established. Studies focusing on the clinical significance of DDIs involving NOACs are very sparse.

PK DDIs involving NOACs are mediated through P-gp, for which all NOACs are substrates, and CYP3A4, which is responsible for liver metabolism of factor Xa inhibitors (especially rivaroxaban and apixaban).

The EHRA has proposed that potential DDIs involving NOACs can be categorized according to recommended handling: (1) do not combine (red in Fig. 7.1.1); (2) reduce the NOAC dose (orange in Fig. 7.1.1); (3) consider dose reduction if two drugs in this category are combined with the NOAC (yellow in Fig. 7.1.1); (4) no interventions or cautions are needed (white in Fig. 7.1.1); and (5) use with caution or avoid (pink in Fig. 7.1.1).[5,6] The categorization is based on available knowledge from drug labels and from PK and clinical DDI studies, and is intended for use in AF patients. The recommendations for specific combinations can be found in Fig. 7.1.1.

Pharmacodynamic drug–drug interactions involving oral anticoagulants

Use of multiple antithrombotic drugs infers a synergistic effect on the bleeding risk. Use of more than one anticoagulant agent is contraindicated, even in the context of bridging. Combined use of an oral anticoagulant and one or more platelet inhibitor (e.g. clopidogrel and low-dose ASA) has the potential to increase the bleeding risk markedly and should only be used if absolutely indicated by guidelines.[7]

Other drugs known to increase the risk of bleeding in the context of oral anticoagulant therapy are NSAIDs (e.g. ibuprofen and high-dose ASA) and antidepressants mediating their action through interference with serotonin reuptake mechanisms [SSRIs, serotonin noradrenaline reuptake inhibitors (SNRIs), and clomipramine].

Statins

Statins (HMG CoA reductase inhibitors) are widely used in the prevention of CV disease. The risk of muscular side effects increases with increasing plasma levels of statins. Very high plasma levels can lead to rhabdomyolysis (muscular necrosis), which is a rare, but much feared, complication of statin therapy. Most cases of statin-associated rhabdomyolysis and myopathy are due to PK DDIs leading to the inhibition of hepatic metabolism of statins.

Concomitant treatment with simvastatin, lovastatin, or atorvastatin and a potent inhibitor of CYP3A4 (see Table 7.1.2) can result in up to a 5-fold increase in the AUC of the given statin.[8] Such combinations should therefore be avoided. Short-term treatment with potent CYP3A4 inhibitors during therapy with simvastatin, lovastatin, or atorvastatin can be handled with a temporary interruption of statin therapy. In cases of long-term therapy with potent CYP3A4 inhibitors, statin therapy should be with a statin not dependent on CYP3A4 metabolism (e.g. rosuvastatin).

Simvastatin and lovastatin are more susceptible to CYP3A4 inhibition than atorvastatin, and even moderate CYP3A4 inhibition might lead to adverse muscular effects. Therefore, the dose of simvastatin and lovastatin should, in contrast to atorvastatin, be reduced when combined with moderate CYP3A4 inhibitors.

Liver metabolism of rosuvastatin through CYP2C9 is negligible. No clinically relevant DDIs between either rosuvastatin or fluvastatin and inhibitors of CYP2C9 have been described.

Other lipid-lowering drugs

There are no known DDIs involving either ezetimibe or any of the PCSK9 inhibitors (evolocumab and alirocumab).

Gemfibrozil serves as an inhibitor of CYP2C9, CYP2C19, and CYP1A2, as well as other metabolizing enzymes. It is contraindicated to use gemfibrozil in combination with dasabuvir and repaglinide. Further, when combined with statins (especially simvastatin), the risk of statin-related side effects is increased.[8]

Bile acid sequestrants, such as colestyramine, bind any kind of acids in the GI tract. These drugs therefore have the potential to decrease the absorption, and thereby the bioavailability, of several drugs (e.g. anticoagulants, digoxin, and thyroxine). Generally, intake of other drugs should be avoided from 1h before to 4h after the administration of a bile acid sequestrant.[8]

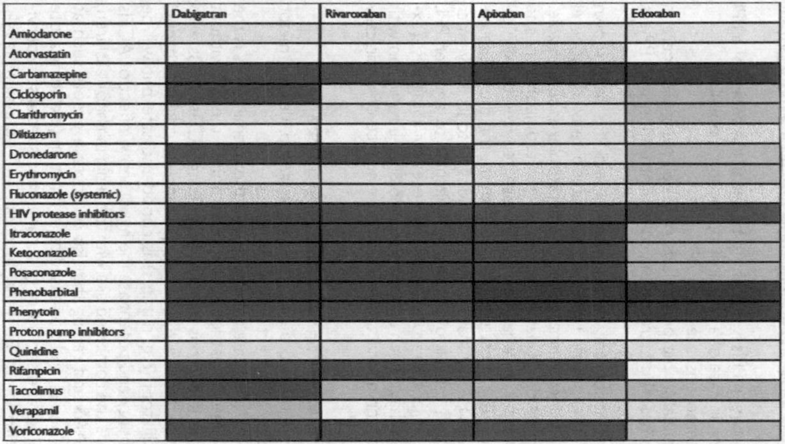

	Dabigatran	Rivaroxaban	Apixaban	Edoxaban
Amiodarone				
Atorvastatin				
Carbamazepine				
Ciclosporin				
Clarithromycin				
Diltiazem				
Dronedarone				
Erythromycin				
Fluconazole (systemic)				
HIV protease inhibitors				
Itraconazole				
Ketoconazole				
Posaconazole				
Phenobarbital				
Phenytoin				
Proton pump inhibitors				
Quinidine				
Rifampicin				
Tacrolimus				
Verapamil				
Voriconazole				

Fig. 7.1.1 Recommended clinical approach in the context of specific drug combinations involving NOACs. Red cells indicate contraindicated combinations. Orange cells indicate that the combination can be used, but the NOAC dose should be reduced. Yellow cells indicate that NOAC dose reduction should be considered when two or more 'yellow drugs' are used concomitantly with NOAC therapy. Pink cells indicate use with caution or avoid. White cells indicate that there is no need for intervention/caution, and grey cells indicate that no data on the combination are available.

Source data from Heidbuchel H, Verhamme P, Alings M *et al.* Updated European Heart Rhythm Association Practical Guide on the use of non-vitamin K antagonist anticoagulants in patients with non-valvular atrial fibrillation. Eur Eur Pacing Arrhythm Card Electrophysiol J Work Groups Card Pacing *Arrhythm Card Cell Electrophysiol Eur Soc Cardiol.* October 2015;17(10):1467–507; and Steffel J, Verhamme P, Potpara TS *et al.* ESC Scientific Document Group. The 2018 European Heart Rhythm Association Practical Guide on the use of non-vitamin K antagonist oral anticoagulants in patients with atrial fibrillation. *Eur Heart J* 2018;39(16):1330–93.

Proton pump inhibitors

PPIs inhibit the secretion of hydrochloric acid in the stomach by specific blockade of the proton pumps (the H^+/K^+-ATPase enzyme) of the parietal cells. PPIs may therefore reduce the absorption of active substances whose bioavailability is dependent on gastric pH (e.g. antifungal medication).

PPIs are almost exclusively metabolized primarily by CYP2C19 and, to a lesser extent, by CYP3A4. In addition to being a substrate, most PPIs also inhibit CYP2C19. Omeprazole and esomeprazole may elicit a more potent inhibition of CYP2C19.

Since the efficacy between PPIs is thought to be equal, the choice of a PPI with less CYP inhibition in case of a potential interaction is possible.

For potential PK interactions, see Table 7.1.2.

Since PPIs are essential in the prophylaxis of GI bleeding disorders in patients receiving antithrombotic treatment, co-administration with PPIs is often seen.

Data on the PK interaction between clopidogrel and PPIs have shown up to 45% reduction in exposure to the active metabolite of clopidogrel when administered concomitantly with omeprazole/esomeprazole. Although this PK interaction is mainly established for esomeprazole and omeprazole, it is not clear to what degree this also reduces the clinical efficacy of clopidogrel. The most plausible mechanism for the PK interaction is inhibition of CYP2C19 that converts clopidogrel to its active metabolite. This interaction can be overcome by switching to another PPI, such as pantoprazole or lansoprazole, or to a H2 receptor antagonist (except cimetidine). There have been concerns of a possible interaction with VKAs, but a recent observational study found no evidence of a clinically meaningful DDI.

ACE inhibitors and angiotensin II receptor blockers

The PD interaction potential is comparable for this group, despite minor differences in the mechanism of action.

ACEIs and ARBs both modulate the RAAS, and the overall effect is the same, causing vasodilatation that leads to a reduction in the BP without activating the sympathetic nervous system. Combining ACEIs/ARBs with other types of antihypertensive drugs (e.g. β-blockers, calcium channel antagonists) or vasodilators (e.g. nitrates) is considered safe but will be expected to act in synergy and potentiate the hypotensive effect of ACEIs and ARBs. A concern is the combined use with the renin inhibitor aliskiren, also acting on the RAAS and raising the risk of adverse events such as hypotension, hyperkalaemia, and decreased renal function (including acute renal failure). Dual blockade should only occur under specialist supervision, with close monitoring of BP, renal function, and potassium levels, and triple blockade with aliskiren and ACEIs/ARBs is contraindicated in patients with diabetes mellitus or renal impairment (GFR <60mL/min/1.73m^2) (see Fig. 7.1.2).

The risk of increased potassium levels is also with the concomitant use of potassium-sparing diuretics or potassium supplements and, in some cases, with the concurrent use of ACEIs and co-trimoxazole.

For NSAIDs, see ➲ Analgesics, pp. 401–2.

A rarer interaction due to the same side effects is an increased risk of angio-oedema in patients taking both an ACEI and an mTOR inhibitor such as sirolimus.

Lithium

ACEIs/ARBs can raise lithium levels, with up to a 7-fold increase in the risk of lithium toxicity and an average rise in serum lithium levels of 35% (from 0.64 to 0.86mmol/L) and with a 26% decrease in lithium clearance after initiating treatment with an ACEI. The mechanism is not fully understood, but theories include inhibition of aldosterone activity, resulting in increased sodium loss by renal tubules and retention of lithium, as well as reduced thirst stimulation and fluid depletion caused by ACEIs. In cases of concomitant use of lithium with ACEIs or ARBs, consider reducing the initial lithium dose and monitoring lithium levels more frequently.

PK interactions differ between the two drug classes, but within the same class, the differences are minor. Despite these differences, PK interactions for both classes are comparably few and rarely clinically relevant. ACEIs are not known to be metabolized via the CYP enzyme system to a clinical relevant extent, and even though some ARBs (losartan, irbesartan, candesartan) are known to be metabolized via CYP2C9, few clinically relevant changes in their plasma levels have been reported when used concomitantly with other drugs also metabolized by CYP2C9 (see Table 7.1.2 and Fig. 7.1.2).

Analgesics

Analgesics are frequently used drugs, for both acute and chronic pain treatment. In this section, interaction with commonly used analgesics will be described.

Paracetamol

Paracetamol is indicated for mild to moderate pain and fever relief. It is usually well tolerated, and its potential for interaction is low. Interaction with warfarin has been proposed, which underscores the importance of close INR monitoring when adding this drug to, or removing it from, warfarin treatment. However, short-term use and single dosages of paracetamol is safe.

Non-steroidal anti-inflammatory drugs

NSAIDs are widely used for musculoskeletal pain relief. Both selective and non-selective NSAIDs increase the risk of various adverse events. GI complications are well known and are largely due to COX-1 inhibition, while CV adverse effects are mostly COX-2-dependent. It is known that NSAIDs, mostly due to COX-2 inhibition, increase the risk of major CV events and the risk is proportional to the dose and the patient's baseline risk. The increased risk appears early and is not attenuated by concomitant aspirin use.[9]

Concerning DDIs, NSAIDs increase BP, thereby potentially inhibiting the BP-lowering effect of antihypertensive drugs. The clinical relevance of such interaction is, however, unresolved. Nevertheless, aspirin used in anti-inflammatory doses (1–2g) has been shown to decrease the antihypertensive effects of captopril and enalapril in about 50% of patients, particularly in low-renin hypertensives. Still, low-dose aspirin (≤100mg daily) does not appear to affect the BP.

The combination of an NSAID with ACEIs and ARBs increases the risk of renal impairment and increased potassium levels, especially in patients with already existing renal impairment.

NSAIDs can interfere with the antiplatelet effect of low-dose aspirin, reducing the cardioprotective effects of aspirin. Additionally, the combination of NSAIDs with aspirin, as well as with other antiplatelet drugs, also increases the bleeding risk.

NSAIDs also increase the bleeding risk when used in combination with warfarin, increasing the GI bleeding risk by 2- to 4-fold. The bleeding risk is also increased with NOACs.

Naproxen and all other NSAIDs, if indicated, should be used at the lowest effective dose for the shortest possible duration.

Opioids

Morphine is recommended for severe pain and also for pain management in patients with ACS. There are several studies reporting a negative impact of morphine on the initial blood concentrations of clopidogrel, but also of ticagrelor and prasugrel. The maximal plasma concentration was generally reduced and delayed by approximately 2h with concomitant use. The suspected mechanism of interaction is reduced gut motility by morphine and impaired absorption. However, larger randomized studies investigating the impact of those findings on clinically relevant endpoints are still lacking.

The impact of other opioids on P2Y12 receptor inhibitors has not been investigated, but since all opioids reduce gut motility, the same effect could be expected.

Methadone is used for pain management and in the maintenance treatment of opioid dependency. Methadone is found to increase the risk of QTc prolongation by blocking potassium ion (hERG) channels in a concentration-dependent manner. Methadone exists most commonly as a racemic formulation, consisting of S- and R-methadone, of which S-methadone is found to be a more potent hERG inhibitor. Risk assessment prior to prescription and ECG monitoring are suggested. Furthermore, methadone is mainly metabolized by CYP3A4, and its concomitant use with CYP3A4 inhibitors (see Table 7.1.2) is contraindicated.

Antibiotics

Bacterial infections are some of the challenges encountered in the treatment of patients with CV disease, because of DDIs, among other reasons. DDIs with antibiotics are based on several mechanisms of interaction. It can be due to inhibition or induction of P-gp and CYP450 enzymes. Depending on how strong that induction or inhibition is, concentrations of the susceptible drugs can vary, leading to an increased risk of toxicity, adverse events, or treatment failure.

However, all antibiotics can lead to a change in the intestinal bacterial flora. This can influence vitamin K synthesis, thereby increasing the bleeding risk in patients on warfarin. Interactions between various antibiotics and warfarin have been reported, with important interactions involving macrolides, quinolones, and sulfonamides, all increasing the risk of bleeding.

Potassium-sparing diuretics/potassium supplements	Potassium retention	Close monitoring of serum potassium levels and renal function
Co-trimoxazole (trimethoprim/sulfamethoxazole)	Potassium retention	**Monitor serum potassium levels**
NSAIDs (not low-dose aspirin)	Inhibition of prostaglandin synthesis	Monitor blood pressure and renal function
Allopurinol	Sodium retention	Use with caution, monitor for signs of hypersensitivity
Lithium	Increase in blood pressure, potassium levels, and renal impairment	Reduce initial lithium dose; titrate slowly; monitor lithium levels; look for signs of lithium toxicity more frequently
Aliskiren	Not fully understood. Risk of hypersensitivity	Contraindicated in diabetics and patients with GFR <60mL/min
Rifampicin	Sodium loss leading to lithium retention	Monitor blood pressure and consider higher doses of losartan
Fluconazole	Decreased lithium excretion	Consider the possibility of an interaction if the blood pressure is undesirably lowered

Fig. 7.1.2 Recommended clinical approach in the context of specific drug combinations involving ACEIs and ARBs. Red cells indicate contraindicated combinations. Orange cells indicate that the combination can be used, but the dose should be reduced. Yellow cells indicate that dose reduction should be considered.

Source data from Heidbuchel H, Verhamme P, Alings M *et al.* Updated European Heart Rhythm Association Practical Guide on the use of non-vitamin K antagonist anticoagulants in patients with non-valvular atrial fibrillation. Eur Eur Pacing Arrhythm Card Electrophysiol J Work Groups Card Pacing Arrhythm Card Cell Electrophysiol Eur Soc Cardiol. October 2015;17(10):1467–507.

Rifampicin is somewhat different and is probably the antibiotic with the greatest ability to cause DDIs, due to its potential to induce many CYP enzymes and P-gp. Rifampicin is not very frequently used in the Western world, but since it can lead to very important interactions, it will be mentioned briefly here. Rifampicin induces, among others, CYP1A2, 2C9, 2C19, 2D6, and 3A4. These enzymes are involved in the metabolism of many CV drugs (see Table 7.1.2). Drugs that are metabolized by these enzymes may have decreased plasma concentrations with concomitant use and also to a clinically relevant level (e.g. simvastatin, atorvastatin, amlodipine, verapamil, diltiazem, digoxin, losartan, metoprolol, dabigatran, rivaroxaban, warfarin, ticagrelor). For prodrugs like clopidogrel, concomitant treatment with rifampicin increases the concentration of the active metabolite.

Importantly, both macrolides and quinolones are reported to cause QTc prolongation, and their combination with other QTc-prolonging drugs should be avoided, if possible, and to be used with caution if not possible. This is particularly evident for erythromycin and moxifloxacin. CV drugs such as verapamil and diltiazem, by inhibiting CYP3A4, increase the concentration of macrolides such as clarithromycin and erythromycin, and an increased concentration of these drugs can further increase the risk of QTc prolongation.

Macrolides are the group of antibiotics that are responsible for most PK interactions with CV drugs, due to their pharmacological properties by inhibiting CYP3A4. Fig. 7.1.3 presents interactions between commonly used CV drugs and macrolides.

Antifungal medications and cardiovascular drugs

Antifungal drugs are widely used for the treatment of local and systemic infections. Azoles are the most commonly used antifungal drugs for systemic therapy and are of great importance in terms of DDIs. Other systemic antifungals, such as nystatin, anidulafungin, and caspofungin, have no significant interactions with the usual CV drugs.

The azoles used for systemic infections, including fluconazole, itraconazole, voriconazole, posaconazole, and ketoconazole, are CYP3A4 inhibitors, particularly itraconazole and ketoconazole which are potent inhibitors. Voriconazole and fluconazole also inhibit CYP2C9. Due to their PK properties, azoles increase considerably the risk of interactions with CV drugs, since many of these drugs are metabolized by CYP3A4 and CYP2C9. However, most published interactions with azoles are with warfarin and statins. There is still a lack of clinical data on DDIs for many other drugs (see Fig. 7.1.4). This calls for caution when azoles are used with drugs that are metabolized via the CYP3A4 and CYP2C9 pathways (see Table 7.1.2), since important theoretical interactions still exist.

Fluconazole is special, since the inhibition of CYP450 enzymes seems to be dose-dependent. Treatment with fluconazole increases the plasma concentrations of fluvastatin and, to a lesser extent, simvastatin and atorvastatin, but dosages below 200mg daily can be used with simvastatin, fluvastatin, and atorvastatin—with close monitoring of adverse events. In cases of short-term treatment with a higher dosage of fluconazole, statin treatment can be adjusted either by temporarily withholding statin therapy or reducing the statin dose. In cases of long-term fluconazole treatment, statin therapy should be changed to a statin that is not dependent on CYP3A4 metabolism (e.g. pravastatin, rosuvastatin). However, statins should not be used with potent CYP3A4 inhibitors; for clinical management, see ➔ Statins, p. 398.

Miconazole is a topical antifungal agent, and clinically important interactions with warfarin through CYP2C9 have been described.

Fig. 7.1.4 shows the most important interactions between azoles and frequently used CV drugs.

	Azithromycin	**Clarithromycin**	**Erythromycin**	**Roxithromycin**
Mechanism of interaction	Possible P-gp inhibitor and impairment of intestinal flora	Substrate for CYP3A4	Moderate inhibitor of CYP3A4 and P-gp Impairment of intestinal flora QTc prolongation Substrate for CYP3A4	Weak inhibitor of CYP3A4 Impairment of intestinal flora
Digoxin Substrate for P-gp				
R-warfarin Substrate for CYP3A4 and impairment of intestinal flora				
Dabigatran Substrate for P-gp and CYP3A4				
Rivaroxaban Substrate for CYP3A4				
Apixaban Substrate for P-gp and CYP3A4				
Edoxaban Substrate for P-gp				

Fig. 7.1.3 Interactions with commonly used cardiovascular drugs and macrolides. Red: contraindicated/not recommended combination. Orange: consider dose reduction. Yellow: monitor for adverse effects and/or consider using a reduced dose; consider other risk factors (elderly, renal impairment). Grey: no data available.

Source data from Heidbuchel H, Verhamme P, Alings M *et al.* Updated European Heart Rhythm Association Practical Guide on the use of non-vitamin K antagonist anticoagulants in patients with non-valvular atrial fibrillation. Eur Eur Pacing Arrhythm Card Electrophysiol J Work Groups Card Pacing *Arrhythm Card Cell Electrophysiol Eur Soc Cardiol.* October 2015;17(10):1467–507; Steffel J, Verhamme P, Potpara TS *et al.* ESC Scientific Document Group. The 2018 European Heart Rhythm Association Practical Guide on the use of non-vitamin K antagonist oral anticoagulants in patients with atrial fibrillation. *Eur Heart J* 2018;39(16):1330–93; and other sources.

	Fluconazole	**Voriconazole**	**Itraconazole, ketoconazole, posaconazole**	**Miconazole (topical)**
Mechanism of interaction	Inhibitor of CYP2C9 and dose-dependent moderate inhibitor of CYP3A4	Inhibitor of CYP3A4 and CYP2C9	Strong inhibitor of CYP 3A4 and P-gp	Inhibitor of CYP3A4 and CYP2C9
Warfarin Substrate CYP2C9				
Dabigatran Substrate of P-gp and CYP3A4.				
Rivaroxaban Substrate of CYP3A4.				
Apixaban Substrate of P-gp and CYP3A4.				
Edoxaban Substrate for P-gp				
Statins Simvastatin, atorvastatin and lovastatin are substrates for CYP3A4. Fluvastatin substrate for CYP2C9.	See text	See text	See text	

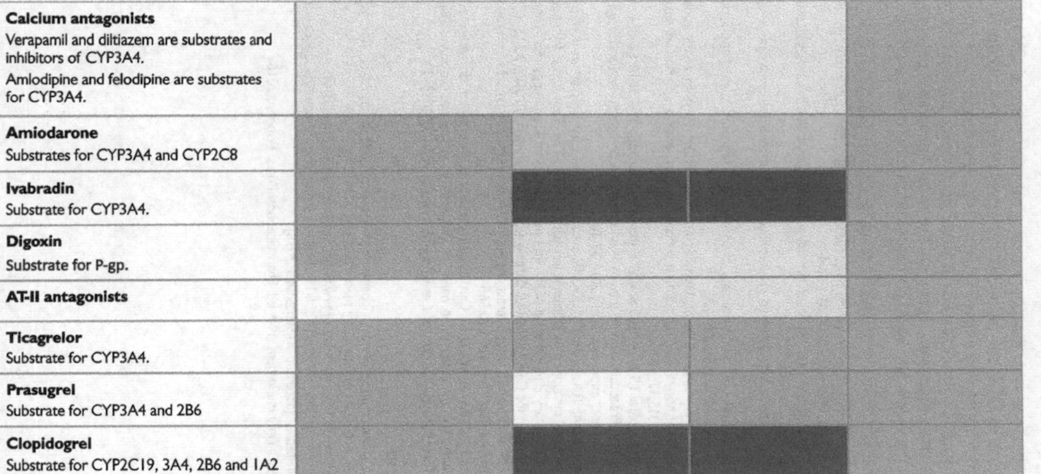

Fig. 7.1.4 Interactions with commonly used cardiovascular drugs and azoles. Red: contraindicated/not recommended combination. Orange: consider dosage reduction. Yellow: monitor for adverse effects and/or consider using a reduced dose; consider other risk factors (elderly, renal impairment). White: no need for intervention/caution. Grey: no data available.

Source data from Heidbuchel H, Verhamme P, Alings M *et al*. Updated European Heart Rhythm Association Practical Guide on the use of non-vitamin K antagonist anticoagulants in patients with non-valvular atrial fibrillation. Eur Eur Pacing Arrhythm Card Electrophysiol J Work Groups Card Pacing *Arrhythm Card Cell Electrophysiol Eur Soc Cardiol*. October 2015;**17**(10):1467–507; Steffel J, Verhamme P, Potpara TS *et al*. ESC Scientific Document Group. The 2018 European Heart Rhythm Association Practical Guide on the use of non-vitamin K antagonist oral anticoagulants in patients with atrial fibrillation. *Eur Heart J* 2018;**39**(16):1330–93; and other sources.

Conclusion

Many drugs can interfere with the pharmacological treatment of CV diseases, but in most cases DDIs can be overcome either by dose reduction or by increased monitoring of side effects. Only in rare cases are the concomitant use of two drugs contraindicated. In order to protect patients from more side effects than necessary, focus on the most vulnerable patients, regular medication reviews, and good communication would be beneficial.

References

1 Howard RL, Avery AJ, Slavenburg S, *et al*. Which drugs cause preventable admissions to hospital? A systematic review. *Br J Clin Pharmacol* 2007;**63**:136–47.
2 Al-Khazaali A, Arora R. P-glycoprotein: a focus on characterizing variability in cardiovascular pharmacotherapeutics. *Am J Ther* 2014;**21**:2–9.
3 Bailey DG, Dresser GK. Interactions between grapefruit juice and cardiovascular drugs. *Am J Cardiovasc Drugs* 2004;**4**:281–97.
4 Holbrook AM, Pereira JA, Labiris R, *et al*. Systematic overview of warfarin and its drug and food interactions. *Arch Intern Med* 2005;**165**:1095–106.
5 Heidbuchel H, Verhamme P, Alings M, *et al*. Updated European Heart Rhythm Association Practical Guide on the use of non-vitamin K antagonist anticoagulants in patients with non-valvular atrial fibrillation. *Europace* 2015;**17**:1467–507.
6 Steffel J, Verhamme P, Potpara TS *et al*. ESC Scientific Document Group. The 2018 European Heart Rhythm Association Practical Guide on the use of non-vitamin K antagonist oral anticoagulants in patients with atrial fibrillation. *Eur Heart J* 2018;**39(16)**:1330–93.
7 Valgimigli M, Bueno H, Byrne RA, *et al*. 2017 ESC focused update on dual antiplatelet therapy in coronary artery disease developed in collaboration with EACTS: The Task Force for dual antiplatelet therapy in coronary artery disease of the European Society of Cardiology (ESC) and of the European Association for Cardio-Thoracic Surgery (EACTS). *Eur Heart J* 2018;**39**:213–60.
8 Neuvonen PJ, Niemi M, Backman JT. Drug interactions with lipid-lowering drugs: mechanisms and clinical relevance. *Clin Pharmacol Ther* 2006;**80**:565–81.
9 Schmidt M, Lamberts M, Olsen A-MS, *et al*. Cardiovascular safety of non-aspirin non-steroidal anti-inflammatory drugs: review and position paper by the working group for Cardiovascular Pharmacotherapy of the European Society of Cardiology. *Eur Heart J* 2016;**37**:1015–23.

Further reading

Brunton LL, Chapner BA, Knollmann BC (eds). *Goodman and Gilman's The Pharmacological Basis of Therapeutics*, 12th ed. McGraw-Hill Education: New York, NY; 2011.

Drugs.com. *Amiodarone*. Available from: http://www.drugs.com [accessed 5 June 2016].

Indiana University. *Drug interactions: Flockhart Table™*. Available from: http://medicine.iupui.edu/clinpharm/ddis/main-table/ [accessed 10 September 2018].

Preston CL (ed). *Stockley's Drug Interactions*, 11th ed. Pharmaceutical Press: London; 2016.

Section 8

Cardiovascular drugs—from A to Z

Section editor

Juan Tamargo

Chapter 8.1

Cardiovascular drugs—from A to Z

Juan Tamargo, Ricardo Caballero, and Eva Delpón

Abciximab

Fab fragment (c7E3 Fab) of the chimeric monoclonal antibody 7E3 directed against the GPIIb/IIIa receptor (see Glycoprotein IIb/IIIa receptor antagonists, pp. [illegible]).

Cardiovascular indications

In addition to unfractionated heparin and ASA for:

- Prevention of ischaemic cardiac complications in patients undergoing PCI (balloon angioplasty, atherectomy, and stent).
- Short-term (1-month) reduction of the risk of MI in patients with UA not responding to full conventional therapy who have been scheduled for PCI.

Mechanism of action

Abciximab inhibits platelet aggregation by preventing the binding of fibrinogen, von Willebrand factor, and other adhesive molecules to GPIIb/IIIa receptor sites on activated platelets. It also binds to the vitronectin receptor (αvβ3) on platelets and endothelial and vascular smooth muscle cells which mediates the procoagulant and proliferative effects. This dual effect may explain why abciximab more effectively blocks the burst of thrombin generation that follows platelet activation. Abciximab also binds to the activated Mac-1 receptor on monocytes and neutrophils (CD11b) and reduces the number of circulating leucocyte–platelet complexes.

The mechanism of action is thought to involve steric hindrance and/or conformational effects to block access of large molecules to the receptor, rather than direct interaction with the RGD (arginine–glycine–aspartic acid) binding site of GPIIb/IIIa. Maximal inhibition of platelet aggregation is obtained when ≥80% of GPIIb/IIIa receptors are blocked. In non-human primates, IV abciximab produced rapid dose-dependent inhibition of platelet function, as measured by ex vivo platelet aggregation in response to ADP or by prolongation of bleeding time. Low levels of GPIIb/IIIa receptor blockade are present for >10 days following cessation of the infusion.

Pharmacokinetics

Following IV bolus administration, abciximab produces a rapid onset of action and a very potent antiplatelet inhibitory effect. Free plasma concentrations decrease rapidly for approximately 6h, and then decline at a slower rate, with an initial t½ <10min and a second-phase t½ of about 30min. Inhibition of platelet aggregation is maximal at 2h after a bolus injection, and platelet function generally recovers over the next 48h. After discontinuation, however, the antibody remains in circulation for up to 15 days or more in a platelet-bound state. Its action can be reversed by platelet transfusion. It is catabolized by proteolytic degradation.

Abciximab

Fab fragment (46.6kDa) of the chimeric monoclonal antibody 7E3 directed against the GPIIb/IIIa receptor (see ➲ Glycoprotein IIb/IIIa receptor antagonists, pp. 613–15).

Cardiovascular indications

In adults, as an adjunct to heparin and ASA for:

- Prevention of ischaemic cardiac complications in patients undergoing PCI (balloon angioplasty, atherectomy, and stent)
- Short-term (1-month) reduction of the risk of MI in patients with UA, not responding to full conventional therapy, who have been scheduled for PCI.

Mechanism of action

Abciximab inhibits platelet aggregation by preventing the binding of fibrinogen, von Willebrand factor, and other adhesive molecules to GPIIb/IIIa receptor sites on activated platelets. It also binds to the vitronectin receptor ($\alpha v\beta 3$) on platelets and endothelial and smooth muscle cells where it exerts procoagulant and proliferative effects. This dual effect may explain why abciximab more effectively blocks the burst of thrombin generation than other GPIIb/IIIa receptor antagonists. Abciximab also binds to the activated Mac-1 receptor on monocytes and neutrophils and reduces the number of circulating leucocyte–platelet complexes.

The mechanism of action is thought to involve steric hindrance and/or conformational effects to block access of large molecules to the receptor, rather than direct interaction with the RGD (arginine–glycine–aspartic acid) binding site of GPIIb/IIIa. Maximal inhibition of platelet aggregation is observed when ≥80% of GPIIb/IIIa receptors are blocked. In non-human primates, IV abciximab produces rapid dose-dependent inhibition of platelet function, measured by *ex vivo* platelet aggregation, in response to ADP or by prolongation of bleeding time. Low levels of GPIIb/IIIa receptor blockade are present for >10 days, following cessation of the infusion.

Pharmacokinetics

Following IV bolus administration, abciximab produces a rapid onset of action and a very potent antiplatelet inhibitory effect. Its free plasma concentrations decrease rapidly for approximately 6h and then decline at a slower rate, with an initial t½ of <10min and a second-phase t½ of about 30min. Inhibition of platelet aggregation is maximal at 2h after a bolus injection, and platelet function generally recovers over the next 48h after discontinuation. However, the antibody remains platelet-bound in circulation up to 15 days or more in a platelet-bound state. Its action can be reversed by platelet transfusion. It is eliminated by proteolytic degradation.

Practical points

1. *Doses*
   - 0.25mg/kg IV bolus over 10–60min before PCI, followed by 0.125mcg/kg/min (maximum 10mcg/min) continuous IV infusion for 12h.
   - ASA should be administered orally (PO) at a daily dose of not less than 300mg.
   - Heparin bolus pre-percutaneous transluminal coronary angioplasty (PTCA): an initial bolus of heparin should be given upon gaining arterial access. If ACT is <150s: administer 70U/kg; if ACT is 150–199s: give 50U/kg. The initial heparin bolus dose should not exceed 7000U.
2. *Side effects*
   - Bleeding: major and minor. Abciximab increases the risk of retroperitoneal bleeding in association with femoral vascular puncture. The use of venous sheaths should be minimized, and only the anterior wall of an artery or vein should be punctured when establishing vascular access. Heparin should be discontinued at least 2h prior to arterial sheath removal.
   - Administration of abciximab may result in human anti-chimeric antibody (HACA) formation that could potentially cause allergic or hypersensitivity reactions, thrombocytopenia, or reduced drug benefit.
   - Factors associated with an increased risk of thrombocytopenia include a history of thrombocytopenia on previous abciximab exposure, re-administration within 30 days, and a positive HACA assay prior to re-administration.
3. *Interactions* (see ➔ Glycoprotein IIb/IIIa receptor antagonists, pp. 613–15)
   - No interactions with other drugs used in the treatment of angina, MI, or hypertension nor with common IV infusion fluids.
4. *Cautions/notes* (see ➔ Glycoprotein IIb/IIIa receptor antagonists, pp. 613–15)
   - Administration of abciximab may result in HACA formation that could potentially cause allergic or hypersensitivity reactions, thrombocytopenia, or reduced benefit.
   - If allergic reactions or anaphylaxis appear, the infusion should be stopped immediately. Adrenaline, dopamine, theophylline, antihistamines, and corticosteroids should be available for immediate use.
   - Its safety and efficacy are uncertain in patients <18 years of age.
   - Major bleeding is commoner in patients weighing ≤75kg.
   - Keep vials cold; use in-line filter for infusion; discard vials after use.
   - To prevent spontaneous GI bleeding, patients should be pre-treated with H2-histamine receptor antagonists or liquid antacids. Antiemetics should be given, as needed, to prevent vomiting.
5. *Contraindications* (see ➔ Glycoprotein IIb/IIIa receptor antagonists, pp. 613–15)
   - Hypersensitivity to murine monoclonal antibodies.
   - Severe renal failure in patients on haemodialysis.

Acenocoumarol

Vitamin K epoxide reductase antagonist.

Indications

- Treatment and prevention of thromboembolic diseases.

Mechanism of action

Vitamin K epoxide reductase complex subunit 1 isoform 1 inhibitor (see ➔ Warfarin, pp. 800–7).

Pharmacodynamics

Acenocoumarol is a coumarin derivative and functions as a VKA. Depending on the initial dosage, acenocoumarol prolongs the thromboplastin time within approximately 36–72h. Following drug withdrawal, the thromboplastin time usually reverts to normal after a few days.

Pharmacokinetics

Acenocoumarol is a racemic mixture of the optical R(+) and S(–) enantiomers. It is extensively metabolized via CYP2C9 [(R)-acenocoumarol via CYP1A2 and CYP2C19]. CYP2C9-related genetic variability accounts for 14% of the inter-individual variability. The total plasma clearance of the R(+) enantiomer, which possesses significantly higher anticoagulant activity, is much lower than that of the S(–) enantiomer (see Table 8.1.1).

Practical points

1. *Doses*
   - Starting dose: 2–4mg/day without loading dose. Treatment may also be initiated with a loading dose of 6mg on the first day, followed by 4mg on the second day. Maintenance dose: 1–8mg/day. Reduce the dose in elderly patients, patients with liver disease or severe HF, those with hepatic congestion, or those who are malnourished. The optimal intensity of anticoagulation or therapeutic range to be aimed at generally lies with INR values of between 2.0 and 3.5.
2. *Side effects* (see ➔ Warfarin, pp. 800–7)
   - Common: haemorrhage. Rare: anorexia, nausea, vomiting, hypersensitivity (urticaria, rash, dermatitis, fever), alopecia.
3. *Interactions* (see ➔ Warfarin, pp. 800–7)
   - It can interact with CYP2C9 inhibitors/inducers (see Table 8.1.2).
4. *Cautions/notes* (see ➔ Warfarin, pp. 800–7)
5. *Pregnancy and lactation*
   - It is contraindicated in women who are, or may become, pregnant because it passes through the placenta, is teratogenic, and may cause fatal fetal haemorrhage *in utero* (Pregnancy category X). Women of childbearing potential should take contraceptive measures during treatment.
6. *Contraindications*
   - Known hypersensitivity to acenocoumarol.
   - Pregnancy.

Table 8.1.1 Pharmacokinetic characteristics of anticoagulants

Drug	F (%)	T_{max} (h)	PPB (%)	Vd (L/kg)	Metabolism	t½ (h)	Renal excretion* (%)
Acenocoumarol	60	3–4	>99	0.28	CYP2C9, 1A2, 2C19	8–11	<1
Apixaban	50	3–4	87	0.3	CYP3A4 (CYP1A2, 2C8, 2C9, 2C19, 2J2)	12 (8–15)	27
Argatroban (IV)	100	1–3	54	0.3	CYP3A4/5	52min	Faeces
Bemiparin (SC)	96	2–3	–	0.1	Desulfation, depolymerization	5–6	–
Bivalirudin (IV)	100	2–5	0		Proteolytic cleavage	25min	
Dabigatran	6.5	2	35	1	Not substrate of CYP450 enzymes	12–14	85
Dalteparin (SC)	87	3–4	<90	0.13	Desulfation, depolymerization	3.5	–
Edoxaban	62	1–2	55	10–14	Hydrolysis, conjugation, CYP3A4	1.52	50
Enoxaparin (SC)	90	1–4	–	0.12	Desulfation, depolymerization	4–5	10
Fondaparinux (SC)	100	0.5	–	0.15	Not metabolized	17–21	77
Nadroparin (SC)	>98	3–4			Desulfation, depolymerization	2–4	<5
Rivaroxaban	80–100**	2–4	92–95	0.65	CYP3A4/5 and CYP2J2, hydrolysis	5–13	66
Tinzaparin (SC)	90	4–6	–	–	Desulfation, depolymerization	3.7	–
Unfractionated heparin (SC)		2–4	–	0.058	Sulfation, depolymerization	25min	<2
Warfarin	95	1.5–3 days	>98	0.14	R-warfarin: CYP1A2, CYP2C19, CYP3A4 S-warfarin: CYP2C9	37 (20–60)	92

F, oral bioavailability; h, hour; IV, intravenous; min, minute; PPB, protein plasma binding; SC, subcutaneous; t½: drug half-life; T_{max}, time to peak plasma levels; Vd, volume of distribution.

* Renal excretion without biotransformation.

** With food.

Table 8.1.2 Substrates, inducers, and inhibitors of some cytochrome P450 isoforms and the P-glycoprotein transporter

CYP1A2 substrates	Agomelatine, amitriptyline, apixaban, clomipramine, clozapine, efavirenz, eltrombopag, erlotinib, febuxostat, fluoroquinolones, haloperidol, imipramine, naproxen, olanzapine, oestradiol, ondansetron, paracetamol, propranolol, retinol, riluzole, ritonavir, rizatriptan, ropivacaine, tacrine, tamoxifen, theophylline, verapamil, R-warfarin, zileuton, zolmitriptan
CYP1A2 inhibitors	Aciclovir, allopurinol, amiodarone, cimetidine, ciprofloxacin, enoxacin, erythromycin, fluvoxamine, mexiletine, norfloxacin, oral contraceptives, peginterferon alfa-2a, verapamil, zafirlukast, zileuton
CYP1A2 inducers	Barbiturates, carbamazepine, lansoprazole, omeprazole, phenytoin, rifampicin, St. John's wort, tobacco
CYP2B6 substrates	Artemisine, bupropion, cyclophosphamide, efavirenz, ifosfamide, ketamine, mepridine, methadone, nevirapine, propofol, selegiline, sertraline, sorafenib, testosterone, ticlopidine
CYP2B6 Inhibitors	Clopidogrel, ticlopidine, voriconazole
CYP2B6 inducers	Carbamazepine, cyclophosphamide, phenobarbital, phenytoin, rifampicin
CYP2C8 substrates	Enzalutamide, montelukast, paclitaxel, repaglinide, sorafenib, torasemide
CYP2C8 inhibitors	Gemfibrozil, montelukast, trimethoprim, zafirlukast
CYP2C8 inducers	Rifampicin
CYP3A4 substrates	Alfentanil, alfuzosin, almotriptan, amiodarone, amlodipine, amprenavir, anastrozole, apatinib, apixaban, aprepitant, aripiprazole, atazanavir, atorvastatin, benzodiazepines, bicalutamide, bosentan, bromocriptine, buprenorphine, bupropion, buspirone, calcium channel blockers, carbamazepine, chloroquine, cilostazol, citalopram, clarithromycin, clopidogrel, colchicine, cyclophosphamide, ciclosporin, dapsone, darunavir, dasabuvir, dasatinib, delavirdine, disopyramide, docetaxel, dofetilide, domperidone, donepezil, doxorubicin, dronedarone, droperidol, edoxaban, efavirenz, eletriptan, eplerenone, enzalutamide, ergot alkaloids, erlotinib, erythromycin, ethinylestradiol, etoposide, everolimus, fentanyl, finasteride, flurazepam, fosamprenavir, galantamine, gefitinib, glucocorticoids, glyburide, granisetron, halofantrine, ifosfamide, imatinib, indinavir, isotretinoin, itraconazole, ketoconazole, lansoprazole, lapatinib, levomethadyl, lidocaine, loperamide, lopinavir, loratadine, losartan, lovastatin, macitentan, methadone, midazolam, mifepristone, miraviroc, mirtazapine, modafinil, montelukast, morphine, nefazodone, nelfinavir, nevirapine, nilotinib, oestradiol, omeprazole, oxybutynin, oxycodone, paclitaxel, pazopanib, phenprocoumon, pimozide, pioglitazone, ponatinib, progesterone, propoxyphene, quetiapine, quinidine, quinine, ranolazine, repaglinide, rifabutin, riociguat, ritonavir, rivaroxaban, saquinavir, sertraline, sibutamine, sildenafil, simvastatin, simeprevir, sirolimus, sitagliptin, sufentanyl, sunitinib, tacrolimus, tadalafil, tamoxifen, tamsulosin, telithromycin, testosterone, tiagabine, tinidazole, tipranavir, tolterodine, topiramate, toremifene, tricyclic antidepressants, troleandomycin, vardenafil, vinblastine, vincristine, R-warfarin, zaleplon, zileuton, ziprasidone, zolpidem, zopiclone

CYP3A4 inhibitors	• Potent: atazanavir, boceprevir, clarithromycin, conivaptan, danoprevir, dasabuvir, elvitegravir, grapefruit juice, indinavir, itraconazole, ketoconazole, lopinavir, nefazodone, nelfinavir, paritaprevir, posaconazole, ritonavir, saquinavir, telaprevir, telithromycin, tipranavir, troleandomycin, voriconazole • Moderate: amiodarone, amprenavir, aprepitant, atazanavir, cimetidine, ciprofloxacin, clotrimazole, crizotinib, ciclosporin, danazol, darunavir, delavirdine, diltiazem, dronedarone, efavirenz, erythromycin, ethinylestradiol, fluconazole, fluoxetine, fluvoxamine, fosamprenavir, imatinib, isoniazid, lapatinib, verapamil, zafirlukast
CYP3A4 inducers	• Strong: carbamazepine, enzalutamide, fosphenytoin, mitotane, modafinil, nevirapine, oxcarbazepine, phenobarbital, phenytoin, primidone, rifabutin, rifampicin, St. John's wort • Moderate: bosentan, dexamethasone, efavirenz, etravirine, modafinil
CYP2C9 substrates	Amiodarone, amitryptiline, angiotensin II receptor antagonists, apixaban, bosentan, carvedilol, celecoxib, diclofenac, etodolac, febuxostat, fluoxetine, fluvastatin, ibuprofen, ifosfamide, ketamine, macitentan, montelukast, naproxen, nateglinide, NSAIDs, phenprocoumon, phenytoin, pitavastatin, propofol, rosiglitazone, rosuvastatin, sildenafil, sulfadiazine, sulfonylureas (gliclazide, glimepiride, glipizide, glyburide), tamoxifen, terbinafine, testosterone, torasemide, treprostinil, S-warfarin, zafirlukast, zidovudine
CYP2C9 inhibitors	• Potent: amiodarone, fluconazole, metronidazole, trimethoprim/sulfamethoxazole • Moderate: capecitabine, clopidogrel, cyclizine, delarvidine, efavirenz, fenofibrate, fluconazole, fluorouracil, fluoxetine, fluvoxamine, fluvastatin, imatinib, lovastatin, miconazole, modafinil, paroxetine, phenylbutazone, phenytoin, promethazine, sertraline, ticlopidine, valproic acid, voriconazole, zafirlukast
CYP2C9 inducers	Aprepitant, barbiturates, bosentan, rifampicin, St. John's wort
CYP2C19 substrates	Amiodarone, antidepressants (amitriptyline, bupropion, clomipramine, citalopram, desipramine, escitalopram, imipramine, moclobemide), antiepileptics (diazepam, phenobarbital, phenytoin, primidone), cilostazol, clopidogrel, clozapine, cyclophosphamide, fluoxetine, gliclazide, glyburide, indomethacin, lapatinib, macitentan, methadone, montelukast, naproxen, nelfinavir, nilutamide, olanzapine, phenytoin, progesterone, propranolol, proton pump inhibitors (lansoprazole, omeprazole), selegiline, sertraline, simeprevir, teniposide, R-warfarin
CYP2C19 inhibitors	• Potent: fluvoxamine, isoniazid, ritonavir • Moderate: cimetidine, clopidogrel, felbamate, fluconazole, fluoxetine, indomethacin, ketoconazole, moclobemide, proton pump inhibitors (lansoprazole, omeprazole, pantoprazole, rabeprazole), ticlopidine, topiramate, voriconazole
CYP2C19 inducers	Artemisinin, barbiturates, carbamazepine, norethisterone, phenytoin, prednisone, primidone, rifampicin, St. John's wort

(*Continued*)

Table 8.1.2 (*Contd.*)

CYP2D6 substrates	Amiodarone, amphetamines, antipsychotics (clozapine, chlorpromazine, haloperidol, risperidone, perphenazine, thioridazine, zuclopenthixol), atomoxetine, atypical antidepressants (duloxetine, fluoxetine, fluvoxamine, mirtazapine, paroxetine, trazodone, venlafaxine), β-blockers (carvedilol, metoprolol, nebivolol, propranolol, timolol), class I antiarrhythmics (flecainide, lidocaine, mexiletine, propafenone), dasabuvir, dexfenfluramine, dextromethorphan, donepezil, loratadine, metoclopramide, ondasetron, opioids (codeine, hydrocodone, methadone, oxycodone, tramadol), perhexiline, pravastatin, ritonavir, rucaparib, tamoxifen, tolterodine, trazodone, tricyclic antidepressants, tropisetron, vernakalant
CYP2D6 inhibitors	• Potent: amiodarone, bupropion, cimetidine, fluoxetine, paroxetine, quinidine, ritonavir, terbinafine • Moderate: buprenorphine, celecoxib, citalopram, clomipramine, cocaine, doxepin, doxorubicin, duloxetine, escitalopram, fluphenazine, fluvoxamine, halofantrine, H1-receptor antagonists (clemastine, chlorphenamine, diphenhydramine, hydroxyzine, promethazine), levomepromazine, mirabegron, metoclopramide, methadone, neuroleptics (chlorpromazine, haloperidol, moclobemide, perphenazine, risperidone, thioridazine), paroxetine, propafenone, quinidine, ritonavir, sertraline, terbinafine, ticlopidine
CYP2D6 inducers	Dexamethasone, glutethimide, haloperidol, rifampicin
P-gp substrates	Aliskiren, ambrisentan, apixaban, atorvastatin, boceprevir, bromocriptine, carbamazepine, carvedilol, cimetidine, colchicine, ciclosporin, daclatasvir, dabigatran etexilate, dasabuvir, dexamethasone, digoxin, diltiazem, dipyridamole, domperidone, doxorubicin, edoxaban, empagliflozin, erythromycin, estradiol, etoposide, everolimus, ezetimibe, fexofenadine, fosamprenavir, imatinib, indinavir, itraconazol, lapatinib, linagliptin, loperamide, losartan, lovastatin, maraviroc, methylprednisolone, methotrexate, morphine, nelfinavir, nilotinib, paclitaxel, paliperidone, phenytoin, posaconazole, pravastatin, quinidine, ranolazine, ritonavir, rivaroxaban, saquinavir, saxagliptin, simvastatin, sirolimus, sitagliptin, sofosbuvir, tacrolimus, talinolol, ticagrelor, telaprevir, tipranavir, tolvaptan, topotecan, vecuronium, verapamil, vinblastine, vincristine
P-gp inhibitors	• Potent: amiodarone, atorvastatin, carvedilol, cimetidine, ciclosporin, dronedarone, everolimus, HIV protease inhibitors, nicardipine, omeprazole, quinidine, sirolimus, tacrolimus, vardenafil, verapamil • Moderate: azithromycin, captopril, clarithromycin, conivaptan, diltiazem, dipyridamole, erythromycin, itraconazole, ketoconazole
P-gp inducers	Carbamazepine, dexamethasone, doxorubicin, nefazodone, phenobarbital, phenytoin, rifampicin, St. John's wort, tenofovir, tipranavir, trazodone, vinblastine

HIV: human immunodeficiency virus; NSAIDs: non-steroidal anti-inflammatory drugs.

Adenosine

Adenosine is an endogenous purine nucleoside, which is present in all cells of the body. It plays an important role in signal transduction pathways as cAMP, a neuromodulator, and a potent coronary vasodilator.

Indications

- IV adenosine is indicated for the rapid conversion to sinus rhythm of narrow complex paroxysmal supraventricular tachycardia (PSVT), including those associated with accessory bypass tracts [Wolff–Parkinson–White (WPW) syndrome].
- Diagnostic tool of broad or narrow complex SVT. Although adenosine does not convert atrial flutter, AF, or VT to sinus rhythm, the slowing of AV conduction helps the diagnosis of atrial activity.
- IV adenosine infusion is a coronary vasodilator for use in conjunction with radionuclide myocardial perfusion imaging in patients who cannot exercise adequately or for whom exercise is inappropriate.

Mechanism of action

Cardiac effects are mediated via the Gi-coupled A1 receptors located in the sinoatrial (SA) node and AVN. Adenosine produces membrane hyperpolarization, through activation of the adenosine-sensitive inward rectifier K^+ channel, and inhibits adenylyl cyclase, decreasing cAMP-mediated Ca^{2+} influx through L-type calcium channels. Hence, adenosine exerts a negative chronotropic effect on the SA node and a negative dromotropic effect on the AVN (prolongs PR), causing transient heart block and interrupting re-entry pathways through the AVN. Stimulation of vascular A2 receptors causes vasodilatation and reduces peripheral vascular resistance (PVR) and BP.

Pharmacodynamics

An IV bolus of adenosine results in a rapid and transient AV nodal block (10–30s when the bolus reaches the heart) and is as effective as IV verapamil or diltiazem for the rapid termination of narrow QRS complex SVT. Adenosine is preferred in infants and neonates, in patients with hypotension, or those treated with IV β-blockers. Adenosine does not convert atrial flutter, AF, or VT to normal sinus rhythm.

In *wide-complex tachycardia* of uncertain origin, adenosine can help to differentiate between VT or SVT (with aberrant conduction). In SVT, adenosine is likely to stop the tachycardia, whereas in the presence of VT, the arrhythmia most probably continues. IV adenosine may be used to unmask *latent pre-excitation* in patients with WPW syndrome. Adenosine usually produces a transient high-grade AVB; in the presence of an anterograde conduction accessory pathway, it shortens the PR interval and widens the QRS without interruption in AV conduction.

Pharmacokinetics

After IV administration, adenosine is rapidly cleared from the circulation via cellular uptake, primarily by erythrocytes and vascular endothelial cells, where it is metabolized to inosine and adenosine monophosphate. Thus, its t½ is <10s. Because adenosine does not require hepatic or renal function for its inactivation, hepatic and renal failure would not be expected to alter its effectiveness (see Table 8.1.3).

Table 8.1.3 Pharmacokinetic characteristics of antiarrhythmic drugs

Drugs	F (%)	T_{max} (h)	PPB (%)	Vd (L/kg)	Metabolism	t½ (h)	Renal excretion* (%)
Adenosine (IV)						10–30s	
Amiodarone	35–65	3–8	99	66	CYP3A4 and 2C8	58 (20–100 days	1
Bisoprolol	90	2.4	30	3.5	CYP3A4	10–12	50
Digoxin	60–75	0.5–2 PO 5–30min IV	25	3.5	No CYP450	35	80
Diltiazem	38	30–60min PO 3min IV	80	3.3	CYP3A4	3.5–5	1–4*
Disopyramide	60–85	1–2.5 (4–7**)	50–60	0.6	CYP3A4	6–9	55
Dofetilide	95	2–3	65	3.4	CYP3A4	7–13	80
Dronedarone	5	3.6	>98	20	CYP3A4	13–19	84
Esmolol (IV)	–	2–10min			Hydrolysis	9min	
Flecainide	95	2.3	40–50	5.5–10	CYP2D6	20 (12–27)	35
Ibutilide (IV)	–		40	11	No CYP3A4/2D6	2–12 (6)	7*
Lidocaine	30	45–90s	70	1.1	CYP1A2 (3A4)	1.5–2	<10
Metoprolol tartrate	40–50	1–2	12	3.5	CYP2D6	3–5 (2.8 EM; 7.5 PM)	3
Mexiletine	85–90	2–3	50–70	5–6	CYP2D6 and 1A2	7–17	10

Procainamide	85	2	15–20	2	Hydrolysis	3–5	60
Propafenone	5–30	2–3.5	95	2.5–4	CYP2D6 (3A4, 1A2)	2–10 EM; 10–32 PM	1
Propranolol	25–35	2	90	2	CYP2D6 (1A2)	2–6	1
Quinidine	70–80	6	80–90	2.7	CYP3A4	6–8	20
Sotalol	90–100	2.5–4	0	1.5–2.5	Not metabolized	12 (7–18)	85
Verapamil	20–35	1.2 PO	90	5	CYP3A4	2–7.5	5
Vernakalant (IV)		1–5min IV	40–55	2.3	CYP2D6	3.1 (1.7–5.4)	14

EM/PM, extensive/poor metabolizers; F, oral bioavailability; h, hours; IV, intravenous; min, minutes; PO, oral administration; PPB, protein plasma binding; s, seconds; t½, drug half-life; T_{max}, time to peak plasma levels; Vd, volume of distribution.

* Renal excretion without biotransformation.

** Slow-release formulation.

Practical points

1. *Doses*
   - First dose: 3mg (0.05–0.25mg/kg) as a rapid IV bolus over 2s, injected as proximal to or as close to the heart as possible), followed by a rapid saline flush. If after 1–2min, the arrhythmia persists, give a 6-mg bolus; if this dose does not result in arrhythmia suppression within 1–2min, a 12-mg bolus can be administered.
   - In children: first bolus of 0.1mg/kg (maximum dose of 6mg). Increments of 0.1mg/kg, as needed, to achieve termination of SVT (maximum dose of 12mg).
   - The initial dose should be reduced to ≤3mg in patients taking verapamil, diltiazem, β-blockers, or dipyridamole, or in elderly people at risk of sick sinus syndrome.
2. *Side effects*
   - Common: facial flushing, shortness of breath/dyspnoea, flushing, bradycardia, sinus pause, AVB, atrial extrasystoles, skipped beats, ventricular excitability disorders, thoracic constriction/oppression, apprehension, degeneration of atrial flutter or PSVT to AF. Atrial and ventricular premature beats may occur and can reinitiate PSVT or AF.
   - Uncommon: headache, light-headedness, apprehension, nausea, chest pressure, and/or burning sensation. In patients with asthma or COPD, adenosine may precipitate bronchospasm that may last >30min.
3. *Interactions*
   - Dipyridamole inhibits the uptake of adenosine and may potentiate its effects; thus, the dose of adenosine should be reduced.
   - The effects of adenosine are antagonized by methylxanthines (theophylline and aminophylline). Higher doses are required when these drugs are co-administered.
   - Digoxin and verapamil, when associated with adenosine, produce synergistic depressing effects on the SA and AV nodes.
   - Carbamazepine may increase the degree of heart block produced by adenosine.
4. *Cautions/notes*
   - Due to the possibility of transient cardiac arrhythmias arising during conversion of SVT to normal sinus rhythm, adenosine should only be used in a hospital setting and cardiorespiratory resuscitation equipment should be available.
   - Adenosine shortens atrial and ventricular refractoriness and may cause transient new arrhythmias at the time of cardioversion. Continuous ECG monitoring during adenosine administration may help to distinguish drug failure to terminate the arrhythmia from successful termination with immediate arrhythmia reinitiating.
   - Adenosine should be used with caution in patients with left main coronary stenosis, uncorrected hypovolaemia, stenotic VHD, left-to-right shunt, pericarditis or pericardial effusion, autonomic dysfunction, or stenotic carotid artery disease with cerebrovascular insufficiency.
   - Patients who develop high-level AVB at a particular dose should not be given further dosage increments.

- Reduced doses of adenosine may be required in the presence of dipyridamole.
- In the presence of atrial flutter or AF, transient slowing of ventricular response may occur, immediately following adenosine administration; when an accessory bypass tract is present, adenosine may develop increased conduction down the anomalous pathway.
- In atrial flutter, adenosine may induce 1:1 conduction and rapid ventricular rate.
- Severe bradycardia would favour the occurrence of TdP, especially in patients with prolonged QT intervals. Adenosine should be used with caution in patients with a prolonged QT interval, whether this is congenital or acquired.
- In patients with asthma or COPD, adenosine may precipitate or aggravate bronchospasm.
- In patients with VT, adenosine produces minimal effects, while verapamil or diltiazem, through myocardial depression and peripheral vasodilatation, can be fatal.
- Adenosine may trigger convulsions in patients who are susceptible to convulsions.

5. *Pregnancy and lactation*
   - Because of the absence of clinical data, adenosine should be used only when absolutely necessary (Pregnancy category C).
6. *Contraindications*
   - Known hypersensitivity to adenosine or to any of the excipients.
   - Sick sinus syndrome, second- or third-degree AVB (except in patients with a functional artificial pacemaker).
   - LQTS.
   - Bronchospasm, asthma.
   - Severe hypotension.
   - UA not successfully stabilized with medical therapy.
   - Decompensated HF.
   - Concomitant use of dipyridamole.

Adrenaline

Catecholamine neurotransmitter of the sympathetic nervous system.

Indications

- Cardiopulmonary resuscitation in adults and children aged >12 years. It should be restricted to patients with persistent hypotension despite adequate cardiac filling pressures and the use of other vasoactive agents, according to resuscitation protocols.
- Emergency treatment of anaphylaxis or acute angioneurotic oedema with airways obstruction, or acute allergic reactions.

Mechanism of action

Adrenaline acts on both α- and β-adrenergic receptors, being more selective for β-receptors (β2 > β1 > α1 = α2).

Pharmacodynamics

A low physiologic infusion rate (<0.01mcg/kg/min) of adrenaline increases the stroke volume and SBP and decreases the PVR and DBP. At >0.2mcg/kg/min, adrenaline stimulates β1-adrenoceptors increasing cardiac contractility, β2-adrenoceptors reducing cardiac afterload, and α-adrenoceptors restoring BP in hypotensive states. It is used when combined inotropic–chronotropic stimulation is urgently needed, as in cardiac arrest or an acutely failing heart. β2-adrenoceptor stimulation produces bronchial smooth muscle relaxation and alleviates bronchospasm, wheezing, and dyspnoea that may occur during anaphylaxis. Adrenaline also produces hyperglycaemia and hypokalaemia. Catecholamine toxicity leads to myocyte necrosis and apoptosis, so that sympathomimetics must be used only as short-term treatment of acute HF. It was suggested that adrenaline would present fewer side effects and lower mortality than dopamine in the treatment of shock.

Pharmacokinetics

When administered IV, adrenaline has a rapid onset and a short duration of action (plasma t½ 2–3min), because it is rapidly inactivated, mostly in the GI mucosa, liver, and neuronal tissues and in the liver by COMT and MAO. When given by SC or intramuscular (IM) injection, local vasoconstriction may delay absorption, so that its effects may last longer than its t½ suggests. Adrenaline binds to plasma proteins (50%) and crosses the placenta. Only 1% of the dose can be recovered unchanged.

Practical points

1. *Doses*
   - HF: 1mg IV bolus; then 0.05–0.5mcg/kg/min.
   - Cardiopulmonary resucitation: 0.5mg SC or IM (0.5mL of 1:1000), or 0.5–1mg into central veins, or 0.1–0.2mg intra-cardiac.
   - Severe allergic reactions: 5–10mcg/kg; higher doses may be necessary.

2. *Side effects*
   - CV: palpitations, tachyarrhythmias, ECG changes, hypertension, pallor, and coldness of extremities. Angina may occur in patients with CAD. Arrhythmias, including fatal VF, can occur, particularly in patients with underlying organic heart disease or receiving drugs that sensitize the heart to arrhythmias and can potentially increase myocardial ischaemia. Rapid increases in BP can produce cerebral haemorrhage, particularly in elderly patients with CV disease, and pulmonary oedema. β2-stimulation also causes hypokalaemia, with an enhanced risk of arrhythmias.
   - Neurological: dizziness, anxiety, confusion, irritability, insomnia, restlessness, tremor, weakness, headache, dizziness, tremors.
   - Other: dyspnoea, sweating, weakness, difficulty in micturition, urinary retention.
3. *Drug interactions*
   - Adrenaline should be administered cautiously in patients taking other sympathomimetic agents or oxytocin, because of possible additive effects.
   - The vasoconstricting and hypertensive effects of adrenaline are antagonized by α-adrenergic-blocking drugs (phentolamine, ergot alkaloids).
   - Severe hypertension and reflex bradycardia may occur with non-selective β-blocking drugs (propranolol) due to α-mediated vasoconstriction.
   - β-blockers, especially non-cardioselective agents, can antagonize the cardiac and bronchodilator effects of adrenaline.
   - Patients treated with digitalis, diuretics, quinidine, and other antiarrhythmics should be monitored for the development of cardiac arrhythmias.
   - Co-administration of adrenaline with some general anaesthetics (i.e. halothane) may result in serious ventricular arrhythmias, including VT/VF.
   - The effects of adrenaline (hypertension and cardiac arrhythmias) can be potentiated by tricyclic antidepressants (imipramine inhibits the reuptake of adrenaline in nerve terminals), MAOIs, levothyroxine, and certain antihistamines (diphenhydramine, tripelennamine, dexchlorpheniramine).
   - Phenothiazines block α-adrenergic receptors. Thus, adrenaline should not be used to counteract circulatory collapse or hypotension caused by these drugs.
   - Adrenaline increases BP and may antagonize the effects of antihypertensive drugs.
   - The hypokalaemia produced by adrenaline can be potentiated by corticosteroids, potassium-depleting diuretics, aminophylline, and theophylline.
   - Adrenaline-induced hyperglycaemia may lead to loss of blood sugar control in diabetic patients treated with insulin or oral hypoglycaemic agents.
   - Adrenaline increases the risk of cardiac adverse effects of levodopa.
   - Entacapone may potentiate the arrhythmogenic effects of adrenaline.

4. *Cautions*
    - IV adrenaline should only be used by those experienced in the use and titration of vasopressors (e.g. anaesthetists, emergency physicians, intensive care doctors).
    - Adrenaline can cause sinus tachycardia and may induce myocardial ischaemia and arrhythmias; thus, ECG monitoring is required.
    - Adverse effects increase in patients with heart disease, hypertension, or hyperthyroidism.
    - In patients with Parkinson's disease, adrenaline may produce psychomotor agitation or a temporary worsening of symptoms.
    - Continuous β1-adrenergic stimulation may lead to decreased receptor expression and a reduced inotropic response.
5. *Pregnancy and lactation*
    - Adrenaline crosses the placenta and produces teratogenicity in animal models (Pregnancy category C) and may cause anoxia to the fetus and fetal palpitations and tachycardia. Adrenaline inhibits spontaneous or oxytocin-induced contractions of the pregnant human uterus and may delay the second stage of labour. There are no data on the excretion of adrenaline into human milk.
6. *Contraindications*

There are not absolute contraindications in life-threatening emergency situations.

- Hypersensitivity to adrenaline, sodium metabisulfite, or other excipients.
- Adrenaline should not be used in fingers, toes, ears, nose, or genitalia, owing to the risk of ischaemic tissue necrosis.
- Presence of shock (other than anaphylactic shock), VF, organic heart disease, cardiac dilatation, organic brain disease, or atherosclerosis.
- Narrow-angle glaucoma.
- During the second stage of labour.
- Avoid if the solution is discoloured.

Alirocumab

Proprotein convertase subtilisin/kexin type 9 (PCSK9) inhibitor.

Indications

- Adults with primary hypercholesterolaemia (heterozygous familial and non-familial) or mixed dyslipidaemia, as an adjunct to diet and maximally tolerated statin therapy: (1) in combination with a statin or a statin with other lipid-lowering therapies in patients unable to reach LDL-C goals with the maximum tolerated dose of a statin, or (2) alone or in combination with other lipid-lowering therapies in patients who are statin-intolerant or for whom a statin is contraindicated.

Mechanism of action

Alirocumab is a fully human IgG1 monoclonal antibody that binds with high affinity and specificity to PCSK9 near the catalytic domain. PCSK9 is a serine protease that binds to LDL-Rs on the surface of hepatocytes to promote LDL-R degradation within the liver. The decrease in LDL-R levels results in higher blood levels of LDL-C. By inhibiting the binding of PCSK9 to LDL-Rs, alirocumab increases the number of LDL-Rs available on the liver cell surface, prevents PCSK9-mediated LDL-R degradation, and lowers plasma LDL-C levels. Conversely, patients with familial hypercholesterolaemia and gain-of-function mutations in the *PCSK9* gene have increased LDL-C levels and a clinical diagnosis of familial hypercholesterolaema.

Pharmacodynamics

Following a single SC administration, alirocumab reduces free PCSK9 in a concentration-dependent manner, and maximal suppression of free PCSK9 occurs within 4–8h. Free PCSK9 concentrations return to baseline when alirocumab concentrations decrease below the limit of quantitation. Alirocumab reduces baseline LDL-C plasma levels by 55–72%, even in patients treated with statins. The LDL-R also binds TG-rich VLDL remnant lipoproteins and intermediate-density lipoprotein (IDL). Thus, alirocumab reduces these remnant lipoproteins, apolipoprotein B (Apo B), lipoprotein (a), non-HDL-C, and TGs. Alirocumab reduces the risk of recurrent ischaemic cardiovascular events in patients who had a previous acute coronary syndrome and who were receiving high-intensity statin therapy.

Pharmacokinetics

After SC administration into the abdomen, upper arm, or thigh, alirocumab reaches peak plasma levels within 3–7 days. The drug is distributed primarily in the circulatory system. At low concentrations, alirocumab is eliminated through saturable binding to its target (PCSK9); at higher concentrations, the elimination of alirocumab is largely through a non-saturable proteolytic pathway to small peptides and individual amino acids. Its t½ is reduced to 12 days when co-administered with a statin. However, this difference does not impact dosing recommendations (see Table 8.1.4).

The safety and efficacy of alirocumab in children and adolescents <18 years of age have not been established.

Table 8.1.4 Pharmacokinetic properties of lipid-modifying drugs

Drugs	F (%)	T_{max} (h)	PPB (%)	Vd (L/kg)	Metabolism	t½ (h)	Renal excretion** (%)
Statins							
Atorvastatin	12	1–2.5	>98	5.4	CYP3A4	14	<2
Fluvastatin	25	0.5–1.5	98	0.35	CYP2C9 (3A4, 2D6)	3	<2
Lovastatin	<5	2–3	95		CYP3A4	2–3	30
Pitavastatin	40–50	1	99	2.11	CYP2C9 (2C8)	12	15
Pravastatin	17	1–1.5	50	0.5	Hydroxylation, sulfoconjugation	1.5–3	20
Rosuvastatin	20	3–5	90	1.9	CYP2C9/19 (minor)	19 (13–20)	5
Simvastatin	<5	2–4	>95		CYP3A4	2	13
Fibrates							
Bezofibrate*	70 (100[a])	1–2	95	0.24	Glucuronoconjugation	1–2	95
Fenofibrate*	60	2–3	99	0.42	Glucuronoconjugation	20–23	65
Gemfibrozil	100	1–2	97	0.15	Hydroxylation, carboxylation	1.5	70
Cholesterol absorption inhibitors							
Ezetimibe	20–30	1.2	>90		Glucuronoconjugation	22	11
PCSK9 inhibitors							
Alirocumab (SC)	85	3–7 days	–	0.04–0.05	Endo-/exonucleases	17–20 days	–
Evolocumab (SC)	72	3–4 days	–	0.04	Endo-/exonucleases	11–17 days	–

CYP, cytochrome P450; F, oral bioavailability; h, hour; PPB, protein plasma binding; SC, subcutaneous; t½, drug half-life; T_{max}, time to peak plasma levels; Vd, volume of distribution.

* Prodrug.

** Renal excretion without biotransformation.

Practical points

1. *Doses*
   - Starting dose: 75mg SC once every 2 weeks, that can be increased to 150mg SC every 2 weeks. Patients requiring larger LDL-C reduction (>60%) may be started on 150mg SC every 2 weeks, or 300mg SC once monthly. No dose adjustment is needed for elderly patients or for patients with mild or moderate hepatic or renal impairment.
2. *Side effects*
   - Local injection site reactions (redness, pain, itching, swelling, pain/tenderness), pruritus, myalgia, muscle spasms, and upper respiratory tract signs or symptoms (sore throat, runny nose, sneezing). Rare, and sometimes serious, allergic reactions, such as hypersensitivity, nummular eczema, urticaria, and hypersensitivity vasculitis, have been reported. Antidrug antibodies appear in up to 4.8% of patients.
3. *Drug interactions*
   - Since alirocumab is a biological medicinal product, no pharmacokinetic effects on other medicinal products and no effect on cytochrome P450 enzymes are anticipated.
   - Statins and other lipid-modifying agents increase the production of PCSK9, increase the clearance, and reduces systemic exposure of alirocumab. However, reduction in LDL-C is maintained during the dosing interval when alirocumab is administered every 2 weeks.
4. *Cautions*
   - Alirocumab should not be injected into areas of active skin disease or injury (i.e. sunburn, skin rashes, inflammation, or skin infections).
   - Avoid co-administration of alirocumab with other injectable medicinal products at the same injection site.
   - No data are available in children and adolescents <18 years of age.
   - Alirocumab has not been tested in patients with severe hepatic or renal impairment.
5. *Pregnancy and lactation*
   - No available data on use in pregnant women, although other IgG antibodies cross the placenta and are present in human milk. US FDA Pregnancy category not assigned.
6. *Contraindications*
   - Hypersensitivity reaction to alirocumab or to any of the excipients.

Aliskiren

A direct renin inhibitor.

CV indications

- Treatment of essential hypertension in adults.

Mechanism of action

Renin catalyses the first rate-limiting step of the RAAS. Both renin and its precursor (prorenin) bind to the (pro)renin receptor and stimulate signalling pathways that may have adverse CV and renal effects independently from angiotensin II synthesis. Aliskiren binds to the active site of renin and inhibits the conversion of angiotensinogen to angiotensin I by renin and the synthesis of angiotensin II without affecting kinin metabolism.

Pharmacodynamics

Aliskiren reduces BP, as do other antihypertensives, but in contrast to other RAAS inhibitors, it fails to reduce the incidence of major CV events, total mortality, cardiac death, MI, or stroke.

Pharmacokinetics

Aliskiren is rapidly absorbed following oral administration, but presents low oral bioavailability (2–3%), reaching peak plasma levels within 1–3h. High-fat meals decreases the AUC and C_{max} to 71% and 85%, respectively. It is approximately 50% protein-bound and has a volume of distribution (Vd) of 1.9L/kg. It is metabolized in the liver via CYP3A4 and eliminated in faeces largely unchanged (78% corresponding to non-absorbed drug), and 0.6% is recovered in the urine. The t½ is 30–40h, and steady-state levels are reached in 5–7 days. It appears to be retained in the kidney, which may explain why its antihypertensive effects last for days or weeks after drug withdrawal.

Practical points

1. *Doses*
   - 150–300mg od. No dose adjustment is required for patients with mild to moderate renal impairment or mild or severe hepatic impairment, but aliskiren is not recommended in those with severe renal impairment (GFR <30mL/min/1.73m^2).
2. *Common side effects*
   - Dizziness, diarrhoea, arthralgia, hyperkalaemia (particularly when used with ACEIs in diabetic patients), hypotension (particularly in volume-depleted patients), rash. Small decreases in haemoglobin and haematocrit. Cases of angio-oedema have been reported.
3. *Interactions*
   - Avoid the concomitant use of aliskiren with potent P-gp inhibitors (e.g. ketoconazole, clarithromycin, erythromycin, amiodarone, atorvastatin, quinidine).
   - Aliskiren reduces furosemide serum concentrations.
   - NSAIDs may reduce the effect of aliskiren and increase the risk of renal impairment.

- Concomitant use with agents that raise serum K^+ levels increases the risk of hyperkalaemia. Monitor serum K^+ levels.
- Aliskiren shows no clinically relevant interactions with warfarin, lovastatin, atenolol, celecoxib, digoxin, or cimetidine.

4. *Cautions/notes*
   - Routine monitoring of urea and electrolytes is recommended in patients with diabetes, kidney disease, or HF.
   - Concomitant use of aliskiren with an ACEI or an ARB is contraindicated in patients with diabetes mellitus or GFR of <60mL/min/1.73m^2 because of the increased risk of hypotension, renal dysfunction, and hyperkalaemia.
   - Aliskiren has not been used in hypertensive patients with GFR of <30mL/min, a history of dialysis, nephrotic syndrome, or renovascular disease.
   - With caution in patients with NYHA class III–IV HF.
5. *Pregnancy and lactation*
   - RAAS inhibitors are associated with fetal malformations and neonatal death (Pregnancy category D). Aliskiren is not recommended in pregnancy and breastfeeding.
6. *Contraindications*
   - Second and third trimesters of pregnancy.
   - History of angio-oedema with aliskiren, hyperkalaemia.
   - Bilateral renal stenosis, severely impaired renal function.

Allopurinol

Inhibitor of xanthine oxidase.

CV indications

- Patients with stable CAD.
- Treatment of patients with signs and symptoms of primary or secondary gout.
- Prophylaxis and treatment of urate/uric acid formation in conditions where urate/uric acid deposition has already occurred.
- Treatment of recurrent mixed calcium oxalate renal stones in the presence of hyperuricosuria.

Mechanism of action

Allopurinol and its main metabolite oxypurinol lower the level of uric acid in plasma and urine by inhibition of xanthine oxidase, the enzyme catalysing the oxidation of hypoxanthine to xanthine and xanthine to uric acid.

Pharmacodynamics

In stable CAD patients, allopurinol reduces vascular oxidative stress and prolongs the time to ST-segment depression and chest pain. In patients with HF, it conserves cardiac ATP levels.

Pharmacokinetics

Orally, allopurinol is rapidly absorbed (bioavailability 67–90%) and reaches C_{max} in 1.5h. Allopurinol is negligibly bound by plasma proteins and presents a Vd of 1.6L/kg, which suggests a relatively extensive uptake by tissues. It is metabolized into oxypurinol (C_{max} in 3–5h) and excreted in the faeces (approximately 20%) and urine (<10% as unchanged drug; oxypurinol is eliminated unchanged in the urine). The elimination t½ is 1–2h (oxypurinol 18–30h). Clearance of allopurinol and oxypurinol is greatly reduced in patients with impaired renal function.

Practical points

1. *Doses*
   - Allopurinol should be introduced at low dosage (100mg/day) to reduce the risk of adverse reactions. Maintenance dose 600mg/day.
2. *Side effects*
   - Gastric discomfort and allergic reactions (mainly rashes with eosinophilia). Potentially fatal skin reactions [Stevens–Johnson syndrome (SJS) and toxic epidermal necrolysis (TEN)] have been reported. The HLA-B*5801 allele has been identified as a genetic risk factor for allopurinol-associated SJS/TEN.
3. *Interactions*
   - Reduce the dose of 6-mercaptopurine and azathioprine when given with allopurinol, because inhibition of xanthine oxidase will prolong their activity.
   - Uricosuric drugs or large doses of salicylate can accelerate the excretion of oxypurinol.
   - Allopurinol can prolong the hypoglycaemic activity of chlorpropamide.

- Allopurinol may increase the plasma levels and toxicity of ciclosporin, adenine arabinoside, cyclophosphamide, and mercaptopurine. Allopurinol may enhance bone marrow depression produced by cyclophosphamide, doxorubicin, bleomycin, procarbazine, and chlormethine. Monitor the clinical response.
- Reduce the dose of didanosine when co-administered with allopurinol; patients should be closely monitored.
- Intake of antacids and allopurinol should be separated by 3h.
- Co-administration of allopurinol and ACEIs may increase the risk of hypersensitivity, especially if there is pre-existing renal failure.
- Allopurinol may increase the effects of warfarin by inhibiting its metabolism. Patients receiving anticoagulants must be carefully monitored.
- Furosemide increases serum urate and plasma oxypurinol levels.

4. *Cautions/notes*
   - Allopurinol should be withdrawn immediately when a skin rash or other evidence of serious sensitivity reactions appear (i.e. SJS, TEN). The frequency of skin rash increases in patients receiving ampicillin or amoxicillin concurrently with allopurinol.
   - Monitor theophylline levels in patients starting or increasing allopurinol therapy.
5. *Pregnancy and lactation*
   - There are no data in pregnant women and nursing mothers (Pregnancy category C). Allopurinol and oxypurinol are excreted into human breast milk.
6. *Contraindications*
   - Known hypersensitivity to the drug

Alprostadil

Alprostadil is a synthetic form of prostaglandin E1 (PGE1).

CV indications

- Palliative therapy to temporarily maintain the patency of the ductus arteriosus until corrective or palliative surgery can be performed in neonates who have congenital heart defects and who depend upon the patent ductus for survival.

Mechanism of action

Alprostadil (PGE1) produces vasodilatation, inhibits platelet aggregation, and stimulates intestinal and uterine smooth muscle.

Pharmacodynamics

Smooth muscle of the ductus arteriosus is especially sensitive to alprostadil. It reopens the closing ductus in infants with congenital defects which restricted the pulmonary or systemic blood flow and who depended on a patent ductus arteriosus for adequate blood oxygenation and lower body perfusion. Congenital heart defects include pulmonary or tricuspid atresia, pulmonary stenosis, tetralogy of Fallot, interruption of the aortic arch, coarctation of the aorta, or transposition of the great vessels with or without other defects. Infants with restricted pulmonary blood flow respond to alprostadil infusion with at least a 10-torr increase in blood pO_2; the best responders are those with low pre-treatment blood pO_2 and who are ≤4 days old. In infants with restricted systemic blood flow, alprostadil often increases pH in those having acidosis and systemic BP, and decreases the ratio of PAP to aortic pressure.

Pharmacokinetics

Following IV administration, the drug binds to plasma proteins (81%) and is very rapidly distributed and metabolized (almost 80% of circulating alprostadil may be metabolized in one pass through the lungs), and the metabolites are excreted renally. The pulmonary extraction ratio of PGE1 (i.e. the fractional efficiency of removal of the drug from pulmonary plasma flow on a single pass) is independent of the dose but dependent on the CO and respiratory status. The t½ of PGE1 is <1min, so that it must be infused continuously.

Practical points

1. *Doses*
   - The starting dose is 0.05–0.1mcg/kg/min. The dose may be titrated to 0.4mcg/kg/min in some patients to maintain an open ductus, monitoring for clinical signs of adequate perfusion (arterial blood pH and PO_2, BP, pulse oximetry, urine output, and echocardiography). In most infants, the ductus will reopen within 30min to 2h after starting PGE1. Once the ductus has opened, the dose can usually be reduced to 0.002–0.005mcg/kg/min.

2. *Side effects*
   - The commonest are apnoea, fever, bradycardia, and/or hypotension. Apnoea is most likely to occur within the first hour of therapy and in infants weighing <2kg and is not observed with doses of <0.01mcg/kg/min.
   - Cortical proliferation appears to involve hyperostosis in the diaphyses of long tubular bones; changes disappear within 6–12 weeks after stopping PGE1.
   - Other: flushing, seizures, tachycardia, diarrhoea, gastric outlet obstruction secondary to antral hyperplasia, anaemia, bleeding, thrombocytopenia.
3. *Interactions*
   - The risk of hypotension increases if co-administered with antihypertensives and vasodilators.
   - No drug interactions have been reported between alprostadil and the therapy standard in neonates with restricted pulmonary or systemic blood flow.
4. *Cautions/notes*
   - Alprostadil should be administered only by well-trained healthcare professionals and in facilities with immediate access to paediatric intensive care. In all neonates, BP, blood oxygenation, and pH should be monitored.
   - Alprostadil inhibits platelet aggregation; caution in neonates at risk of bleeding.
   - Alprostadil may result in gastric outlet obstruction secondary to antral hyperplasia.
   - Alprostadil should not be used in neonates with respiratory distress syndrome.
5. *Pregnancy and lactation*
   - There are no data in pregnant women and nursing mothers (Pregnancy category C), but it is excreted in breast milk.
6. *Contraindications*
   - Hypersensitivity to alprostadil or other prostaglandins.

Alteplase

A single-chain tissue plasminogen activator (tPA) produced by recombinant DNA technology (rt-PA, 70kDa, 527 amino acids) from a human melanoma cell line (see ➔ Thrombolytic agents, pp. 774–6).

CV indications

- Treatment of acute MI.
- Treatment of acute ischaemic stroke.
- Acute PE accompanied by haemodynamic instability.

Mechanism of action

tPA is a naturally occurring enzyme that binds to fibrin in the thrombus and converts the entrapped plasminogen to plasmin. Alteplase is more active on fibrin-bound plasminogen than on plasma plasminogen (i.e. clot-selective). This initiates local fibrinolysis with limited systemic proteolysis. rtPA is not antigenic and is indicated in patients allergic to streptokinase or likely to have antibodies to streptokinase.

Pharmacodynamics

(See ➔ Thrombolytic agents, pp. 774–6).

Pharmacokinetics

Alteplase is rapidly cleared from plasma, with an initial t½ of 4–8min. So it should be given as an IV bolus, followed by an infusion. The very short t½ mandates co-therapy with IV heparin to avoid reocclusion. The initial Vd is 0.1L/kg. The drug is eliminated primarily by the liver, and <2% is excreted in the urine.

Practical points

1. *Doses*
   - Acute MI: two regimens of alteplase are used.
     —Accelerated infusion for patients in whom treatment can be started within 6h after symptom onset; 15mg as an IV bolus, followed by 50mg infused over the next 30min, and then 35mg over 60min, until the maximal dose of 100mg.
     —3-h infusion in patients in whom treatment can be started between 6 and 12h after symptom onset: 10mg as an IV bolus; 50mg as an infusion over the first hour, followed by infusions of 10mg over 30min, until the maximal dose of 100mg over 3h.
     —Lower doses in elderly people and in patients with a body weight of <65kg.
   - *Acute ischaemic stroke*: 0.9mg/kg infused over 60min, with 10% of the total dose administered as an initial IV bolus over 1min. Total dosage not to exceed 90mg.
   - *Acute PE*: 100mg administered by IV infusion over 2h.
2. *Common side effects* (see ➔ Thrombolytic agents, pp. 774–6)
   - Bleeding: GI, genitourinary, ecchymosis, retroperitoneal, epistaxis, and gingival; haemorrhagic stroke (0.7%).
   - Allergic reactions: <1%

3. *Interactions* (see ➲ Thrombolytic agents, pp. 774–6)
   - Glyceryl trinitrate appears to impair the thrombolytic effects of tPA.
   - Diltiazem, combined with tPA, appears to increase the risk of cerebral haemorrhage.
4. *Cautions and contraindications* (see ➲ Thrombolytic agents, pp. 774–6)
   - Hypersensitivity to alteplase or any component of the formulation. Gentamicin sensitivity because gentamicin is used in the preparation of alteplase.

Ambrisentan

Endothelin ET_A receptor antagonist.

CV indications

- Treatment of PAH in adult patients with WHO functional classes II–III, including use in combination treatment. Efficacy has been shown in idiopathic PAH (IPAH) and in PAH associated with connective tissue disease.
- In combination with tadalafil to reduce the risks of disease progression and hospitalization for worsening PAH and to improve exercise ability.

Pharmacodynamics

Ambrisentan improves haemodynamics (increases cardiac index and reduces PAP and pulmonary vascular resistance) and exercise capacity, and delays clinical worsening.

Pharmacokinetics

Oral absorption is rapid, but bioavailability uncertain, reaching peak plasma levels at approximately 1.5–2h. Food does not affect its bioavailability. Ambrisentan is highly bound to plasma proteins (99%), is metabolized by CYP3A4 (less by 3A5 and 2C19) and uridine 5′-diphosphate glucuronosyltransferases (UGTs), and is excreted in the urine (22%; 3% unchanged) and faeces. The terminal t½ is 9–15h.

Practical points

1. *Doses*
   - 5mg od initially; increase to 10mg PO od if 5mg/day tolerated; do not chew, crush, or split the tablet. When used in combination with tadalafil, ambrisentan should be titrated to 10mg od. No dose adjustment in renal impairment; it has not been studied in individuals with hepatic impairment.
2. *Side effects*
   - Headache, peripheral oedema, anaemia (reduction in haemoglobin concentrations and haematocrit), dizziness, hypotension, flushing, epistaxis, dyspnoea, upper respiratory tract congestion, sinusitis, nasopharyngitis, rhinitis, abdominal pain, constipation, palpitations, and HF. Liver aminotransferase elevations >3 times the upper limit of normal (ULN) (0.8–2.8%). Lower-extremity oedema is more frequent (29%) and severe in patients >65 years of age.
3. *Cautions and contraindications*
   - Similar to bosentan.
4. *Pregnancy and lactation*
   - Ambrisentan may produce serious birth defects if used by pregnant women, and its use is contraindicated (Pregnancy category X). Pregnancy testing should be performed before the initiation of treatment, monthly while on treatment, and for 1 month after stopping treatment.
5. *Contraindications*
   - Similar to bosentan.

Amiloride

Potassium-sparing diuretic.

Indications

- Diuretic used alone or as an adjunct to other diuretics in the treatment of oedema and hypertension.
- Bartter syndrome.

Mechanism of action

Amiloride inhibits Na^+ reabsorption after binding to renal epithelial Na^+ channels (ENaCs) located in the luminal membrane of the principal cells of the distal tubule and collecting duct, perhaps by competing with Na^+ for negative charges within the channel pore. The reduction in Na^+ reabsorption hyperpolarizes the apical membrane of the tubule and reduces the electrochemical gradient, K^+ secretion from the principal cells, and H^+ secretion via the H^+-ATPAse from the intercalated cells. The reduction in K^+ secretion decreases H^+ secretion via K^+/H^+ ATPase, which can cause metabolic acidosis. The net effect is an increase in Na^+ excretion and a decrease in K^+ and H^+ excretion. However, unlike spironolactone, amiloride is effective, regardless of the level of circulating aldosterone.

Pharmacodynamics

In monotherapy, amiloride produces mild (compared with thiazide diuretics) natriuretic effects and is rarely used in monotherapy to treat oedema or hypertension. Its natriuretic effect increases in patients with hyperaldosteronism (e.g. with cirrhosis and ascites or HF). Thus, amiloride is primarily used in combination with thiazide or loop diuretics, either to prevent the urinary loss of K^+ and magnesium ions (Mg^{2+}) or to increase net diuresis in patients with low-renin hypertension, resistant hypertension, or refractory oedema due to secondary hyperaldosteronism.

Amiloride is effective in patients with polyuria and polydipsia due to lithium-induced nephrogenic diabetes insipidus. Amiloride is also indicated in patients with Liddle syndrome and those with some ENaC mutations.

Pharmacokinetics

(See Table 8.1.5.)

Practical points

1. *Doses*
    - Initially 5mg bd or 10mg od (maximum dose 20mg daily). If combined with an ACEI/ARB, the doses will be reduced to 2.5 and 10–20mg, respectively. Cirrhosis with ascites: 5mg daily. The safety of amiloride in children under 18 years of age has not been established.
2. *Side effects*
    - Hyperkalaemia, hyponatraemia, polyuria, dehydration, nausea, vomiting, abdominal pain, anorexia, headache, fatigue, dizziness, skin rash.

Table 8.1.5 Pharmacokinetic properties of diuretics

Drugs	F (%)	T_{max} (h)	PPB (%)	Vd (L/kg)	Metabolism	t½ (h)	Renal excretion* (%)
Loop diuretics							
Bumetanide	80–95	1–2 (30–45min IV)	97	0.15–0.28	Oxidation	1–3.5	36–69
Furosemide	45–65	1–2	95	0.2	Glucuronidation	0.5—2	80
Torasemide	90	1–2 (15–30min IV)	99	0.09—0.3	CYP2C8	3–6	20
Potassium-sparing diuretics							
Amiloride	15–25	6–10	–	5–7	Not metabolized	6–9	50
Eplerenone	70	1.5–2	50	0.7 (0.6–1.3)	CYP3A4	3–6	5
Spironolactone	80–90	48–72h	90	10	Sulfur-containing metabolities	1.4 (metabolites 13–24)	<1
Triamterene	50	2–3	60–70	2.2–3.7	Sulfoconjugation	2–4.5	50
Thiazide-like diuretics							
Bendroflumethiazide	95	2	96	1–1.5	Minor metabolism	3–4	30
Chlortalidone	65	3–6	98**	0.14	Minor metabolism	47 (40–60)	65
Hydrochlorothiazide	60	1–3	68	0.83	Minor metabolism	6–14	>95
Indapamide	95	1–4	79		CYP3A4	14–24	7
Metolazone	65	2–4	96	1–1.5	Minor metabolism	14 (8–24)	80
Xipamide	75–95	1	98	0.14	Glucuronidation	5–8	50

F, oral bioavailability; h, hours; IV, intravenous; min, minute; PPB, protein plasma binding; t½, drug half-life; T_{max}, time to peak plasma levels; Vd, volume of distribution.

* Renal excretion without biotransformation.

** Binding to erythrocytes.

3. *Drug interactions*
   - Amiloride increases the risk of hypotension when combined with antihypertensive drugs, nitrates, hydralazine, alprostadil, general anaesthetics, antidepressants (tricyclics, MAOIs), phenothiazines, and alcohol.
   - Additive diuretic effects when administered with a thiazide or loop diuretic, but amiloride decreases the urinary excretion of K^+ and Mg^{2+}.
   - Increased risk of hyperkalaemia when co-administered with RAAS inhibitors, potassium supplements, or ciclosporin. These combinations should be used with caution, with monitoring of serum K^+ levels.
   - Amiloride increases the risk of nephrotoxicity induced by NSAIDs. Indometacin and possibly other NSAIDs increase the risk of hyperkalaemia with potassium-sparing diuretics. Indometacin and ketorolac antagonize the diuretic effect.
   - The antiarrhythmic activity of quinidine can be opposed by amiloride.
   - Carbamazepine and chlorpropamide increase the risk of hyponatraemia.
   - Amiloride may reduce the renal clearance of lithium and increases the risk of lithium toxicity. Monitor serum lithium levels, and adjust the lithium dosage.
   - Oral contraceptives and oestrogens may antagonize the diuretic effect. Increased risk of hyperkalaemia with trilostane.
   - Muscle relaxants: enhanced hypotensive effect with baclofen and tizanidine.
   - Amiloride antagonizes the ulcer-healing effect of carbenoxolone.
   - Amiloride blocks the tubular secretion of creatinine, leading to falsely high measurements of creatinine clearance (CrCl).
4. *Cautions*
   - To reduce the risk of hyperkalaemia, patients should restrict dietary potassium and reduce or avoid potassium supplements without consulting the prescribing physician. Careful monitoring of blood K^+ levels.
   - In patients with renal impairment, amiloride should be administered under careful and frequent monitoring of serum electrolytes, creatinine, and blood urea nitrogen (BUN) levels.
5. *Pregnancy and lactation*
   - Amiloride is a folic acid antagonist and should be avoided during pregnancy.
6. *Contraindications*
   - Anuria, renal impairment (GFR <30mL/min/1.73m^2, CKD stages 4–5).
   - Hyperkalaemia (serum K^+ levels >5.5mEq/L), hyponatraemia.
   - Hypersensitive to this product.
   - Addison's disease.

Amiodarone

Class III antiarrhythmic drug with multiple mechanisms of action.

Indications

1. Oral amiodarone is indicated for the treatment of tachyarrhythmias not responding to other AADs or when other treatments cannot be used, including tachyarrhythmias associated with WPW syndrome, atrial flutter/AF, and all types of tachyarrhythmias, including supraventricular, nodal, and ventricular.
2. Treatment and prophylaxis of life-threatening recurrent ventricular arrhythmias (VT and/or VF) not responding to other treatments or other AADs, particularly in patients with structural heart disease (i.e. HF, MI, hypertension, or cardiomyopathies) or after cardiac surgery.
   - *Amiodarone* is the preferred IV antiarrhythmic agent for incessant VT or frequent VT episodes and severe LV dysfunction. If given during incessant VT, the response will be a gradual slowing of the VT cycle length, with eventual termination. However, amiodarone has no benefit on SCD or total mortality.
3. AF/flutter. Amiodarone is the most effective AAD to prevent recurrences of paroxysmal AF or flutter (maintenance of sinus rhythm). It is also effective for the conversion of atrial flutter/AF to sinus rhythm, although it has the disadvantage of a slow onset of action. Additional advantages of amiodarone are that it also slows the heart rate and, unlike other AADs, can be administered in patients with structural heart disease and has no risk of post-conversion ventricular arrhythmias.
   - Alone or in combination with β-blockers, amiodarone reduces the risk of post-operative AF.
   - It is effective for rhythm control in patients with a history of HF or with LV systolic dysfunction. For patients with NYHA class IV, in addition to treatment for acute HF, an IV bolus of amiodarone should be considered to reduce the ventricular rate.

Because of its potentially serious extra-cardiac side effects, in many arrhythmias, amiodarone becomes the last option.

Mechanism of action

Amiodarone is a 'wide-spectrum' AAD, which presents class I, II, III, and IV activity. It blocks Na^+, L-type Ca^{2+} and several K^+ currents [transient (I_{to}), ultrarapid (I_{Kur}), rapid (I_{Kr}), and slow (I_{Ks}) components of the delayed rectifier, inward rectifier (I_{K1}), and acetylcholine-activated (I_{KAch})]. It also inhibits inactivated Na^+ channels at high stimulation rates, reducing cardiac excitability and conduction velocity. Amiodarone also produces a non-competitive inhibition of α- and β-adrenergic receptors and a vasodiator effect mediated via the L-type Ca^{2+} current and β-adrenergic blockade.

Pharmacodynamics

Amiodarone exhibits class III antiarrhythmic effects, lengthening the action potential duration (APD) and refractoriness in all cardiac tissues, including bypass tracts. Thus, it can suppress arrhythmias with a short excitable gap.

Amiodarone prolongs the ventricular APD (QT interval) but makes the ventricular APD more uniform, reducing heterogeneity of repolarization and possible re-entry. Despite the fact that amiodarone prolongs the QT interval, the risk of TdP is less than with other AADs, possibly because it produces a more homogenous ventricular repolarization and blocks L-type Ca^{2+} channels and β-adrenoceptors.

Amiodarone reduces the slope of phase 4 diastolic depolarization in automatic cells, decreasing the sinus rate, and suppresses the ectopic pacemaker activity, as well as the triggered activity induced by early and delayed after-depolarizations. It also slows AV nodal conduction (prolongation of the PR interval). In chronic treatments and at fast driving rates, amiodarone decreases cardiac excitability and conduction velocity and increases the VF threshold. In patients with AF, amiodarone prolongs the refractory periods in the pulmonary veins and slows conduction through the AVN; in experimental models, it prevents atrial remodelling.

After oral dosing, it does not appear to cause a reduction in LVEF, even in patients with reduced LVEF, possibly because its vasodilator effect reduces LV afterload. However, after acute IV administration, amiodarone may exert a mild negative inotropic effect.

Amiodarone may be considered:

1. Prior to and following successful electrical cardioversion of atrial flutter/AF to maintain sinus rhythm and following cardioversion to maintain the sinus rhythm and prevent recurrences of the arrhythmias.
2. IV amiodarone is recommended when episodes of VT or VF are frequent and can no longer be controlled by successive electrical cardioversion or defibrillation. At the lowest possible dose, it can be administered in selected patients with refractory ventricular arrhythmias in which an ICD is not appropriate.
3. To acutely suppress recurrent haemodynamically relevant ventricular arrhythmias in patients with ACS. Amiodarone does not reduce SCD in post-MI patients with preserved LVEF but reduces arrhythmic episodes.
4. In symptomatic ventricular tachyarrhythmias in patients with HF, amiodarone is the AAD of choice because it does not increase mortality.
5. For symptomatic, but not life-threatening, arrhythmias (premature ventricular beats or short and slow NSVT), as amiodarone does not worsen the prognosis.
6. To prevent VT in patients with or without an ICD. In the ICD era, amiodarone (plus β-blockade) inhibits repetitive, unpleasant ICD shocks in spite of optimal device programming or allows termination by anti-tachycardia pacing. If amiodarone is added to an ICD, the defibrillation threshold increases and must be rechecked prior to discharge from hospital.
7. In patients with DCM with an ICD who experience recurrent appropriate shocks in spite of optimal device programming.
8. In patients with ARVC and frequent premature ventricular beats or NSVT who are intolerant of, or have contraindications to, β-blockers to improve symptoms.
9. IV amiodarone is recommended for the treatment of polymorphic VT.

Pharmacokinetics

Food increases the rate of absorption and the exposure of amiodarone. Peak plasma levels are reached after 6–8h, but steady-state effects are obtained after several weeks, unless large loading doses are used. Amiodarone binds to plasma proteins (99%) and is widely distributed (Vd 70L/kg) to adipose tissue, the liver, the heart, and the lungs; the concentration in the myocardium is 10–15 times that in plasma. This wide distribution means that amiodarone must fill all these peripheral tissue depots before achieving adequate blood and cardiac concentrations, accounting for its slow onset of action. Amiodarone is extensively metabolized in the liver by CYP450 3A4 and 2C8, leading to various active metabolites (desethylamiodarone) and excreted primarily via the hepatic and biliary routes, with almost no elimination via the renal route; amiodarone is not dialysable. Following drug withdrawal, amiodarone is slowly eliminated from peripheral tissues, so that its t½ is 20–100 days. Therapeutic plasma levels: 1–2.5mcg/mL. (See Table 8.1.3.)

Practical points

1. *Doses*
   - *PO*: when rapid control of an urgent arrhythmia is needed, the initial loading regimen is up to 1600mg in 2–4 divided doses, usually given for 7–14 days, which is then reduced to 400–800mg/day for a further 1–3 weeks. Loading doses of 200mg td continued for 1 week can be given in less urgent settings; the dosage should then be reduced to 200mg bd for a further week. *Maintenance dose*: 200–400mg od.
     —Chronic oral drug therapy to prevent recurrence of AF: 600mg daily in divided doses for 4 weeks. Then 200mg od; at these low doses amiodarone may be very effective with little risk of side effects.
   - *IV: Loading dose*: 5–7mg/kg over 20min to 2h (diluted in 5% glucose). This can be followed by up to 1200mg (15mg/kg) in 5% glucose for 24h; higher doses can produce hypotension. Do not use concentrations higher than 3mg/mL to prevent phlebitis. In extreme clinical emergencies: a slow (3–5min) injection of 2.5–5mg/kg in 10–20ml 5% glucose under close monitoring.
   - *Maintenance dose*: 10–20mg/kg in physiological glucose solution every 24h (600–800mg/24h up to a maximum of 1200mg/24h) for a few days. Do not add other medicinal products to the infusion fluid.
     —Rate control in AF: 300mg IV diluted in 250mL 5% glucose over 30–60 min (preferably via central venous cannula); then, if needed, 900mg IV over 24h diluted in 500–1000mL.
     —Pharmacological cardioversion of AF: 5–7mg/kg over 1–2h, followed by 50mg/h to a maximum of 1g over 24h.
     —Ventricular arrhythmias: 150–350mg IV bolus diluted in 20mL 5% glucose; a further dose of 2.5mg/kg can be considered if the VF persists.

Dose adjustments may be required during prolonged therapy to avoid development of side effects while maintaining optimal antiarrhythmic effect. Maintenance doses for atrial flutter or AF are generally lower than those needed for serious ventricular arrhythmias.

2. *Side effects*

Extra-cardiac side effects are very common with amiodarone. They occur in up to 75% of patients, causing discontinuation in 7–18%; some side effects may be potentially fatal. This explains why amiodarone is reserved as the last antiarrhythmic option. Thus, the benefit must be balanced against the cost of side effects, which may be reduced at low doses (100–200mg daily).

- Reversible corneal microdeposits usually only discernable under slit-lamp examination, requiring discontinuation due to halos or blurred vision; photosensitivity may persist for many months after discontinuation and optic neuropathy/neuritis. Periodic eye examinations are recommended.
- *CV*: sinus bradycardia (elderly), AVB, conduction disturbances, HF, QT prolongation, and occasional TdP, VT, and VF. TdP are rare but may occur in patients with hypokalaemia or bradycardia, or those receiving QT-prolonging drugs. Hypotension is observed when given IV.
- *Endocrine*: amiodarone produces hypothyroidism (TSH >10mU/L) or hyperthyroidism (TSH <0.35mU/L). Hyperthyroidism can induce cardiac arrhythmias and should be excluded if new arrhythmias appear during amiodarone therapy. Thyrotoxicosis may be much commoner in iodine-deficient areas. Testicular dysfunction.
- *Skin*: blue/grey skin discoloration (slowly reverses after 18 months but may not disappear); rashes and photosensitivity. Avoid sun exposure, and use a sunscreen ointment with ultraviolet A (UVA) and UVB protection.
- *GI*: nausea, vomiting, constipation, and anorexia. Nausea can occur in 25% of patients with CHF. Reversible increase in transaminase levels, hepatitis, and cirrhosis.
- *Neurological*: proximal muscle weakness, fatigue, headache, peripheral neuropathy, ataxia, tremors, nightmares, and sleep disturbances. Neurological (tremor, ataxia, and peripheral neuropathy) and GI (nausea and vomiting) side effects are common during loading with high daily doses and usually improve once maintenance doses are begun.
- *Pulmonary*: chronic interstitial pneumonitis, potentially leading to pulmonary fibrosis, occurs in patients receiving chronic doses of ≥400mg/day, which may be fatal in 10% of those affected. Pulmonary toxicity may be dose-related and very rarely occurs with low doses (200mg daily). Risk factors include pre-existing lung disease.
- Amiodarone can increase creatinine plasma levels due to partial inhibition of the tubular organic cationic transporter system, rather than a decline in renal function. In fact, the drug does not affect the GFR, renal blood flow, and Na^+ or K^+ excretion.

3. *Interactions*

Amiodarone is metabolized by CYP3A4 and is a substrate for P-gp and presents multiple drug interactions. Due to its long t½, the interactions may last several months after drug discontinuation.

- Additive proarrhythmic effects with QT-prolonging drugs.
- Amiodarone and its metabolite desethylamiodarone inhibit several CYP450 isoenzymes (CYP1A1/2, CYP3A4, CYP2C9, CYP2D6) and some transporters such as Pgp and organic cation transporter 2

(OCT2), which can result in unexpectedly high plasma levels and increased adverse effects of drugs metabolized by these CYP450 enzymes or which are substrates of P-gp (see Table 8.1.2). The doses of these drugs should be reduced.

- Combination with digoxin, β-blockers (propranolol), verapamil, or diltiazem increases the risk of bradycardia and AVB; with verapamil or diltiazem increases the risk of bradycardia, hypotension, and HF.
- Amiodarone increases the plasma digoxin concentration; decrease the dose of digoxin by 50%, and monitor digoxin plasma levels.
- Amiodarone prolongs the PT and may increase the risk of bleeding in patients on warfarin; decrease the dose of warfarin by 30–50%, and monitor the INR.
- Amiodarone may decrease the antiplatelet activity of clopidogrel.
- Antihypertensive drugs can increase the risk of hypotension, particularly following the IV administration of amiodarone.
- Amiodarone increases the plasma levels of flecainide; reduce the dose of flecainide, and monitor the patient.
- Amiodarone increases the plasma levels of phenytoin, and phenytoin enhances the conversion of amiodarone to desethylamiodarone.
- Colestyramine and colestipol decrease the absorption of amiodarone.
- Cimetidine increases the plasma levels and adverse effects of amiodarone.
- Combination with atorvastatin, rosuvastatin, or simvastatin may increase the risk of myopathy and rhabdomyolysis. Doses of lovastatin and simvastatin should not exceed 40mg/day and 20mg/day, respectively.
- Higher IV doses of dopamine and dobutamine are needed in patients receiving amiodarone.
- Rifampicin and St John's wort decrease the plasma levels of amiodarone, thus decreasing its therapeutic effect.
- Amiodarone decreases the metabolism of methotrexate and increases its adverse effects.
- Nelfinavir and ritonavir increase amiodarone plasma levels and the risk of adverse effects.
- Amiodarone increases the plasma levels of quinidine, disopyramide, and procainamide. Avoid the combination with class IA AADs.
- The combination with vardenafil increases the risk of serious ventricular arrhythmias.
- Grapefruit increases exposure to amiodarone (50–80%). Avoid drinking grapefruit.
- Potentially severe complications have been reported in patients taking amiodarone undergoing general anaesthesia: bradycardia unresponsive to atropine, hypotension, disturbances of conduction and decreased CO.
- Severe bradycardia when amiodarone is combined with sofosbuvir and daclatasvir. Monitor heart rate during the first 48h.

4. *Cautions/notes*

- Amiodarone can cause serious adverse reactions affecting the eyes, heart, lung, liver, thyroid gland, skin, and peripheral nervous system. Thus, patients on long-term treatment should be carefully supervised every 6 months, with physical examination of the skin, eyes, and peripheral nerves if symptoms develop. As undesirable effects are usually dose-related, the minimum effective maintenance dose should be given.

- Amiodarone increases aspartate aminotransferase (AST) and alanine aminotransferase (ALT) and inhibits the peripheral conversion of T4 to T3, decreases serum T3, increases serum T4, and can increase creatinine plasma levels.
- IV amiodarone should be initiated and monitored only under hospital or specialist supervision.
- Amiodarone injection contains benzyl alcohol, which may cause toxic and allergic reactions in infants and children up to 3 years old. Medications containing benzyl alcohol given to newborns or premature neonates have been associated with fatal 'gasping syndrome'.
- Caution when combined with drugs which may also cause hypokalaemia and/or hypomagnesaemia: diuretics, systemic corticosteroids, tetracosactide, IV amphotericin, and laxatives. Hypokalaemia increases the risk of TdP.
- Caution when amiodarone is co-administered with dabigatran, due to the risk of bleeding. Adjust the dosage of dabigatran as per its label.

5. *Pregnancy and lactation*

- Amiodarone and desethylamiodarone cross the placenta, and hypo-/hyperthyroidism, growth retardation, VSDs, bradycardia, and prolonged QT interval can be observed in some amiodarone-newborns (Pregnancy category D). Amiodarone is excreted in breast milk; avoid amiodarone during breastfeeding.

6. *Contraindications*

- Sinus bradycardia and SA heart block, second- or third-degree heart block (unless a pacemaker is present).
- Cardiogenic shock.
- Severe chronic lung disease.
- Lactation; pregnancy (except in exceptional circumstances).
- Evidence or history of thyroid dysfunction.
- In combination with other drugs that may cause TdP.
- Known hypersensitivity to amiodarone or to iodine.

Amlodipine

Dihydropyridine derivative L-type CCB (see ➔ Calcium channel blockers, pp. 504–9).

CV indications

- Treatment of hypertension.
- Symptomatic treatment of chronic stable angina.
- Treatment of vasospastic angina (Prinzmetal's variant angina).
- Patients with recently documented CAD without HF or an LVEF of <40% to reduce the risk of hospitalization due to angina and the risk of a coronary revascularization procedure.

Mechanism of action

Amlodipine presents a slow rate of association and dissociation from its receptor site in the L-type Ca^{2+} channel, resulting in a gradual onset and long duration of its effects. Amlodipine also exhibits antioxidant and antiproliferative effects.

Pharmacokinetics

Oral bioavailability is unaffected by food. The AUC increases 40–60% in elderly patients and patients with hepatic insufficiency (t½ of up to 56h) or HF (see Table 8.1.6).

Practical points

1. *Doses*
   - 5–10mg od. In the elderly or in patients with hepatic insufficiency, start with 2.5mg od.
2. *Side effects* (see ➔ Calcium channel blockers, pp. 504–9)
   - Peripheral oedema appears in approximately 10% of patients at 10mg/day (more frequent in women).
3. *Interactions* (see ➔ Calcium channel blockers, pp. 504–9)
   - Amlodipine has been safely used with thiazide diuretics, β-blockers, ACEIs, long-acting nitrates, sublingual glyceryl trinitrate, digoxin, warfarin, cimetidine (in contrast to verapamil and nifedipine), NSAIDs, antacids, phenytoin, sildenafil, grapefruit juice, and oral hypoglycaemic drugs.
   - Co-administration with CYP3A inhibitors increases exposure to amlodipine and may require dose reduction (see Table 8.1.2). Monitor BP.
   - Amlodipine increases the systemic exposure of simvastatin. Limit the dose of simvastatin to 20mg/day.
   - Amlodipine may increase the systemic exposure of ciclosporin or tacrolimus in renal transplant patients. Frequent monitoring of BP, and adjust the dose as appropriate.
4. *Cautions/notes*
   - Caution in patients with impaired hepatic function and the elderly.
5. *Pregnancy and lactation* (see ➔ Calcium channel blockers, pp. 504–9)
6. *Contraindications* (see ➔ Calcium channel blockers, pp. 504–9)

Table 8.1.6 Pharmacokinetic properties of L-type calcium channel blockers

Drugs	F (%)	T_{max} (h)	PPB (%)	Vd (L/kg)	Metabolism	t½ (h)	Renal excretion* (%)
Amlodipine	60–90	6–12	95	16	CYP3A4	35–45	5
Diltiazem	45	1–2	80	3.3 (8–11)**	CYP3A4	4–7	1–4
Felodipine	15	2.5–5	99	10	CYP3A4	17–31	<0.5
Lacidipine	10	1–2	98	4–8	CYP3A4	13–19	1
Lercanidipine	10	1.5–3	98	2.5	CYP3A4	2–5	1
Nicardipine	30	1–2	98	1.2	CYP3A4	4–6	0
Nifedipine SR	45–55	1.5–5.4	95	0.78	CYP3A4	6–11	2
Verapamil	25	1.2 (7.6)**	90	4.4	CYP3A4	3–7	<1

F, oral bioavailability; h, hour; PPB, protein plasma binding; SR, slow-release formulation; t½, drug half-life; T_{max}, time to peak plasma levels; Vd, volume of distribution.

* Renal excretion without biotransformation.

** Slow release formulation.

Andexanet alfa

Genetically modified variant of human factor Xa (alanine is substituted for serine) that is unable to cleave and activate prothrombin and cannot assemble into the prothrombinase complex.

Indications

- For patients treated with factor Xa inhibitors, when reversal of anticoagulation is needed due to life-threatening or uncontrolled bleeding.

Mechanism of action

Andexanet alfa acts as a decoy, binding to factor Xa inhibitors and neutralizing their anticoagulant effect. Based on its mechanism of action, andexanet alfa is expected to reduce the anti-factor Xa activity of direct (apixaban, betrixaban, edoxaban, rivaroxaban) and indirect (enoxaparin, fondaparinux) factor Xa inhibitors. Andexanet alfa exerts procoagulant effects by binding and sequestering the FXa inhibitors and binding and inhibiting the activity of tissue factor pathway inhibitor (TFPI); this latter effect can increase tissue factor-initiated thrombin generation. To reduce the risk of thrombosis, resume anticoagulant therapy as soon as appropriate after dose.

Pharmacodynamics

Andexanet alfa produces a rapid decrease in anti-FXa activity corresponding to the IV bolus that was sustained through the end of the continuous infusion. Approximately 50% of patients experience >90% decrease from baseline anti-FXa activity. Following the infusion, there is an increase in anti-FXa activity, which peaks 4h after infusion; then, the anti-FXa activity decreases at a rate similar to the clearance of the FXa inhibitors.

Pharmacokinetics

Following its IV administration the effect is immediate. Presents a low Vd (0.05L/kg) and presents an elimination t½ of 5–7h (pharmacodynamic t½ ≈ 1h).

Practical points

1. *Doses*
    - Low-dose regimen. Patients taking rivaroxaban ≤10mg or apixaban ≤5mg per dose: 400mg IV bolus of andexanet alfa, followed by a 4mg/min infusion for up to 2h.
    - High-dose regimen. Patients taking rivaroxaban >10mg or apixaban >5mg per dose: 800mg IV bolus dose of andexanet alfa, followed by an 8mg/min continuous infusion for up to 2h if the last dose was <8h before starting andexanet alfa. If the last dose was ≥8h before starting andexanet alfa, the low-dose regimen should be used. If the dose and/or timing since the last dose of the factor Xa inhibitor is unknown, the high-dose regimen should be used. Safety and efficacy of an additional dose has not been established.

2. *Side effects*
   - Risk of thromboembolic events (ischaemic stroke, DVT, PE, and acute MI), bleeding and infusion-related reactions (urinary tract infections and pneumonia), sudden cardiac death, cardiogenic shock, HF. Low titres of neutralizing antibodies against andexanet alfa were detected in 17% of patients.
3. *Cautions*
   - Monitor for arterial and venous thromboembolic events, ischaemic and cardiac events, including sudden death.
4. *Pregnancy and lactation*
   - Safety during pregnancy and breastfeeding has not been evaluated.
5. *Contraindications*
   - None.

Angiotensin II AT1 receptor blockers

(See ➲ Candesartan (cilexetil), p. 510; ➲ Irbesartan, p. 630; ➲ Losartan, pp. 651–2; ➲ Olmesartan (medoxomil), p. 688; ➲ Telmisartan, p. 766; ➲ Valsartan, p. 791.)

Indications

- Treatment of hypertension.
- Treatment of HF to reduce the risk of: (1) HF hospitalization and CV death in symptomatic patients unable to tolerate an ACEI (patients should also receive a β-blocker and an MRA), and (2) HF hospitalization and death in patients who are symptomatic despite treatment with a β-blocker who are unable to tolerate an MRA.
- Slow the progression of nephropathy caused by T2DM.

Mechanism of action

ARBs inhibit the RAAS by antagonizing the effects of angiotensin II mediated via stimulation of AT1 receptors, including vasoconstriction, endothelial dysfunction, cell growth and proliferation, fibrosis, oxidative stress, sodium and water retention, and aldosterone release. Moreover, in the presence of an ARB, angiotensin II can stimulate AT2 receptors that are not blocked, producing vasodilator, antiproliferative, and natriuretic effects. Thus, the effects of ARBs are due to blockade of AT1 receptors and the stimulation of AT2 receptors. ARBs avoid the bradykinin-related side effects (cough, angio-oedema) of ACEIs.

Pharmacodynamics

(See ➲ Candesartan (cilexetil), p. 510; ➲ Irbesartan, p. 630; ➲ Losartan, pp. 651–2; ➲ Olmesartan (medoxomil), p. 688; ➲ Telmisartan, p. 766; ➲ Valsartan, p. 791.)

- *Hypertension*: a meta-analysis of 50 trials found that ARBs produced a BP reduction similar to ACEIs. The antihypertensive effect is independent of age and gender but is reduced in black patients (usually a low-renin population). ARBs are indicated in hypertensives with ACEI-related cough or intolerance, HF or LV dysfunction, LV hypertrophy, microalbuminuria, T2DM, chronic renal disease, and MetS. ARBs are better tolerated than ACEIs and all other antihypertensive drug classes, and thus promote adherence.
- *HF and post-MI patients*: ACEIs and ARBs have similar efficacy in chronic HF, as well as in patients after acute MI with signs of HF or LV dysfunction. ARBs are indicated in symptomatic patients intolerant to ACEIs, to improve morbidity and mortality.
- *Renal protection*: ARBs reduce proteinuria and slow the progression of glomerular sclerosis and loss of renal function in chronic renal disease, with or without T2DM. In proteinuric renal disease, with or without diabetes, ARBs and ACEIs similarly reduced proteinuria.

Practical points

1. *Doses* (see ➲ Candesartan (cilexetil), p. 510; ➲ Irbesartan, p. 630; ➲ Losartan, pp. 651–2; ➲ Olmesartan (medoxomil), p. 688; ➲ Telmisartan, p. 766; ➲ Valsartan, p. 791)
2. *Side effects*
   - Adverse effects are comparable to placebo.
   - (1–10%): dizziness, vertigo; fatigue; hypotension; hyperkalaemia, rise in urea and creatinine levels.
   - Others: nausea, vomiting; chest infection; headache; angio-oedema has been reported with some ARBs.
3. *Interactions*
   - Antihypertensive effects of ARBs are enhanced by other antihypertensives and vasodilators (nitrates), tricyclic antidepressants and antipsychotics, baclofen.
   - Prior treatment with high-dose diuretics may result in volume depletion and a risk of hypotension when initiating therapy with an ARB.
   - NSAIDs and sympathomimetics can attenuate the antihypertensive effects.
   - Concomitant use of ARBs and NSAIDs may lead to an increased risk of worsening of renal function, including acute renal failure, and an increase in serum K^+ levels, especially in the elderly and in patients dehydrated or those with poor pre-existing renal function.
   - The antihypertensive effect of ARBs is potentiated by thiazides and loop diuretics or a low-salt diet; ARBs compensate the hypokalaemia produced by diuretics.
   - The risk of hyperkalaemia increases with renal impairment, and especially with concomitant use of ACEIs, potassium-sparing diuretics, eplerenone, β-blockers, NSAIDs, heparin, or potassium supplements. Monitor serum K^+ levels, if combined.
   - ARBs increase serum lithium concentrations and toxicity; avoid the combination. If it is not possible, careful monitoring of serum lithium levels is recommended.
   - Patients taking concomitant an mTOR inhibitor (e.g. temsirolimus, sirolimus, everolimus) may be at increased risk for angio-oedema.
   - No interaction has been found with cimetidine, digoxin, furosemide, or warfarin.
4. *Cautions*
   - Dual blockade of the RAAS with ARBs, ACEIs, or aliskiren increases the risk of hypotension, hyperkalaemia, and renal impairment (including acute renal failure), compared to monotherapy. Closely monitor BP, renal function, and electrolytes. ACEIs and ARBs should not be used concomitantly in patients with diabetic nephropathy.
   - ARBs should be used with caution in those with a history of angio-oedema, particularly if induced by ACEIs.
   - In the absence of diuretic co-therapy, there is relative resistance to the antihypertensive effects of ARBs in black patients.
   - In patients with impaired renal function, periodic monitoring of serum K^+ and creatinine levels is recommended.

- Symptomatic hypotension, especially after the first dose, may be seen in patients who are volume-deplete or with vigorous diuretic therapy, dietary salt restriction, diarrhoea, or vomiting. These patients should be closely monitored, particularly those with severe HF. The risk of hypotension may be minimized by discontinuing the diuretic; if is not possible to discontinue the diuretic, the starting dose of the ARB should be reduced.
- As with other vasodilators, use with caution in patients with aortic or mitral valve stenosis, obstructive HCM, or constrictive pericarditis.
- Monitor serum K^+ levels, especially in patients with diabetes or renal insufficiency and those on potassium-sparing diuretics or potassium supplements.
- There is an increased risk of hypotension and renal failure in those with renovascular disease, e.g. bilateral renal artery stenosis or artery stenosis of a single functioning kidney. This is usually reversible on stopping therapy.
- As with any antihypertensive agent, excessive BP decrease in patients with ischaemic cardiopathy or ischaemic CV disease could result in an MI or stroke.

5. *Pregnancy and lactation*
   - Treatment with an ARB is not recommended during pregnancy. When pregnancy is diagnosed, treatment with ARBs should be stopped immediately, and, if appropriate, alternative therapy should be started (Pregnancy category D). Because of the lack of information, ARBs are not recommended during breastfeeding.
6. *Contraindications*
   - History of hereditary or idiopathic angio-oedema; previous ACEI-related angio-oedema.
   - Hyperkalaemia.
   - Hyperaldosteronism.
   - Hypotension.
   - Biliary obstruction.
   - Pregnancy and breastfeeding.
   - Severe renal failure (CrCl <30mL/min), anuria.
   - Renal artery stenosis in a solitary kidney or significant bilateral renal artery stenosis.
   - Concomitant use of ARBs with aliskiren-containing products is contraindicated in patients with diabetes mellitus or renal impairment (GFR <60mL/min/1.73m^2).

Angiotensin-converting enzyme inhibitors

For example: captopril, enalapril, lisinopril, perindopril, ramipril, trandolapril.
Others: benazepril, cilazapril, fosinopril, imidapril, moexipril, quinapril.

Indications

- Treatment of hypertension.
- Treatment of HF, at all stages, to reduce CV death and hospitalizations.
  - ACEIs are recommended in patients with asymptomatic LV systolic dysfunction and a history of MI, in order to prevent or delay the onset of HF and reduce mortality.
  - ACEIs are recommended, in addition to a β-blocker, for symptomatic patients with HFrEF, to reduce the risk of HF hospitalization and death.
  - ACEIs should be considered in patients with stable CAD, even if they do not have LV systolic dysfunction, in order to prevent or delay the onset of HF.
- Treatment of haemodynamically stable patients with acute MI within 24h, acute phase for high-risk patients, and post-infarct LV dysfunction.
- Diabetic nephropathy.
- Slow progression of renal disease in patients with T1DM with microalbuminuria.
- Secondary CV protection (ramipril, perindopril, trandolapril).

Mechanism of action

ACEIs prevent the conversion of angiotensin I to angiotensin II. As a consequence, ACEIs decrease the synthesis of angiotensin II, leading to arteriovenous vasodilator effects, improve endothelial dysfunction, decrease cardiac, vascular, and renal remodelling (neointimal proliferation, hypertrophy, fibrosis, dilatation) and oxidative stress, and exert antiproliferative, anti-inflammatory, antiarrhythmic, and antiaggregant effects. Furthermore, angiotensin II increases the sympathetic tone and the synthesis and release of aldosterone, vasopressin, and ET1, leading to potent vasoconstriction, oxidative stress, and proliferative, proarrhythmic, and prothrombotic effects. All these adverse effects are inhibited by ACEIs. Additionally, ACE is identical to kininase II, so that ACEIs inhibit the breakdown of bradykinin. Bradykinin stimulates its endothelial B2 receptors and promote the release of NO and vasodilatory prostaglandins (I_2 and E_2), which exert vasodilatory, antiaggregant, and antiproliferative effects. Additionally, ACEIs inhibit platelet aggregation and the release of tPA and inhibits plasminogen activator inhibitor-1 (PAI-1), effects which increase fibrinolysis.

Pharmacodynamics

(See ➲ Captopril, pp. 514–16; ➲ Enalapril, p. 570; ➲ Lisinopril, p. 644; ➲ Perindopril, p. 694; ➲ Ramipril, pp. 720–1; ➲ Trandolapril, p. 783.)

1. *Hypertension*: ACEIs produce arterial and venous vasodilatation via multiple mechanisms: (1) inhibition of angiotensin II synthesis, (2) inhibition of the sympathetic tone and the release of aldosterone, ET1, and vasopressin, and (3) an increase in the release of kinins, NO,

and prostaglandins I_2 and E_2. ACEIs improve endothelial dysfunction and peripheral (skeletal muscle, coronary, and cerebral) blood flow, reduce LVH, and increase arterial distensibility but do not alter glucose, lipid, or uric acid plasma levels or increase the risk of new-onset diabetes.

ACEIs are indicated in hypertensives with HF or LV dysfunction, post-MI, T1DM, nephropathy, microalbuminuria or proteinuria, MetS, and asymptomatic atherosclerosis. They are more effective in white patients but are less so in black patients, possibly because of a higher prevalence of low-renin states in the black hypertensive population. ACEIs are also effective in mild to moderate hypertension, even when plasma renin is not high. In acute severe hypertension, sublingual (chewed) captopril rapidly brings down BP.

A particularly effective combination is with thiazide (or loop) diuretics, because they increase circulating renin activity and angiotensin II levels, effects with are inhibited by ACEIs. The combination enhances the antihypertesive effects but increases the risk of hypotension, so that the diuretic dose is usually halved before starting ACEIs. This combination decreases hyperkalaemia induced by thiazides and loop diuretics. The combination of ACEIs plus spironolactone or eplerenone increases the risk of hyperkalaemia and creatinine serum levels.

2. *HF*. ACEIs reduce pre-/afterload; improve signs, symptoms, haemodynamics (increase CO, reduce PCWP and LV end-diastolic pressure), exercise tolerance, functional capacity, and coronary, skeletal muscle, and kidney blood flow, and diuresis; and decrease hospitalization, progression of disease, and mortality. Furthermore, ACEIs inhibit neurohumoral activation, decreasing the plasma levels of angiotensin II, noradrenaline, adrenaline, and vasopressin, slow the progression of disease, and decrease LV remodelling.

Therefore, they are recommended: (1) in addition to a β-blocker, for symptomatic patients with HFrEF to reduce the risk of HF hospitalization and death; (2) as initial therapy in the absence of fluid retention and in patients with fluid retention together with diuretics; (3) in patients with signs or symptoms of HF after the acute phase of MI, even if the symptoms are transient, to improve survival and reduce reinfarctions and hospitalization for HF; and (4) in asymptomatic patients with documented LV systolic dysfunction to prevent the development of overt CHF.

3. *Early-phase AMI*. ACEIs orally administered for overt LV failure or LV dysfunction starting on the first day produce a modest, but significant, reduction in mortality. Best results are obtained in higher-risk patients, i.e. those with large infarcts, LVEF of <35%, diabetes, chronic renal disease, tachycardia, or overt LV failure. ACEIs also attenuate LV remodelling and reduce the risk of subsequent MI or HF. The best approach is to start ACEI therapy as soon as the patient is haemodynamically stable, with close monitoring of BP and renal function. Because of the risk of hypotension, IV administration of ACEIs is not recommended.
4. *Renal diseases*. ACEIs produce preferential vasodilatation of the renal efferent glomerular arteriole, reduce intraglomerular pressure, and thus protect against progressive glomerulosclerosis. They can

produce hyperkalaemia, especially in the presence of pre-existing renal dysfunction and diabetes complicated by type 4 renal tubular acidosis, or when combined with potassium-retaining agents.

5. *Diabetes mellitus.* In type 1 diabetic nephropathy, ACEIs reduce proteinuria and slow the progression of glomerular sclerosis and loss of renal function, reducing the risk of death, dialysis, and renal transplantation. ACEIs also delay the onset of microalbuminuria and its progression towards albuminuria. These renoprotective effects are independent of BP reduction.
6. *CV protection in high-risk patients.* In patients at high risk of CAD, the addition of ramipril to standard therapy provides substantial cardioprotection. ACEIs are not direct anti-anginal agents but might have an indirect anti-ischaemic effect, as they reduce cardiac afterload and preload, LV wall stress, and myocardial oxygen demands and improve coronary oxygen supply, reduce the sympathetic tone, and improve endothelial function. In patients with hypertension or HF, ACEIs prevent/reduce LV remodelling and attenuate further LV chamber enlargement.

There is a lower prevalence of AF among patients treated with ACEIs, probably due to reversal of atrial remodelling (hypertrophy, fibrosis, and dilatation). They also reduce sudden death in patients with CHF, particularly post-MI.

Practical points

1. *Doses* (see ➲ Captopril, pp. 514–16; ➲ Enalapril, p. 570; ➲ Lisinopril, p. 644; ➲ Perindopril, p. 694; ➲ Ramipril, pp. 720–1; ➲ Trandolapril, p. 783)
   - ACEIs should be initiated under specialist supervision in patients with severe HF, receiving multiple or high-dose diuretics or those with hypovolaemia, hyponatraemia (<130mmol/L), pre-existing hypotension (SBP <90mmHg), unstable HF, concomitant high-dose vasodilator therapy, and known renovascular disease. If possible, the diuretic should be discontinued 2–3 days before beginning therapy with an ACEI, to avoid hypotension.
2. *Side effects*
   - (1 15%): dry, non-productive cough (thought to be due to an increased production of bradykinin and prostaglandins), hyperkalaemia (especially in patients with renal impairment or diabetes), blurred vision, dizziness, headache, pruritic rash, loss of taste, and GI disturbances, including diarrhoea and vomiting.
   - Hypotension is not uncommon, particularly in high-renin states (chronic HF, renal artery stenosis, hyponatraemia related to diuretic use, or increased creatinine serum levels of 1.5–3mg/dL or 135–265micromol/L). To avoid hypotension, discontinue or halve the dose of diuretics 1–2 days before the initial dose.
   - Angio-oedema of the face, extremities, lips, tongue, glottis, and/or larynx are more frequent in blacks and can be occasionally fatal. Warning signs are facial swelling, unilateral facial oedema, or periorbital oedema.

- Anaphylactoid reactions have been reported in patients dialysed with high-flux membranes (e.g. AN69), LDL apheresis with dextran sulfate, and during desensitization.
- Deterioration of renal function. Preferential vasodilatation of glomerular efferent arterioles reduces the intraglomerular pressure and GFR and may cause an increase in creatinine serum levels initially. Specifically, ACEIs can induce or exacerbate renal impairment in patients with renal artery stenosis, particularly if treated with NSAIDs or diuretics, or in the presence of hypotension, severe sodium and volume depletion, or low renal blood flow (severe CHF or renal artery stenosis). Rarely, irreversible renal failure occurs in patients with bilateral renal artery stenosis.
- Others. Neutropenia/agranulocytosis, thrombocytopenia, and anaemia have been reported. ACEIs should be used with extreme caution in patients with collagen vascular disease or immunosuppressant therapy, those on treatment with allopurinol or procainamide, or if there is pre-existing impaired renal function. In these patients, periodic monitoring of white blood cell counts is advised and patients should be instructed to report any sign of infection. Very rarely, ACEIs can produce a syndrome that starts with cholestatic jaundice and progresses to fulminant necrosis and (sometimes) death.

3. *Interactions*
   - The risk of hyperkalaemia increases in patients with renal impairment or diabetes, and especially with concomitant use of potassium-sparing diuretics, ARBs, eplerenone, β-blockers, heparin, or potassium supplements. Careful monitoring of serum K^+ levels is critical, because hyperkalaemia is potentially lethal.
   - The antihypertensive effects of ACEIs are enhanced when used with other antihypertensives and vasodilators (e.g. nitrates), alcohol, certain anaesthetic agents, tricyclic antidepressants, and antipsychotics. ACEIs compensate the hypokalaemia produced by thiazides and loop diuretics.
   - The antihypertensive effect of ACEIs is reduced by ciclosporin and sympathomimetics.
   - NSAIDs, especially indometacin, inhibit the antihypertensive effect and increase the risk of hyperkalaemia. Reduced renal flow induced by NSAIDs can also rarely contribute to renal failure, particularly in the elderly or dehydrated patients. Thus, if an NSAID has to be used, frequent checks of renal function are required.
   - ACEIs decrease the GFR and renal clearance of other renally excreted drugs (atenolol, nadolol, sotalol, flecainide, disopyramide, procainamide).
   - Concomitant use of ACEIs with lithium may increase lithium exposure and toxicity; this combination should be avoided. If the combination proves necessary, careful monitoring of serum lithium levels should be performed.
   - It is possible that concomitant use of ACEIs with oral antidiabetic agents may cause an increased glucose-lowering effect, with a risk of hypoglycaemia.
   - Higher doses of erythropoietin are needed in dialysed patients on ACEIs.

- Nitritoid reactions (flushing, nausea, dizziness, and hypotension) can be observed following injectable gold (i.e. sodium aurothiomalate) in patients receiving ACEI therapy.
- The combined use of ACEIs, ARBs, or aliskiren is associated with a higher frequency of adverse events such as hypotension, hyperkalaemia, and decreased renal function (including acute renal failure), compared with monotherapy with any of these agents.

4. *Cautions*
   - Symptomatic hypotension is more likely to occur in volume-depleted patients (e.g. by diuretic therapy, dietary salt restriction, dialysis, diarrhoea, or vomiting), with hyponatraemia, severe renin-dependent hypertension, or severe HF. In patients at increased risk of symptomatic hypotension, initiation of therapy and dose adjustment should be closely monitored. A transient hypotensive response is not a contraindication to further doses.
   - The risk of hypotension and renal failure (azotaemia, oliguria, or rarely acute renal failure) increases in individuals with renovascular disease, e.g. bilateral renal artery stenosis or artery stenosis of a single functioning kidney. In these patients, treatment should be started under close medical supervision with low doses and careful dose titration.
   - Excessive BP decrease in patients with ischaemic cardiopathy or ischaemic CV disease could result in MI or stroke.
   - Use with caution in malignant hypertension, mitral valve stenosis, obstruction in the outflow of the left ventricle such as aortic stenosis or HCM, and constrictive pericarditis.
   - Check serum K^+ levels, BP, and renal function periodically during treatment, especially in patients with diabetes or renal insufficiency and those on potassium-sparing diuretics or potassium supplements.
   - ACEIs and ARBs should not be used concomitantly in patients with diabetic nephropathy.
   - Avoid the use of an ACEI in patients with acute MI and those with haemodynamic compromise, particularly if SBP is <100mmHg or the creatinine level is >177micromol/L, and discontinue if renal failure (creatinine >203micromol/L or 2.3mg/dL) or if the creatinine level doubles after initiation. During the first 3 days, reduce the dose if SBP is <120mmHg.
   - Monitor glucose plasma levels during the first few months in diabetic patients treated with oral hypoglycaemic agents and/or insulin, due to the increased risk of hypoglycaemia.
5. *Pregnancy and lactation*
   - ACEIs should not be initiated during pregnancy (Pregnancy category D), due to an increased risk of fetotoxicity (decreased renal function, oligohydramnios, skull ossification, retardation) and neonatal toxicity (hyperkalaemia, hypotension, and renal failure). Ultrasound check of renal function and the skull should be arranged in the event of exposure to ACEIs in the second trimester. When pregnancy is diagnosed, treatment with ACEIs should be stopped immediately. Use of lisinopril is not recommended during breastfeeding.

6. *Contraindications*
   - History of hereditary or idiopathic angio-oedema; previous ACEI-related angio-oedema.
   - Hypotension (SBP <95mmHg).
   - Pregnancy and breastfeeding.
   - Hyperkalaemia (requires caution or cessation).
   - Severe renal failure (serum creatinine levels >2.5–3 mg/dL or >225–265micromol/L).
   - Renal artery stenosis (bilateral or unilateral with a solitary functioning kidney).
   - Partial contraindications: severe cough, severe aortic stenosis, or obstructive cardiomyopathy.

Apixaban

Selective inhibitor of factor Xa, the serine protease located in the final common pathway of the coagulation cascade, and prothrombinase activity.

Indications

- Prevention of stroke and systemic embolism in adult patients with NVAF, with one or more risk factors such as prior stroke or TIA, age ≥75 years, hypertension, diabetes mellitus, and symptomatic HF (NYHA class ≥ II).
- Treatment of deep vein thrombosis (DVT) and PE, and prevention of recurrent DVT and PE in adults.

Mechanism of action

Apixaban is an oral, potent, reversible, direct, and highly selective active site inhibitor of factor Xa that does not require antithrombin III for its antithrombotic activity. It inhibits both free and clot-bound factor Xa and prothrombinase activity. Apixaban has no direct effects on platelet aggregation, but by inhibiting factor X, apixaban indirectly inhibits platelet aggregation induced by thrombin.

Pharmacodynamics

Selective factor Xa inhibitors interrupt the intrinsic and extrinsic pathways of the blood coagulation cascade and inhibit free and prothrombinase-bound factor Xa, reducing the formation of thrombin, a reaction leading to fibrin clot formation and the development of thrombus formation.

Although selective factor Xa inhibitors do not require routine monitoring, plasma levels measured with a calibrated quantitative chromogenic anti-factor Xa assay may be useful in some situations, e.g. overdose and emergency surgery. Selective factor Xa inhibitors prolong clotting tests such as PT, INR, and activated partial thromboplastin time (aPTT), but changes in these tests are subject to a high degree of variability, and not useful in monitoring the anticoagulation effect of these drugs.

Pharmacokinetics

(See Table 8.1.1.)

Practical points

1. *Doses*
   - Prevention of stroke and systemic embolism in patients with NVAF: 5mg bd. Reduce to 2.5mg bd in patients with NVAF and at least two of the following characteristics: age ≥80 years, body weight ≤60kg, or creatinine serum levels ≥1.5mg/dL (133micromol/L).
   - Treatment of acute DVT and PE: 10mg bd for the first 7 days, followed by 5mg bd. Short duration of treatment (at least 3 months) should be based on transient risk factors (e.g. recent surgery, trauma, immobilization).

     —*Prevention of recurrent DVT and PE*: 2.5mg bd. When prevention of recurrent DVT and PE is indicated, 2.5mg bd should be initiated, following completion of 6 months of treatment with apixaban 5mg bd or with another anticoagulant.

- Apixaban should be discontinued at least 48h prior to elective surgery or invasive procedures with a moderate or high risk of unacceptable or clinically significant bleeding. Discontinue at least 24h prior to elective surgery or invasive procedures with a low risk of bleeding or where bleeding would be non-critical in location and easily controlled.
- Switching from parenteral anticoagulants to apixaban (and vice versa) can be done at the next scheduled dose, but these medicinal products should not be administered simultaneously.
- Switching from VKA therapy to apixaban: VKA therapy should be discontinued and apixaban started when the INR is <2.
- Switching from apixaban to warfarin: apixaban should be continued for at least 2 days after beginning VKA therapy. Co-administration of apixaban and VKA therapy should be continued until the INR is ≥2.
- Switching from apixaban to anticoagulants other than warfarin: discontinue apixaban, and take the new anticoagulant at the usual time of the next dose of apixaban.
- Switching anticoagulants other than warfarin to apixaban: discontinue the anticoagulant, and begin taking apixaban at the usual time of the next dose of the anticoagulant.
- Renal impairment. No dose adjustment is necessary in patients with mild or moderate renal impairment. In patients with severe renal impairment (CrCl 15–29mL/min): 2.5mg bd. Apixaban is not recommended in patients with CrCl<15mL/min. No dose adjustment is required in patients with mild or moderate hepatic impairment; avoid in severe hepatic impairment.

2. *Side effects*
   - The commonest reason for treatment discontinuation is bleeding that can appear in any location. Anaemia, contusion, epistaxis, haematuria, menorrhagia, haematoma, gingival bleeding, thrombocytopenia, and hypotension. Mucosal bleeding (i.e. epistaxis, gingival, GI, genitourinary) and anaemia occur more frequently during long-term treatment, as compared with VKA treatment. Increased risk of thrombotic events after premature discontinuation.
     —Post-procedural haemorrhage or haematoma, wound haemorrhage, vessel puncture site haematoma, and catheter site haemorrhage. Ecchymosis, skin haemorrhage, petechiae.
     —If life-threatening bleeding occurs, delay the next dose or discontinue the drug. For serious bleeding, andexanet alfa (a selective factor Xa antidote; see ➔ Andexanet alfa, pp. 454–5), activated prothrombin complex concentrates (aPCCs) or recombinant activated factor VII may be considered.
   - Other: dizziness, headache, hypotension, allergic reactions, tachycardia, increase in transaminase levels. Nausea, increases in blood alkaline phosphatase, blood bilirubin, aspartate aminotransferase, and gamma-glutamyltransferase levels.
3. *Drug interactions*
   - Apixaban is a substrate of CYP3A4, P-gp and breast cancer resistance protein (BCRP).
   - Co-administration of antiplatelet agents, fibrinolytics, anticoagulants, aspirin, chronic NSAIDs, dipyridamole, dextran, and sulfinpyrazone

increases the risk of bleeding. A 50–60% increase in anti-factor Xa activity was observed when apixaban was co-administered with enoxaparin or naproxen.

- In healthy subjects, apixaban did not meaningfully alter the pharmacokinetics of digoxin, naproxen, atenolol, prasugrel, or ASA.
- Avoid the concomitant use of apixaban with strong inhibitors of both CYP3A4 and P-gp inhibitors: abiraterone, aprepitant, crizotinib, enzalutamide, HIV-protease inhibitors, idelalisib, imatinib, itraconazole, ketoconazole, posoconazole or voriconazole.
- Caution (reduce the dose to 2.5mg bd) if apixaban is co-administered with amiodarone, clarithromycin, ciclosporin, diltiazem, erythromycin, lapatinib, naproxen, nilotinib, paclitaxel, pazopanib, prednisone, quinidine, sirolimus, tacrolimus, tamoxifen or temserolimus. These drugs increase apixaban exposure and the risk of bleeding.
- Strong dual inducers of CYP3A4 and P-gp (dexamethasone, doxorubicin, rifampicin, St John's wort, sunitinib, vandetanib, vermurafenib, vinblastine) decrease the exposure to apixaban and its anticoagulant activity, increasing the risk of stroke and other thromboembolic events. Avoid the combination.

4. *Cautions*
   - The risk of bleeding increases in patients with: congenital or acquired bleeding disorders, concomitant use of drugs that increase the risk of bleeding, uncontrolled severe hypertension, active or recent GI ulceration, other GI diseases without active ulceration that can potentially lead to bleeding complications (e.g. known or suspected oesophageal varices, inflammatory bowel disease, oesophagitis, gastritis, and gastroesophageal reflux disease), presence of malignant neoplasms, vascular retinopathy, recent intracranial or intracerebral haemorrhage, intraspinal or intracerebral vascular abnormalities, recent brain, spinal, or ophthalmic surgery, and hepatic (Child–Pugh B) and renal impairment (CrCl <30mL/min). Patients need to be carefully observed for signs of bleeding. Caution is recommended under conditions with an increased risk of bleeding.
   - When neuraxial anaesthesia (spinal/epidural anaesthesia) or spinal/epidural puncture is employed, patients are at risk of developing an epidural or a spinal haematoma, which can result in long-term or permanent paralysis. Wait at least 18h after the dose, before removing the catheter, and do not give the next dose until at least 6h after catheter removal.
   - Because of their short t½, it is critically important to educate the patient about the importance of strict adherence to treatment. Apixaban should not be discontinued, because of the rapid decline of the protective anticoagulation effect. In patients in whom low compliance is suspected, a VKA is preferred.
   - Patients with elevated liver aminotransferases (>2 times ULN or total bilirubin ≤1.5 times ULN) were excluded in clinical trials.
   - Tablets can be swallowed or may be crushed and suspended in 60mL of water and promptly delivered through an NG tube.
   - Laboratory testing of haemoglobin/haematocrit could be of value to detect occult bleeding.

5. *Pregnancy and lactation*
    - Apixaban should be used during pregnancy only if the benefit outweighs the risks (Pregnancy category B). It is unknown whether apixaban is excreted in human milk.
6. *Contraindications*
    - Hypersensitivity to the active substance or to any of the excipients.
    - Impaired haemostasis.
    - Clinically significant active bleeding.
    - Hepatic disease associated with coagulopathy and clinically relevant bleeding risk, including cirrhotic patients with Child–Pugh B and C.
    - Caution in conditions considered a significant risk factor for major bleeding: current or recent GI ulceration, presence of malignant neoplasms, recent brain or spinal injury, recent brain, spinal, or ophthalmic surgery, recent intracranial haemorrhage, known or suspected oesophageal varices, arteriovenous malformations, vascular aneurysms, or major intraspinal or intracerebral vascular abnormalities.
    - Patients with prosthetic heart valves.
    - Uncontrolled severe hypertension.
    - Severe renal impaiment (CrCl<15mL/min).
    - Pregnant and breastfeeding women.
    - Concomitant treatment with any other anticoagulants, except under specific circumstances of switching oral anticoagulant therapy or when UFH is given at doses necessary to maintain an open central venous or arterial catheter.

Argatroban

Synthetic L-arginine derivative acting as a highly selective direct thrombin inhibitor (molecular weight 526Da).

Indications

- Anticoagulation in adults with HIT type II who require parenteral antithrombotic therapy. The diagnosis should be confirmed by the heparin-induced platelet activation assay (HIPAA) or an equivalent test.

Mechanism of action

Argatroban is a direct thrombin inhibitor that reversibly binds to the thrombin active site, independently of antithrombin III. Argatroban exerts its anticoagulant effects by inhibiting thrombin-catalysed reactions, including fibrin formation, activation of coagulation factors (V, VIII, and XIII) and protein C, and platelet aggregation. Argatroban inhibits both free and clot-associated thrombin, but it does not interact with heparin-induced antibodies. Anticoagulant parameters return to baseline within 2–4h after drug discontinuation. There was no evidence of formation of antibodies against argatroban in patients who received multiple doses of argatroban.

Pharmacodynamics

Argatroban reduces the incidence of individual endpoints (mortality, new thrombosis, amputation) in patients with HIT type II, without and with thromboembolic complications. At doses of up to 40mcg/kg/min, argatroban increases, in a dose-dependent fashion, the aPTT, ACT, INR, and thrombin time (TT) in healthy volunteers and cardiac patients.

Pharmacokinetics

Upon initiation of argatroban IV infusion, anticoagulant effects reached steady-state levels within 1–3h and are maintained until the infusion is discontinued or the dosage adjusted. It is metabolized by hydroxylation and aromatization in the liver via CYP3A4/5. An active metabolite (M1) exerts 40-fold weaker anticoagulant effects than argatroban. Argatroban is excreted primarily in the faeces, presumably through biliary secretion. Its t½ is approximately 52min. No dose adjustment is necessary by age or renal function, but argatroban is contraindicated in patients with severe hepatic impairment. Upon cessation of argatroban infusion in hepatically impaired patients, full reversal of anticoagulant effects may require longer than 4h due to decreased drug clearance. (See Table 8.1.1.)

Practical points

1. *Doses*
   - Initial dosage: 2mcg/kg/min, administered as a continuous IV infusion (maximum dose: 10mcg/kg/min). Before its administration, heparin therapy should be discontinued and a baseline aPTT value obtained. The maximum recommended duration of treatment is 14 days.
   - Therapy is monitored using the aPTT (target range for steady-state aPTT is 1.5–3.0 times the initial baseline value, but not exceeding 100s). The aPTT should be checked 2h after the start of the infusion to confirm that the aPTT is within the desired therapeutic range.

If the aPTT is >100s, the infusion should be discontinued until the aPTT is within the desired range, and the infusion restarted at one half of the previous infusion rate. Thereafter, the aPTT should be monitored at least once daily.

2. *Side effects*
   - Common: anaemia, DVT, nausea, purpura. Haemorrhage can occur at any site of the body. An unexplained fall in haematocrit, a fall in BP, or any other unexplained symptom should lead to consideration of a haemorrhagic event.
   - Other: headache, diarrhoea, abdominal pain, hypotension, bradycardia, cardiac arrest, myocardial ischaemia, arterial thrombosis, and AF.
   - Allergic reactions: coughing, dyspnoea, rash, vasodilatation. They occurred in patients who concomitantly received thrombolytic therapy (e.g. streptokinase) or contrast media.
3. *Drug interactions*
   - If argatroban is to be initiated after cessation of heparin therapy, allow sufficient time for the effect of heparin on the aPTT to decrease (about 1–2h) before initiation of argatroban therapy.
   - Concomitant use of argatroban and warfarin prolongs the PT/INR.
   - Concomitant use with antiplatelet agents, thrombolytics, and other anticoagulants may increase the risk of bleeding.
   - There are no interactions between argatroban and aspirin, paracetamol, or erythromycin.
   - Argatroban contains ethanol; possible interaction with metronidazole or disulfiram.
4. *Cautions*
   - Use with caution in patients with hepatic failure and clinical circumstances with an increased risk of haemorrhage: severe hypertension; diabetic retinopathy; immediately following a lumbar puncture; spinal anaesthesia; major surgery, especially involving the brain, the spinal cord, or the eye; haematological conditions associated with increased bleeding tendencies such as congenital or acquired bleeding disorders, and GI lesions such as ulcerations.
   - Parenteral anticoagulants should be discontinued before administration of argatroban. Concomitant use with oral anticoagulants may result in prolongation of the PT/INR beyond that produced by oral anticoagulants alone.
   - Caution in patients with hepatic disease; start with a lower dose, and monitor the aPTT closely in patients with hepatic failure, and adjust the dosage as clinically indicated.
   - In patients who underwent PCI, arterial and venous sheaths were removed no sooner than 2h after discontinuation of argatroban and when the ACT is <160s.
   - Obtain an ACT before dosing, 5–10min after bolus dosing, following adjustments in the infusion rate, and at the end of a PCI procedure. Additional ACTs should be determined every 20–30min during a prolonged procedure.
   - Avoid in patients with rare hereditary problems of fructose intolerance.
   - There is no specific antidote to argatroban.

- Measure the INR daily while argatroban and warfarin are co-administered. Argatroban injection can be discontinued when the INR is >4. After argatroban is discontinued, repeat the INR measurement in 4–6h. If the repeat INR is below the desired therapeutic range, resume the infusion of argatroban injection, and repeat the procedure daily until the desired therapeutic range on warfarin alone is reached.

5. *Pregnancy and lactation*
   - There are no adequate data in pregnant women and on the passage of argatroban into human milk (Pregnancy category B).
6. *Contraindications*
   - Uncontrolled bleeding.
   - Patients with a history of hypersensitivity to argatroban.
   - Severe hepatic impairment.

Aspirin (acetylsalicylic acid)

COX inhibitor.

CV indications

- Secondary prevention of MI. Reduces the combined risk of death and non-fatal MI in patients with a previous MI or UA.
- Prevention of CV morbidity in patients with chronic stable angina. In patients with a history of UA, except during the acute phase.
- Prevention of graft occlusion after CABG.
- Coronary angioplasty, except during the acute phase.
- Secondary prevention of TIAs and ischaemic CVAs, provided intracerebral haemorrhages have been ruled out.
- Treatment of acute and/or recurrent pericarditis.
- Aspirin is recommended in all patients with CAD, unless contraindicated.

At concentrations much higher than those currently used for secondary prevention, aspirin has analgesic, antipyretic, and anti-inflammatory actions due to its inhibitory effect on prostaglandin synthesis. As an NSAID, it is also used in pericarditis, rheumatic fever, and Kawasaki's disease.

Mechanism of action

Aspirin irreversibly blocks COX-1, the rate-limiting enzyme that catalyses the conversion of arachidonic acid into prostaglandin H2, which is further modified by tissue-specific isomerases into bioactive lipids (prostanoids), including PGI2 (prostacyclin), D2, E2, and F2α, and thromboxane A2 (TXA2). Platelets contain only COX-1, which converts arachidonic acid to TXA2, which activates thromboxane (TP) receptors, causes changes in platelet shape, and induces platelet aggregation by increasing the expression GPIIb/IIIa receptors in the cell membrane of platelets.

Aspirin inhibits TXA2-dependent platelet aggregation by irreversibly acetylating Ser^{529} of COX-1 and Ser^{516} of COX-2, but is approximately 170-fold more potent in inhibiting COX-1 than COX-2. As a result, aspirin decreases the production of PGI2 and TXA2. These effects are observed before ASA is detectable in peripheral blood, due to presystemic acetylation of platelet COX and inhibition of TXA2 formation in the portal circulation. However, endothelial cells regenerate active COX-1 within hours, while mature platelets are unable to synthesize COX-1, so that the antiplatelet effects of aspirin last for the duration of the platelet life (approximately 7–10 days). Although it may take 10 days to renew the total platelet population and to restore normal COX activity, if as little as 20% of platelets have normal COX activity, haemostasis may be normal.

Pharmacodynamics

Due to a favourable benefit/risk ratio and its low cost, low-dose aspirin (75–150mg/day) remains the cornerstone of pharmacological prevention of arterial thrombosis, being the antiplatelet drug of choice in all patients with chronic stable angina, UA, or MI in whom it is not contraindicated. In patients with unstable angina, aspirin reduces the incidence of MI or sudden death and major vascular events (vascular events, vascular death, all-cause mortality, stroke). A single dose of 100mg of aspirin effectively abolishes the production of TXA2, but the maximum antithrombotic effect occurs after 48h; thus, higher doses (140–450mg) should be given at the onset of symptoms of acute MI or UA. In patients with acute MI, aspirin reduces 5-week vascular mortality.

A meta-analysis of 16 secondary prevention trials showed that long-term aspirin in a wide range of patients with high CV risk (previous history of MI, stroke or TIAs, or some major CV events) produces a significant reduction in the incidence of new CV events.

Pharmacokinetics

Aspirin is rapidly and almost completely absorbed in the stomach and small intestine (bioavailability 25–45%) and reaches the C_{max} within 15–20min, and platelet function is inhibited within 1h. Absorption is delayed by the presence of food but is increased by antacids. Aspirin is rapidly biotransformed by plasma and liver esterases into salicylic acid, being undetectable 1–2h after dosing (t½ of approximately 15–20min). Low-dose enteric-coated aspirin is often prescribed to avoid GI side effects; this delivers aspirin to the duodenum, rather than the stomach, and decreases oral bioavailability, with a risk of suboptimal clinical response. Salicylic acid reaches peak plasma levels within 1–2h, binds to plasma proteins (90–99%), and is widely distributed (Vd 0.1–0.2L/kg), reaching the CNS, fetal tissues, and breast milk. At low doses (<250mg), salicylic acid is glucoconjugated in the liver with glycine (salicyluric acid) and, to a lesser extent, with glucuronic acid and several other metabolites that are excreted in the urine (salicyluric acid 75%, free salicylic acid 10%); the elimination t½ is 2–4h. Urinary excretion of salicylic acid is markedly pH-dependent; there is a 10- to 20-fold increase in renal clearance (from 5% to >80%) when the urine pH is increased from 5 to 8. (See Table 8.1.7.)

Practical points

1. *Doses*
   - Recommended dose: 75–160mg od. In some circumstances, a higher dose (up to 300mg) may be appropriate. In post-coronary bypass surgery, aspirin should be started within 48h of surgery and continued indefinitely.
   - Secondary prevention of TIA and ischaemic CVAs, provided intracerebral haemorrhages have been ruled out: 75–325mg od.
   - Acute MI: a loading dose of 150–450mg as soon as possible after onset of symptoms.
   - NSTEMI: aspirin is recommended for all patients without contraindications, with an initial oral loading dose of 150–300mg (in aspirin-naïve patients) and a long-term maintenance dose of 75–100mg/day, regardless of the treatment strategy.
   - Acute pericarditis: 500–1000mg every 6–8h (1.5–4g/day).
2. *Common side effects*
   - Inhibition of the COX-1-mediated production of prostaglandins in gastric mucosal cells increases the risk of GI adverse effects: dyspepsia, nausea, vomiting, heartburn, gastritis, GI ulcers, and bleeding. Even at low doses (50–75mg/day), aspirin increases the

Table 8.1.7 Pharmacokinetic characteristics of platelet anti-aggregants

Drugs	F (%)	T_{max} (h)	PPB (%)	Vd (L/kg)	Metabolism	t½ (h)	Renal excretion (%)
Aspirin	25–45	2–4	90–99	0.1–0.2	Hydrolysis	0.25	85–90
Cangrelor (IV)	–	2min	98	0.01	Dephosphorylation	2.5–6min	51
Cilostazol		2.7	95–98	–	CYP3A4 (2C19, 1A2)	11–13	<2
Clopidogrel	30–50	1	94–98	5.3–8.5	CYP1A2, 2B6, 2C9, 2C19, 3A4/5	6	50
Dipyridamole	60%	1.5–2	97–98	1.3	Glucoconjugation	10–15	5
Prasugrel	>79	0.5	98	0.6–1	CYP3A4, 2B6 (2C9, 2C19)	7	68
Ticagrelor	36	1.5–5	99	1.25	CYP3A4	7–10	<1
Ticlopidine	>80		98	–	Extensive	4–5 days	60
Vorapaxar	100	1-2	>99	6	CYP3A4, CYP2J2	187 (115–317)	0

F, oral bioavailability; h, hour; IV, intravenous; min, minute; PPB, protein plasma binding; t½, drug half-life; T_{max}, time to peak plasma levels; Vd, volume of distribution.

risk of upper GI events by 2- to 4-fold; the risk can be partly reduced with buffered or enteric-coated preparations or by taking aspirin with food. The risk of GI adverse effects increases in the elderly and in patients with a history of prior GI events, or when aspirin is co-administered with other NSAIDs, clopidogrel, or warfarin or with 'natural' supplements with COX-2-inhibiting properties (i.e. garlic extracts, curcumin, bilberry, pine bark, ginkgo, fish oil, resveratrol, genistein, quercetin, or resorcinol).

- Major (haemorrhagic stroke) and minor bleeding (epistaxis, haematuria, melaena, bruising) occurs frequently in patients taking aspirin. Thrombocytopenia, anaemia.
- Others: dizziness, tinnitus, bruising, water and salt retention; hyperuricaemia, deterioration in renal function.
- Allergic responses to aspirin (hives, facial swelling, anaphylactic shock, skin rash, and asthmatic reactions) are rare. Aspirin may precipitate bronchospasm in patients with asthma or NSAID-precipitated bronchospasm. Risk factors are existing asthma, hay fever, nasal polyps, chronic respiratory diseases, or a history of allergic reactions to other substances. Serious skin reactions, including SJS, have been rarely reported. Discontinue aspirin at the first appearance of any sign of hypersensitivity.
- Aspirin inhibits renal prostaglandin synthesis and can cause hyperkalaemia by inducing a hyporenin–hypoaldosteronic state.

3. *Interactions*
   - The risk of bleeding is increased when aspirin is co-administered with warfarin, heparin, antiplatelets, alcohol, corticosteroids, other NSAIDs, SSRIs (sertraline, paroxetine), and venlafaxine. If GI bleeding or ulceration occurs, treatment should be withdrawn.
   - Aspirin inhibits the synthesis of prostaglandins and can decrease the antihypertensive effects of ACEIs, ARBs, thiazides, spironolactone, and β-blockers. Aspirin inhibits the increase in renal prostaglandins produced by ACEIs and loop diuretics.
   - Aspirin impairs the renal excretion of digoxin and lithium, increasing their plasma concentrations. Monitoring of plasma concentrations and dose adjustment of digoxin and lithium are recommended.
   - Aspirin can displace a number of drugs from their protein-binding sites in blood, including antidiabetic drugs (increase the risk of hypoglycaemia), warfarin, phenytoin, valproic acid, and other NSAIDs.
   - Aspirin displaces methotrexate from plasma proteins and reduces its renal excretion. Thus, the use of methotrexate (at doses of >15mg/week) with aspirin 75mg is contraindicated.
   - Aspirin reduces the renal excretion of uric acid and may exacerbate hyperuricaemia and precipitate gout, especially in combination with thiazide diuretics.
   - Aspirin may reduce the efficacy of uricosuric drugs (i.e. sulfinpyrazone).
   - Liver enzyme inducers (see Table 8.1.2) decrease the efficacy of aspirin.
   - The hypoglycaemic effect of sulfonylureas and insulins may be enhanced by aspirin.

- Co-administration of aspirin with ciclosporin or tacrolimus may increase the risk of nephrotoxicity. Monitor the renal function.
- The excretion of aspirin may be increased by alkaline urine, which can occur with some antacids.

4. *Cautions/notes*
   - Aspirin resistance, defined as the inability of aspirin to reduce platelet production of TXA2, and thereby platelet activation and aggregation, can appear in up to 25% of patients and may correlate with an increasing risk of CV events. Potential causes include poor patient compliance, inadequate dose, drug interactions, type of aspirin used (e.g. enteric versus non-enteric-coated), genetics (polymorphisms in COX-1 and other genes involved in TXA2 biosynthesis), upregulation of non-platelet sources of TXA2 biosynthesis, increased platelet turnover, and drug interactions (e.g. ibuprofen).
   - There is an increased risk of haemorrhage, particularly during or after operative procedures (even a tooth extraction). Use with caution before surgery, and temporary discontinuation of treatment may be necessary.
   - Caution in patients receiving concomitant medications which could increase the risk of ulceration (oral corticosteroids, SSRIs, deferasirox).
   - Aspirin is not recommended during menorrhagia, as it may increase menstrual bleeding.
   - Aspirin may increase the risk of haemorrhagic stroke, and patients with haemophilia or other bleeding tendencies should not take aspirin.
   - Aspirin can cause haemolytic anaemia in people who have the genetic disease glucose-6-phosphate dehydrogenase (G6PD) deficiency.
   - In patients who develop GI side effects while taking aspirin and in those with an increased risk of GI bleeding, a PPI should be used.
   - Aspirin has been associated with Reye's syndrome in children. Children and teenagers should not use aspirin for chickenpox or flu symptoms before a doctor is consulted.
   - Avoid aspirin in patients with CrCl of <10mL/min and with severe hepatic impairment.
   - Aspirin inhibits the kidney's ability to excrete uric acid, and thus, it should not be prescribed in patients with hyperuricaemia or gout.
   - Some NSAIDs (e.g. ibuprofen, naproxen) may reversibly block COX-1, preventing the irreversible inhibition by aspirin and cardioprotection and stroke prevention and causing potentially prothrombotic effects via COX-2 inhibition. This combination should be avoided.
   - Aspirin should be administered with caution in patients with asthma or NSAID-induced bronchospasm, dyspepsia, or iron deficiency anaemia.
   - Elderly patients who are more prone to adverse events.
   - With caution in dehydrated patients because NSAIDs may deteriorate renal function.
   - Aspirin tablets contain lactose. Avoid in patients with galactose intolerance, Lapp lactase deficiency, or glucose–galactose malabsorption.
   - Low doses of aspirin are not suitable as an antipyretic, anti-inflammatory agent, or analgesic.

5. *Pregnancy and lactation*
    - Aspirin should be avoided in pregnancy and lactation (Pregnancy category D). Aspirin produces alterations in maternal and neonatal haemostasis, decreases birthweight, and increases perinatal mortality, and because of the risk of premature closure of the ductus arteriosus *in utero*, it should be avoided in the third trimester of pregnancy. It should be avoided 1 week before labour and delivery, because it may increase the risk of haemorrhage; additionally, it may delay the onset and prolong labour. Aspirin is excreted into breast milk.
6. *Contraindications*
    - Active, or a history of, recurrent peptic ulcer and/or gastric/GI haemorrhage or other kinds of bleeding such as cerebrovascular haemorrhages, haemorrhagic diathesis, and coagulation disorders (i.e. haemophilia and thrombocytopenia).
    - Severe renal and hepatic impairment.
    - Hypersensitivity to salicylic acid compounds or prostaglandin synthetase inhibitors and to any of the excipients.
    - Late pregnancy and lactation. Doses of >100mg/day during the third trimester of pregnancy.
    - Gout.
    - Methotrexate used at doses of >15mg/week.

Atenolol

Cardioselective β1-adrenergic receptor antagonist (see also ➲ Beta-adrenergic blocking agents, pp. 485–94).

CV indications

Treatment of hypertension, angina pectoris, cardiac dysrhythmias, and MI (early intervention in the acute phase and improvement of long-term prognosis following MI).

Pharmacokinetics

Oral bioavailability is decreased by 20% when taken with food. The duration of action is longer (approximately 24h) than its t½. Reduce the dose in patients with renal and hepatic impairment. (See Table 8.1.8.)

Practical points

1. *Doses*
   - PO: 50–100mg od or 50mg bd for hypertension or angina; dose adjusted to achieve a resting heart rate of 50–60bpm.
   - IV (cardiac arrhythmias): 2.5–5mg over 10min, under careful monitoring. The dose can be repeated at 5-min intervals, until a response is observed or a maximum dosage of 10mg.
   - MI: within 12h of the onset of MI, give 5–10mg IV (1mg/min), followed by 50mg PO 15min later. Another 50mg PO 12h after the IV dose, and then 12h later by 100mg PO od. If bradycardia and/or hypotension appear, atenolol should be discontinued.
2. *Side effects* (see ➲ Beta-adrenergic blocking agents, pp. 485–94)
3. *Interactions* (see ➲ Beta-adrenergic blocking agents, pp. 485–94)
4. *Cautions/notes* (see ➲ Beta-adrenergic blocking agents, pp. 485–94)
5. *Pregnancy and lactation* (see ➲ Beta-adrenergic blocking agents, pp. 485–94)
   - Atenolol crosses the placenta and appears in cord blood. Controlled data in human pregnancy exist only for atenolol in the second and third trimesters of pregnancy (Pregnancy category D). Atenolol is excreted in breast milk.
6. *Contraindications* (see ➲ Beta-adrenergic blocking agents, pp. 485–94)

Table 8.1.8 Pharmacokinetic properties of beta-adrenergic blockers

Drug	F (%)	T_{max} (h)	PPB (%)	Vd (L/kg)	Metabolism	t½ (h)	Renal excretion* (%)
Acebutolol	40	1–4	25	1–3	Carboxylesterase 2 and CYP2C19	11	40
Atenolol	55	2–4	<5	0.7–1.2	Poor metabolism	6–9	90
Bisoprolol	90	2–4	30	3	CYP3A4 (2D6)	9–12	50
Carvedilol	25	1–3	95–99	1.5–2	CYP2D6, CYP2C9 (minor CYP3A4, 2C19, 1A2, 2E1)	6–10	16
Esmolol (IV)	–	2min	55	3.4	Erythrocyte esterases	9min	<1
Labetalol	25	1–2	90	3.2–13.5	Conjugation	6–8	<5
Metoprolol	40–50	1.5–2	12	3.5	CYP2D6	3–5	3
Nadolol	30	2–4	30	2	Not metabolized	20–24	75
Nebivolol	12–96	1.5–4	98	1.5	CYP2D6	10	<1
Oxprenolol	25–60	0.5–1.5	80–90	1.3	*O*-glucuronidation	1–3	<5
Propranolol	25	2	90	4	CYP2D6, CYP1A2	3–4 (8–11**)	<1
Sotalol	90–100	2.5–4	0	1.5–2.5	Not metabolized	7–18	75
Timolol	50–75	0.4–3	10	1.8–3.5	CYP2D6	3–5	20

F, oral bioavailability; h, hour; IV, intravenous; min, minute; PPB, protein plasma binding; SC, subcutaneous; t½, drug half-life; T_{max}, time to peak plasma levels; Vd, volume of distribution.

* Renal excretion without biotransformation.

** Slow-release formulation.

Atorvastatin

Oral HMG CoA reductase inhibitor (see also ➲ Statins (3-hydroxy-3-methylglutaryl-coenzyme A reductase inhibitors), pp. 760–3).

Specific indications

- Hypercholesterolaemia as an adjunct to diet to reduce:
  - Elevated total cholesterol (total-C), LDL-C, Apo B, and TG in adults, adolescents, and children aged 10 years or older with primary hypercholesterolaemia, including familial hypercholesterolaemia (heterozygous familial and non-familial) or combined (mixed) hyperlipidaemia (Fredrickson types IIa and IIb) when the response to diet and other non-pharmacological measures is inadequate.
  - Total-C and LDL-C in adults with homozygous familial hypercholesterolaemia as an adjunct to other lipid-lowering treatments (e.g. PCSK9 inhibitors, LDL apheresis) or if such treatments are unavailable.
- Prevention of CV events in adult patients estimated to have a high risk for a first CV event, as an adjunct to correction of other risk factors.

Pharmacodynamics

At doses of 10–80mg/day, atorvastatin reduces LDL-C (22–55%), total-C (17–55%), and TG (12–25%) levels and increases HDL-C levels (3–10%). Blood lipid levels should be checked 2–4 weeks after starting therapy, and the dosage adjusted accordingly.

Pharmacokinetics

Atorvastatin is rapidly absorbed but presents low bioavailability (approximately 12%), due to presystemic clearance in the GI mucosa and/or hepatic first-pass metabolism. Antacids can decrease drug absorption. Atorvastatin is also a substrate of intestinal P-gp, which pumps the drug back into the intestinal lumen during drug absorption. It is metabolized by CYP450 3A4 into active metabolites, which explains why the inhibitory activity for HMG CoA reductase is longer (approximately 20–30h) than the pharmacokinetic t½ of atorvastatin. Plasma concentrations are markedly increased in chronic alcoholic liver disease and in patients with Child–Pugh B disease. In patients aged >65 years, the mean AUC and C_{max} values are higher (40% and 30%, respectively) and show a greater pharmacodynamic response to atorvastatin. (See Table 8.1.4.)

Practical points

1. *Doses*
   - Primary hypercholesterolaemia and combined (mixed) hyperlipidaemia: 10mg od at any time of the day, with or without food (maximum: 80mg daily). Doses may be individualized, according to baseline LDL-C levels, the goal of therapy, and patient response. Dose adjustments should be made at intervals of 4 weeks or more. No dose adjustment is needed in patients with renal dysfunction or haemodialysis.
   - Homozygous familial hypercholesterolaemia: 10–80mg/day.
   - Prevention of CV disease: 10–80mg/day. Because advanced age (≥65 years) is a predisposing factor for myopathy, atorvastatin should be prescribed with caution in the elderly.

2. *Side effects* (see ➔ Statins (3-hydroxy-3-methylglutaryl-coenzyme A reductase inhibitors), pp. 760–3)
   - Elevated serum ALT levels are reported in 0.4–1.3%. Clinically important (>3 times ULN) elevations in serum ALT occurred in 0.7%.
   - Elevated serum CPK levels (>3 times ULN in 2.5%; >10 times ULN in 0.4%).
3. *Interactions* (see ➔ Statins (3-hydroxy-3-methylglutaryl-coenzyme A reductase inhibitors), pp. 760–3)
   - Administer atorvastatin with caution in patients treated with potent CYP3A4 inhibitors (see Table 8.1.2). The starting dose of atorvastatin should be 10mg od, and the maximum dose 20mg od.
   - In patients taking HIV PIs (nelfinavir, tipranavir) or hepatitis C PIs (boceprevir), the maximum dose of atorvastatin should be limited to 40mg.
   - In patients treated with ciclosporin, fibrates, erythromycin, or telaprevir, atorvastatin should be avoided. Do not administer with tipranavir/ritonavir.
   - Efavirenz and etravirine decrease atorvastatin's AUC.
   - Cases of myopathy, including rhabdomyolysis, when atorvastatin is co-administered with colchicine.
   - Atorvastatin increase the plasma levels of digoxin. Monitor plasma digoxin levels.
   - Atorvastatin increases the plasma levels of some oral contraceptives (norethindrone and ethinylestradiol).
   - There is no interaction with warfarin or clopidogrel.
4. *Cautions/notes* (see ➔ Statins (3-hydroxy-3-methylglutaryl-coenzyme A reductase inhibitors), pp. 760–3)
   - An appropriate clinical assessment for any signs or symptoms of muscle pain, tenderness, or weakness is recommended in patients receiving CYP34A inhibitors (see Table 8.1.2), particularly during initial titration, to ensure that the lowest dose of atorvastatin is employed.
   - Avoid doses of atorvastatin of >10mg/day when co-administered with ciclosporin, tacrolimus, everolimus, or sirolimus, without close monitoring of CPK and signs/symptoms of myopathy.
5. *Contraindications* (see ➔ Statins (3-hydroxy-3-methylglutaryl-coenzyme A reductase inhibitors), pp. 760–3)

Atropine

Indications

- Treatment of haemodynamically compromising bradycardia and/or AVB due to excessive vagal tone in emergency situations.
- Cardiopulmonary resuscitation: to treat symptomatic bradycardia and AVB.
- As a pre-anaesthetic medication to prevent vagal reactions associated with tracheal intubation and surgical manipulation.
- To block the muscarinic effects of neostigmine, when given post-surgically to counteract non-depolarizing muscle relaxants.
- As an antidote for CV collapse following an overdose of anticholinesterase inhibitors, e.g. anticholinesterases, organophosphorus, carbamates, and muscarinic mushrooms.

Mechanism of action

Atropine competitively antagonizes the effects of acetylcholine on smooth and cardiac muscles, exocrine glands, and the CNS. Peripheral effects include tachycardia (up to 90bpm, sometimes preceded by an initial transient bradycardia), increased AV conduction, decreased production of saliva, sweat, and bronchial, nasal, lacrimal, and gastric secretions, decreased intestinal motility, and inhibition of micturition. Atropine does not modify cardiac contractility and BP but relaxes bronchial smooth muscle, producing bronchodilatation.

Pharmacokinetics

After IV injection of atropine, a peak increase in the heart rate occurs within 2–4min; peak plasma levels after IM administration are reached within 30min, but peak effects on the heart, sweating, and salivation may occur after 1h. Atropine is rapidly and widely distributed, crosses the placental barrier, and enters the fetal circulation. It binds poorly (20%) to plasma proteins and is hydrolysed mainly in the liver, and 50% of the dose is excreted unchanged in the urine. The elimination t½ is 2–5h (increases in children under 2 years and in the elderly). Atropine is not removed by dialysis.

Practical points

1. *Doses*
   - Treatment of haemodynamically compromising bradycardia, AVB, and cardiopulmonary resuscitation. Sinus bradycardia: 0.5mg IV every 2–5min until the desired heart rate is achieved. AVB: 0.5mg IV every 3–5min (maximum dose 3mg). Cardiac resuscitation: 0.5mg IV, repeated at 5-min intervals until the desired heart rate is achieved. In asystole, 3mg may be given IV as a single dose.
   - Pre-anaesthetic medication: 0.3–0.6mg IM 30–60min before surgery or the same dose IV immediately before surgery.
   - To control the muscarinic side effects of neostigmine: 0.6–1.2mg IV.
   - Anticholinesterase poisoning: 1–2mg IM or IV, repeated every 5–60min until signs and symptoms disappear.

2. *Common side effects*
   - Common: dry mouth (a dose-limiting effect) and skin, blurred vision, mydriasis, photophobia, tachycardia, palpitations, flushing, constipation, nausea, and urinary retention.
   - Restlessness, disorientation, confusion; at high doses: hallucinations, restlessness, and delirium. Mental confusion and/or excitement may occur, especially in the elderly.
   - Reduced bronchial secretions may cause the formation of thick bronchial plugs that are difficult to eject from the respiratory tract. Anaphylaxis, urticaria, and rash, occasionally progressing to exfoliation, may develop in some patients.
   - These adverse effects can be antagonized with physostigmine.
3. *Interactions*
   - The adverse effects of atropine are enhanced by drugs with anticholinergic activity: tricyclic antidepressants, antispasmodics, some anti-parkinsonian drugs and antihistamines (diphenhydramine), phenothiazines, disopyramide, and quinidine.
   - By delaying gastric emptying, atropine may alter the absorption of other drugs.
4. *Cautions*
   - In patients with prostatic enlargement, atonia in the elderly, pyloric stenosis.
   - Renal or hepatic insufficiency.
   - COPD because reduction in bronchial secretions may lead to the formation of bronchial plugs.
   - Elderly patients are more susceptible to adverse effects.
   - Avoid in patients with myasthenia gravis (unless given with anticholinesterase).
   - Atropine should not delay external pacing for unstable patients, particularly those with high-degree (Mobitz type II second-degree or third-degree) block.
   - Atropine should thus be used with caution in patients with tachyarrhythmias, CHF, CAD, or hyperthyroidism.
5. *Pregnancy and lactation*
   - It is not known whether atropine can cause fetal harm when given to a pregnant woman or can affect reproduction capacity (Pregnancy category C).
6. *Contraindications*
   - Hypersensitivity to atropine.
   - Risk of urinary retention because of prostatic or urethral disease.
   - Achalasia of the oesophagus, paralytic ileus, toxic megacolon.
   - Closed-angle glaucoma.
   - Other contraindications are not applicable to the use of atropine in life-threatening emergencies.

Bendroflumethiazide

Oral thiazide diuretic.

CV and other indications

(See ➔ Thiazide and related diuretics, pp. 768–73.)

- Treatment of essential hypertension alone or as an adjunct to other antihypertensive drugs.
- Treatment of oedema of cardiac, renal, or hepatic origin, iatrogenic oedema, and premenstrual syndrome.

Pharmacodynamics

A low dose (1.25mg od) of bendroflumethiazide reduces BP without metabolic side effects. Doses above 2.5mg od do not increase the antihypertensive effects but increase adverse effects. In the Medical Research Council (MRC) Trial, bendroflumethiazide (10mg) reduced the rate of stroke and all CV events in patients with mild hypertension but significantly increased glucose intolerance, impotence, gout, headache, constipation, dizziness, and nausea.

Pharmacokinetics

(See Table 8.1.5.)

Practical points

1. *Doses*
   - For hypertension: 1.25–5mg od in the morning. Higher doses are rarely necessary.
   - For HF: initial dose of 2.5mg od, up to 10mg od.
   - For oedema: initially 5–10mg od in the morning. Maintenance dose: 2.5–5mg 2–3 days in the week.
2. *Side effects* (see ➔ Thiazide and related diuretics, pp. 768–73)
3. *Interactions* (see ➔ Thiazide and related diuretics, pp. 768–73)
   - Bendroflumethiazide prolongs the INR when co-administered with warfarin.
4. *Cautions and contraindications* (see ➔ Thiazide and related diuretics, pp. 768–73)

Beta-adrenergic blocking agents

(See also ➜ Atenolol, p. 478; ➜ Bisoprolol, p. 496; ➜ Carvedilol, pp. 517–18; ➜ Esmolol, pp. 582–3; ➜ Labetalol, p. 636; ➜ Metoprolol, pp. 660–1; ➜ Nadolol, p. 671; ➜ Nebivolol, pp. 673–4; ➜ Propranolol, pp. 713–15; ➜ Sotalol, pp. 754–6.)

β-adrenergic receptor antagonists (β-blockers) bind to, and block, the effects of noradrenaline and adrenaline produced via the stimulation of β-adrenoceptors.

Effects of β-blockers vary, depending on their cardioselectivity, lipophilicity, and ancillary properties. First-generation β-blockers were relatively *non-selective agents*: carteolol, nadolol, penbutolol, propranolol, sotalol, or timolol; they block both β1- and β2-adrenoceptors. By blocking β2-receptors, they may cause vascular and bronchial smooth muscle contraction, increasing the risk of bronchospasm in predisposed individuals. This same quality might, however, explain their benefit in migraine when vasoconstriction could inhibit the attack.

Second-generation β-blockers are the so-called cardioselective agents (acebutolol, atenolol, betaxolol, bisoprolol, celiprolol, or metoprolol). When given in low doses, they are relative selective for the β1- (largely cardiac) receptors. They are preferable in patients with chronic respiratory diseases, those with insulin-requiring diabetes mellitus, and in stroke prevention. Nevertheless, cardioselectivity is lost at high doses, and no β-blocker is safe in an asthmatic patient.

Third-generation vasodilatory agents have added properties, acting chiefly via two mechanisms: (1) direct vasodilatation, possibly mediated by the release of NO, as for carvedilol and nebivolol, (2) stimulation of β2-adrenoceptors or added α-adrenergic blocking properties, as for labetalol and carvedilol. Endothelial β3-receptors mediate vasodilatation induced by NO in response to nebivolol. Nebivolol and carvedilol present additional advantages, as they produce minimal effect on glucose and lipid levels.

Indications

1. *Main CV indications* (see individual drugs)
   - Long-term management of chronic stable angina.
   - Post-MI. Early phase of acute MI: atenolol, metoprolol. During follow-up: carvedilol, metoprolol, propranolol, timolol.
   - Treatment of hypertension (all β-blockers).
     —Severe urgent hypertension: labetalol.
     —Severe perioperative hypertension: esmolol.
     —Hypertensive disorders during pregnancy: labetalol.
   - Treatment of supraventricular and ventricular arrhythmias.
     —Urgent sinus tachycardia, SVT, perioperative tachyarrhythmias: IV esmolol.
     —Sinus node re-entry or in some automatic ATs.
     —Rate control in patients with atrial flutter/AF.
     —Recurrences of AF or atrial flutter: sotalol.
     —Life-threatening ventricular arrhythmias.
   - Treatment of HFrEF, β-blockers are recommended:
     —In patients with asymptomatic LV systolic dysfunction and a history of MI, in order to prevent or delay the onset of HF or prolong life.

—In addition an ACEI (or ARB), for patients with stable, symptomatic HFrEF to reduce the risk of HF hospitalization and death.
- Reduction of early mortality and improvement of long-term prognosis following acute MI.

2. *Other cardiac indications*
   - Hypertrophic obstructive cardiomyopathy: high-dose propranolol.
   - MS with sinus rhythm: β-blockers decrease resting and exercise heart rates, prolong the diastolic filling time, and improve exercise tolerance. In mitral valve prolapse, β-blockers control the associated arrhythmias.
   - Aortic dissecting aneurysms. In the hyperacute phase, propranolol has been replaced by esmolol. Thereafter, oral β-blockade is continued.
   - Marfan's syndrome with aortic root involvement.
   - Fallot's tetralogy: propranolol is effective against the cyanotic spells, probably acting by inhibition of RV contractility.
   - Acquired/congenital LQTS. β-blockers are the first-choice drugs. They are theoretically most effective when the underlying mutation affects K^+ channel-modulated outward currents.
   - CPVT.
   - Neurocardiogenic (vasovagal) syncope to control the episodic adrenergic reflex discharge.
   - Postural tachycardia syndrome (POTS): low doses of propranolol (20mg).
3. *Other indications*
   - Central: glaucoma; essential tremor (propranolol).
   - Thyrotoxicosis: propranolol.
   - Anxiety states. Propranolol (and probably other β-blockers) reduce the peripheral manifestations of anxiety such as tremor and tachycardia.
   - Glaucoma. β-blockers (betaxolol, carteolol, levobunolol, metipranolol, timolol) are indicated in patients with chronic open-angle glaucoma or ocular hypertension.
   - Migraine. Propranolol is used prophylactically to reduce the incidence of migraine attacks.
   - Alcohol withdrawal: atenolol, propranolol.
   - Oesophageal varices. β-blockers (propranolol) may prevent bleeding by reducing portal pressure.
   - Phaeochromocytoma: propranolol in patients treated with an α-blocker.

Mechanism of action

β1-adrenergic receptors are G_s-coupled receptors and, within the heart, mediate positive chronotopic, inotropic, and dromotropic effects in response to stimulation by noradrenaline and adrenaline. By antagonizing these effects, cardioselective β1-blockers reduce heart rate, cardiac contractility, CO and MVO_2, and slow AV nodal conduction velocity. In addition, the decrease in heart rate increases the diastolic filling time and improves cardiac perfusion. Stimulation of β1-adrenoceptors also increase renin release from juxtaglomerular cells, lipolysis in adipose tissue, aqueous humour production, and cardiac apoptosis.

β-adrenergic agonists interact with the β-adrenergic receptor coupled to a G_s, activate adenylyl cyclase, and increases the formation of cAMP. cAMP activates protein kinase A (PKA) to phosphorylate the L-type Ca^{2+} channel, increasing its open probability and extracellular Ca^{2+} entry via the slow inward Ca^{2+} current (I_{CaL}). The entry of Ca^{2+} ions further produce the release of more Ca^{2+} ions from the sarcoplasmic reticulum (SR), leading to a positive inotropic effect. In the SA node, β1-agonists increase the pacemaker current (I_f); this effect, together with the increase in I_{CaL}, produces a positive chronotropic effect. In the AVN, the increase in I_{CaL} accelerates the passage of impulses from the atria to the ventricles (positive dromotropic effect). Additionally, β1-agonists increase the rate of relaxation (lusitropic effect), due to: (1) the phosphorylation of phospholamban by PKA, so that its inhibitory effect on the SR calcium pump (SERCA) is lost and more Ca^{2+} is incorporated in the SR; and (2) the phosphorylation of troponin I, so that the interaction between the myosin heads and actin ends more rapidly. Paradoxically, formation of cAMP in vascular smooth muscle decreases intracellular Ca^{2+}, producing a vasodilator effect. Thus, during exercise, an increase in sympathetic tone makes the heart pump faster and more forcefully, while the coronary blood flow increases.

Pharmacodynamics

- *Hypertension*. β-blockers are no longer recommended as first-line treatment for hypertension in patients without CV risk factors, as they produce modest CV disease reductions and little or no effects on mortality and have been relegated to specific concomitant conditions for secondary prevention. Indeed, β-blockers are less effective than other antihypertensive drugs at preventing major CV events, especially stroke, and, when combined with thiazide diuretics, predispose to new-onset diabetes. Older hypertensives, especially black hypertensives, respond less well to β-blocker monotherapy. β-blockers are also less effective than diuretics, and losartan in elderly hypertensives, especially those with LVH, possibly because at equivalent brachial artery pressures, β-blockers reduce the central aortic pressure less than other agents. Vasodilator β-blockers (carvedilol and nebivolol) did not present this disadvantage. In addition, patients on β-blockers are more likely to discontinue treatment due to adverse effects than those on diuretics and RAAS inhibitors. Nevertheless, β-blockers are still first-choice drugs in hypertensive patients with CAD, HF, AF, tachyarrhythmias, and phaeochromocytoma (in conjunction with an α-blocker).

The mechanism of the antihypertensive effects of β1-blockers are unknown, but several possible mechanisms have been proposed: (1) blocking of prejunctional β2-adrenoceptors that decreases the release of noradrenaline from sympathetic nerve terminals and adrenergic-mediated vasoconstriction; (2) a central effect leading to a decrease in peripheral sympathetic tone; (3) inhibition of renin release from renal juxtaglomerular cells and the activation of the RAAS; and (4) reduction in CO (due to a decrease in heart rate and contractility), although this effect can produce a compensatory reflex rise in PVR.

- *Angina*. β-blockers are the standard therapy for effort and unstable angina. All β-blockers are potentially equally effective in chronic stable angina, but drugs recommended are long-acting, cardioselective drugs without intrinsic sympathomimetic activity. β-blockers reduce MVO_2 during exercise by lowering heart rate, BP, and myocardial contractility. Additionally, β-blockers switch the heart from using oxygen-wasting fatty acids towards oxygen-conserving glycolysis. Although β-blockers would be expected to produce coronary vasoconstriction and decrease coronary blood flow, they decrease heart rate during exercise and prolong the diastolic time (due to their negative chronotropic effects), improving the subendocardial coronary blood flow to ischaemic areas during diastole.

In patients with chronic stable angina, β-blockers are effective in controlling exercise-induced angina, improve exercise capacity, and reduce both symptomatic and asymptomatic ischaemic episodes. A meta-analysis of 90 studies found that β-blockers and CCBs present similar efficacy and safety, but β-blockers were better tolerated. β-blockers are also very effective in reducing the frequency and number of episodes of silent ischaemic attacks that can be precipitated by minor elevations in the heart rate. However, β-blockers are not indicated in vasospastic angina, due to a predominance of α-mediated coronary vasoconstriction.

β-blockers are often combined with nitrates and CCBs in the therapy of angina. Their combination with diltiazem or verapamil should be avoided, because of the increased risk of bradycardia, AVB, hypotension, and HF; however, the combination of β-blockers with long-acting dihydropyridines is well tolerated.

- *ACS*. Early initiation of β-blocker treatment is indicated in all patients with ACS who do not have contraindications. In non-ST-segment elevation ACS (NSTE-ACS), β-blocker treatment reduces mortality in the first week following MI; β-blockers also reduce chest pain, MVO_2, hypertension, and tachycardia. However, the evidence favouring the use of β-blockers in UA is limited to the borderline benefits results of metoprolol in one placebo-controlled trial. In general, it is recommended to start half-dose oral β-blockade on day 2 (assuming haemodynamic stability), followed by dose increase to the full or the maximum tolerated dose, followed by long-term post-MI β-blockade. Early administration of β-blockers should be avoided if the LV function is unknown and in patients with symptoms possibly related to coronary vasospasm or cocaine use, as they might favour spasm by leaving α-mediated vasoconstriction unopposed by β-mediated vasodilatation.

Some β-blockers (carvedilol, metoprolol succinate, or bisoprolol) are recommended for all post-MI patients with an LVEF of ≤40%, unless contraindicated, to reduce reinfarction and CV mortality in a wide spectrum of patients, including diabetics. The mechanisms concerned are multiple and include a protective effect *from catecholamine myocyte toxicity* as a result of their antihypertensive, anti-ischaemic, and antiarrhythmic properties (prevent SCD). However, most of the trials in post-MI patients were performed before the implementation of other secondary prevention therapies, such as statins and ACEIs, leaving uncertainty regarding their efficacy when added to modern therapeutic strategies.

- *Heart failure.* All patients with chronic HFrEF should receive a β-blocker, unless contraindicated. In patients with HF (NYHA classes III–IV) and LVEF of <35% treated with diuretics and RAAS inhibitors, some β-blockers (bisoprolol, carvedilol, metoprolol, and nebivolol) reduce all-cause mortality and sudden death mortality rates. The benefit is observed, independent of age and gender and in older adults, diabetics, and black patients. Propranolol and atenolol have not been well studied in HF. In patients with haemodynamically stable HF, β-blocker therapy should be started at low doses, which will be gradually increased after at least 2 weeks, up to the target doses from the relevant clinical trials, if tolerated. Several mechanisms have been proposed to explain their beneficial effect in patients with HFrEF:
    - *Improved β-adrenergic signalling.* In CHF, β1-receptors are downregulated in response to high circulating catecholamine levels and the β-adrenergic inotropic response is diminished. However, during sustained β-blocker therapy, the number of β-receptors and the activity of adenylyl cyclase increases (i.e. β-blockers may indirectly increase the formation of cAMP), while the expression of GRK2 decreases. This can explain why long-term β-blockade can improve systolic function in HF, while at the beginning of the treatment, they can produce a negative inotropic effect.
    - *The hyperphosphorylation hypothesis* proposes that the continued excess adrenergic stimulation leads to hyperphosphorylation of the ryanodine receptor (RyR2) on the SR, leading to a Ca^{2+} leak during diastole and cytosolic Ca^{2+} overload. Additionally, the SR Ca^{2+}-ATPase (SERCA) that regulates Ca^{2+} uptake into the SR is downregulated. These changes lead to decreased contraction and delayed relaxation. β-blockers inhibit the hyperphosphorylation of the SR, normalize SERCA expression, and increase the uptake of Ca^{2+} by the SR.
    - *Bradycardia.* Slow heart rates may improve coronary blood flow, decrease MVO_2, and improve LVEF.
    - *Protection from catecholamine-induced cardiotoxicity and cardiac remodelling.* The high circulating concentrations of noradrenaline found in patients with severe HF may exert direct toxic effects on the myocardium, an effect partly mediated through Ca^{2+} overload.
    - *Metabolic modulation.* β-blockers switch the heart from using oxygen-wasting fatty acids to oxygen-conserving glucose.
    - *Antiarrhythmic effects.* β-blockers inhibit ventricular arrhythmias in patients with HF.
    - *Antiapoptotic effects.* Coupling of the β2-receptor to the inhibitory G protein G_i may be antiapoptotic.
    - *Inhibition of the RAAS.* β-blockers reduce renin release and RAAS activation.
- *Arrhythmias.* β-blockers are effective and generally safe AADs and can be considered the mainstay of AAD therapy. They inhibit sympathetic influences on cardiac electrical activity (class II effects) and the release of Ca^{2+} from the ryanodine receptor channel. As a consequence, they: (1) reduce the sinus rate, decrease conduction velocity, and increase the effective refractory period in the AVN, i.e. they produce negative chronotropic and dromotropic effects; (2) decrease the

dispersion of ventricular repolarization and increase the VF threshold in the ischaemic myocardium; and (3) inhibit sympathetically mediated triggering mechanisms.

β-blockers are effective in the prophylaxis of SVTs by inhibiting initiating atrial ectopic beats and in the treatment of SVT by slowing conduction through the AVN and reducing the ventricular response rate. The inhibitory effect on the AVN is the basis for the use of β-blockers to effectively reduce the ventricular response in patients with AF or atrial flutter, being more effective that verapamil, diltiazem, or digoxin. Furthermore, short-term therapy with β-blockers decreases the incidence of post-operative AF. *IV esmolol* has challenged the previously standard use of verapamil or diltiazem in the treatment of SVT, but adenosine is still preferred. Treatment with β-blockers improves rate control, ventricular function, and survival in patients with persistent AF and LV dysfunction. However, they are ineffective in the cardioversion of AF to sinus rhythm or to enhance the success of cardioversion. β-blockers exhibit moderate efficacy in preventing AF recurrence (maintain sinus rhythm) or reducing the frequency of paroxsymal AF and may be dangerous in patients with WPW syndrome by blocking the AVN and redirecting impulses down the bypass tract.

β-blockers are effective in suppressing ventricular ectopic beats and ventricular tachyarrhythmias and are the most effective drugs to prevent SCD in a wide spectrum of cardiac disorders in patients with and without HF. β-blockers are effective as monotherapy in severe recurrent VT not obviously ischaemic in origin and in sustained ventricular tachyarrhythmias. The combination of β-blockers with amiodarone may be effective in treating episodes of 'electrical storm' and may reduce cardiac mortality. β-blockers titrated to the maximally tolerated dose are the first-line therapy in patients with ARVC and frequent ventricular premature beats (VPBs) and NSVT. Oral metoprolol, propranolol, or verapamil are recommended for long-term management of idiopathic sustained VT. Treatment with β-blockers is also recommended in symptomatic patients with idiopathic left VT and mitral and tricuspid annular tachycardia and/or papillary muscle tachycardia.

β-blockers should be considered during hospital stay and continued thereafter for the prevention/treatment of recurrent VT/VF and SCD in patients with ACS. In post-MI patients with depressed LV function and ventricular arrhythmias, β-blockers reduce all-cause mortality and arrhythmic deaths. In acute MI complicated by stress-induced hypokalaemia, non-selective blockers are preferred to β1-selective blockers and reduce MI mortality. The general arguments for β-blockade include: (1) the role of sympathetic-mediated triggered activity in precipitating some arrhythmias; (2) the increased sympathetic activity in patients with sustained VT or acute MI; (3) the key role of cAMP, the second messenger of β-adrenergic activity, in the causation of ischaemia-related VF; and (4) the antihypertensive and anti-ischaemic effects of these drugs. However, a registry in patients with STEMI or NSTEMI found that in patients with two or more risk factors for shock, the risk of shock or death was significantly increased in those treated with β-blockers.

β-blockers are very effective against any supraventricular and ventricular arrhythmias associated with an increase in sympathetic β-adrenergic activity: stress, anxiety, HF, CAD, hyperthyroidism, phaeochromocytoma, anaesthesia, digitalis intoxication, cardiac surgery, post-operative states, exercise-induced arrhythmias, or increased cAMP- and calcium-dependent triggered arrhythmias.

β-blockers are recommended in patients with a clinical diagnosis of LQTS and in carriers of a causative LQTS mutation and normal QT interval. Long-acting β-blockers (e.g. nadolol) are recommended. They are also recommended in all patients with a clinical diagnosis of CPVT and in genetically positive family members, even after a negative exercise test.

Pharmacokinetics

β-blockers are rapidly absorbed following PO administration. Hydrophilic β-blockers (atenolol, acebutolol, bisoprolol, nadolol, sotalol) present low plasma protein binding and low brain penetration and are excreted mainly unchanged by the kidneys. Thus, as renal blood flow falls, the doses should be reduced. Conversely, the most lipophilic drugs (carvedilol, metoprolol, propranolol) are largely metabolized by the GI tract and the liver (first-pass), so that they present lower oral bioavailability and higher protein binding and tissue distribution (cross the blood–brain barrier). They are biotransformed in the liver to active metaboites, and their metabolism depends on hepatic blood flow and metabolism. Thus, their t½ increases in the elderly and in patients with severe hepatic impairment, while they can be prescribed in patients with renal impairment. The pharmacodynamic t½ is much longer than the pharmacokinetic t½, so that twice-daily dosage of standard propranolol is effective, even in angina pectoris. Longer-acting drugs (carvedilol, nadolol, sotalol, atenolol) and slow-release or extended-release formulations are the preferred formulations for hypertension and effort angina. (See Table 8.1.8.)

Practical points

1. *Doses* (see ➲ Atenolol, p. 478; ➲ Bisoprolol, p. 496; ➲ Carvedilol, pp. 517–18; ➲ Esmolol, pp. 582–3; ➲ Labetalol, p. 636; ➲ Metoprolol, pp. 660–1; ➲ Nadolol, p. 671; ➲ Nebivolol, pp. 673–4; ➲ Propranolol, pp. 713–15; ➲ Sotalol, pp. 754–6)
2. *Side effects*
   - *CV*: bradycardia, AVB, deterioration of HF (at the beginning of treatment), postural hypotension, dizziness, syncope, cold extremities, and worsening of claudication. β-blockers reduce exercise tolerance and increases the sense of fatigue. The rate of CV side effects increases with non-selective drugs.
   - *Respiratory*: bronchospasm, asthma. The risk of bronchospasm is higher with non-selective β-blockers.
   - *Neurological*: confusion, depression, insomnia, paraesthesiae, headache, nightmares. The CNS side effects are more frequent with lipid-soluble β-blockers that presumably penetrate the CNS more readily, while they are less frequent with cardioselective β1-blockers.
   - *GI*: nausea, vomiting, constipation, abdominal cramps, dry mouth.
   - *Endocrine*: β-blockers impair insulin sensitivity, can mask hypoglycaemia signs (tremor, tachycardia; sweating can increase), and may increase the incidence of new-onset T2DM. Vasodilatory β-blockers (carvedilol and nebivolol) have a better metabolic profile than cardioselective agents.

- *Metabolic*. β-blockers reduce HDL-C and increase TG plasma levels and may worsen MetS. Vasodilatory β-blockers (carvedilol, nebivolol) cause less metabolic adverse effects.
- *Dermatological*: rash. β-blockers can aggravate skin reactions in patients with psoriasis.
- *Others*: dry eyes, blurred vision, hypokalaemia, and impotence (changing to nebivolol may improve erection).
- Cardioselective β1-blockers are thought to cause fewer CNS side effects and have less risk of bronchospasm than non-selective β-blockers.

3. *Interactions*
   - Risk of hypotension increases when β-blockers are co-administered with antihypertensives, nitrates, tricyclic antidepressants, MAOIs, anaesthetics (e.g. halothane, enflurane), alcohol, and benzodiazepines. Conversely, NSAIDs, glucocorticoids, and oral contraceptives can antagonize their antihypertensive effects.
   - The co-administration of β-blockers with diltiazem and verapamil increases the risk of hypotension, bradycardia, and AVB and can precipitate HF. Close ECG and BP monitoring is recommended. The combination of β-blockers with long-acting dihydropyridines is better tolerated.
   - There may be an increased risk of myocardial depression when β-blockers are given with antiarrhythmic agents. Increased risk of bradycardia and AV block and myocardial depression when given with amiodarone, and of myocardial depression and bradycardia with class I antiarrhythmics. Close ECG monitoring is recommended.
   - Risk of ventricular arrhythmias increased when used with tricyclic antidepressants or antipsychotics (e.g. phenothiazines).
   - β-blockers reduce the hepatic blood flow and increase the plasma levels and the risk of lidocaine toxicity.
   - β-blockers can produce hyperkalaemia and increase that produced by ACEIs, ARBs, and potassium-sparing diuretics.
   - β-blockers with α-antagonist activity (carvedilol) or releasing NO (nebivolol) may be more prone to cause postural hypotension but have a better metabolic profile than other β-blockers.
   - β-blockers increase the risk of AVB and bradycardia, and antagonize the inotropic effect of digoxin.
   - In insulin-requiring diabetes, non-selective β-blockers may increase blood glucose levels (1–1.5mmol/L), can mask certain symptoms of hypoglycaemia (tremor, tachycardia), and may prolong the hypoglycaemic response to insulin (and oral antidiabetic drugs). Use carvedilol or nebivolol.
   - β-blocker and diuretics increase the risk of new-onset T2DM. Thus, this combination is not recommended as initial therapy in those prone to diabetes or with MetS.
   - Co-administration with α-adrenergic receptor antagonists (terazosin or doxazosin) increases the risk of hypotension, tachycardia, and palpitations.
   - Clonidine: increased risk of hypertension on withdrawal.
   - Sympathomimetics: risk of severe hypertension and bradycardia.

- Inhalational anaesthetics: synergistic negative inotropic and hypotensive effects.
- Mefloquine: increased risk of bradycardia.
- Fingolimod: potentiates the risk of bradycardia, with possible fatal outcomes.

4. *Cautions/notes*
   - β-blockers antagonize the bronchodilator effects of β-agonist bronchodilators and should be avoided in patients with asthma and severe COPD, due to the risk of bronchospasm, unless a compelling indication is present and under close surveillance. Cardioselective β1-blockers in low doses are best for patients with reversible bronchospasm.
   - In HF patients, β-blockers should be initiated in clinically stable patients at a low dose and gradually uptitrated to the maximum tolerated dose. In patients admitted due to acute HF, β-blockers should be cautiously initiated in hospital, once the patient is stabilized.
   - Abrupt withdrawal of β-blockers (especially in patients with CAD) may result in exacerbation of angina (sometimes resulting in MI), rebound hypertension, ventricular arrhythmias, and SCD. Consequently, β-blockers should be withdrawn gradually over 1–2 weeks.
   - β-blockers are less effective in reducing coronary events in smoking men.
   - β-blockers can mask symptoms of hyperthyroidism.
   - β-blockers should also not be initiated in patients with phaeochromocytoma, without prior α-blockade.
   - In patients with renal impairment, avoid or reduce the dose of β-blockers excreted predominantly in the urine (atenolol, sotalol).
   - In patients with liver impairment, avoid β-blockers with higher hepatic clearance (acebutolol, carvedilol, metoprolol, propranolol, timolol). Use agents with low clearance (atenolol, nadolol, sotalol).
   - β-blockers may increase the sensitivity towards a variety of allergens and lead to more severe anaphylactic reactions that are less responsive to adrenaline. They may exacerbate psoriatic rashes and unmask or potentiate a myasthenic condition.
   - After chronic therapy with non-selective β-blockers, the administration of adrenaline may develop uncontrolled hypertension due to α-receptor stimulation.
   - In patients with cold extremities, Raynaud's phenomenon, and absent pulses: avoid non-selective agents; consider carvedilol and nebivolol.
   - In acute MI complicated by stress-induced hypokalaemia, non-selective β-blockers theoretically should be better antiarrhythmics than β1-selective blockers.
5. *Pregnancy and lactation* (see also ➲ Atenolol, p. 478; ➲ Bisoprolol, p. 496; ➲ Carvedilol, pp. 517–18; ➲ Esmolol, pp. 582–3; ➲ Labetalol, p. 636; ➲ Metoprolol, pp. 660–1; ➲ Nadolol, p. 671; ➲ Nebivolol, pp. 673–4; ➲ Propranolol, pp. 713–15; ➲ Sotalol, pp. 754–6)

β-blockers should be avoided during pregnancy or breastfeeding, except in women with hypertensive disorders during pregnancy (pregnancy category C). In general, β-blockers reduce placental perfusion and may result in IUGR and immature and premature deliveries. Neonatal adverse effects (e.g. bradycardia, respiratory depression, hypotension, and hypoglycaemia) may also occur in the fetus and newborn infant. If treatment with β-blockers is necessary, β1-selective blockers are preferable.

6. *Contraindications*
   - Severe bradycardia (<45bpm), sinus node disease, and second- or third-degree heart block (unless a pacemaker is present).
   - Hypotension (<100/60mmHg); cardiogenic shock.
   - Vasospastic (Prinzmetal-type) angina.
   - Unstable HF.
   - Acute phase of MI (avoid if bradycardia, hypotension, LV failure).
   - Severe peripheral vascular disease with rest ischaemia.
   - Untreated phaeochromocytoma.
   - Severe depression (avoid propranolol).
   - Metabolic acidosis.
   - Asthma and severe obstructive airway diseases.

Bezafibrate

Oral PPAR-α receptor agonist (see also ➔ Fibrates, pp. 590–2).

CV indications

As an adjunct to diet and other non-pharmacological treatment for the treatment of severe hypertriglyceridaemia, with or without low HDL-C, and of mixed hyperlipidaemia when a statin is contraindicated or not tolerated.

Pharmacodynamics

At a daily dose of 600 mg, it lowers total-C (17%) and LDL-C (19.6%), VLDL-C (44.3%), TGs (13.7%), and Apo B (24.0%) and increases HDL-C (15.3%) plasma levels. In patients with impaired glucose tolerance, bezafibrate reduces fasting blood glucose and may delay progress to diabetes. In patients with CAD and T2DM, bezafibrate attenuates the development of insulin resistance and the progressive failure of pancreatic β-cell function.

Pharmacokinetics

Modified release: oral bioavailability is approximately 70%, reaching peak plasma levels 4h after ingestion. Protein binding is approximately 95%; elimination t½ is approximately 1–2h and slower in renal dysfunction. Excretion is almost exclusively (95%) renal, so that the elimination t½ is longer in patients with renal impairment and dose adjustments may be necessary. Significant hepatic disease (other than fatty infiltration) is a contraindication to the use of bezafibrate. (See Table 8.1.4.)

Practical points

1. *Doses*
    - Standard preparation: 200mg bd or tds, after meals. Slow-release formulation: 400mg od. It is contraindicated in patients on dialysis. Treatment should be withdrawn if an adequate response has not been achieved within 3–4 months.
2. *Side effects* (see ➔ Fibrates, pp. 590–2)
3. *Interactions* (see ➔ Fibrates, pp. 590–2)
    - MAOIs (with hepatotoxic potential) should not be administered together with bezafibrate.
4. *Cautions/notes*
    - The dose of warfarin should be reduced by up to 50%.
    - Dose should be adjusted according to renal function. GFR 40–60mL/min: 400mg daily; GFR 15–40mL/min: 200mg daily or every 2 days; GFR <15mL/min: contraindicated.
    - Modified-release is not appropriate in patients with renal dysfunction or on dialysis.
5. *Pregnancy and lactation* (see ➔ Fibrates, pp. 590–2)
6. *Contraindications* (see ➔ Fibrates, pp. 590–2)

Bisoprolol

(See also ➔ Beta-adrenergic blocking agents, pp. 485–94.)

Selective β1-adrenergic receptor antagonist with high lipid solubility.

CV indications

- Treatment of hypertension.
- Treatment of angina pectoris.
- Treatment of stable chronic HFrEF, in addition to ACEs and diuretics, and optionally cardiac glycosides.

Mechanism of action

Bisoprolol exhibits greater cardioselectivity than other cardioselective β-blockers.

Pharmacokinetics

(See Tables 8.1.3 and 8.1.8.)

Practical points

1. *Doses*
   - Angina: 5–10mg od; maximum dose 20mg daily.
   - Hypertension: 2.5–40mg od.
   - HF: initially 1.25mg od (uptitrated at intervals of 2 weeks to a maximum of 10mg od).
2. *Side effects, interactions, cautions, and contraindications* (see ➔ Beta-adrenergic blocking agents, pp. 485–94)

Bivalirudin

A specific and reversible direct thrombin (factor IIa) inhibitor.

Indications

- As an anticoagulant in adult patients undergoing PCI, including patients with STEMI undergoing PPCI.
- Treatment of adult patients with UA/NSTEMI planned for urgent or early intervention.
  Bivalirudin should be administered with ASA and clopidogrel.

Bivalirudin is also licensed for patients with, or at risk of, HIT and heparin-induced thrombocytopenia and thrombosis syndrome (HITTS) who are undergoing PCI.

Mechanism of action

Bivalirudin is a short synthetic peptide (20 amino acids) that produces a potent, highly specific, and reversible inhibition of both free circulating and clot-bound thrombin by specifically binding both to the catalytic site and to the anion-binding exosite. It inhibits thrombin-induced conversion of fibrinogen to fibrin and inactivates fibrin-bound, as well as fluid-phase, thrombin. As bivalirudin does not bind to plasma proteins, its anticoagulant effect is more predictable than that of UFH.

Pharmacodynamics

In patients undergoing routine PTCA, IV bivalirudin produces an immediate anticoagulant effect and prolongs the ACT, aPTT, TT, and PT in a concentration-dependent manner. The dose and anticoagulant activity of bivalirudin correlate well with aPTT and ACT values. Coagulation times return to baseline of approximately 1h, following cessation of bivalirudin administration. In ACS with planned PCI, bivalirudin alone gave similar outcome rates to UFH plus GPIIb/IIIa inhibition, with less bleeding. In patients with moderate- to high-risk ACS and planned early catheterization, bivalirudin with upstream aspirin is superior to UFH or enoxaparin plus GPIIb/IIIa antagonists, with less bleeding and similar clinical outcomes.

Pharmacokinetics

Bivalirudin exhibits linear pharmacokinetics following IV administration. It does not bind to plasma proteins (other than thrombin) or to red blood cells and is cleared from plasma by a combination of renal mechanisms and proteolytic cleavage, with a t½ of 25min. Total body clearance is reduced by 20% in patients with moderate to severe renal impairment. Approximately 25% of the drug can be cleared by haemodialysis. (See Table 8.1.1.)

Practical points

1. *Doses*
   - *Patients undergoing PCI, including patients with STEMI undergoing PPCI.* In patients undergoing PCI: IV bolus of 0.75mg/kg, followed immediately by an IV infusion at a rate of 1.75mg/kg for at least the duration of the procedure. The infusion may be continued for up to

4h post-PCI and at a reduced dose of 0.25mg/kg for an additional 4–12h, if clinically necessary. In STEMI patients, the infusion of 1.75mg/kg/h should be continued for up to 4h post-PCI and continued at a reduced dose of 0.25mg/kg/h for an additional 4–12h, as clinically necessary.

- *Patients with UA/NSTEMI.* The recommended starting dose for medically managed patients with ACS is an IV bolus of 0.1mg/kg, followed by an infusion of 0.25mg/kg/h. Patients who are to be medically managed may continue the infusion of 0.25mg/kg/h for up to 72h. If the medically managed patient proceeds to PCI, an additional bolus of 0.5mg/kg should be administered before the procedure and the infusion increased to 1.75mg/kg/h for the duration of the procedure. Following PCI, the reduced infusion dose of 0.25mg/kg/h may be resumed for 4–12h, as clinically necessary.
  —For patients who proceed to CABG surgery off-pump: the IV infusion of bivalirudin should be continued until the time of surgery. Just prior to surgery, a 0.5mg/kg bolus dose should be administered, followed by a 1.75mg/kg/h infusion for the duration of the surgery.
  —For patients proceeding to CABG surgery on-pump: the IV infusion of bivalirudin should be continued until 1h prior to surgery, after which the infusion should be discontinued and the patient treated with UFH. Five minutes after the bolus, ACT should be checked, and if <225s, an additional bolus of 0.3mg/kg should be administered. Once the ACT value is >225s, no further monitoring is required, provided the 1.75mg/kg/h infusion dose is properly administered.
  —The arterial sheath can be removed 2h after discontinuation of the bivalirudin infusion without anticoagulation monitoring.

Patients can be started on bivalirudin 30min after discontinuation of UFH given IV, or 8h after discontinuation of LMWH given SC.

2. *Side effects*
   - Very common: minor haemorrhage at any site.
     Common: thrombocytopenia, decreases in haematocrit and haemoglobin, ecchymosis. Bivalirudin causes relatively less bleeding than UFH or heparin plus a GPIIb/IIIa inhibitor in unselected patients undergoing PCI.
   - Uncommon: nausea, vomiting, thrombocytopenia, anaemia, hypersensitivity (including anaphylactic reaction and shock), headache, haematoma or pain at the injection site, rash, urticaria, hypotension, back pain.
   - Rare: MI, bradycardia, coronary stent thrombosis, cardiac tamponade, pericardial haemorrhage, angina pectoris, VT.
3. *Drug interactions*
   - Co-administration of bivalirudin with heparins, platelet inhibitors, warfarin, or thrombolytics increases the risk of major bleeding events. When bivalirudin is combined with a platelet inhibitor or an anticoagulant, clinical and biological parameters of haemostasis should be regularly monitored.

4. *Cautions*
   - The bolus dose should be administered by a rapid IV push to ensure that the entire bolus reaches the patient before the start of the procedure. The infusion dose should be initiated immediately after the bolus is administered. IV infusion lines should be primed with bivalirudin to ensure continuity of drug infusion after delivery of the bolus. An increase in the ACT may be used as an indication that the patient has received bivalirudin.
   - Bivalirudin is contraindicated in patients with severe renal insufficiency (GFR <30mL/min). If the CrCl is between 30 and 59mL/min, keep the bolus dose, but reduce the infusion rate to 1.4mg/kg/h. No dose adjustment is needed in patients with hepatic impairment. In the elderly, dose adjustments should be based on the basis of renal function.
   - Patients should be carefully monitored following PPCI for signs and symptoms consistent with myocardial ischaemia.
5. *Pregnancy and lactation*
   - There are limited data in pregnant women (Pregnancy category B), and it is unknown whether bivalirudin is excreted in human milk. With caution during pregnancy and in breastfeeding mothers.
6. *Contraindications*
   - Active bleeding or increased risk of bleeding.
   - Hypersensitivity to bivalirudin or its components.
   - Severe uncontrolled hypertension.
   - Subacute bacterial endocarditis.
   - Severe renal impairment and in dialysis-dependent patients.

Bosentan

Specific, competitive dual endothelin ETA and ETB receptor antagonist, with relatively greater affinity for ETA receptors.

CV indications

- Treatment of PAH to improve exercise capacity and symptoms in patients with WHO functional class III. Efficacy has been shown in primary (idiopathic and heritable) PAH, PAH secondary to scleroderma without significant interstitial pulmonary disease, and PAH associated with congenital systemic-to-pulmonary shunts and Eisenmenger's physiology.
- Some improvements have also been shown in patients with PAH WHO functional class II.
- To reduce the number of new digital ulcers in patients with systemic sclerosis and ongoing digital ulcer disease.

Mechanism of action

ET1 is the most potent human endogenous vasoconstrictor. It also exerts profibrotic, proliferative, hypertrophic, and pro-inflammatory effects. ET1 binds to two homologous G protein-coupled receptor subtypes—endothelin type A (ETA) and B receptors (ETB). ETA and ETB receptors are variably distributed in vessels, bronchi, and alveoli. ETA receptors are expressed in airway smooth muscle, smooth muscle cells of large human pulmonary arteries, and cardiac myocytes. ETB receptors are expressed on endothelial cells where ETA receptors are not expressed as well as in airway smooth muscle and alveolar wall tissue and capillaries. The activation of ETA receptors produces vasoconstriction and proliferation of vascular smooth muscle cells. Activation of ETB receptors results in vasodilatation due to the release of both NO and prostacyclin, and inhibition of apoptosis and is involved in the clearance of ET1. Human lungs are also the major site for both the production and clearance of circulating ET1 and remove about 50% of circulating ET1 via ETB receptors and release a similar amount into circulation.

Patients with PAH exhibit endothelial dysfunction, with a decrease in vasodilators and an increase in vasoconstrictors. ET1 expression, production, and concentration in plasma and lung tissue are elevated in these patients, and levels of ET1 correlate with disease severity and prognosis of PAH. These findings confirm that endothelin plays a role in the development and progression of PAH and is the basis for the administration of endothelin receptor antagonists.

Pharmacodynamics

Bosentan reduces pulmonary vascular resistance and improves exercise capacity, functional class, haemodynamics (increases cardiac index, reduces pulmonary arterial and right atrial pressures and pulmonary vascular resistance), functional class, exercise capacity, and symptoms, compared to placebo. In patients with Eisenmenger's syndrome, bosentan improves exercise capacity and quality of life and decreases PVR after 16 weeks of treatment in WHO functional class III patients; however, an effect on mortality remains uncertain.

Pharmacokinetics

Oral bioavailability (50%) is unaffected by food, reaching peak plasma levels within 3–5h. Bosentan is highly protein-bound (98%), present a large Vd

(18L/kg), and is eliminated by biliary excretion following metabolism in the liver by CYP450 2C9 and CYP3A4; <3% of an administered oral dose is recovered in urine. Elimination t½ is 5.4h. Drug effects are not altered in patients with renal impairment. However, bosentan is contraindicated in patients with moderate to severe liver dysfunction (i.e. Child–Pugh classes B and C).

Practical points

1. *Doses*
   - Treatment should only be initiated and monitored by a physician experienced in the treatment of PAH. If the decision to withdraw bosentan is taken, it should be done gradually, while an alternative therapy is introduced.
   - The starting dose is 62.5mg PO bd for 4 weeks; then increase to 125mg PO bd indefinitely. Doses above 125mg bd do not appear to confer sufficient benefit to offset the risk of hepatic injury. When used in children with PAH aged 1 year and older, the recommended starting and maintenance dose is 2mg/kg morning and evening.
2. *Side effects*
   - Very common: headache, oedema, fluid retention, and dose-dependent increases in liver aminotransferases. Elevation of aminotransferases usually progresses slowly and mostly occurs asymptomatically, although there have been rare reports of unexplained liver cirrhosis and liver failure. Liver function testing should be performed monthly, and therapy should be discontinued if liver aminotransferase elevations are accompanied by clinical symptoms of hepatotoxicity (i.e. nausea, vomiting, fever, abdominal pain, jaundice, fatigue) or increases of ≥2 times ULN are observed.
   - Bosentan decreases haemoglobin concentration (approximately 1g/dL in 57% of patients) and haematocrit, particularly during the first weeks of treatment; changes stabilize after 3–4 months of treatment. Thus, haemoglobin concentrations should be checked after 1 and 3 months, and every 3 months thereafter.
   - Common: flushing, anaemia, erythema, palpitations, flushing, hypotension, upper respiratory tract infections/nasopharyngitis, gastro-oesophageal reflux, diarrhoea, hypersensitivity reactions (including dermatitis, pruritus, and rash). Endothelin antagonists may cause testicular atrophy and male infertility.
3. *Interactions*
   - Bosentan is an inducer of CYP3A and CYP2C9; thus, plasma concentrations of drugs metabolized by these isoenzymes will be reduced when co-administered with bosentan (see Table 8.1.2). Bosentan is also metabolized by these enzymes, so that their inhibition may increase the plasma concentration of bosentan.
   - Co-administration with potent CYP3A4 or CYP2C19 inhibitors increases bosentan plasma levels, while CYP3A and 2C19 inducers may increase the metabolism of bosentan and decrease its plasma levels (see Table 8.1.2). These combinations are not recommended.
   - Bosentan is a substrate of OATP. Ritonavir inhibits OATP, and co-administration of bosentan and lopinavir/ritonavir increases the plasma levels of bosentan. Monitor patient tolerability to bosentan.

- Fluconazole inhibits CYP2C9 and CYP3A4 and increases plasma concentrations of bosentan. The combination is not recommended.
- Amiodarone increases bosentan plasma levels considerably; this combination is contraindicated.
- Tacrolimus and sirolimus may increase the plasma concentrations of bosentan.
- Co-administration of bosentan and ciclosporin decreases the plasma concentrations of ciclosporin (50%) but markedly increases bosentan plasma levels. This combination is contraindicated.
- Bosentan increases the plasma levels of apixaban and rivaroxaban.
- The combination of bosentan and glibenclamide increases hepatic aminotransferases, and bosentan decreases the hypoglycaemic effect of glibenclamide. This combination is contraindicated.
- Bosentan decreases (40%) the plasma concentrations of simvastatin, lovastatin, and atorvastatin (they are metabolized by CYP3A). Monitor LDL-C plasma levels.
- Bosentan decreases the exposure to oral contraceptives containing norethindrone and ethinylestradiol; thus, hormonal contraceptives are not considered as reliable methods of contraception, and females should practise additional methods of contraception.
- Bosentan decreases the plasma concentrations of both S-warfarin (a CYP2C9 substrate) and R-warfarin (a CYP3A substrate) by 29% and 38%, respectively. Monitor the INR, but dose adjustment is usually unnecessary.
- Bosentan reduces sildenafil plasma concentrations (60%), and sildenafil increases bosentan plasma concentrations by 50%. Dose adjustments are not necessary.

4. *Cautions/notes*
    - Bosentan should be avoided in patients with moderate to severe hepatic impairment. However, many patients with PAH have mild hepatic impairment, and it may still be appropriate to try bosentan with caution under specialist supervision.
    - Bosentan should only be initiated if SBP is >85mmHg.
    - If signs of pulmonary oedema occur during bosentan administration, the possibility of associated veno-occlusive disease should be considered.
    - The benefit/risk balance of bosentan has not been established in patients with WHO functional class I PAH.
5. *Pregnancy and lactation*
    - Bosentan is expected to cause fetal harm and is not recommended in pregnancy and breastfeeding (Pregnancy category X). Pregnancy should be excluded before treatment with bosentan and advice regarding contraception sought. It is unknown whether bosentan is excreted into human breast milk.
6. *Contraindications*
    - Hypersensitivity to the active substance or to any of the excipients.
    - Moderate to severe hepatic impairment. Elevated baseline levels of hepatic aminotransferases (>3 times ULN).
    - Concomitant use of ciclosporin.
    - Pregnancy; women of childbearing age not using reliable contraception.

Bumetanide

Loop diuretic (see ➔ Furosemide, pp. 601–2).

CV indications

- Treatment of oedema associated with CHF, cirrhosis of the liver, and renal disease including the nephrotic syndrome.

Pharmacodynamics

In comparison to furosemide, 1mg bumetanide is equivalent to 40mg furosemide, with a similar pattern of water and electrolyte excretion.

Pharmacokinetics

(See Table 8.1.5.)

Practical points

1. *Doses*
   - PO: 1mg increased to 5mg od or bd, according to response. A dose of 0.5mg daily may be sufficient in some elderly patients.
2. *Common side effects* (see ➔ Furosemide, pp. 601–2)

Severe, generalized musculoskeletal pain, sometimes associated with muscle spasm, occurring 1–2h after administration and lasting up to 12h; can occur at high doses in patients with severe chronic renal failure. All patients recovered fully, and there was no deterioration in their renal function.

3. Interactions *and cautions* (see ➔ Furosemide, pp. 601–2)
4. *Pregnancy and lactation* (see ➔ Furosemide, pp. 601–2)
   - No teratogenic effects have been seen in animals (Pregnancy category C). It is not known whether bumetanide is excreted in breast milk.
5. *Contraindications* (see ➔ Furosemide, pp. 601–2)

Calcium channel blockers

Ca^{2+} influx through voltage-gated L-type cardiac Ca^{2+} channels located in the cell membrane of cardiac and vascular smooth muscle cells is responsible for the depolarization (phase 0) of action potentials generated in the SA and AV nodal cells, regulates SA node firing rate, and determines the conduction velocity and refractoriness in the AVN. Ca^{2+} entry during the plateau phase of the cardiac action potential is responsible for the excitation–contraction coupling via the release of Ca^{2+} ions from the SR (Ca^{2+}-induced Ca^{2+} release). In vascular smooth muscle cells, Ca^{2+} influx increases vascular tone and PVR.

Calcium channel blockers: classification

CCBs are a heterogenous group of drugs that block the entry of extracellular Ca^{2+} through L-type channels. Based on their chemical structures, they can be classified into two subgroups:

1. Dihydropyridines: amlodipine, barnidipine, felodipine, isradipine, lacidipine, lercanidipine, manidipine, nicardipine, nifedipine, nimodipine, nisoldipine, nitrendipine.
2. Non-dihydropyridines: diltiazem, verapamil.

(See also ➔ Amlodipine, p. 452, ➔ Felodipine, p. 588, ➔ Lercanidipine, p. 638, ➔ Nifedipine, pp. 678–9, ➔ Diltiazem, pp. 547–8, and ➔ Verapamil, pp. 792–5.)

CV indications

(See individual drugs for specific indications.)

- Essential hypertension (all CCBs, except nimodipine).
- Chronic stable and vasospastic angina (Prinzmetal's or variant angina): amlodipine, diltiazem, nifedipine, verapamil.
- UA: verapamil.
- Prophylaxis and treatment of PSVT and control of ventricular rate in atrial flutter/AF: diltiazem and verapamil (class IV AADs).
- CAD without HF or LVEF of <40% to reduce the risk of hospitalization due to angina and coronary revascularization: amlodipine.
- Post-MI protection in the absence of prior LV failure: verapamil and diltiazem.
- Treatment of ischaemic neurological deficits following aneurysmal subarachnoid haemorrhage: nimodipine.
- HCM: verapamil and diltiazem may be helpful to improve diastolic relaxation.
- Raynaud's phenomenon: amlodipine, nifedipine, verapamil. These CCBs produce a vasodilator effect, suppress blood vessel spasms that block blood flow to the fingers, toes, ears, and nose, decrease the frequency and severity of the episodes, and can help to heal skin ulcers.
- Patients with idiopathic PAH: amlodipine, diltiazem, nifedipine.

Mechanism of action

CCBs selectively inhibit the entry of Ca^{2+} into excitable cells through the voltage-gated L-type Ca^{2+} channels located in cardiac, vascular, and non-vascular smooth muscles and cardiac SA and AV nodes. CCBs bind to a receptor located at different points in the pore-forming α subunit of the channel. However, their binding affinity is modulated by the conformational state of the channel. L-type Ca^{2+} channels exist in three main conformational states: rested, open-activated, and inactivated. Channels are closed at resting membrane potentials. After membrane depolarization, they activate-open and allow an influx of Ca^{2+} ions into the cell, and then move to the inactivated-closed state. The inactivated channel state is favoured at depolarized membrane potentials and at fast driving rates. Finally, inactivated channels return to the rested state, a process known as reactivation of the channel.

At therapeutic concentrations, CCBs exhibit higher affinity for the inactivated than for the rested and activated states. This explains why CCBs exhibit a greater inhibitory effect on vascular smooth muscle than on cardiac muscle (i.e. they present vascular selectivity), and their effects are more marked in depolarized tissues that generate Ca^{2+}-dependent action potentials (SA and AV nodes) than in less depolarized cardiac tissues that generate sodium-dependent action potentials (atrial and ventricular muscle, His–Purkinje system). CCBs differ in their relative selectivity for cardiac and vascular L-type Ca^{2+} channels. Thus, dihydropyridines have higher selectivity for vascular channels than diltiazem and verapamil.

Pharmacodynamics

1. *Antihypertensive effects*. CCBs are potent arteriolar vasodilators that reduce PVR and BP. The rapid and potent reduction of BP can increase modestly the heart rate and CO, plasma renin activity, and noradrenaline and angiotensin II plasma levels. These changes suggest that arteriolar vasodilatation is accompanied by a baroreflex-mediated increase in sympathetic tone and activation of the RAAS which increases heart rate, AV nodal conduction, and cardiac contractility that counteract the direct negative chronotropic, dromotropic, and inotropic effects of dihydropyridines. Verapamil and diltiazem are less potent vasodilators and produce less baroreflex activation and more depression of cardiac function. Thus, the final net effect depends on the CCB used, but in hypertensive patients with normal cardiac function, they produce minimal cardiodepressant effects.

In hypertensive patients, BP reduction correlates with the baseline levels (no change is observed in normotensive individuals) but is independent from Na^{+} intake (possibly because CCBs exert a mild diuretic effect) and is not modified by NSAIDs. CCBs decrease BP without altering plasma glucose, lipid, potassium, or uric acid levels and do not produce postural hypotension or bronchoconstriction. Thus, CCBs are the drugs of choice in patients with isolated systolic hypertension (elderly), angina pectoris, LVH, carotid/coronary atherosclerosis, peripheral artery disease, Raynaud's phenomenon, and pregnancy and are equally effective in blacks as in non-black hypertensives. Compared with other antihypertensives, CCBs have the same effect on CV death and total mortality, reduce new-onset diabetes, and provide more effective protection against stroke, but present a reduced ability to protect against the incidence of HF. Verapamil and diltiazem, but not dihydropyridines, inhibit AV nodal conduction and are the first-choice drugs for ventricular rate control in hypertensives with supraventricular arrhythmias.

2. *Anti-anginal effects*. CCBs reduce PVR (afterload) and MVO_2 and produce coronary vasodilatation and relief of exercise-induced vasoconstriction, increasing coronary oxygen supply. They also reduce coronary vascular tone and suppress coronary vasospasm. In addition, verapamil and diltiazem decrease the heart rate (and slow the heart rate during exercise) and cardiac contractility, which further reduces MVO_2. These effects are the basis for the use of CCBs in patients with chronic stable and vasospastic angina pectoris. Compared to placebo, CCBs reduce the frequency of anginal attacks, improve exercise tolerance, and increase the total duration of exercise, time to onset of angina, and time to ≥1-mm ST-segment depression in patients with stable chronic angina. However, only verapamil is recommended for UA.

This combination of dihydropyridines and β-blockers provides greater anti-anginal efficacy than either agent alone and has the advantage of preventing the reflex tachycardia caused by dihydropyridines. The combination of diltiazem or verapamil with β-blockers is only recommended under close medical monitoring, due to an increased risk of bradycardia, AVB, and a decrease in cardiac contractility.

3. *HF*. CCBs are not recommended in HF patients because of their direct negative inotropic effects. This direct negative inotropic effect is partly counteracted by their peripheral vasodilator effects that reduce LV afterload, but the cardiodepressant effects of CCBs can be unmasked in patients treated with β-adrenergic blockers or myocardial diseases (HF, previous MI). Interestingly, when HF is caused by SVTs, diltiazem and verapamil may restore sinus rhythm or decrease the ventricular rate, leading to haemodynamic improvement.

In patients with HF, amlodipine or felodipine, added to standard therapy (including enalapril and diuretics), does not modify all-cause or cardiac morbidity, NYHA classification, or hospitalization rates, as compared with placebo. Thus, both CCBs may be cautiously added in patients with HF on standard therapy with uncontrolled hypertension or angina. In post-MI patients, verapamil may be used if β-blockers are not tolerated or contraindicated, provided that there is no HF. Dihydropyridines lack good evidence for safety and efficacy in post-MI patients.

4. *Electrophysiological and antiarrhythmic effects*. CCBs do not alter excitability, conduction velocity, or refractoriness in atrial or ventricular muscle or in Purkinje fibres that generate sodium-dependent action potentials. At therapeutic concentrations, dihydropyridines do not cause significant changes in heart rate and contractility, AV conduction, or the QRS complex, PR, PQ, and HV intervals.

Non-dihydropyridine CCBs (e.g. diltiazem, verapamil) stabilize the L-type channel in its inactivated state and prolong the reactivation of the channel from inactivation, so that their effects on the SA and AV nodes increase at fast rates (use-dependent block) and at depolarized membrane potentials (voltage-dependent block). As a consequence, at fast heart rates, diltiazem and verapamil decrease the sinus rate and prolong the refractory period and slow conduction through the AVN (prolong the PR and A-H intervals), so that the action potentials arrive at the AVN when the channels are still in the inactivated state and cannot be conducted. This is the basis for their use to terminate or prevent re-entrant SVT where the circuit involves the AVN (AVNRT, AVRT) and to control the ventricular rate in patients with AF or flutter. However, diltiazem or verapamil are not recommended for the cardioversion of AF to sinus rhythm or for the maintenance of sinus rhythm. In SVTs, including atrial flutter and AF, the presence of a bypass tract contraindicates the use of diltiazem or verapamil.

In SVTs, verapamil terminates intranodal re-entry and stops tachycardia, but it has been replaced by adenosine and the ultra-short-acting β-blocker esmolol. Verapamil is the drug of choice in the treatment of VT with LBBB morphology in patients without structural heart disease arising in the RVOT or with a left axis deviation and an RBBB pattern re-entry occurring in or near the left posterior fascicle. Diltiazem and verapamil exert anti-ischaemic effects that can also suppress some ventricular arrhythmias in patients with CAD.

Diltiazem and verapamil also suppress abnormal automaticity generated in depolarized cardiac cells (abnormal automatism) and the triggered activity induced by early after-depolarizations responsible for the induction of TdP. Therefore, verapamil and diltiazem, but not dihydropyridines, are classified as Vaughan–Williams class IV antiarrhythmic agents.

5. *Anti-atherogenic effects*. Some CCBs (amlodipine, nifedipine, and lacidipine) slow the progression of carotid hypertrophy and atherosclerosis. In patients with angiographically documented CAD, amlodipine has no effect on the progression of coronary atherosclerosis or the risk of major CV events but significantly reduces hospitalizations for UA and revascularizations and slows the progression of carotid artery atherosclerosis. In patients with stable symptomatic effort angina, nifedipine GI therapeutic system (GITS) added to β-blocker therapy reduces the need for coronary angiography and bypass surgery.
6. *Pulmonary hypertension*. High doses of nifedipine, diltiazem, and amlodipine are recommended in patients with idiopathic PAH, heritable PAH, and drug-induced PAH who are responders to acute vasoreactivity testing. Nifedipine and amlodipine are selected in patients with a relative bradycardia; a relative tachycardia favours diltiazem or verapamil.
7. *Renal effects*. CCBs produce a preferential vasodilator effect of afferent arterioles, increase renal blood flow, while GFR remains unchanged, and exert mild diuresis, natriuresis, and kaliuresis. CCBs also protect against acute renal failure produced by radiocontrast agents, aminoglycoside antibiotics, chemotherapy, or ciclosporin nephrotoxicity. In hypertensive patients with renal damage, both dihydropyridines and non-dihydropyridines reduce BP to a similar extent, but dihydropyridines does not reduce proteinuria, whereas verapamil and diltiazem exert a protective effect in the presence or absence of diabetes. Thus, non-dihydropyridines, alone or in combination with an ACEI (or ARB), are the preferred agents to lower BP in hypertensive patients with diabetic nephropathy associated with proteinuria.

Pharmacokinetics

CCBs are metabolized primarily in the liver and the AUC and t½ of CCBs increase in elderly patients and in patients with hepatic disease or HF that reduces the hepatic clearance. In these patients the starting dose should be lower and increased slowly. However, no dosage adjustment is required in patients with renal impairment. Pharmacokinetics vary widely between formulations and brands. To ensure consistency of response, once it is established, it is not advisable to substitute different brands for another. Short-acting preparations of CCBs can cause a rapid drop in BP, reflex tachycardia, and neurohumoral activation and are not recommmended for long-term management. Long-acting, once-daily dose formulations are currently recommended. (See Table 8.1.6.)

Practical points

1. *Doses* (see individual drugs)
   - There are marked differences among the different preparations of each drug, so that patients may require different doses.
   - CCBs are metabolized primarily by the liver and the AUC and t½ of CCBs increase in elderly patients and in those with hepatic disease or HF which reduces the hepatic clearance. In patients with liver dysfunction, the starting dose should be lower and increased slowly. However, no dosage adjustment is required in patients with renal impairment.
2. *Adverseeffects*
   - General: somnolence, dizziness, headache, fatigue, flush (especially on initiation of treatment), ankle oedema (due to precapillary vasodilatation). Non-dihydropyridines produce less flushing or headaches or pedal oedema.
   - CV: sinus bradycardia, palpitations, first-degree AVB, fatigue, hypotension, nasal congestion. At high doses or in patients with prior myocardial damage: bradyarrhythmias, second- and third-degree AVB, transient asystole, HF. Diltiazem and verapamil produce more cardiac adverse effects, and dihydropyridines more vascular adverse effects.
   - Central: paraesthesiae.
   - GI: abdominal pain, nausea, dyspepsia, and constipation (very frequent with verapamil and in the elderly). Transient increase in liver transaminases and isolated cases of hepatitis (reversible after treatment withdrawal).
   - Others: light-headedness, giddiness, weakness, gingival hyperplasia, facial pain, skin rashes (diltiazem: exfoliative dermatitis, erythema multiforme, vasculitis), impotence, polyuria.
   - There is no evidence that CCBs increase cancer, bleeding, and all-cause mortality.
3. *Interactions*
   - Co-administration of CCBs with other antihypertensive agents, vasodilators (long-acting nitrates), phenothiazines, or alcohol produce an additive BP-lowering effect.
   - Efficacy of dihydropyridine CCBs may be reduced by CYP3A4 inducers and increased by CYP3A4 inhibitors (see Table 8.1.2). Avoid combinations with potent CYP3A4 inhibitors and/or inducers.

- Co-administration of CCBs with other drugs metabolized by CYP3A4 (see Table 8.1.2) leads to an increase in their plasma levels; thus, the doses of these drugs may need to be reduced. Plasma levels of ciclosporin and tacrolimus should be closely monitored.
- Co-administration of β-blockers with dihydropyridine CCBs is usually well tolerated in patients with hypertension or angina, even when the combination may increase the likelihood of CHF, severe hypotension, bradycardia, or AVB.
- CCBs potentiate the depression of cardiac heart rate and contractility and AV conduction and the vasodilatation produced by general anaesthetics.
- High doses of vitamin D and/or high intake of Ca^{2+} salts leading to elevated serum Ca^{2+} levels may reduce the response to CCBs.

4. *Cautions/notes*
    - Verapamil and diltiazem alone, and particularly when combined with β-blockers, can occasionally produce marked bradycardia, AVB, and worsening of cardiac function. Thus, their combination should be used under close medical supervision. To avoid pharmacokinetic interactions, dihydropyridines are best combined with atenolol or nadolol that are excreted via the renal route than with β-blockers that are metabolized in the liver (carvedilol, metoprolol, propranolol).
    - In patients preserved LV function, verapamil and diltiazem do not exert a negative inotropic effect, while in patients with ventricular dysfunction, they deteriorate LV function, worsening HF. Amlodipine and felodipine are an option in these patients to control BP levels and angina pectoris.
    - Diltiazem can be combined with dihydropyridines in patients with resistant coronary artery vasospasm. This benefit can be explained because they bind to different receptor sites on the Ca^{2+} channel.
5. *Pregnancy and lactation* (see individual drugs)
    - Some CCBs produce teratogenic effects in animals, but there are no well-controlled studies in pregnant women. Thus, CCBs should be used during pregnancy only if the potential benefit justifies the potential risk to the fetus (Pregnancy category C).
6. *Contraindications* (see individual drugs)
    - Hypersensitivity to the drug.
    - Hypotension (SBP <90mmHg) or cardiogenic shock.
    - Bradycardia (<50bpm), sick sinus syndrome, second or third-degree AVB, and sick sinus syndrome (unless a functioning pacemaker is present).
    - AF/atrial flutter associated with an accessory pathway (WPW syndrome).
    - UA, acute phase of MI (avoid if bradycardia, hypotension, LV failure), and pulmonary congestion documented on admission.
    - Decompensated HF, LV dysfunction (LVEF <40%).
    - Pregnancy and lactation, unless the clinical condition of the woman requires treatment with a CCB (i.e. hypertensive disorders during pregnancy).
    - Because they reduce cardiac afterload, CCBs should not be given to patients with severe aortic stenosis or obstructive cardiomyopathy.

Candesartan (cilexetil)

Angiotensin AT1 receptor blocker (see ➔ Angiotensin II AT1 receptor blockers, pp. 456–8).

Indications

- Treatment of essential hypertension.
- Treatment of HFrEF (NYHA classes II–IV), when ACEIs are not tolerated, to reduce CV deaths and HF hospitalization.

Pharmacokinetics

Following oral administration, candesartan cilexetil is converted to its active metabolite candesartan. The absolute bioavailability of candesartan varies according to the formulation (14–40%) and is not significantly affected by food. Serum concentrations peak at 3–4h and increase linearly with increasing doses in the therapeutic dose range. Candesartan is highly bound to plasma protein (>99%), with an apparent Vd of 0.1L/kg. Candesartan is mainly eliminated unchanged via urine (33%), bile (77%), and, to a minor extent, by hepatic metabolism (CYP2C9). Renal elimination of candesartan is by both glomerular filtration and active tubular secretion. The terminal t½ is approximately 9h. Candesartan is not removed by dialysis. (See Table 8.1.9.)

Practical points

1. *Doses*
   - Initial dose: 4mg od (for HF) or 8mg od (for hypertension); maximum dose 32mg od.
   - Reduce the initial dose to 2mg od in patients with hepatic impairment and 4–6mg od in those with renal impairment.
2. *Side effects, interactions, cautions, and contraindications* (see ➔ Angiotensin II AT1 receptor blockers, pp. 456–8).

Table 8.1.9 Pharmacokinetic properties of angiotensin AT1 receptor blockers and sacubitril/valsartan

Drug	F (%)	T_{max} (h)	PPB (%)	Vd (L/kg)	Metabolism	t½ (h)	Renal excretion** (%)
Candesartan cilexetil*	42	3–4	99	0.1	CYP2C9	9	26
Eprosartan	15	0.5–3	98	13	Not CYP	5–7	2
Irbesartan	60-80	1.5–2	96	0.7–1.2	Glucoconjugation, CYP2C9	11–15	20
Losartan	33	0.5–2	99	0.6	CYP3A4, 2C9, 2C10	2	35
Olmesartan medoxomil*	25	1.5–2.5	99	0.24	Ester hydrolysis	13	40
Sacubitril/valsartan	>60/23	1–2	94–97	1.47/1.07	Sacubitril: carboxylesterases	1.43/9.9	50–68/13
Telmisartan	50	1–2	99	0.48	No CYP metabolism	24	2
Valsartan	23	1–2	94–97	0.25	Minimally metabolized	6–9	13

F, oral bioavailability; h, hour; PPB, protein plasma binding; t½, drug half-life; T_{max}, time to peak plasma levels; Vd, volume of distribution.

* Prodrug.

** Renal excretion without biotransformation.

Cangrelor

IV nonthiepyridine, direct P2Y12 platelet receptor antagonist.

Indications

- Co-administered with aspirin, cangrelor is indicated for the reduction of thrombotic CV events in adult patients with CAD undergoing PCI who have not received an oral P2Y12 inhibitor prior to the PCI procedure and in whom oral therapy with P2Y12 inhibitors is not feasible or desirable.
- NSTEMI: cangrelor may be considered in P2Y12 inhibitor-naïve patients undergoing PCI.

Mechanism of action

Cangrelor binds selectively and reversibly to the P2Y12 receptor to prevent further signalling and platelet activation.

Pharmacodynamics

Cangrelor is a rapid-acting (within 2min), reversible, potent, competitive inhibitor of the P2Y12 receptor, causing an almost complete inhibition of ADP-induced platelet aggregation. Irrespective of the dose, platelet function returns to normal within 1h of stopping the infusion.

Unlike clopidogrel, which is a prodrug, cangrelor is an active drug that does not require metabolic conversion to an active metabolite.

Pharmacokinetics

IV cangrelor reaches peak plasma levels within 2min. Following cessation of its administration, normal platelet function is restored within 1h. The pharmacokinetics of cangrelor are not affected by gender, age, or renal or hepatic status. (See Table 8.1.7.)

Practical points

1. *Doses*
   - The starting dosage is a 30mcg/kg IV bolus, followed by a 4mcg/kg/min IV infusion for at least 2h. The bolus and infusion should be initiated prior to the procedure and continued for the duration of the procedure, whichever is longer. To maintain platelet inhibition, a loading dose of an oral P2Y12 platelet inhibitor should be administered immediately following discontinuation of the cangrelor infusion. Alternatively, a loading dose of ticagrelor or prasugrel, but not clopidogrel, may be administered up to 30min before the end of the infusion. No dose adjustment in patients with renal or hepatic impairment.
2. *Side effects*
   - The commonest are bleeding events that can occur at any site, mainly at the site of arterial puncture. In phase III trials, intracranial haemorrhage and moderate and mild bleeding events were commoner in patients treated with cangrelor than in those treated with clopidogrel.

- Haematoma, ecchymosis, anaemia, hypotension, fall in haematocrit and haemoglobin levels. In patients undergoing PCI, dyspnoea occurred more commonly in patients treated with cangrelor than clopidogrel.
- Risk of hypersensitivity reactions (rash, pruritus, urticaria, anaphylactic reactions/shock, and angio-oedema). Increase in creatine plasma levels and hypersensitivity reactions.

3. *Drug interactions*
   - When clopidogrel is administered during infusion of cangrelor, the expected inhibitory effect of clopidogrel on platelets is not achieved. No interaction was observed when clopidogrel was administered immediately after discontinuation of the cangrelor infusion. However, cangrelor and prasugrel or ticagrelor can be administered concomitantly.
   - No interactions were observed with aspirin, heparin, bivalirudin, LMWH, fondaparinux, and GPIIb/IIIa inhibitors or glyceryl trinitrate.
   - Metabolism of cangrelor is not dependent on CYPs, and CYP isoenzymes are not inhibited by therapeutic concentrations of cangrelor or its major metabolites.
4. *Cautions*
   - Patients can be transitioned from cangrelor to prasugrel when prasugrel is administered immediately following discontinuation of the cangrelor infusion or up to 1h before, optimally at 30min before the end of the cangrelor infusion, to limit the recovery of platelet reactivity.
   - Cangrelor should be used with caution in disease states associated with an increased bleeding risk or when taking medicines that may increase the risk of bleeding.
   - Cangrelor is contraindicated in patients with any history of stroke/TIA.
   - Cangrelor may increase the risk of cardiac tamponade.
   - In patients with severe renal impairment (CrCl 15–30mL/min), a higher rate of worsening in renal function was reported in the cangrelor group, compared to clopidogrel. Cangrelor should be used with caution in these patients.
   - This product contains sorbitol. Avoid in patients with rare hereditary problems of fructose intolerance.
5. *Pregnancy and lactation*
   - There are no adequate and well-controlled studies of cangrelor in pregnant women (Pregnancy category C). It is unknown whether cangrelor is excreted in human milk.
6. *Contraindications*
   - Significant active bleeding or increased risk of bleeding.
   - History of stroke or TIA.
   - Hypersensitivity to the drug.

Captopril

Orally active ACEI (see ➔ Angiotensin-converting enzyme inhibitors, pp. 459–64).

Indications

- Treatment of hypertension.
- Treatment of CHF.
- Treatment post-MI: (1) short-term treatment (4 weeks) in any clinically stable patient within the first 24h of MI; and (2) long-term treatment for the prevention of symptomatic HF in clinically stable patients with asymptomatic LV dysfunction.
- Treatment of macroproteinuric diabetic nephropathy in patients with T1DM.

Pharmacokinetics

(See Table 8.1.10.)

Practical points

1. *Doses*
   - *Hypertension*: starting dose is 25–50mg bd; reduce the dose in patients at risk of hypotension. Maximum dose: 100–150mg/day bd. A once-daily dosing regimen may be appropriate when combined with a thiazide diuretic.
   - *HF*: 6.25–12.5mg bd or tds, titrated up to daily maximum of 50mg tds, based on responses.
   - *Post-MI*: (1) short term: 6.25mg test dose, followed by 12.5mg 2h afterwards and a 25mg dose 12h later. From the following day, captopril should be administered at 100mg/day bd for 4 weeks; (2) chronic treatment: once the patient is stable, start with 6.25mg, followed by 12.5mg tds for 2 days, and then 25mg tds. The maintenance dose is 75–150mg/day in 2–3 doses.
   - In patients with impaired renal function, the following daily doses are recommended.

CrCl	Starting dose	Maximum daily dose
>40mL/min/1.73m²	25–50mg	150mg
21–40mL/min/1.73m²	25mg	100mg
10–20mL/min/1.73m²	12.5mg	75mg
10mL/min/1.73m²	6.25mg	37.5mg

2. *Side effects* (see ➔ Angiotensin-converting enzyme inhibitors, pp. 459–64)
   - At high doses: neutropenia, especially in collagen vascular renal disease. Proteinuria (especially in the presence of pre-existing renal disease), skin reactions, loss of taste, oral lesions.
3. *Interactions* (see ➔ Angiotensin-converting enzyme inhibitors, pp. 459–64)

Table 8.1.10 Pharmacokinetic characteristics of angiotensin-converting enzyme inhibitors

Drugs	F (%)	T_{max} (h)	PPB (%)	Vd (L/kg)	Metabolism	t½ (h)	Renal excretion** (%)
Captopril	75	1.5	25–30		Disulfide dimers	2	40–50
Enalapril*	60	1	60	1.7	Carboxylesterases	11	40
Lisinopril	25	7	0	2.4	Not metabolized	12	88–100
Perindopril*	65–70	1	20	0.2	Carboxylesterases, UDP-glucuronosyltransferase	17	4–12
Quinapril*	≤60	2	97	–	Carboxylesterases	2–4	96
Ramipril*	45	1	60	–	Carboxylesterases	13–17	60
Trandolapril*	40–60	0.5–1	>85	0.25	Carboxylesterases, UDP-glucuronosyltransferase	15–23	33

F, oral bioavailability; h, hour; PPB, protein plasma binding; t½, drug half-life; T_{max}, time to peak plasma levels; Vd, volume of distribution.

* Prodrug.

** Renal excretion without biotransformation.

4. *Cautions* (see ➲ Angiotensin-converting enzyme inhibitors, pp. 459–64)
   - Captopril has a rapid onset of action; the risk of hypotension increases in patients with HF.
   - Co-administration with allopurinol may increase the risk of hypersensitivity reactions (SJS, skin eruptions, anaphylaxis, fever, and arthralgias).
   - Captopril should be used with extreme caution in patients with collagen vascular disease, those on immunosuppressant therapy, and those on treatment with allopurinol or procainamide, especially if there is pre-existing impaired renal function. Some of these patients developed serious infections which, in a few instances, did not respond to intensive antibiotic therapy.
   - Monitor neutrophil counts in patients with pre-existing collagen vascular disease.
5. *Pregnancy and lactation* (see ➲ Angiotensin-converting enzyme inhibitors, pp. 459–64)
6. *Contraindications* (see ➲ Angiotensin-converting enzyme inhibitors, pp. 459–64)

Carvedilol

Vasodilator, non-selective, lipid-soluble β-adrenergic receptor antagonist with α-antagonism and antioxidant properties (see ➲ Beta-adrenergic blocking agents, pp. 485–94).

CV indications

- Essential hypertension.
- Chronic stable angina pectoris.
- Adjunctive treatment of moderate to severe stable chronic HF.

Pharmacodynamics

(See ➲ Beta-adrenergic blocking agents, pp. 485–94.)

Carvedilol is an α- and β-adrenergic blocker with vasodilatory, antiproliferative, and antioxidant activity. Renal blood flow and renal function, as well as peripheral blood flow, remain normal; therefore, cold extremities, often observed with β-blockers, are rarely seen. Metabolically, carvedilol may increase insulin sensitivity.

Pharmacokinetics

In patients with liver cirrhosis, the systemic availability of carvedilol is increased 80% due to reduced first-pass effect. Drug accumulation in patients with renal impairment is unlikely. Plasma levels appear approximately 50% higher in the elderly. (See Table 8.1.8.)

Practical points

1. *Doses*
   - HF: 3.125mg bd (uptitrated by doubling at intervals of 2 weeks to the highest tolerated dose or a maximum of 25mg bd).
   - Hypertension and chronic angina: 12.5mg od (increase after 2 days to 25mg od, up to a maximum of 50mg od or bd).
   - In general, there is no dose adjustment in the elderly or those with renal impairment.
2. *Side effects* (see ➲ Beta-adrenergic blocking agents, pp. 485–94)
3. *Interactions* (see ➲ Beta-adrenergic blocking agents, pp. 485–94)
   - Carvedilol may prolong AV conduction time when given with digoxin and increases trough levels of digoxin. Monitor digoxin levels when initiating or adjusting carvedilol doses.
   - Care when combined with CYP2D6/CYP2C9 inducers or inhibitors (see Table 8.1.2). Cimetidine may increase carvedilol plasma levels.
   - Modest increases in ciclosporin plasma levels (20%) may require an approximately 30% reduction in dosage and close monitoring of ciclosporin plasma levels.
   - Amiodarone may increase carvedilol plasma levels, resulting in further slowing of the heart rate and cardiac conduction.
   - Carvedilol may enhance the hypoglycaemic effects of insulin and oral antidiabetics. Regular monitoring of blood glucose levels is necessary.
4. *Cautions/notes* (see ➲ Beta-adrenergic blocking agents, pp. 485–94)
   - HF: monitor for hypotension (SBP <100mmHg), worsening renal function, or HF before dose increase. If transient worsening of HF, adjust the doses of diuretics and ACEIs (ARBs) or temporarily stop carvedilol.

5. *Pregnancy and lactation*
   - Inadequate data in pregnant women (Pregnancy category C). Carvedilol is excreted in breast milk in animals, and therefore, mothers receiving carvedilol should not breastfeed.
6. *Contraindications* (see ➔ Beta-adrenergic blocking agents, pp. 485–94)
   - Carvedilol contains lactose monohydrate and sucrose. Avoid in patients with galactose/fructose intolerance, Lapp lactase deficiency, or glucose–galactose malabsorption.

Chlortalidone

Oral thiazide diuretic (see ➲ Thiazide and related diuretics, pp. 768–73).

CV and other indications

- Treatment of arterial hypertension, essential or nephrogenic or isolated systolic hypertension.
- Treatment of stable, chronic HF (NYHA class II or III).
- Oedema of specific origin: ascites due to cirrhosis of the liver in stable patients under close control and oedema due to nephrotic syndrome.
- Diabetes insipidus.

Mechanism of action

BP reduction with chlortalidone (12.5–25mg od) decreases the risk of stroke, CV endpoints, as well as all-cause mortality, but at the cost of increased hyperglycaemia and hypokalaemia. The reduction in the risk of HF may be greater with chlortalidone, compared with the ACEI lisinopril or the CCB amlodipine.

Pharmacokinetics

Its oral bioavailability is approximately 65%. Following absorption, chlortalidone is approximately 98% bound to erythrocytes where it binds carbonic anhydrase, reaching 7–10 times greater concentrations than in plasma, and its Vd is 0.14L/kg. It has a long t½ of 40–60h and 65% of the dose is excreted unchanged in the urine. The diuretic effect begins within 2.5h and reaches peak plasma levels within 3–6h, and the duration of action is up to 72h. Renal dysfunction does not alter the pharmacokinetics of chlortalidone. (See Table 8.1.5.)

Practical points

1. *Doses*
    - Hypertension and oedema: 12.5–50mg od.
    - HF: 25–50mg od, increased up to 100–200mg/day.
    - Diabetes insipidus: 100mg bd, reduced to 50mg daily.
2. *Side effects, interactions, cautions/notes, and contraindications* (see ➲ Thiazide and related diuretics, pp. 768–73)
3. *Pregnancy and lactation*
    - Chlortalidone crosses the placental barrier and passes into breast milk (Pregnancy category C). Levels in fetal whole blood are about 15% of those found in maternal blood.

Colestyramine

Oral bile acid sequestrant.

CV indications

As adjunctive therapy to diet and exercise in:

- Primary prevention of CAD in individuals aged between 35 and 59 years and with primary hypercholesterolaemia who have not responded to diet and other appropriate measures.
- Reduction in plasma cholesterol levels in hypercholesterolaemia, particularly in those patients who have been diagnosed with Fredrickson type IIa (high plasma cholesterol levels with normal or slightly elevated TG levels).

Non-CV indications

- Relief of pruritus associated with partial biliary obstruction and primary biliary cirrhosis.
- Relief of diarrhoea associated with ileal resection, Crohn's disease, vagotomy, and diabetic vagal neuropathy.
- Management of radiation-induced diarrhoea.

Mechanism of action

Bile acids are synthesized in the liver from cholesterol and are released into the intestinal lumen, but most of the bile acid is returned to the liver from the terminal ileum via active absorption. Colestyramine adsorbs and combines with bile acids in the intestine to form an insoluble complex that is not reabsorbed but excreted in the faeces. The increased faecal loss of bile acids leads to increased oxidation of cholesterol to bile acids and hepatic depletion of cholesterol. This increases the expression LDL-Rs and the activity of HMG CoA reductase in hepatocytes. Both effects increase the clearance of LDL-C from blood and decrease total-C and LDL-C plasma levels. Serum TG levels, however, may remain unchanged or increase.

In partial biliary obstruction, a reduction in serum bile acid levels reduces the amount of bile acids deposited in dermal tissue, leading to a decrease in pruritus.

Pharmacodynamics

Primary hypercholesterolaemia: colestyramine reduces plasma total-C and LDL-C levels (8.5% and 12.6% greater than placebo, respectively). It reduces CAD death and/or non-fatal MI in middle-aged men with primary hypercholesterolaemia and the progression of CAD, compared to placebo. Its combination with a statin reduces LDL-C levels by an additional 10–20%.

Pharmacokinetics

Colestyramine is not absorbed from the digestive tract.

Practical points

1. *Doses*

Colestyramine should be taken with water or other fluids.

- *Primary hypercholesterolaemia*: 4g od or bd (maximum daily dose 36g). Treatment should only be continued if a reduction in LDL-C levels of at least 10–15% has been achieved after 1–2 months.
- *To relieve pruritus*: 4g or 8g daily.
- *To relieve diarrhoea*: dose as for reduction of cholesterol; if a response is not seen within 3 days, alternative therapy should be initiated.

2. *Side effects*
   - Constipation (frequently disappears on continued use), abdominal discomfort, flatulence, nausea, vomiting, diarrhoea, heartburn, dyspepsia, and steatorrhoea. These adverse effects can be attenuated by beginning treatment at low doses and ingesting ample fluid with the drug.
   - Increased bleeding tendency due to hypoprothrombinaemia associated with vitamin K deficiency (usually responds to parenteral vitamin K).
   - Others: skin irritation, taste disturbance.
3. *Interactions*
   - Colestyramine may delay or reduce the absorption of many drugs (warfarin, digoxin, thiazide diuretics, propranolol, tetracycline, oral contraceptives containing ethinylestradiol and norethindrone, levothyroxine, and glibenclamide). These drugs should be taken either at least 1h before or 4–6h after colestyramine.
4. *Cautions/notes*
   - Colestyramine may interfere with the absorption of fat-soluble vitamins and folic acid. Patients may require supplementation with vitamins A, D, and K and folic acid.
   - Colestyramine can increase TG levels in patients with TG levels of >3.4mmol/L.
   - Caution in patients with dysphagia, swallowing disorders, severe GI motility disorders, inflammatory bowel disease, liver failure, or major GI tract surgery.
   - Long-term use of high doses of colestyramine may produce hyperchloraemic acidosis.
   - Monitor ciclosporin plasma levels, and adjust the doses if combined with colestyramine.
   - Colestyramine reduces the absorption of vitamin K and interferes with the effect of warfarin. Monitor the INR.
   - Colestyramine can affect the bioavailability of the oral contraceptive pill when administered simultaneously.
5. *Pregnancy and lactation*
   - Safety has not been established in pregnant women (Pregnancy category C). The possibility of interference with the absorption of fat-soluble vitamins should be considered.
6. *Contraindications*
   - Hypersensitivity to any of its product ingredients.
   - Complete biliary obstruction (as colestyramine cannot be effective).

Cilostazol

Phosphodiesterase type 3 (PDE-3) inhibitor.

Indications

- To improve the maximal and pain-free walking distances in patients with intermittent claudication, who do not have rest pain and who do not have evidence of peripheral tissue necrosis (peripheral arterial disease Fontaine stage II).
- Second-line use in patients in whom lifestyle modifications (including stopping smoking and exercise programmes) and other appropriate interventions have failed to sufficiently improve their intermittent claudication symptoms.

Mechanism of action

Cilostazol and several of its metabolites are PDE-3 inhibitors that increase cAMP levels in platelets and blood vessels.

Pharmacodynamics

Cilostazol reversibly inhibits platelet aggregation induced by a variety of stimuli and produces greater vasodilatation in femoral beds than in vertebral, carotid, or superior mesenteric arteries. In patients with stable intermittent claudication, cilostazol improves the maximal walking distance, as compared with placebo or pentoxifylline. Its long-term effects on limb preservation and hospitalization have not been evaluated. Cilostazol reduces restenosis after endovascular therapy but increases the risk of bleeding.

Pharmacokinetics

Cilostazol is absorbed after oral administration, and its C_{max} and AUC increase with a fat meal. It is extensively metabolized by hepatic cytochrome P450 enzymes, mainly 3A4 (to a lesser extent by 2C19 and 1A2), and its metabolites (some active) are largely excreted in urine (74%). Cilostazol and its active metabolites have an apparent elimination t½ of 11–13h. (See Table 8.1.7.)

Practical points

1. *Doses*
   - 100mg bd taken at least 0.5–1h before or 2h after breakfast and dinner. Reassess the patient after 3 months, and discontinue cilostazol where an inadequate effect is observed or symptoms have not improved. No special dosage requirements for the elderly or in patients with mild hepatic disease or CrCl of >25mL/min.
2. *Side effects*
   - The most frequent are: headache, palpitations, tachycardia, hypotension, dizziness, flush symptoms, and diarrhoea. Other: asthenia, chest pain, oedema, anorexia, rhinitis, rash, pruritus, ecchymosis, dyspepsia, flatulence, abdominal pain, angina pectoris, ventricular extrasystoles, and NSVT. Rare/very rare: thrombocytopenia, leucopenia, agranulocytosis, pancytopenia, and aplastic anaemia.

3. *Drug interactions*
    - Strong CYP3A4 inhibitors/inducers (see Table 8.1.2) reduce/increase cilostazol plasma levels.
    - Co-administration with aspirin increases the inhibition of ADP-induced platelet aggregation.
    - Diltiazem and erythromycin increase cilostazol exposure. Smoking decreases cilostazol exposure by about 20%.
4. *Cautions*
    - Co-administration with antiplatelet drugs and oral anticoagulants increases the risk of bleeding.
    - Reduce the dose to 50mg bd if co-administered with strong or moderate CYP3A4 inhibitors or with CYP2C19 inhibitors (see Table 8.1.2).
    - Patients who may be at increased risk for serious cardiac adverse events as a result of tachycardia (stable CAD) should be closely monitored during treatment with cilostazol.
    - Caution when prescribing cilostazol in patients with atrial or ventricular ectopy and AF or flutter.
    - Because cilostazol inhibits platelet aggregation and may increase the risk of bleeding, it should be stopped 5 days prior to surgery.
5. *Pregnancy and lactation*
    - Cilostazol is only recommended during pregnancy when there are no alternatives and benefit outweighs risk (Pregnancy category C). There are no data on the excretion of cilostazol into human milk.
6. *Contraindications*
    - Known or suspected hypersensitivity to any of its components.
    - Patients with any known predisposition to bleeding: active peptic ulceration, recent (within 6 months) haemorrhagic stroke, proliferative diabetic retinopathy, or poorly controlled hypertension.
    - CHF.
    - Moderate or severe hepatic impairment.
    - Severe renal impairment (CrCl ≤25mL/min).
    - Pregnancy.
    - Patients with any history of VT, VF, or multifocal ventricular ectopics and in patients with prolongation of the QTc interval.
    - Patients treated concomitantly with two or more additional antiplatelet or anticoagulant agents.
    - Patients with UA, MI, or a coronary intervention in the last 6 months.
    - Patients with rare hereditary problems of fructose intolerance should not take this medicine.

Clopidogrel

Thienopyridine derivative acting as an irreversible inhibitor of the platelet ADP P2Y12 receptor.

CV indications

DAPT with aspirin and clopidogrel is recommended for:

1. *Prevention of atherothrombotic events*:
   - Adult patients with MI (from a few days until <35 days), ischaemic stroke (from 7 days until <6 months), or established peripheral arterial disease to reduce the rate of a combined endpoint of new ischaemic stroke (fatal or not), new MI (fatal or not), and other vascular death.
   - Adult patients suffering from ACS:
     —NSTE-ACS (UA/NSTEMI), including patients undergoing a stent placement following PCI. Clopidogrel decreases the combined endpoint of CV death, MI, stroke, or refractory ischaemia.
     —STEMI in medically treated patients eligible for thrombolytic therapy. Clopidogrel reduces the rate of death from any cause and the rate of a combined endpoint of death, reinfarction, or stroke.
2. *Prevention of atherothrombotic and thromboembolic events in AF*:
   - In adult patients with AF who have at least one risk factor for vascular events, who are not suitable for treatment with VKAs, and who have a low bleeding risk, clopidogrel is indicated in combination with ASA for the prevention of atherothrombotic and thromboembolic events, including stroke.

Mechanism of action

Platelets release ADP, a pro-aggregant agonist. The binding of ADP to its G_i-coupled P2Y12 receptor leads to the inhibition of adenylyl cyclase and lowers platelet cAMP levels. This inhibits cAMP-mediated phosphorylation of vasodilator-stimulated phosphoprotein (VASP), which is closely related to the inhibition of GPIIb/IIIa receptor activation.

Clopidogrel is a prodrug that must be metabolized in the liver by CYP450 enzymes to an active metabolite that competitively and irreversibly inhibits the binding of ADP to its platelet P2Y12 receptor and the subsequent ADP-mediated activation of the GPIIb/IIIa complex. Because the inhibition is irreversible, platelets exposed to clopidogrel are affected for their lifespan (7–10 days). Clopidogrel also inhibits the platelet aggregation induced by agonists other than ADP by blocking the amplification of platelet activation by released ADP.

Pharmacodynamics

Clopidogrel inhibits approximately 40–60% of ADP-induced aggregation, reaching steady-state effects after 5–7 days and increases the bleeding time. A 600-mg oral loading dose of clopidogrel achieves maximal inhibition of platelet aggregation after 2h, compared with 24–48h with a 300-mg loading dose. This is the basis for the administration of a high loading dose, followed by a low maintenance dose. Platelet aggregation and bleeding time gradually return to baseline values about 5 days after drug discontinuation.

Pharmacokinetics

Clopidogrel is an inactive prodrug. It is rapidly absorbed after oral administration (bioavailability 30–50%), a process that is not influenced by food, reaching peak plasma levels after 45–60min. It is extensively metabolized in the liver by mulltiple CYP450 isoforms (CYP3A4, 2C19, 1A2, and 2B6), firstly to 2-oxo-clopidogrel and then to an active metabolite that binds rapidly and irreversibly to the platelet P2Y12 receptors to inhibit platelet aggregation. The C_{max} of this active metabolite is twice as high, following a loading dose of 300mg of clopidogrel. The onset of the antiplatelet effect is within 2–8h and reaches steady state within 3–7 days. Clopidogrel and its active metabolite are highly protein-bound (98% and 94%, respectively) and excreted in urine (50%) and faeces (50%). The plasma t½ is approximately 6h (longer in the elderly), but due to the irreversible blockade of the P2Y12 receptor, clopidogrel effects last for the whole lifespan of the platelet (7–10 days). (See Table 8.1.7.)

Inhibition of ADP-induced platelet aggregation induced by clopidogrel decreases (25%) in patients with moderate to severe renal impairment. In patients with severe hepatic impairment, inhibition of ADP-induced platelet aggregation was similar to that observed in healthy subjects.

Clopidogrel pharmacokinetics and antiplatelet effects may differ according to polymorphisms of the gene encoding the P2Y12 receptor or CYP2C19 or CYP3A4. The CYP2C19*1 allele corresponds to fully functional metabolism, while the CYP2C19*2 and *3 alleles are non-functional and account for the majority of reduced-function alleles in white (85%) and Asian (99%) poor metabolizers. Frequencies for poor CYP2C19 metabolizer genotypes are approximately 2% for whites, 4% for blacks, and 14% for Chinese. The CYP2C19*2 allele is associated with increased rates of ischaemic events and stent thrombosis after PCI. There is currently no recommendation to perform genetic testing in patients with stable CAD.

Practical points

1. *Doses*
    - UA/NSTEMI: a single 300–600mg oral loading dose, followed by 75mg od as maintenance dose; clopidogrel is given in combination with aspirin (75–325mg od). The optimal duration of treatment has not been formally established. Clinical trial data support use up to 12 months, and the maximum benefit was seen at 3 months. Clopidogrel is recommended for patients who cannot receive ticagrelor or prasugrel or who require oral anticoagulation.
    - Patients with STEMI: 300mg loading dose in combination with ASA (100mg/day) and with or without thrombolytics, followed by 75mg od. In patients over 75 years of age, avoid the loading dose of clopidogrel. Combined therapy should be started as early as possible after symptoms start and continued for at least 4 weeks.
    - In patients with AF, clopidogrel should be given as a single daily dose of 75mg. ASA (75–100mg/day) should be initiated and continued in combination with clopidogrel.

- After implantation of a BMS, clopidogrel should be continued at 75mg/daily for 4–6 weeks, and after a DES for 12 months (aspirin must be kept on indefinitely).

Clopidogrel (75mg/day) is chosen in patients intolerant to aspirin. PPIs are recommended if gastric intolerance to aspirin or clopidogrel.

2. *Side effects*
   - Common: bleeding at the puncture site, haematoma, epistaxis, bruising, GI (haemorrhage, diarrhoea, abdominal pain, dyspepsia). The absolute risk of major bleeding associated with clopidogrel is approximately 3.7%, and 0.7% of GI bleeds requiring hospitalization, but there is less major GI bleeding than with aspirin.
   - Uncommon: thrombocytopenia, leucopenia, eosinophilia, headache, paraesthesiae, dizziness, intracranial bleeding, rash, pruritus, skin bleeding (purpura), haematuria, and GI (gastric and duodenal ulcer, gastritis, vomiting, nausea, constipation, flatulence). Rare: neutropenia. Very rare: thrombotic thrombocytopenic purpura, pancytopenia, agranulocytosis, severe thrombocytopenia, hypersensitivity reactions, confusion, taste disturbances, serious haemorrhages at multiple sites, hypotension, abnormal LFTs, arthritis, arthralgia, increases in blood creatinine levels, and fever.
   - The percentage of 'low responders' or 'resistant' patients ranges from 5% to 40% across studies. High platelet reactivity on clopidogrel treatment results from multiple factors: non-compliance, accelerated platelet turnover, drug interactions, patient characteristics (such as age, gender, diabetes), and single-nucleotide polymorphisms [cytochrome P450 2C19 (CYP2C19*2), ATP-binding cassette subfamily B member 1 (ABCB1)]. One strategy to overcome non-responsiveness is use of higher-than-currently-approved loading and maintenance doses of clopidogrel.
3. *Interactions*
   - The risk of bleeding increases when clopidogrel is co-administered with warfarin, NSAIDs, anticoagulants, antiplatelet agents, or thrombolytics because of independent effects on haemostasis. Therefore, concomitant use should be undertaken with caution.
   - Clopidogrel inhibits CYP2C9 and may interfere with the metabolism of phenytoin, tamoxifen, tolbutamide, warfarin, torasemide, fluvastatin, and many NSAIDs. Caution is thus required when these drugs are co-administered with clopidogrel.
   - Clopidogrel is metabolized to its active metabolite partly by CYP2C19. Potent CYP2C19 inhibitors (see Table 8.1.2) reduce the levels of the active metabolite and should be administered with caution.
   - CYP2D6 inhibitors (see Table 8.1.2) reduce plasma levels of the active metabolite of clopidogrel and its clinical efficacy and should be avoided.
   - Omeprazole or esomeprazole decreases exposure of the active metabolite and reduces inhibition of platelet aggregation. Lansoprazole and pantoprazole had less effect on the antiplatelet activity of clopidogrel.

- Both selective SSRIs and SNRIs affect platelet activation and may increase the risk of bleeding when given with clopidogrel.
- Atorvastatin and omeprazole competitively inhibit hepatic activation of clopidogrel, reducing clopidogrel responsiveness.
- Clopidogrel may increase exposure to CYP2C8 substrate drugs (repaglinide, paclitaxel), and co-administration should be undertaken with caution.
- No interaction with H2 blockers or antacids, atenolol, digoxin, oestrogens, nifedipine, phenytoin, and tolbutamide.

4. *Cautions/notes*
   - Limitations of clopidogrel include its delayed onset of action, important inter-individual variability in the formation of the active metabolite, and irreversibility of its inhibitory effect. Prasugrel or ticagrelor can be given, instead of clopidogrel, in carriers of the CYP2C19*2 allele.
   - Due to its long t½, discontinuation 5–7 days before CABG may be recommended.
   - Experience is limited in patients with moderate hepatic disease who may have bleeding diatheses and in patients with renal impairment.
   - Clopidogrel should not be used in children because of efficacy concerns.
5. *Pregnancy and lactation*
   - Animal studies do not indicate any harmful effects with respect to pregnancy (Pregnancy category B). Clopidogrel is excreted in breast milk in animals; thus, breastfeeding should not be continued during treatment.
6. *Contraindications*
   - Active pathological bleeding (e.g. intracranial haemorrhage or GI bleed).
   - Severe hepatic impairment.
   - Hypersensitivity to clopidogrel or any of the excipients.

Colchicine

Anti-inflammatory drug.

CV indications

- Acute pericarditis, as an adjunct to aspirin/NSAID therapy, to improve response and prevent recurrences.
- Treatment of acute gout and for short-term prophylaxis of gout attack during initiation of therapy with allopurinol and uricosuric drugs.

Mechanism of action

Colchicine inhibits neutrophil-mediated inflammatory responses and disrupts the polymerization of β-tubulin into microtubules, thereby preventing the activation, degranulation, and migration of neutrophils to sites of inflammation. It also interferes with the inflammasome complex found in neutrophils and monocytes that mediates IL-1β activation.

Pharmacokinetics

Oral colchicine is readily absorbed (bioavailability 45%), reaching C_{max} in 0.5–2h. It binds to plasma proteins by 39%, presents a Vd of 5–8L/kg, and crosses the placenta. Colchicine is metabolized by CYP3A4 and is a substrate of P-gp. Colchicine and its metabolites are excreted in the urine (40–65% unchanged) and faeces. Colchicine is not effectively removed by haemodialysis. Elimination t½ is 22–50h.

Practical points

1. *Doses*
   - Acute pericarditis: 0.5mg od (<70kg) or 0.5mg bd (≥70kg) for ≥6 months.
2. *Side effects*
   - Common: nausea, vomiting, and abdominal pain. Larger doses may cause profuse diarrhoea, GI haemorrhage, skin rashes, and renal and hepatic damage. Rare: peripheral neuritis, myopathy, rhabdomyolysis, alopecia, inhibition of spermatogenesis, and, with prolonged treatment, bone marrow suppression.
3. *Interactions*
   - Increased risk of colchicine toxicity when given with clarithromycin or erythromycin in patients with pre-existing renal impairment.
   - Reduce dosage or interrupt colchicine treatment in patients with normal renal or hepatic function if co-administered with strong P-gp or CYP3A4 inhibitors (see Table 8.1.2).
   - Colchicine increases the risk of nephrotoxicity and myotoxicity in patients on ciclosporin.
   - The absorption of vitamin B12 may be impaired by chronic administration of high doses of colchicine; requirements may be increased.
   - Co-administration of colchicine and statin therapy may produce synergistic muscle-related toxicity. Inhibition of P-gp by atorvastatin or lovastatin may further increase serum colchicine levels. In patients with renal impairment, reduced doses of colchicine should be considered when co-administered with a statin.

4. *Cautions/notes*
   - Myelosuppression, leucopenia, and aplastic anaemia have been reported.
   - Concomitant use of colchicine with CYP3A4 and P-gp inhibitors (see Table 8.1.2) can result in life-threatening or fatal colchicine toxicity.
   - Reduce the dose of atorvastatin, simvastatin, and lovastatin when co-administered with colchicine, given the potential for interactions via CYP3A4 and P-gp pathways.
   - Neuromuscular toxicity and rhabdomyolysis when administered in patients with impaired renal function and elderly patients.
5. *Pregnancy and lactation*
   - Do not use in pregnancy, as there is a risk of fetal chromosome damage (Pregnancy category C). Avoid during breastfeeding.
6. *Contraindications*
   - Patients with renal or hepatic impairment should not be given colchicine with drugs that inhibit both P-gp and CYP3A4 inhibitors.

Colesevelam

Oral bile acid sequestrant.

CV indications

- Co-administration with a statin is indicated as adjunctive therapy to diet, to provide an additive reduction in LDL-C levels in adults with primary hypercholesterolaemia who are not adequately controlled with a statin alone.
- As monotherapy is indicated as adjunctive therapy to diet for reduction of elevated total-C and LDL-C levels in adults with primary hypercholesterolaemia, in whom a statin is considered inappropriate or is not well tolerated.
- In combination with ezetimibe, with or without a statin, in adults with primary hypercholesterolaemia, including patients with familial hypercholesterolaemia.

Mechanism of action

(See ➔ Colestyramine, pp. 520–1.)

Colesevelam is a non-absorbed, lipid-lowering polymer that binds bile acids in the intestine, impeding their reabsorption. As the bile acid pool becomes depleted, the hepatic cholesterol 7α-hydroxylase is upregulated, increasing the conversion of cholesterol to bile acids. This causes an increased demand for cholesterol in the hepatocytes, resulting in an increase in the transcription and activity of HMG CoA reductase and in the number of hepatic LDL-Rs, which, in turn, results in decreased serum LDL-C levels. Serum TG levels may increase.

In patients with T2DM, colesevelam improves glycaemic control and reduces HbA1c; this effect reached steady state after 12–18 weeks of treatment.

Pharmacokinetics

Colesevelam is not absorbed from the GI tract.

Practical points

1. *Doses*
   - Hyperlipidaemia: combination therapy (with statin): 4–6 tablets (2.5–3.75g) od or bd. Monotherapy: 6–7 tablets (3.75–4.375g) per day.
2. *Side effects*
   - Common: constipation, dyspepsia, nausea, asthenia, pharyngitis, raised TG levels.
   - Uncommon: isolated transaminase elevations, myalgia.

Combination with statins did not result in any frequent unexpected adverse reactions, compared to statins alone.

3. *Interactions* (see ➔ Colestyramine, pp. 520–1)
   - Colesevelam decreases exposure of ciclosporin, glimepiride, glipizide, glyburide, levothyroxine, metformin, and oral contraceptives containing ethinylestradiol and norethindrone. These drugs should be administered 4h prior to colesevelam to minimize the risk of any interaction. Monitor the ciclosporin plasma levels, and adjust its dose accordingly.

- Colesevelam decreased phenytoin plasma levels and reduced the INR in patients on warfarin therapy. Colesevelam also reduced the absorption of vitamin K. Thus, the INR should be monitored.
- Colesevelam increases exposure of metformin. Monitor glucose plasma levels.

4. *Cautions/notes* (see ➔ Colestyramine, pp. 520–1)
   - Colesevelam should be taken orally with a meal and liquid.
   - Colesevelam can induce or worsen present constipation. This should especially be considered in patients with CAD and angina pectoris.
   - Safety and efficacy have not been established in patients with TG levels of >3.4mmol/L (they were excluded from the clinical studies) or in children/adolescents.
5. *Pregnancy and lactation*
   - There are no well-controlled studies of colesevelam in pregnant women (Pregnancy category B). Colesevelam is not expected to be excreted in human milk.
6. *Contraindications*
   - Hypersensitivity to the active substance or excipients.
   - History of bowel or biliary obstruction.

Dabigatran etexilate

Dabigatran etexilate is an oral prodrug that is rapidly converted to dabigatran, a potent, direct competitive inhibitor of thrombin (factor IIa).

CV indications

- Prevention of stroke and systemic embolism in adult patients with NVAF, with one or more risk factors such as prior stroke or TIA, age ≥75 years, HF (NYHA class ≥II), diabetes mellitus, and hypertension.
- Treatment of DVT and PE, and prevention of recurrent DVT and PE in adults.

Mechanism of action

Thrombin is a serine protease that plays a key role on the coagulation cascade, as it activates the clotting factors V, VIII, and XI, facilitates the conversion of fibrinogen to fibrin, and is the most potent stimulus for platelet activation. Dabigatran binds directly to exosite 1 on thrombin, a site specific for fibrin, preventing the cleavage of fibrinogen to fibrin, thus preventing the final step of the coagulation cascade and thrombus development. Dabigatran reversibly inhibits fibrin-bound thrombin and free circulating fibrin, providing more effective thrombin inhibition than heparins (which block mainly free thrombin). It also inhibits platelet activation induced by thrombin and activation of clotting factors V, VIII, and XI by thrombin.

Pharmacodynamics

Dabigatran has a predictable anticoagulant effect. It prolongs the aPTT, ecarin clotting time (ECT), and TT. When the extent of anticoagulation needs to be assessed, the calibrated quantitative diluted TT (dTT) test provides an estimation of dabigatran plasma concentrations. The ECT can provide a direct measure of the activity of direct thrombin inhibitors. However, the aPTT test has limited sensitivity and is not suitable for precise quantification of the anticoagulant effect, especially at high plasma concentrations of dabigatran. The INR test is unreliable in patients on dabigatran, and false-positive INR elevations have been reported.

The efficacy and safety of dabigatran have not been established for DVT/PE patients with active cancer.

Pharmacokinetics

Dabigatran etexilate is a prodrug that is rapidly absorbed and rapidly hydrolysed by unspecific plasma and hepatic esterases to the active form (bioavailability 6.5%) dabigatran, which reaches peak plasma concentrations within 2h (6h following administration in the post-operative period due to anaesthesia, GI paresis, and surgical effects). Absorption is unrelated to food but may be decreased with co-administration of PPIs. Dabigatran binds to plasma proteins (35%) and is rapidly distributed (Vd 1L/kg). The cytochrome P450 system did not play a major role in the metabolism of dabigatran, but it is a substrate of P-gp. Both the exposure and t½ increase in patients with renal insufficiency, so that in patients with CrCl of ≥30 to <50mL/min, the t½ of the drug is 18h and C_{max} increases 3.2 times. No changes in dabigatran exposure have been found in patients with moderate hepatic impairment (Child–Pugh B). Avoid in patients with severe hepatic impairment (Child–Pugh C). Dabigatran is dialysable. (See Table 8.1.1.)

Practical points

1. *Doses*
   - Prevention of stroke and systemic embolism in adult patients with NVAF with one or more risk factors [stroke prevention in AF (SPAF)]: 150mg bd, after 5–10 days of parenteral anticoagulation. Therapy should be continued long term.
   - Reduction of risk of stroke and systemic embolism in NVAF: 150mg bd taken PO.
   - Treatment of DVT and PE, and prevention of recurrent DVT and PE in adults: 150mg bd, following treatment with a parenteral anticoagulant for at least 5 days. The duration of therapy should be individualized after careful assessment of the treatment benefit against the risk for bleeding. Short duration of therapy (at least 3 months) should be based on transient risk factors (e.g. recent surgery, trauma, immobilization), and longer durations should be based on permanent risk factors or idiopathic DVT or PE.
   - SPAF, DVT/PE: the recommended daily dose is 110mg bd in patients ≥80 years, moderate renal impairment, gastritis, oesophagitis or gastro-oesophageal reflux, or other patients at increased risk of bleeding or who receive concomitant verapamil (dabigatran and verapamil should be taken at the same time).
   - Prophylaxis of VTE following total knee replacement surgery: 110mg bd (>75 years, 75mg bd) 1–4h after surgery; then 220mg (elderly over 75 years, 150mg) od for 9 days.
   - Prophylaxis of VTE following total hip replacement surgery: 110mg bd (elderly over 75 years, 75mg) 1–4h after surgery and after haemostasis has been achieved; then 220mg (elderly over 75 years, 150mg) od for 27–35 days.
   - Converting from warfarin to dabigatran: discontinue warfarin and start dabigatran when the INR is below 2.0.
   - Converting from dabigatran to warfarin: adjust the starting time of warfarin, as follows:
     - —For CrCl of ≥50mL/min, start warfarin 3 days before discontinuing dabigatran.
     - —For CrCl of 30–50mL/min, start warfarin 2 days before discontinuing dabigatran.
   - *Converting from or to parenteral anticoagulants*: start dabigatran 0–2h before the time that the next dose of the parenteral drug was to have been administered or at the time of discontinuation of a continuously administered parenteral drug (e.g. IV UFH).
   - *From dabigatran to parenteral anticoagulant*: wait 12h after the last dose before initiating treatment with a parenteral anticoagulant.
   - No dose adjustment is necessary in patients with mild renal impairment (CrCl >50mL/min). Patients with CrCl of 30–50mL/min: 150mg bd or 110mg bd for patients with high risk of bleeding. Dabigatran

is not recommended for patients with severe renal impairment (CrCl <30mL/min) or those on dialysis. Patients with elevated liver enzymes >2 times ULN were excluded in the main trials.

- Reduce the dose to 110mg bd in: patients aged ≥80 years and those receiving concomitant verapamil. Some patients may need 110 or 150mg bd: patients between 75 and 80 years, those with moderate renal impairment, gastritis, oesophagitis, or gastro-oesophageal reflux, or those at increased risk of bleeding.

2. *Side effects*
   - The most serious adverse reactions are related to bleeding (higher incidence in patients ≥75 years), and the most frequent adverse reactions leading to dabigatran discontinuation were bleeding and GI events. Risk factors for bleeding include advanced age and use of drugs that increase the risk of bleeding in general (e.g. antiplatelet agents, anticoagulants, heparins, and chronic use of NSAIDs).
   - Common (>3%): dyspepsia (including upper abdominal pain, abdominal pain, abdominal discomfort, nausea, and diarrhoea) and gastritis-like symptoms (including gastritis, gastro-oesophageal reflux disease, oesophagitis, erosive gastritis, and gastric haemorrhage).
   - Others: constipation, pyrexia, wound secretion, hypotension, insomnia, peripheral oedema, anaemia, thrombocytopenia, dizziness, diarrhoea, and headache.
   - Moderate increases in ALT of >3 times ULN have a 2% frequency after 12 months.
   - Hypersensitivity reactions: urticaria, rash, and pruritus; allergic oedema, anaphylactic reactions. The hard capsules contain the colourant sunset yellow (E110), which may cause allergic reactions.
3. *Interactions*
   - Anticoagulants, antiplatelet drugs, and thrombolytics, as well as NSAIDs, SSRIs or SNRIs, or other drugs that impair haemostasis, increase the risk of bleeding. Close observation for signs of bleeding is recommended.
   - UFH can be administered at doses necessary to maintain a patent central venous or arterial catheter.
   - In the RE-LY trial, concomitant use of ASA or clopidogrel approximately doubled the major bleeding rates with both dabigatran etexilate and warfarin.
   - Co-administration of aspirin and dabigatran increased the risk of major bleeding, without any evidence of benefit in reducing stroke and other serious vascular events.
   - The risk of haemorrhage increases notably with NSAIDs, with elimination t½ of >12h.
   - Dabigatran etexilate and dabigatran are not metabolized by the cytochrome P450 system; thus, related medicinal product interactions are not expected.
   - However, because of its low oral bioavailability, dabigatran can present pharmacokinetic drug interactions with significant clinical impact.
   - Avoid the concomitant use of dabigatran with abiraterone, ciclosporin, crizotinib, dronedarone, enzalutamide, HIV-1 protease inhibitors, ibrutinib, imatinib, itraconazole, ketoconazole, tacrolimus or voriconazole.

- Caution (reduce the dose to 110mg bd) if co-administered with amiodarone, clarithromycin, erythromycin, lapatinib, nilotinib, quinidine, posoconazole, tamoxifen, ticagrelor or verapamil (no interaction if verapamil is given 2h after dabigatran). These drugs increase dabigatran exposure and the risk of bleeding.
- The co-administration of dabigatran with P-gp inhibitors should be avoided in patients with CrCl of <50mL/min.
- P-gp inducers decrease dabigatran exposure: carbamazepine, dexamethasone, doxorubicin, phenytoin, rifampicin, St John's wort, sunitinib, vandetanib, vemurafenib, or vinblastine. Avoid the combination.

4. *Cautions/notes*
   - Assess renal function prior to initiation of treatment and periodically during treatment, and adjust dabigatran dose accordingly. Discontinue dabigatran in patients with CrCl of <30mL/min.
   - Renal function should be assessed during treatment with dabigatran at least once a year or more frequently when it is suspected that the renal function could decline or deteriorate (e.g. hypovolaemia, dehydration, concomitant use of nephrotoxic drugs).
   - Careful administration in the presence of significant risk factors for major bleeding, i.e. elderly, body weight <50kg, current or recent GI ulceration, presence of malignant neoplasms, recent brain or spinal injury, recent brain, spinal, or ophthalmic surgery, recent intracranial haemorrhage, known or suspected oesophageal varices, arteriovenous malformations, vascular aneurysms or major intraspinal or intracerebral vascular abnormalities, uncontrolled hypertension, bacterial endocarditis, severe liver disease, and anaesthesia with post-operative indwelling epidural catheter (risk of paralysis; give initial dose at least 2h after catheter removal, and monitor for neurological signs).
   - Increased risk of thrombotic events after premature discontinuation and thromboembolic and bleeding events in patients with prosthetic heart valves.
   - When rapid reversal of the anticoagulation effect of dabigatran is required, the specific reversal agent idarucizumab should be administered. Dabigatran can be re-initiated 24h after administration of idarucizumab.
   - Instruct patients to swallow the capsules of dabigatran with a full glass of water. Oral bioavailability of etexilate increases by 75% when the pellets are taken without the capsule shell; therefore, capsules should not be broken, chewed, or opened before administration.
   - Patients with elevated liver enzymes >2 ULN were excluded from clinical trials.
   - Dabigatran can increase the INR. Thus, the INR will better reflect warfarin's effect only after dabigatran has been stopped for at least 2 days.

- Patients on dabigatran etexilate who undergo surgery or invasive procedures are at an increased risk for bleeding; thus, treatment should be temporarily discontinued, taking into consideration renal function.

Renal function (CrCl in mL/min)	Estimated t½ (h)	Stop dabigatran before elective surgery	
		High risk of bleeding or major surgery	Standard risk
≥80	Approximately 13	2 days before	24h before
≥50 to <80	Approximately 15	2–3 days before	1–2 days before
≥30 to <50	Approximately 18	4 days before	2–3 days before (>48h)

- When rapid reversal of the anticoagulation effect is required, the specific reversal agent idarucizumab should be administered. Dabigatran can be reinitiated 24h after administration of idarucizumab.
- Surgery/intervention should be delayed, if possible, until at least 12h after the last dose; if this cannot be delayed, the risk of bleeding may be increased.
- *Elective surgery*: dabigatran etexilate should be discontinued at least 24h before invasive or surgical procedures. In patients at higher risk of bleeding or in major surgery where complete haemostasis may be required, consider stopping dabigatran etexilate 2–4 days before surgery (4 days in patients with CrCl of ≥30 to <50mL/min).
- *Spinal anaesthesia/epidural anaesthesia/lumbar puncture*: may require complete haemostatic function. The risk of spinal or epidural haematoma may be increased in cases of traumatic or repeated puncture and by the prolonged use of epidural catheters. After removal of a catheter, an interval of at least 2h should elapse before administration of the first dose of dabigatran etexilate. These patients require frequent observation for neurological signs and symptoms of spinal or epidural haematoma.
- *Post-operative phase*: dabigatran etexilate should be restarted after an invasive procedure or surgical intervention as soon as possible.

5. *Pregnancy and lactation*
   - Because there are no adequate and well-controlled studies in pregnant women, dabigatran should not be given to pregnant women (Pregnancy category C). Breastfeeding should be discontinued during treatment.
6. *Contraindications*
   - Active clinically significant bleeding, including: GI ulceration, presence of malignant neoplasms at high risk of bleeding, recent brain or spinal injury, recent brain, spinal, or ophthalmic surgery, recent

intracranial haemorrhage, known or suspected oesophageal varices, arteriovenous malformations, vascular aneurysms, or major intraspinal or intracerebral vascular abnormalities.

- Severe renal failure (CrCl <30mL/min).
- Severe hepatic impairment or liver disease expected to have any impact on survival.
- Concomitant treatment with systemic ketoconazole, ciclosporin, itraconazole, and dronedarone.
- Prosthetic heart valves requiring anticoagulant treatment.
- Concomitant treatment with any other anticoagulants, except under specific circumstances of switching anticoagulant therapy or when UFH is given to maintain an open central venous or arterial catheter.
- Hypersensitivity to any component of the product.

Dalteparin

LMWH fraction (average molecular weight 5500–6400Da) produced from porcine-derived heparin sodium (see ➲ Enoxaparin, pp. 571–4).

CV indications

- Treatment of VTE presenting clinically as DVT, PE, or both.
- Prevention of clotting in the extracorporeal circulation during haemodialysis or haemofiltration, in patients with chronic renal insufficiency or acute renal failure.
- UA and non-Q wave MI, administered concurrently with aspirin.
- Peri- and post-operative surgical thromboprophylaxis.
- Extended use: dalteparin may be used beyond 8 days in patients awaiting angiography/revascularization procedures.
- Patients with solid tumours: extended treatment of symptomatic VTE and prevention of its recurrence.

Mechanism of action

(See ➲ Enoxaparin, pp. 571–4.)

Pharmacodynamics

In patients with UA or NSTEMI, the rate of death, MI, recurrence of angina or revascularization procedures is similar in those assigned to dalteparin or dose-adjusted IV infusion of UFH; thus, dalteparin may be an alternative to UFH.

Pharmacokinetics

(See Table 8.1.1.)

Practical points

1. *Doses*
   - *Treatment of VTE presenting clinically as DVT, PE, or both*: (1) 200IU/kg SC od (maximum daily dose 18,000IU); (2) 100IU/kg SC bd can be used for patients with an increased risk of bleeding. Recommended plasma levels are between 0.5 and 1.0IU (anti-factor Xa)/mL. Simultaneous anticoagulation with oral vitamin K; at least 5 days of combined treatment is normally required.
   - *Prevention of clotting during haemodialysis and haemofiltration*: (1) long-term haemodialysis or haemofiltration (>4h): IV bolus injection of 30–40IU (anti-factor Xa)/kg, followed by an infusion of 10–15IU/kg/h; (2) short-term haemodialysis or haemofiltration (<4h): as described or a single IV bolus of 5000IU. The plasma anti-factor Xa levels should be within 0.2–0.4IU (anti-factor Xa)/mL.
     —In acute or chronic renal failure in patients with a high risk of bleeding: IV bolus of 5–10IU/kg, followed by an infusion of 4–5IU/kg/h. The plasma anti-factor Xa levels should be within 0.2–0.4IU (anti-factor Xa)/mL.
   - *Unstable CAD*: 120IU/kg SC every 12h for up to 8 days. The maximum dose is 10,000IU/12h.

- *Patients needing treatment beyond 8 days, while awaiting angiography/revascularization*: 5000IU (women <80kg and men <70kg) or 7500IU (women ≥80kg and men ≥70kg) every 12h. Treatment will continue until the day of the revascularization procedure (PTCA or CABG), but not for >45 days.
- *Patients with solid tumours*: month 1: 200IU/kg total body weight SC od for the first 30 days of treatment. The total daily dose should not exceed 18,000IU. Months 2–6: 150IU/kg SC od using a fixed dose according to body weight. In patients who experience platelet counts of between 50,000 and 100,000/mm^3, the daily dose should be reduced by 2500IU until the platelet count recovers to ≥100,000/mm^3. In patients who experience platelet counts of <50,000/mm^3, dalteparin should be discontinued until the platelet count recovers to above 50,000/mm^3.

2. *Common side effects* (see ➔ Enoxaparin, pp. 571–4)
3. *Interactions* (see ➔ Enoxaparin, pp. 571–4)
4. *Cautions/notes* (see ➔ Enoxaparin, pp. 571–4)
   - Dalteparin is given as a deep SC injection. Due to the risk of haematoma, IM injection of other medical preparations should be avoided when the 24h dose of dalteparin exceeds 5000IU.
   - In severe renal impairment (CrCl <30mL/min), the dose should be adjusted, based on anti-factor Xa activity, if the anti-factor Xa level is below or above the desired range.
   - Insertion or removal of an epidural or spinal catheter should be postponed to 10–12h after dalteparin doses have been administered for thrombosis prophylaxis; in patients receiving higher doses (100–120IU/kg every 12h or 200IU/kg od), the interval should be a minimum of 24h.
   - Dalteparin is not recommended to prevent valve thrombosis in patients with prosthetic heart valves.
5. *Pregnancy and lactation* (see ➔ Enoxaparin, pp. 571–4)
   - Dalteparin does not cross the placenta, and it can be used during pregnancy if needed (Pregnancy category B). It has been used without apparent harmful effects in the nursing infant.
6. *Contraindications* (see ➔ Enoxaparin, pp. 571–4)

Diazoxide

Benzothiadiazine derivate with antihypertensive and hyperglycaemic activities.

CV indications

- Hypertensive emergencies (IV preparation).
- Hypoglycaemia due to hyperinsulinism (idiopathic hypoglycaemia in infancy, inoperable islet cell adenoma or carcinoma, extra-pancreatic neoplasms producing hypoglycaemia, or hypoglycaemia of unknown origin).

Mechanism of action

Diazoxide binds to the SUR1 subunit of K^+ channels sensitive to ATP (K_{ATP}) and to the large-conductance Ca^{2+}-activated K^+ channels in vascular smooth muscle cells; this results in hyperpolarization of the resting membrane potential, decrease in the open probability of L-type Ca^{2+} channels, arteriolar vasodilatation, and decreases in PVR and BP. Diazoxide stabilizes K_{ATP} channels present in pancreatic β-cells in the active-open state, so that cells remain hyperpolarized, the release of insulin decreases, and blood glucose levels increase. Diazoxide inhibits active Cl^- reabsorption in the early distal tubule via the Na-Cl co-transporter, resulting in an increase in the excretion of Na^+, Cl^-, and water. This results in an increase in K^+ excretion via the Na^+–K^+ exchange mechanism.

Pharmacodynamics

Via the IV route, diazoxide lowers BP very rapidly, achieving its maximum effect in 2–5min and the effect persists for 2–12h. Diazoxide produces a dose-related increase in blood glucose levels. It also increases the heart rate and serum uric acid levels and decreases sodium and water excretion. Small controlled studies suggested a role of a mini-bolus of diazoxide in patients with hypertensive crises in labour. However, experience with diazoxide remains limited and meta-analyses do not support its use in hypertensive crises in pregnancy.

Pharmacokinetics

Diazoxide is fully absorbed following oral administration. It binds to plasma proteins (>90%) and crosses the placenta, so that fetal plasma levels are similar to those of the mother. It is metabolized in the liver by oxidation and sulfate conjugation and is excreted in the urine by glomerular filtration as unchanged drug (50%) and metabolites. Its t½ is approximately 28h (9–24h in children; longer in patients with impaired renal function).

Practical points

1. *Doses*
   - PO: 3mg/kg every 8–12h; maintenance dose 3–8mg every 8–12h.
   - IV: 1mg/kg every 8h; maintenance: 3–8mg/kg daily in 2–3 doses, given every 8–12h.
2. Side effects
   - Common (>1%): transient hyperglycaemia (due to inhibition of insulin release from the pancreas), hypotension, anorexia, nausea, vomiting, headache, dizziness, weakness, palpitations, tachycardia, and sodium and fluid retention.
   - Others: hyperuricaemia, hyperlipidaemia, diabetic ketoacidosis, hyperosmolar non-ketotic coma. Thrombocytopenia, neutropenia, eosinophilia. Diplopia, transient loss of taste, hirsutism.

- Pulmonary hypertension has been described in newborns and infants with hypoglycaemia treated with diazoxide; treatment should be discontinued if symptoms appear. Monitoring infants with risk factors for pulmonary hypertension.

3. *Interactions*
   - Diazoxide can potentiate the effects of other antihypertensives and vasodilator drugs.
   - It displaces warfarin from plasma proteins, increasing their plasma levels; monitor the INR.
   - Co-administration of diazoxide and diphenylhydantoin may result in loss of seizure control.
   - Co-administration with thiazides potentiates the hyperglycaemic and hyperuricaemic effects of diazoxide.
   - Diazoxide should not be administered within 6h of hydralazine, reserpine, alphaprodine, methyldopa, β-blockers, prazosin, minoxidil, nitrites, and other papaverine-like compounds.
4. *Cautions/notes*
   - As diazoxide causes transient hyperglycaemia, blood glucose levels should be carefully monitored until the patient's condition has stabilized. It should be used with caution in patients with diabetes mellitus.
   - Diazoxide may interfere with certain laboratory tests (such as glucagon test), possibly causing false test results.
   - Diazoxide causes sodium and fluid retention, and repeated injection may precipitate CHF; fluid retention responds to conventional diuretics in patients with normal renal function.
   - Diazoxide can increase serum uric acid levels and should be administered with caution in patients with hyperuricaemia or a history of gout.
   - Diazoxide increases heart rate and CO and should be used with care in patients with coronary or cerebrovascular insuficiency, HF, or aortic aneurysm.
   - Diazoxide is ineffective against hypertension due to phaeochromocytoma.
   - When used for the management of hypertensive crises in pregnancy, diazoxide can cause delay in the second stage of labour. Thus, it should only be used when other agents (hydralazine or labetalol) are ineffective.
   - Ketoacidosis and non ketotic hyperosmolar coma reported in patients treated with recommended doses usually during intercurrent illness.
   - Due to high alkalinity, care should be taken to ensure administration directly into a vein, and not the surrounding tissue.
5. *Pregnancy and lactation*
   - Diazoxide crosses the placenta, and it should only be used to treat hypertensive crises in pregnant women when hypertension is considered life-threatening (Pregnancy category C). Diazoxide causes cessation of labour in eclamptic patients, although oxytocin will reverse this effect. Excretion in breast milk is unknown; diazoxide is not recommended in nursing mothers.
6. *Contraindications*
   - Compensatory hypertension (e.g. coarctation of the aorta), acute aortic dissection.
   - Patient's hypersensitivity to diazoxide, other thiazides, or other sulfonamide-derived drugs.

Digoxin

Positive inotropic drug.

CV indications

- Digoxin may be considered in symptomatic patients with HFrEF in sinus rhythm despite treatment with an ACEI (or ARB), a β-blocker, and an MRA, to reduce the risk of hospitalization (both all-cause and HF hospitalizations).
- Control of ventricular response rate in adult patients with chronic AF, particularly when uncontrolled ventricular response despite β-blockers or when β-blockers are not tolerated or contraindicated.

Digoxin presents a very narrow therapeutic–toxic window and numerous drug interactions which have relegated its use in clinical practice.

Mechanism of action

Digoxin inhibits the sarcolemmal Na^+-K^+ ATPase (sodium pump), leading to an increase in intracellular Na^+ levels, which, in turn, activates the Ca^{2+}/Na^+ exchange system, leading to an increase in intracellular Ca^{2+} concentrations. This increase in intracellular Ca^{2+} allows more Ca^{2+} to be released from the SR, thereby increasing the availability for binding to troponin C and cardiac contractility. Within vascular smooth muscle, this mechanism and depolarization resulting from Na^+-K^+ ATPase inhibition may contribute to vascular smooth muscle contraction and vasoconstriction.

Digoxin decreases neurohumoral activation, even before any observed haemodynamic changes, which may play an important role in its effects in CHF. It increases the vagal tone but inhibits sympathetic outflow, the release of renin from the kidney, and the plasma levels of renin and angiotensin II. Moreover, digoxin increases CO, which counteracts neurohumoral activation, resulting in vasodilatation and afterload reduction. However, at toxic doses, digoxin increases central and peripheral sympathetic tone.

Digoxin slows the SA node and, in the AVN, slows conduction and increases the refractory period, thus reducing the ventricular rate in patients with AF. These effects are due to an increase in cardiac vagal tone, a decrease in sympathetic activity, and a direct depressant effect.

Pharmacodynamics

1. *HF.* Digoxin reduces signs and symptoms, improves haemodynamics (increases stroke volume and CO, reduces PCWP and LV end-diastolic pressure), inhibits neurohumoral activation, and reduces HF-related hospitalizations and emergency care, while having no effect on mortality. Digoxin use in patients already optimally treated by a combination of mortality-reducing drugs, such as β-blockers, ACEIs (or ARBs), and mineralocorticoid receptor blockers, has never been tested.

Digoxin is indicated in patients with CHF, third heart sound gallop (S3), crepitants, and LVEF <35%; also in patients with hypotension (SBP <100mmHg) where vasodilators are contraindicated. A poor response is expected in low- (valvular stenosis, chronic pericarditis) and high-output states (cor pulmonale, thryrotoxicosis) and in conditions increasing digoxin sensitivity (hypokalaemia, post-MI, chronic pulmonary disease, acute hypoxaemia, myocarditis).

2. *Electrophysiological effects.* Digoxin decreases the slope of phase 4 depolarization in the SA node and increases automaticity of ectopic pacemakers. The increase in $[Ca^{2+}]_i$ predisposes to Ca^{2+}-dependent delayed after-depolarization. Digoxin shortens atrial and ventricular APD and refractoriness and depolarizes the resting membrane potentials, decreasing intra-cardiac conduction velocity; both effects facilitate the appearance of re-entrant arrhythmias. At therapeutic doses, digoxin increases cardiac vagal tone, predisposing to sinus bradycardia and AVB, and exerts a 'direct' depressive effect on both nodal tissues. At the AVN, digoxin slows intra-cardiac conduction and prolongs refractoriness. This is the basis of reduced ventricular rate in patients with AF, particularly in elderly sedentary people. It should be combined with β-blockers, verapamil, or diltiazem for ventricular rate control during exercise. IV administration of cardiac glycosides may be considered for ventricular rate control if the response to β-blockers is not sufficient. Digoxin is not indicated when AF occurs without HF or when AF is due to thyrotoxicosis, and it is ineffective for pharmacologic cardioversion of AF to sinus rhythm.

Digoxin prolongs the PR interval and depresses the ST-segment on the ECG; it may also produce false-positive ST–T changes during exercise testing. These changes are not indicative of toxicity.

Pharmacokinetics

Digoxin has an oral bioavailability of 60–75%. In 10% of patients, the intestinal flora converts digoxin to an inactive metabolite. The onset of its effect occurs within 1–3h and reaches maximum effect at 2–6h. Food delays the absorption, although the total amount absorbed is unchanged. Steady-state levels are reached within 5–7 days. Following IV administration, it produces its pharmacological effects within 5–30min and the maximal effect within 1–5h. Digoxin has a large Vd (6L/kg), indicating that it is extensively bound to body tissues, with the highest concentrations in the heart, liver, kidney, and skeletal muscle. Digoxin (approximately 25%) binds to plasma proteins and crosses the blood–brain barrier and is primarily excreted through the kidneys unchanged (70%) and 30% via non-renal routes (faeces, hepatic metabolism). Its t½ is 35–48h (70h in elderly people; 80–140h in renal failure). Since digoxin is mainly stored in tissues, it is not eliminated by haemodialysis. (See Table 8.1.3.)

Therapeutic plasma levels: 0.5–2ng/mL (1.3–2.6nmol/L). In patients with HF, all-cause mortality was modestly decreased in patients with digoxin plasma levels of between 0.5 and 0.9nmol/L, whereas higher levels were associated with a mortality increase of 12%. Determination of serum digoxin levels should be made no earlier than 6h after the last dose of digoxin.

Practical points

1. *Doses*

They should be titrated according to the patient's age, lean body weight, renal function, concomitant disease states, concurrent medications, or other factors likely to alter the pharmacokinetic or pharmacodynamic profile of digoxin.

- *Chronic HF*: rapid oral loading dose: 0.75–1.5mg as a single dose. Slow oral loading: 0.25–0.76mg daily for 1 week, followed by an appropriate maintenance dose (0.125–0.25mg daily). Reduce the dose in patients with increased sensitivity to the adverse effects of digoxin.
- *Acute HF*: 0.25–0.5mg IV (0.0625–0.125mg in moderate to severe renal dysfunction.
- *Supraventricular tachyarrhythmias*: rapid digitalization can be achieved with a single dose of 0.75–1.5mg or the dose is given in divided doses 6h apart, assessing clinical response before giving each additional dose.
- IV: 0.75–1.25mg as an infusion over 2h or more, depending on age, renal function, and body weight.

2. *Side effects*
   - CV: conduction disturbances, bigeminy, trigeminy, sinus bradycardia, supraventricular tachyarrhythmia, AT, junctional tachycardia, VPBs, VT, and VF.
   - Others: anorexia, nausea, vomiting, diarrhoea, blurred or yellow vision, skin rashes of urticarial or scarlatiniform character, dizziness, headache.
   - Very rare: intestinal ischaemia or necrosis, gynaecomastia, weakness.

Treatment of digoxin toxicity: stop digoxin; discontinue diuretics and drugs increasing digoxin plasma levels; normalize hypokalaemia; check the dose used and correlate with weight, age, and CrCl. With dangerous arrhythmias and hypokalaemia, potassium chloride may be infused IV (0.5–1mEq/min into a large vein through a plastic catheter to avoid tissue necrosis and decrease local irritation and pain); potassium is contraindicated if AVB is present. *Activated charcoal* (50–100g) and colestyramine increase faecal excretion of digoxin. Digoxin-specific antibodies are the most effective treatment in patients with life-threatening ventricular tachyarrhythmias or hypokalaemia. *Tachyarrhythmias*: lidocaine that does not impair AV conduction or cardiac contractility. *Bradyarrhythmias*: atropine and implantation of a temporary pacemaker.

3. *Interactions*
   - With class IA and IC antiarrhythmics: increases the risk of bradycardia, intracardiac conduction block, and arrhythmias.
   - Amiodarone and propafenone reduce the clearance of digoxin and increase digoxinaemia (25–75%); decrease the dose of digoxin by 50%.
   - β-blockers, diltiazem, and verapamil increase the risk of bradycardia and AVB.
   - Some CCBs (diltiazem, felodipine, nicardipine, nifedipine, verapamil) increase digoxin plasma levels.
   - Thiazides and loop diuretics induce hypokalaemia (which sensitizes the heart to digoxin toxicity).
   - Calcium and vitamin D, if administered rapidly, can precipitate arrhythmias in patients on digoxin.
   - ACEIs, NSAIDs, and spironolactone decrease renal elimination and increase serum digoxin levels. Spironolactone falsely increases digoxin assay.
   - Hydralazine and nitroprusside increase the renal excretion of digoxin.

- Digoxin should not be combined with dronedarone.
- Amphotericin, β2-adrenergic agonists, carbenoxolone, glucocorticoids, insulin, laxatives, lithium salts, loop diuretics, and thiazides cause hypokalaemia and increase sensitivity to digoxin.

Drugs that increase or decrease serum digoxin levels are listed below.

Increase digoxin levels	Decrease digoxin levels
NSAIDs, alprazolam, amiloride, amiodarone, atorvastatin, carvedilol, ciclosporin, epoprostenol, flecainide, gentamicin, indometacin, itraconazole, macrolide antibiotics (e.g. clarithromycin, erythromycin), prazosin, propafenone, propantheline, quinidine, quinine, spironolactone, tetracycline, triamterene, trimethoprim, verapamil	Acarbose, adrenaline, antacids, bulk laxatives, colestyramine, cimetidine, colestipol, kaolin-pectin, metoclopramide, neomycin, phenytoin, rifampicin, salbutamol, sulfasalazine, St John's wort

4. *Cautions/notes*
   - Lower doses should be administered in the elderly due to decreased renal function; this, together with low lean body mass, leads to an increased risk of digoxin toxicity.
   - Acute hypoxaemia, severe myocarditis, acute MI, hypokalaemia, hypomagnesaemia, and hypercalcaemia sensitize the heart to cardiac glycosides. Hypokalaemia induced by diuretics also increases cardiac sensitivity to digoxin. Conversely, hyperkalaemia, hypocalcaemia, and hyperthyroidism decreases sensitivity.
   - Monitor serum electrolytes and renal function periodically during treatment with digoxin.
   - Hyperkalaemia increases the risk of AVB.
   - Digoxin doses should be reduced in patients with hypothyroidism, while in hyperthyroidism, there is relative digoxin resistance and the dose may have to be increased. During treatment of hyperthyroidism, the dosage should be gradually reduced as thyroid function comes under control.
   - Digoxin is useful in patients with AVNRT and SBP of <110mmHg in whom β-blockers, verapamil, or diltiazem may cause symptomatic hypotension or bradycardia.
   - Patients with malabsorption syndrome or GI reconstructions may require larger doses of digoxin.
   - Digoxin should be withheld for 24h before cardioversion. In emergencies, the lowest effective energy should be applied when attempting cardioversion. DC cardioversion is inappropriate in the treatment of digitalis-induced arrhythmias.
   - Digoxin is contraindicated in patients with WPW syndrome, because it may enhance antegrade conduction through the accessory pathway.
   - Rapid IV digoxin can cause vasoconstriction, hypertension, and/or reduced coronary flow. Thus, administer the drug at a slow injection rate in hypertensive patients with HF and acute MI.

- Avoid digoxin in patients with HF associated with cardiac amyloidosis, myocarditis, hypertrophic obstructive cardiomyopathy, or constrictive pericarditis (unless it is used to control the ventricular rate of AF or to improve systolic dysfunction).
- Digoxin is uneffective in patients with beri beri and HF, unless the underlying thiamine deficiency is not treated concomitantly.

5. *Pregnancy and lactation*
   - There are no controlled data in pregnant women (Pregnancy category C). Breastfeeding is not contraindicated, although small amounts of digoxin can be detected in breast milk.
6. *Contraindications*
   - Digitalis toxicity.
   - Bradycardia, sick sinus syndrome, or advanced AVB (unless a functioning pacemaker is inserted).
   - WPW syndrome with AF. Digoxin accelerates antegrade conduction over the accessory pathway and may precipitate VT/VF.
   - VPBs, VT/VF.
   - Hypertrophic obstructive cardiomyopathy.
   - Marked hypokalaemia.
   - Acute pulmonary oedema. Acute digoxin is undesirable in view of the prevailing arrhythmogenic environment, unless there is uncontrolled AF.

Diltiazem

Non-dihydropyridine CCB with class IV antiarrhythmic activity (see ➲ Calcium channel blockers, pp. 504–9).

CV indications

- Treatment of hypertension, alone or in combination with other antihypertensives.
- Treatment of chronic stable and vasospastic angina pectoris.
- Treatment and prophylaxis of PSVT and to control the ventricular rate in atrial flutter/AF.

Mechanism of action

(See ➲ Calcium channel blockers, pp. 504–9.)

Pharmacodynamics

(See ➲ Calcium channel blockers, pp. 504–9.)

Diltiazem produces antihypertensive, anti-anginal, and antiarrhythmic effects.

Pharmacokinetics

Pharmacokinetics vary widely between preparations and brands. Diltiazem is available in a range of formulations, including standard (onset of action 15min, peak plasma concentrations after 1–4h, and plasma t½ of 4–7h) and longer-acting (peak plasma concentrations approximately 8–11h after dosing, and average plasma t½ of 6–8h). (See Table 8.1.6.)

Practical points

1. *Doses*

Diltiazem is available in a variety of preparations from different manufacturers, and due to different pharmacokinetics, once established on a particular modified-release formulation, it is not advisable to substitute different brands for another. Product information should be consulted for details regarding specific extended-release formulation dosing.

- *Hypertension*. Modified-release formulations: initial daily dose of 180mg od or bd, up to a daily dose of 240–360mg od, depending on formulation and manufacturer.
- *Chronic angina*. Extended-release: 120–240mg od; maximum dose 540mg/day.
- *Rate control in patients with AF/atrial flutter*: IV 0.25–0.35mg/kg over 2min, monitoring BP and ECG; the dose can be repeated after 15min. Maintenance dose: 5–15mg/h IV, for up to 24h, or 120–360mg PO daily in divided doses.
- *PSVT*: 0.25mg/kg as a bolus administered over 2min. After 15min, a second bolus of 0.35mg/kg may be used, if necessary. Maintenance dose: 5mg/h, increased in 5mg/h increments, up to 15mg/h; maximum duration: 24h.

2. *Side effects* (see ➲ Calcium channel blockers, pp. 504–9)

- In post-MI patients with pre-existing poor LV function, diltiazem increases mortality.

- Rare: gingival hyperplasia (disappearing on cessation of treatment); exfoliative dermatitis, angioneurotic oedema, erythema multiforme, vasculitis, transient increased liver transaminases, and isolated cases of clinical hepatitis resolving after withdrawing treatment.

3. *Interactions* (see ➔ Calcium channel blockers, pp. 504–9)

Diltiazem inhibits the CYP3A4 isoenzyme, which explains the multiple possible drug interactions.

- Co-administration with β-blockers, antiarrhythmics, or cardiac glycosides may increase the risk of bradycardia, AVB, and hypotension and should be avoided.
- Diltiazem can be combined with dihydropyridines in patients with resistant coronary artery vasospasm. Diltiazem plus a β-blocker may be used with caution due to the risk of bradycardia, AVB, or hypotension.
- Unlike verapamil, diltiazem does not interact with digoxin.
- Diltiazem increases blood levels of carbamazepine, ciclosporin, ketoconazole, lovastatin, quinidine, and sildenafil. Conversely, cimetidine increases diltiazem plasma levels. The dose of simvastatin should not exceed 10mg/day in patients taking diltiazem.
- Diltiazem increases the bioavailability of oral propranolol.
- Diltiazem increases the risk of lithium-induced neurotoxicity. Dose adjustments are needed.
- Diltiazem increases exposure of buspirone, midazolam, and triazolam, so dose adjustment is needed.
- Concurrent use of diltiazem and dantrolene increases toxicity of each other and can produce CV collapse and marked hyperkalaemia; thus, it is contraindicated.

4. *Cautions/notes* (see ➔ Calcium channel blockers, pp. 504–9)

- Diltiazem should be used with caution in patients with reduced LV function, mild bradycardia, first-degree AVB, or prolonged PR interval; under close supervision, doses should not be increased if bradycardia (heart rate <50bpm) occurs.
- In patients with ventricular dysfunction, diltiazem deteriorates LV function, worsening HF.
- Diltiazem is not recommended to reduce BP in patients with HFrEF because of their negative inotropic action and risk of worsening HF.
- IV β-blockers should be discontinued during therapy with diltiazem.

5. *Contraindications* (see ➔ Calcium channel blockers, pp. 504–9)

Dipyridamole

Platelet aggregation inhibitor.

CV indications

- As an adjunct to anticoagulation for prophylaxis of thromboembolic complications of cardiac valve replacement.
- In combination with aspirin for the prophylaxis of: (1) DVT as an alternative to SC heparin, other than in hip surgery; (2) recurrent venous thrombosis resistant to oral anticoagulation; and (3) occlusion following prosthetic arterial grafts and CABG.
- As an adjunct to oral anticoagulation for prophylaxis of thromboembolism associated with prosthetic heart valves.

Mechanism of action

Dipyridamole inhibits the uptake of adenosine into platelets, endothelial cells, and erythrocytes. This inhibition results in an increase in local concentrations of adenosine, which, acting on the platelet A2 receptor, stimulates platelet adenylyl cyclase and increases platelet cAMP levels. The increase in platelet cAMP levels inhibits platelet aggregation in response to various stimuli such as platelet activating factor, ADP, and collagen. Dipyridamole also inhibits cyclic-3′,5′-guanosine monophosphate-PDE (cGMP-PDE), thereby augmenting the increase in cGMP produced by NO. Dipyridamole also stimulates the synthesis and release of prostacyclin by the endothelium. The increase in adenosine and prostacyclin explains the vasodilatory effect of dipyridamole.

Dipyridamole produces marked vasodilatation of healthy coronary arteries, whereas stenosed arteries remain narrowed, leading to a coronary 'steal' effect associated with chest pain in patients with CAD.

Pharmacodynamics

In patients undergoing surgical placement or a prosthetic heart valve, dipyridamole, in combination with warfarin, significantly decreased the incidence of post-operative thromboembolic events, compared with warfarin treatment alone.

Pharmacokinetics

(See Table 8.1.7.)

Practical points

1. *Doses*
   - *Oral*: 300–600mg/day in 3–4 doses.
   - *Dipyridamole stress echocardiography protocol*: IV infusion of 0.84mg/kg over 10min in two separated infusions (0.56mg/kg over 4min, followed by 4min of no dose; if still negative, an additional dose of 0.28mg/kg over 2min).
2. *Common side effects*
   - Diarrhoea, nausea, vomiting, dizziness, headache, rash, hypotension, palpitations, and fatigue. It may increase ischaemia and produce anginal pain due to coronary steal. Elevations of hepatic enzymes and hepatic failure have been reported.

3. *Interactions*
   - Dipyridamole increases the risk of bleeding when co-administered with heparins, platelet anti-aggregant, or riociguat.
   - Dipyridamole increases the plasma levels and effects of adenosine; thus, the dose of adenosine should be halved.
   - Dipyridamole may counteract the effect of cholinesterase inhibitors, thereby potentially aggravating myasthenia gravis.
4. *Cautions/notes*
   - Dipyridamole should be used with caution in patients with severe CAD or hypotension.
   - Safety and effectiveness in the paediatric population have not been established.
5. *Pregnancy and lactation*
   - Dipyridamole should be used during pregnancy only if clearly needed (Pregnancy category B). Dipyridamole is excreted in human milk.
6. *Contraindications*
   - Hypersensitivity to dipyridamole and any of the other components.
   - Patients with known cardiac conduction abnormalities or cardiac arrhythmias.

Disopyramide

Oral Na^+ channel blocker with class IA antiarrhythmic properties (see ➔ Quinidine, pp. 716–19).

Indications

- Prevention and treatment of arrhythmias occurring after MI.
- Maintenance of normal rhythm following cardioversion of AF or atrial flutter. It is also indicated in vagal-induced AF.
- Persistent ventricular extrasystoles.
- Suppression of arrhythmias during surgical procedures, e.g. cardiac catheterization.
- Prevention of PSVT.
- Treatment of LVOT obstruction in patients with HCM.

Pharmacodynamics

(See ➔ Quinidine, pp. 716–19.)

Disopyramide exerts a negative inotropic effect and can be used in patients with HCM and significant outflow tract obstruction.

Pharmacokinetics

(See Table 8.1.3.)

Practical points

1. *Doses*
   - *Oral*. Immediate-release: 150mg every 6h; controlled-release 200–400mg bd. A dose reduction is recommended in the elderly and in patients with renal and hepatic impairment. CrCl 15–30mL/min: 100mg bd; CrCl <15mL/min: 100mg od.
2. *Common side effects*
   - Anticholinergic effects: urinary retention, blurred vision, dry mouth, abdominal pain, constipation. Erectile dysfunction, anorexia, diarrhoea, dizziness, headache, bradycardia, and hypotension. Rapid infusion may cause profuse sweating.
   - CV effects: AVB, atrial flutter, monomorphic VT, occasional TdP.
3. *Interactions*
   - Combinations with other AADs should be avoided.
   - Disopyramide prolongs the QT interval. Use with caution with other QT-prolonging drugs.
   - CYP3A4 inducers/inhibitors decrease/increase the plasma levels of disopyramide (see Table 8.1.2).
   - Drugs that induce hypokalaemia potentiate the risk of proarrhythmia.
   - Atropine and other anticholinergic drugs potentiate the atropine-like effect of disopyramide; pyridostigmine (90–180mg tds) reduces these anticholinergic effects.
   - Disopyramide increases the negative inotropic effects and AV nodal depressant effects of diltiazem, verapamil, digoxin, and β-blockers.
   - Risk of hypotension if associated with β-blockers, diltiazem, or verapamil.

4. *Cautions/notes*
   - Disopyramide is not recommended in patients with structural heart disease.
   - Treatment should always be initiated in hospital.
   - The ECG should be monitored and disopyramide discontinued if excessive widening of QRS, bradycardia, or other features of cardiotoxicity occur.
   - Due to its negative inotropic effects, disopyramide should be used with caution in patients with HF. In decompensated HF secondary to an arrhythmia, careful monitoring is required.
   - Monitor blood glucose levels due to the risk of hypoglycaemia.
   - In patients with a family history of glaucoma, intraocular pressure should be measured before initiating therapy.
   - Use with special care in patients with myasthenia gravis.
   - Rare cases of hypoglycaemia with disopyramide have been reported, particularly in patients with HF, malnutrition, hepatic or renal impairment, or treated with β-blockers.
   - Disopyramide is ineffective in patients with hypokalaemia. Plasma K^+ levels should be corrected before starting therapy and monitored due to the risk of exacerbation of arrhythmias.
5. *Pregnancy and lactation*
   - Safety of disopyramide in pregnancy has not been established (Pregnancy category C). The drug crosses the placenta and may induce labour. It is also secreted in breast milk. Thus, in either pregnancy or breastfeeding, it should be used with caution.
6. *Contraindications* (see ➔ Quinidine, pp. 716–19)
   - Patients with glaucoma, myasthenia gravis, hypotension, and symptomatic prostatism.
   - The sustained controlled-release form is contraindicated in liver or renal impairment.
   - Congenital or acquired long QT syndrome.

Diuretics

Diuretics are drugs that increase the renal excretion of Na^+ (and Cl^-) and water from the filtrate (natriuresis) due to direct action at different tubular sites of the nephron. They also modify the renal handling of other cations and anions and uric acid, and sometimes renal haemodynamics.

Diuretics can be classified in three groups, according to their chemical structure, their major site of action within the nephron, and the type of diuresis that they elicit:

1. Loop diuretics: furosemide, bumetanide, piretanide, torasemide.
2. Thiazide diuretics: bendroflumethiazide, chlortalidone, hydrochlorothiazide, indapamide, metolazone, polythiazide.
3. Potassium-sparing agents.
   - MRAs: eplerenone, spironolactone.
   - ENaC blockers: amiloride and triamterene.

Because each type of diuretic acts at a different site of the nephron, a combination of diuretics acting at a different site to produce a *sequential nephron blockade* allows to obtain an additive diuretic effect in patients with severe HF or refractory oedema. This combination requires careful monitoring of fluid status and serum electrolyte levels to avoid dehydration, hypokalaemia, hyponatraemia, hypovolaemia, or renal dysfunction.

Pharmacokinetics

(See Table 8.1.5.)

Practical points

1. *Doses*
   - The dose of the diuretic must be adjusted according to the individual needs over time, to avoid the risk of dehydration and renal dysfunction and to prevent the recurrence of volume overload. In asymptomatic euvolaemic/hypovolaemic patients, the use of a diuretic drug might be (temporarily) discontinued. Patients can be trained to self-adjust their diuretic dose, based on monitoring of symptoms/signs of congestion and daily weight measurements. In cases of sudden, unexpected weight gain of >2kg in 3 days, patients should contact their clinician.
   - The use of inappropriately low doses of diuretics will result in fluid retention, while the use of high doses of diuretics will lead to volume contraction, which can increase the risk of hypotension and renal insufficiency, particularly in combination with ACEIs and ARBs. In general, diuretic doses for HF are higher than for the treatment of hypertension.
   - Low doses may be sufficient in the elderly.
   - Twice-daily doses should be given early in the morning and mid afternoon to avoid nocturia.
   - Combination of a loop diuretic with thiazide-type diuretics or spironolactone may be considered in patients with resistant oedema or insufficient symptomatic response.
   - Acute HF: it is recommended to give diuretics either as intermittent boluses or as a continuous infusion, and the dose and duration should

be adjusted according to the patient's symptoms and clinical status (urine output, renal function, and electrolytes). In patients with acute HF and signs of hypoperfusion, diuretics should be avoided before adequate perfusion is attained.

Diuretic resistance

In some patients, oedema persists despite adequate diuretic therapy (diuretic resistance). Several factors can contribute to diuretic resistance:

- The dosing intervals exceed the time when effective amounts of the diuretic reach its site of action. So at the end of the dosing interval, the nephron avidly reabsorbs sodium, which can counteract the prior natriuresis until the next dose is administered. More frequent administration of the diuretic (bd, tds, or IV infusion) avoids salt retention by reducing the drug-free interval.
- Reduced renal blood flow due to hypovolaemia, low CO, and hypotension. It is necessary to reduce the diuretic dose.
- Neurohumoral activation, as occurs in patients with CHF. Loop diuretics present a short duration of action (approximately 6h), and the initial natriuresis is followed by post-diuretic Na^+ reabsorption in the nephron (breaking) in the distal tubuli, mediated by activation of the RAAS and sympathetic tone, which can counteract the previous natriuresis, especially if sodium intake is not restricted. The breaking can be prevented by increasing the frequency of dosing, avoiding the intake of sodium at the end of the dosing intervals, and using long-acting loop diuretics, i.e. torasemide that can be administered once daily.
- During chronic loop diuretic administration, the distal nephron is exposed to a high Na^+ load that causes aldosterone-induced hypertrophy of distal convoluted tubule cells, which react by reabsorbing more Na^+. Thiazide diuretics inhibit distal tubular hypertrophy, which supports the combined thiazide–loop therapy.
- Reduced secretion of the diuretic into the tubular lumen in patients with renal impairment or HF.
- Decreased oral absorption due to bowel oedema or intestinal hypoperfusion. These patients respond to IV drug administration.
- Incorrect use of diuretics: excessive doses, combination of two drugs from the same class, poor compliance, or use of thiazides when GFR is <20–30mL/min. Check doses and drug compliance.
- Increased dietary sodium intake. Check fluid and sodium intake.
- Concomitant therapy with drugs that antagonize the effects of the diuretics, i.e. NSAIDs. Discontinue NSAIDs.

Other suggested actions to avoid diuretic resistance include:

- Adjust the dose of the diuretic in patients with renal impairment or HF; give the loop diuretic twice daily or on an empty stomach.
- Continuous IV infusion of a loop diuretic avoids post-diuretic salt retention and may succeed where other treatments have failed.
- Combination of loop diuretic with either a thiazide-type diuretic or spironolactone (dual nephron blockade) may be considered in patients with insufficient response.
- In patients refractory to loop diuretics and thiazides, add dopamine (renal vasodilatation) or dobutamine.

Dobutamine

Synthetic analogue of dopamine, used as a positive inotropic agent.

CV indications

- In adults as inotropic support in the short-term treatment of conditions characterized by low-output HF, e.g. MI, open heart surgery, cardiomyopathies, septic shock, and cardiogenic shock. It can also increase or maintain CO during PEEP ventilation.
- Echocardiographic stress testing (as an alternative to exercise in patients in whom routine exercise cannot be satisfactorily performed).

Mechanism of action

Dobutamine directly stimulates β1-adrenergic receptors; it also has mild β2- and α1-adrenergic receptor agonist effects (β1 > β2 > α). Unlike dopamine, dobutamine does not cause renal or mesenteric vasodilatation or a release of endogenous catecholamines.

Pharmacodynamics

Acute HF: dobutamine increases cardiac contractility and CO and improves signs, symptoms, and haemodynamics, but it produces less increase in the heart rate than dobutamine. It reduces SVR, but SBP is usually stable; however, stimulation of β2-receptors may lead to a fall in DBP and reflex tachycardia. Dobutamine increases coronary blood flow and MVO_2 due to enhanced myocardial contractility. The improved diuresis observed with dobutamine is the result of increased renal blood flow in response to improved CO. Dobutamine does not reduce (or even increases) the risk of hospitalization and death in patients with CHF. IV dobutamine in controlled trials did not extend beyond 48h of repeated boluses and/or continuous infusions.

Dobutamine facilitates AV conduction and shortens or causes no important change in intraventricular conduction. The risk of cardiac arrhythmias may be slightly less than that with dopamine and is considerably less than that with isoprenaline.

Pharmacokinetics

Dobutamine is given by IV infusion; the onset of action occurs within 2min, and peak plasma concentrations and effects are reached within 10min. Due to its short t½ (2min), the effects of dobutamine cease shortly after discontinuation of the infusion. Dobutamine is mainly metabolized in the liver and other tissues by COMT and by conjugation with glucuronic acid. Inactive metabolites are excreted in the urine and, to a minor extent, in faeces.

Practical points

1. *Doses*
   - Because of its short t½, dobutamine is administered as a continuous IV infusion. After dilution, it should be administered using an IV drip chamber or other suitable metering device to control the rate of flow.
   - Starting dose 0.5–1mcg/kg/min, titrated at intervals of a few minutes up to 40mcg/kg/min, according to the patient's heart rate, BP, urine output, and, if available, CO. It is recommended that treatment

with dobutamine should be discontinued gradually. Gradual tapering (i.e. decrease in dosage by steps of 2mg/kg/min) and simultaneous optimization of oral therapy are essential.

- *Cardiac stress testing*: 5mcg/kg/min, with incremental increases of 5mcg/kg/min, up to 15–20mcg/kg/min. Continuous cardiac monitoring is essential, and the infusion should be terminated if the following occur: ST-segment depression, development of ventricular tachyarrhythmias, maximum heart rate is achieved, or SBP >220mmHg.

2. *Side effects*
   - *CV*: palpitations, tachyarrhythmias, hypertension, hypotension, anginal pain, myocardial ischaemia, coronary artery spasm, and vasoconstriction in patients treated with β-blockers.
   - *Others*: nausea, headache, hypokalaemia, dyspnoea, exanthema, fever, asthma, bronchospasm, phlebitis at the injection site.
   - *Serious/life-threatening*: cardiac rupture, LVOT obstruction, VT/VF, MI.
3. *Interactions*
   - Cyclopropane and halogenated anaesthetics: increased risk of ventricular arrhythmias.
   - Increased risk of arrhythmias when dobutamine is co-administered with quinidine.
   - Hypertension and an increased risk of arrhythmias when given to patients receiving tricyclic antidepressants. Avoid the use of dobutamine in patients treated with MAOIs or within 14 days of its termination.
   - β-blockers can antagonize the inotropic effect of dobutamine. Co-administration with a non-selective β-blocker can result in hypertension (due to stimulation of α-adrenoceptors) and reflex bradycardia.
   - Carvedilol, an α- and β-receptor blocker, may cause hypotension when co-administered with dobutamine due to vasodilatation caused via stimulation of β2-receptors.
   - Potential for hypotension and tachycardia when dobutamine is co-administered with α-adrenergic antagonists.
   - Co-administration with digoxin increases the risk of arrhythmias.
   - Cimetidine inhibits the metabolism of dobutamine and increases the degree and duration of its action.
   - An increased risk of hypertension when dobutamine is co-administered with doxapram.
   - The effects of dobutamine may be enhanced by entacapone.
   - Concomitant administration of sympathomimetics and ergotamine, ergonovine, or methysergide can produce a marked pressor effect.
   - Oxytocin may enhance the pressor effects of dobutamine.
   - Avoid concomitant use of dobutamine with rasagiline.
4. *Cautions/notes*
   - During the administration of dobutamine, ECG, BP, PCWP, and CO should be continuously monitored.
   - With prolonged infusion (>48–72h), partial tolerance develops, requiring higher doses.

- Metabolic acidosis, hypoxia, hypercapnia, and hypovolaemia should be corrected before and during dobutamine treatment.
- In patients with atrial flutter or AF, dobutamine facilitates AV conduction, which may lead to rapid ventricular responses.
- Care is required with dobutamine use in patients with acute MI, as increases in heart rate or BP may intensify ischaemia.
- Dobutamine does not improve haemodynamics in patients with impaired ventricular filling or outflow caused by mechanical obstruction or those with reduced ventricular compliance (includes cardiac tamponade, valvular AS, and idiopathic hypertrophic subaortic stenosis).
- Care is needed when considering cardiac stress testing in patients with a recent MI, as cardiac rupture is a potential complication, especially in those with a dyskinetic or thinned ventricle. Dobutamine is not recommended for exercise testing in patients with any cardiac condition that could make them unsuitable for exercise stress testing.
- Caution in patients with CV disease, such as CAD, acute HF, arrhythmia, or tachycardia, and occlusive vascular disorders, including arteriosclerosis, hypertension, or aneurysms.
- Use with caution in cardiogenic shock complicated by severe hypotension.
- Anginal pain may be precipitated in patients with CAD, particularly after MI.
- Care is also required when sympathomimetic agents are given to patients with diabetes mellitus or closed-angle glaucoma.
- Hypovolaemia should be corrected, if necessary, before administering dobutamine. If arterial BP remains low or decreases progressively during administration of dobutamine, despite adequate ventricular filling pressure and CO, a concomitant peripheral vasoconstrictor agent (dopamine or noradrenaline) may be needed.
- Partial tolerance develops with continuous infusions of dobutamine over >48–72h.
- Dilute dobutamine in sterile water, glucose, or saline solution, not in alkaline solutions, with other drugs in the same solution or with other agents or diluents containing both sodium bisulfite or ethanol. Use the prepared solution within 24h.

5. *Pregnancy and lactation*
   - There are no well-controlled studies in pregnant women (Pregnancy category B). It is not known whether dobutamine crosses the placenta or is distributed into breast milk. Thus, dobutamine should not be used during pregnancy, unless the potential benefits outweigh the potential risks to the fetus.
6. *Contraindications*
   - Sympathomimetic agents should be used with caution in patients particularly susceptible to their effects, i.e. hyperthyroidism or phaeochromocytoma.
   - Known hypersensitivity to dobutamine (sulfites in dobutamine may cause allergic-type reactions, including anaphylactic symptoms and asthmatic episodes).

- Dobutamine should not be used for detection of myocardial ischaemia and of viable myocardium in cases of:
  —Recent MI (within the last 30 days), UA, stenosis of the main left coronary artery.
  —Haemodynamically significant LV outflow obstruction, including hypertrophic obstructive cardiomyopathy or haemodynamically significant cardiac valvular defect.
  —Severe HF (NYHA class III or IV).
  —History of cardiac arrhythmias, particularly recurrent persistent VT.
  —Acute pericarditis, myocarditis, or endocarditis, aortic dissection, aortic aneurysm.
  —Inadequately treated/controlled arterial hypertension.
  —Hypovolaemia.
  —Previous experience of hypersensitivity to dobutamine.

Dopamine

Dopamine is an endogenous catecholamine and the precursor of noradrenaline and adrenaline.

CV indications

In adults for the correction of haemodynamic imbalance present in:

- Low-perfusion circulatory insufficiency associated with MI, trauma, septicaemia, cardiac failure, and open heart surgery.
- As an adjunct after open heart surgery where there is persistent hypotension after correction of hypovolaemia.
- Acute exacerbations of chronic HF with low CO.

Mechanism of action

Dopamine is the precursor of noradrenaline in the sympathetic nerves and a neurotransmitter in certain areas of the CNS (i.e. nigrostriatal tract) and in some peripheral sympathetic nerves. Dopamine stimulates dopaminergic (DA1/DA2) receptors, β1/β2-receptors, and α-receptors. Stimulation of these receptors varies with the dose.

It is believed that the α-adrenergic effects result from inhibition of adenylyl cyclase and a reduction in the cellular levels of cAMP, whereas the β-adrenergic effects result from stimulation of adenylyl cyclase activity and an increase in cAMP levels. In cardiac myocytes, the increase in cAMP levels increases intracellular Ca^{2+} levels, leading to an increase in heart rate and contractility; in vascular smooth muscle cells, cAMP decreases intracellular Ca^{2+} levels, leading to a vasodilator response.

Pharmacodynamics

At doses of 0.5–2mcg/kg/min, dopamine stimulates predominantly dopaminergic receptors. Stimulation of DA1 receptors in renal, mesenteric, coronary, and intracerebral vascular beds causes vasodilatation; stimulation of presynaptic DA2 receptors decreases the release of noradrenaline from terminal sympathetic endings and renin from juxtaglomerular cells. In patients with renal hypoperfusion and failure, these doses of dopamine increase renal blood flow, GFR, sodium excretion, urine flow, and the response to diuretic agents. This diuretic effect appears only under conditions of fluid retention and can be related to a direct effect on DA1 receptors located in the renal tubular cells where dopamine stimulation opposes the effects of antidiuretic hormone (ADH).

At doses of 2–5mcg/kg/min, dopamine activates β1-adrenergic receptors and also increases the release of noradrenaline from storage sites in sympathetic nerve terminals, which counteracts the effects on DA2 receptors. Both effects increase heart rate and contractility, CO, and SBP, with either no effect or a slight increase in DBP. Dopamine improves signs, symptoms, and haemodynamics in patients with acute HF but does not reduce (or even increases) the risk of hospitalization and death.

At higher doses, dopamine activates α1-adrenoceptors, producing a combined inotropic and vasoconstrictor effect that increases BP and counteracts the renal effects of dopamine (vasodilatation and natriuresis). At these high doses, dopamine also increases the risk of cardiac arrhythmias. Thus, high doses of dopamine should be reserved for patients who require an increase in CO and a pressor effect.

Pharmacokinetics

Dopamine is given by continuous IV infusion. Following an IV bolus, its t½ is approximately 2min (much longer if MAOIs are present). Its effects reach steady state within 5min and, on termination of the infusion, persist for <10min. It is widely distributed (Vd 1.8–2.45L/kg) but does not cross the blood–brain barrier, and it is metabolized within minutes in the liver, kidney, and plasma by MAO and COMT to inactive compounds [homovanillic acid (HVA) and 3,4-dihydroxyphenyl acetic acid (DOPAC)] that are excreted in the urine. About 25% of a dose of dopamine is stored in adrenergic nerve terminals where it is hydroxylated to noradrenaline.

Practical points

1. *Doses*
   - Starting dose: 0.5–1mcg/kg/min, increased gradually in 5–10mcg/kg/min increments, up to 20–50mcg/kg/min, according to the patient's response (urine flow rate, heart rate). When discontinuing the infusion, it may be necessary to gradually decrease the dose of dopamine, while expanding blood volume with IV fluids, to avoid unnecessary hypotension.
2. *Side effects*
   - *CV*: ectopic heartbeats, tachycardia, AF, anginal pain, palpitations, hypotension, vasoconstriction, aberrant conduction, bradycardia, widened QRS complex, hypertension. Fatal ventricular arrhythmias can occur on rare occasions.
   - *Others*: nausea, vomiting, headache, anxiety, dyspnoea, azotaemia, mydriasis, piloerection.
   - Dopamine extravasation may cause necrosis and sloughing of surrounding tissue; thus, the infusion site should be continuously monitored for free flow. Gangrene of extremities has occurred when high doses were administered for prolonged periods or in patients with pre-existing vascular disease.
   - Dopamine may have undesirable side effects such as depression of ventilation and increased pulmonary shunting, which may require supplemental oxygen.
3. *Interactions*
   - When dopamine is administered with halogenated hydrocarbon anaesthetics, ventricular arrhythmias and hypertension may occur. Avoid the combination.
   - The cardiac effects of dopamine are antagonized by β-adrenergic blockers, while peripheral vasoconstriction is antagonized by α-adrenergic blockers.
   - Phenytoin, in combination with dopamine, results in hypotension and bradycardia; avoid this combination, if possible.
   - Co-administration of low-dose dopamine and diuretic agents may produce an additive effect on urine flow.
   - Tricyclic antidepressants may potentiate the pressor response to dopamine.
   - Use of vasoconstricting agents (ergot alkaloids) and some oxytocic drugs may result in severe hypertension.

- MAOIs intensify and prolong the effects of dopamine. In patients treated with MAOIs, the initial dose of dopamine should be reduced to at least one-tenth of the usual dose.
- Dopaminergic drugs (entacapone) may enhance the effects of dopamine.
- Doxapram may cause hypertension in patients receiving dopamine.

4. *Cautions/notes*
   - Use an infusion pump to control flow rate. Titrate the dosage to the desired haemodynamic values or optimal urine flow. Dopamine infusion should be withdrawn gradually, to avoid unnecessary hypotension.
   - Continuous monitoring of BP, urinary flow, ECG, and haemodynamic response (including CO and PCWP, if possible) is required.
   - Hypovolaemia should be corrected, where necessary, prior to dopamine infusion.
   - Dopamine should be used with care in AS or MI.
   - In patients with AF, dopamine may facilitate conduction through the AVN and increase ventricular rate.
   - β2-adrenergic stimulation causes hypokalaemia with an enhanced risk of arrhythmias; serum K^+ levels should be checked to minimize arrhythmias.
   - In the presence of a decline in urine flow rate, tachycardia, or development of new arrhythmias, consider decreasing or temporarily suspending the dosage.
   - Dopamine in 5% glucose should be infused Into a large vein, whenever possible, to prevent the possibility of infiltration of perivascular tissue adjacent to the infusion site. Extravasation may cause necrosis and sloughing of the surrounding tissue.
   - Patients with a history of peripheral vascular disease should be closely monitored for changes in colour or temperature of the skin of the extremities; these changes may be reversed by decreasing the rate or discontinuing the infusion.
   - Dopamine should not be diluted in alkaline solutions. Glucose solutions should be used with caution in patients with known subclinical or overt diabetes mellitus.
   - Safety and effectiveness of dopamine in children have not been established.
5. *Pregnancy and lactation*
   - The effects of dopamine on the human fetus is unknown (Pregnancy category C). It is not known if dopamine is excreted in breast milk.
6. *Contraindications*
   - Patients with phaeochromocytoma or hyperthyroidism.
   - Presence of atrial or ventricular tachyarrhythmias or VF.
   - Cyclopropane and halogenated hydrocarbon anaesthetics should be avoided.

Doxazosin

Selective post-synaptic competitive α1-adrenoreceptor blocker.

CV indications

- Treatment of hypertension, alone or in combination with other antihypertensives.
- Treatment of urinary outflow obstruction and symptoms associated with benign prostatic hyperplasia.

Mechanism of action

Doxazosin antagonizes the vasoconstrictor effect of sympathetic stimulation of vascular α1-adrenoceptors, producing arteriolar and venous vasodilatation, being relatively more effective under conditions of elevated sympathetic activity (e.g. stress, phaeochromocytoma). α1-adrenoreceptor antagonists inhibit platelet aggregation induced by adrenaline, collagen, or ADP.

Pharmacodynamics

- *Hypertension:* doxazosin lowers total plasma cholesterol, LDL-C, and TG levels, increases HDL-C levels, and improves insulin resistance. It is particularly useful in hypertensive patients with benign prostatic hyperthrophy, MetS, and diabetes mellitus.
- *HF*: the doxazosin arm in the Antihypertensive and Lipid Lowering Treatment to Prevent Heart Attack Trial (ALLHAT) was prematurely terminated because of an excess in combined CV endpoints, mainly admissions for HF.

Pharmacokinetics

Doxazosin-XL (mesylate) is rapidly absorbed after oral administration (bioavailability approximately 60%) and reaches peak plasma levels 8–9h after dosing. It is protein-bound (approximately 98%), extensively metabolized in the liver, and excreted predominantly in faeces, with <5% excreted as unchanged drug in the urine. Terminal elimination t½ is approximately 22h. Drug exposure is increased with hepatic impairment.

Practical points

1. *Doses*
   - 1mg od (maximum 16mg od). Doxazosin-XL: 4mg (maximum 8mg od). It should be administered with caution in patients with impaired liver function. No dose adjustment is needed in patients with impaired renal function. Initiation at the lowest possible doses at bedtime and gradual uptitration may help limit the incidence of adverse effects.
2. *Common side effects*
   - Dizziness (>10% of patients); first-dose hypotension (due to loss of reflex vasoconstriction upon standing), orthostatic hypotension, and fainting, especially in the elderly; drowsiness, headache, syncope, vertigo; tachycardia and palpitations.

- Others: oedema, fatigue, general malaise; nausea, diarrhoea; rhinitis, nasal congestion. Urinary incontinence, especially in females, often resulting in drug discontinuation. Oedema may explain the excess of HF in the doxazosin arm of the ALLHAT study.
- In the Treatment of Mild Hypertension Study (TOMHS), impotence was lowest in patients receiving doxazosin.

3. *Interactions*
   - Doxazosin should be used cautiously with other antihypertensives and PDE-5 inhibitors due to the potential for hypotension and rarely syncope. Monitor BP.
   - Avoid intake of alcohol or other sedating medications to prevent excessive drowsiness and dizziness.
   - Doxazosin does not present drug interactions with thiazide diuretics, furosemide, β-blockers, NSAIDs, antibiotics, oral hypoglycaemic drugs, uricosuric agents, or anticoagulants.
4. *Cautions/notes*
   - Dizziness, light-headedness, or vertigo (or syncope) can occur, especially at initiation of therapy or when the dose increases. Avoid getting up too fast from a sitting or lying position to prevent a fall.
   - Tolerance, due to Na^+ and fluid retention, may develop during chronic therapy, requiring the addition of diuretics. If tachycardia is excessive, a β-blocker can be added.
   - Intraoperative floppy iris syndrome has been observed in patients on α-blockers (predominantly tamsulosin) undergoing cataract surgery.
   - Caution in patients with impaired hepatic function.
   - It is not recommended to reduce BP in HFrEF patients because of safety concerns (neurohumoral activation, fluid retention, worsening HF).
5. *Pregnancy and lactation*
   - No data on human pregnancy are available (Pregnancy category B). Due to accumulation in breast milk, doxazosin is contraindicated in breastfeeding.
7. *Contraindications*
   - Known hypersensitvity to quinazolines (e.g. doxazosin, prazosin).
   - History of orthostatic hypotension.
   - Benign prostatic hyperplasia and concomitant congestion of the upper urinary tract, chronic urinary tract infection, or bladder stones.
   - Patients with a history of GI obstruction, oesophageal obstruction, or any degree of decreased lumen diameter of the GI tract.
   - Lactation.

Dronedarone

Non-iodinated benzofuran amiodarone-like AAD, which presents with class I, II, III, and IV actions. A lack of the iodine moiety minimizes the risk of thyroid toxicity, and the addition of a methylsulfonamide group reduces lipophilicity and the risk of neurotoxic effects.

CV indications

For maintenance of sinus rhythm after successful cardioversion in clinically stable adult patients with paroxysmal or persistent AF.

Mechanism of action

Dronedarone exhibits multiple mechanisms of action. It blocks Na^+, L-type Ca^{2+}, and several K^+ currents [transient (I_{to}), ultrarapid (I_{Kur}), rapid (I_{Kr}), and slow (I_{Ks}) components of the delayed rectifier, inward rectifier (I_{K1}), and acetylcholine-activated (I_{KACh})]. It also produces non-competitive inhibition of α- and β-adrenergic receptors and produces a vasodilator effect mediated via L-type Ca^{2+} current blockade and activation of the NO pathway.

Pharmacodynamics

Dronedarone prolongs the APD and refractoriness in all cardiac tissues, an effect independent of the rate of stimulation, and reduces transmural dispersion of repolarization. Dronedarone slows SA nodal automaticity and AV nodal conduction and prolongs the RR, PR, and QTc intervals on the ECG. Dronedarone decreases BP, myocardial contractility, and MVO_2.

Pharmacokinetics

Oral dronedarone is well absorbed, but it undergoes an extensive first-pass metabolism, so that oral bioavailability is approximately 5% (15% when administered with a high-fat meal). Dronedarone is extensively metabolized to an active *N*-debutyl metabolite. Dronedarone and its active metabolite are widely distributed, crossing the blood–brain and placental barriers. No pharmacokinetic difference was observed in patients with mild to severe renal impairment or moderate hepatic impairment. (See Table 8.1.3.)

Practical points

1. *Doses*
   - 400mg bd.
2. *Side effects*
   - Frequent: GI disorders (diarrhoea, nausea, abdominal pain, vomiting, dyspepsia), LFT abnormalities, asthenia, bradycardia, and QT prolongation.
   - Uncommon: skin reactions (rashes, pruritus, eczema, dermatitis, allergic dermatitis, photosensitivity), and dysgeusia. Dronedarone increases serum creatinine levels due to partial inhibition of the tubular organic cationic transporter system, but the drug does not affect the GFR.
3. *Interactions*
   - Dronedarone is a moderate inhibitor of CYP3A4, a mild inhibitor of CYP2D6, and a potent inhibitor of P-gp. It can interact with substrates of P-gp, CYP3A4, or CYP2D6 (see Table 8.1.2).

- Dronedarone is primarily metabolized by CYP3A4. Potent CYP3A4 inhibitors/inducers significantly increase/decrease, respectively, exposure of dronedarone and should be avoided (see Table 8.1.2).
- Reduce the dose of dronedarone when co-administered with moderate CYP3A4 inhibitors (see Table 8.1.2).
- Co-administration of dronedarone with β-blockers, verapamil, or diltiazem increases the depressant effects on SA and AV nodes. Monitor the ECG.
- Dronedarone increases lovastatin and simvastatin plasma levels and the risk of myopathy; the dose of lovastatin and simvastatin should be limited to 20mg/day and 10mg/day, respectively.
- Class I or III antiarrhythmics increase the risk of proarrhythmia and should be avoided.
- Dronedarone inhibits P-gp and increases (1.7- to 2.5-fold) digoxin plasma levels and the risk of bradycardia and AVB. In patients with recently decompensated HF [Antiarrhythmic Trial with Dronedarone in Moderate to Severe CHF Evaluating Morbidity Decrease (ANDROMEDA) trial] or with permanent AF [Permanent Atrial Fibrillation Outcome Study Using Dronedarone on Top of Standard Therapy (PALLAS)], the use of digoxin was associated with an increased risk of arrhythmia or sudden death in dronedarone-treated patients, compared to placebo. Thus, the dose of digoxin should be halved and digoxin plasma levels carefully monitored.
- Dronedarone inhibits CYP2D6 and slightly increases exposure of CYP2D6 substrates (see Table 8.1.2).
- Drugs that prolong the QTc interval and induce TdP are contraindicated.
- The INR should be closely monitored in patients taking VKAs.
- MAOIs might decrease the clearance of the active metabolite of dronedarone and should therefore be used with caution.
- Dronedarone may increase the plasma levels of tacrolimus, sirolimus, everolimus, and ciclosporin. Monitor their plasma concentrations, and adjust doses as appropriate.
- Dronedarone increases the exposure of dabigatran. Avoid this combination.
- There are no interactions between dronedarone and theophylline, metformin, omeprazole, pantoprazole, and clopidogrel.

4. *Cautions/notes*
   - Hypokalaemia increases the incidence of dronedarone-induced QT prolongation.
   - Dronedarone is not recommended for rhythm control in patients with AF and symptomatic HF (NYHA classes II–IV) because of an increased risk of hospital admissions for CV causes and an increased risk of premature death.
   - The combination of Na^+ channel blockers and dronedarone to treat ventricular arrhythmias is not recommended in patients with DCM.
5. *Pregnancy and lactation*
   - Dronedarone may cause fetal harm and is contraindicated in women who are, or may become, pregnant (Pregnancy category X). It should also be avoided in nursing mothers.

6. *Contraindications*
 - Patients with LV systolic dysfunction or with current or previous HF.
 - Second- or third-degree AVB, complete bundle branch block, distal block, sinus node dysfunction, atrial conduction defects, or sick sinus syndrome, except when used in conjunction with a functioning pacemaker.
 - Bradycardia of <50bpm.
 - Permanent AF with an AF duration of ≥6 months (or duration unknown).
 - Patients with unstable haemodynamic conditions.
 - Concomitant use of a strong CYP3A inhibitor, QT-prolonging drugs, and QTc Bazett interval of ≥500ms.
 - Severe hepatic impairment; severe renal impairment (CrCl <30mL/min).
 - Co-administration with dabigatran.
 - Patients with liver and lung toxicity related to previous use of amiodarone.
 - Hypersensitivity to the active substance or to any of the excipients.

Edoxaban

Highly selective, direct, and reversible inhibitor of factor Xa.

Indications

- Prevention of stroke and systemic embolism in adult patients with NVAF with one or more risk factors such as CHF, hypertension, age ≥75 years, diabetes mellitus, and prior stroke or TIA.
- Treatment of DVT and PE, and prevention of recurrent DVT and PE in adults.

Mechanism of action

(See ➲ Apixaban, pp. 465–8.)

Pharmacodynamics

The pharmacodynamic effects, measured by chromogenic anti-factor Xa assays, are predictable and correlate with the dose and concentration of edoxaban.

Pharmacokinetics

Edoxaban is a substrate for the efflux transporter P-gp, but not for uptake transporters such as organic anion transporter polypeptide OATP1B1, organic anion transporters OAT1 or OAT3, or organic cation transporter OCT2.

Age and gender have no effect on edoxaban pharmacokinetics. Patients with mild or moderate hepatic impairment (Child–Pugh A or B) exhibit similar pharmacokinetics and pharmacodynamics; there is no clinical experience in patients with severe hepatic impairment. In patients with CrCl of >50 to <80mL/min, 30–50mL/min, and <30 mL/min, or those undergoing peritoneal dialysis, edoxaban exposure increased by 32%, 74%, 72%, and 93%, respectively, relative to subjects with CrCl of ≤80mL/min. (See Table 8.1.1.)

Practical points

1. *Doses*
   - *Prevention of stroke and systemic embolism*: 60mg od. Therapy with edoxaban in NVAF patients should be continued long term.
   - *Treatment of DVT and PE, and prevention of recurrent DVT and PE (VTE)*: 60mg od, following initial use of parenteral anticoagulant for at least 5 days. Edoxaban and initial parenteral anticoagulant should not be administered simultaneously. The duration of therapy for treatment of DVT and PE (VTE) and prevention of recurrent VTE should be individualized and based on transient risk factors (e.g. recent surgery, trauma, immobilization), and longer durations should be based on permanent risk factors or idiopathic DVT or PE.
   - For NVAF and VTE, the recommended dose is 30mg edoxaban od in patients with one or more of the following clinical factors: moderate or severe renal impairment (CrCl 15–50mL/min), body weight ≤60kg, or concomitant use of the following P-gp inhibitors—ciclosporin, dronedarone, erythromycin, or ketoconazole.
   - *Switching from VKAs to edoxaban*: discontinue VKAs and start edoxaban when the INR is ≤2.5.

- *Switching from oral anticoagulants other than VKAs to edoxaban*: discontinue dabigatran, rivaroxaban, or apixaban, and start edoxaban at the time of the next dose of the oral anticoagulant.
- *Switching from parenteral anticoagulants to edoxaban*: these medicinal products should not be administered simultaneously. (1) SC (i.e. LMWH, fondaparinux): discontinue SC anticoagulants, and start edoxaban at the time of the next scheduled SC anticoagulant dose; (2) IV UFH: discontinue the infusion, and start edoxaban 4h later.
- *Switching from edoxaban to VKAs*: (1) oral: in patients on 60mg edoxaban, reduce the dose to 30mg od, together with an appropriate VKA dose. For patients currently on 30mg od (for one or more of the following clinical factors: CrCl 15–50mL/min, low body weight, or use of P-gp inhibitors), administer a dose of 15mg od, together with an appropriate VKA dose. Patients should not take a loading dose of VKA in order to promptly achieve a stable INR of between 2 and 3. Once a stable INR of ≥2.0 is achieved, edoxaban should be discontinued and warfarin continued. Concomitant use of edoxaban and VKA can increase the INR by up to 45%; (2) parenteral: discontinue edoxaban, and administer a parenteral anticoagulant and VKA at the time of the next scheduled edoxaban dose. When a stable INR of ≥2.0 is achieved, the parenteral anticoagulant should be discontinued and the VKA continued.
- *Transition from edoxaban to oral anticoagulants other than VKA*: discontinue edoxaban, and start the other oral anticoagulant at the time of the next dose of edoxaban.
- *Transition from edoxaban to parenteral anticoagulants*: discontinue edoxaban, and start the parenteral anticoagulant at the time of the next dose of edoxaban. In patients with ESRD (CrCL <15mL/min) or on dialysis, edoxaban is not recommended. No dose adjustment is required in patients with mild or moderate hepatic impairment; avoid edoxaban in patients with severe hepatic impairment.

2. *Side effects* (see ➔ Apixaban, pp. 465–8)
   - Bleeding is the commonest reason for treatment discontinuation.
   - Others: rash, abnormal LFTs.
3. *Drug interactions*
   - Co-administration of anticoagulants, antiplatelet drugs, and thrombolytics may increase the risk of bleeding. Evaluate any signs or symptoms of blood loss if patients are treated concomitantly with anticoagulants, aspirin, other platelet aggregation inhibitors, and/or NSAIDs. Edoxaban can be co-administered with low-dose ASA (≤100mg/day).
   - Avoid the concomitant use of edoxaban with abiraterone, aprepitant, crizotinib, enzalutamide, HIV-1 protease inhibitors, imatinib, or vermurafenib. With caution in patients treated with axitinib. Patients on retroviral therapy (indinavir, nelfinavir, ritonavir, saquinavir) or ciclosporin were excluded from trials.
   - Reduce the dose (30mg od) of edoxaban if co-administered with: amiodarone, clarithromycin, dronedarone, ciclosporin, enzalutamide, erythromycin, itraconazole, ketoconazole, lapatinib, nilotinib, quinidine, tacrolimus, tamoxifen, or voriconazole. These drugs increase edoxaban exposure and the risk of bleeding.

- Dexamethasone, doxorubicin, carbamazepine, phenytoin, rifampicin, St John's wort, sunitinib, vandetanib and vinblastine decrease edoxaban exposure and its anticoagulant activity. Avoid the combination.

4. *Cautions*
   - Patients need to be carefully observed for signs of bleeding, and caution is recommended under conditions with an increased risk of haemorrhage.
   - Discontinue edoxaban at least 24h before invasive/surgical procedures because of the risk of bleeding. Edoxaban can be restarted after the surgical or other procedure as soon as adequate haemostasis has been established, noting that the time to onset of pharmacodynamic effects is 1–2h.
   - Patients on antiretroviral therapy (ritonavir, nelfinavir, indinavir, saquinavir), as well as ciclosporin, were excluded from the Hokusai VTE study.
5. *Pregnancy and lactation*
   - There are no adequate and well-controlled studies in pregnant women (Pregnancy Category C). It is not known if edoxaban is excreted in human milk.
6. *Contraindications* (see ➔ Apixaban, pp. 465–8)

Enalapril

Orally active ACEI (see ➔ Angiotensin-converting enzyme inhibitors, pp. 459–64).

Indications

- Treatment of hypertension.
- Treatment of HF.
- Prevention of symptomatic HF in patients with asymptomatic LV dysfunction (LVEF ≥35%).

Pharmacodynamics

(See ➔ Angiotensin-converting enzyme inhibitors, pp. 459–64.)

Pharmacokinetics

Following absorption, enalapril is rapidly and extensively de-esterified to enalaprilat, a potent and active ACEI, the levels of which peak within 4h of enalapril administration. Drug exposure is increased in renal impairment and especially when CrCl is <30mL/min. Enalapril can be removed by dialysis. (See Table 8.1.10.)

Practical points

1. *Doses*
   - Hypertension: 5–10mg od initially; maximum dose 40mg od.
   - HF/asymptomatic LV dysfunction: starting dose 2.5mg bd; doses are progressively increased. The maximum dose is 40mg daily in two divided doses.

Due to potential accumulation in renal impairment, doses should be reduced accordingly. CrCl 30–80mL/min: 5–10mg/day; 10 to ≤30mL/min: 2.5mg/day; ≤10mL/min: 2.5mg on dialysis days. In severe liver disease, the dose may have to be increased (impaired conversion of enalapril to enalaprilat).

2. *Side effects* (see ➔ Angiotensin-converting enzyme inhibitors, pp. 459–64)
3. *Interactions* (see ➔ Angiotensin-converting enzyme inhibitors, pp. 459–64)
4. *Cautions/notes* (see ➔ Angiotensin-converting enzyme inhibitors, pp. 459–64)
5. *Contraindications* (see ➔ Angiotensin-converting enzyme inhibitors, pp. 459–64)

Enoxaparin

Enoxaparin is an LMWH of 4500Da obtained by alkaline depolymerization.

CV indications

- Prophylaxis of thromboembolic disorders of venous origin, in particular those which may be associated with orthopaedic or general surgery.
- Prophylaxis of VTE in medical patients bedridden due to acute illness.
- Treatment of VTE presenting with DVT, PE, or both.
- Treatment of UA and non-Q-wave MI, administered concurrently with aspirin.
- Treatment of acute STEMI, including patients to be managed medically or with subsequent PCI, in conjunction with thrombolytic drugs (fibrin- or non-fibrin-specific).
- Prevention of thrombus formation in the extracorporeal circulation during haemodialysis.

Mechanism of action

LMWHs inhibit the coagulation process through binding to antithrombin (AT) III via a pentasaccharide sequence that are most commonly found in LMWH than in UFH. This binding leads to a conformational change of AT III, which accelerates its inhibition of activated factor X (factor Xa). However, AT III activated by LMWH cannot inhibit thrombin (factor IIa), so that inhibition of thrombin is less powerful than that of heparin. Thus, LMWHs have greater anti-Xa:IIa ratios, compared with UFH.

LMWHs present several advantages over UFH: (1) they appear not to be inactivated by platelet factor 4 and exhibit less unspecific binding to plasma or vascular proteins (and therefore they present greater bioavailability) and a longer plasma t½ than UFH, so that they can be given SC in a fixed dose, according to body weight; (2) a predictable level of anticoagulation without the need for aPTT monitoring; (3) greater capacity to release tissue factor-pathway inhibitor; and (4) less propensity to stimulate platelet aggregation and lower risk of HIT. Therefore, LMWHs are much easier to use than UFH. LMWHs have a more predictable dose–effect relationship than UFH and cause HIT less frequently.

Pharmacodynamics

At recommended doses, enoxaparin does not significantly influence platelet adhesion and aggregation or binding of fibrinogen to platelets, and clotting tests, such as PT, TT, or aPTT, are unsuitable for monitoring their anticoagulant effect. Drug monitoring is generally not necessary but can be performed with a functional anti-factor Xa assay.

Enoxaparin is superior to UFH for STEMI; even when enoxaprin increases the risk of bleeding, this increase is offset by a reduction in death and reinfarction. In patients undergoing major hip or knee operations, enoxaparin has been displaced by NOACs.

Pharmacokinetics

Enoxaparin is rapidly and completely absorbed following SC injection, and maximum plasma anti-Xa activity occurs within 1–4h. It is metabolized in the liver by desulfation and/or depolymerization to lower-molecular weight derivatives, with much reduced biological potency, and only 10% of the administered dose is eliminated in the urine. Elimination t½, based on anti-factor Xa activity, is 4–5h after a single SC dose but increases (7h) after repeated dosing and in the elderly.

A decreased clearance of enoxaparin is observed in patients with mild to moderate renal impairment (CrCl 30–50mL/min). In patients with severe renal impairment (CrCl <30mL/min), the AUC increases by 65% after repeated 40mg od doses. Therefore, enoxaparin (and LMWHs) are contraindicated in patients with CrCl <30mL/min. The effect of hepatic impairment on the exposure to enoxaparin is unknown. Anti-Xa exposure increases in low-weight individuals. (See Table 8.1.1.)

Practical points

1. *Doses*
   - *Prophylaxis of VTE*. In patients with low to moderate risk: 20mg (2000IU) od SC for 7–10 days or until the risk of thromboembolism has diminished. In patients undergoing surgery, the initial dose should be given approximately 2h preoperatively. In patients at higher risk (in orthopaedic, abdominal, or pelvic surgery): 40mg (4000IU) daily SC, with the initial dose administered approximately 12h before surgery.
   - *Prophylaxis of VTE in medical patients*: 40mg (4000IU) od SC for 6 days and continued until the return to full ambulation, for a maximum of 14 days.
   - *Treatment of VTE*: 1.5mg/kg (150IU/kg) od SC for at least 5 days and until adequate oral anticoagulation is established.
   - *Treatment of UA and non-Q-wave MI*: 1mg/kg SC every 12h with oral aspirin (100–325mg od) for a minimum of 2 days and continued until clinical stabilization (up to 8 days).
   - *Treatment of acute STEMI*: single IV bolus of 30mg plus a 1mg/kg SC dose, followed by 1mg/kg administered SC every 12h (maximum 100mg for the first two doses only).
     - —When administered in conjunction with a thrombolytic, enoxaparin should be given 15min before, and 30min after, the start of fibrinolytic therapy. Patients should receive aspirin (75–325mg od), unless contraindicated. The duration of enoxaparin treatment is 8 days or until hospital discharge, whichever comes first.
     - —For patients managed with PCI: if the last SC dose of enoxaparin was given <8h before balloon inflation, no additional dosing is needed. If the last SC administration was given >8h before balloon inflation, an IV bolus of 0.3mg/kg of enoxaparin should be administered.
     - —In elderly patients ≥75 years of age: 0.75mg/kg SC bd without an initial bolus (maximum 75mg for each of the first two SC doses).
     - —Renal impairment (if CrCl <30mL/min): 1mg/kg SC od, without an initial bolus.
   - *Prevention of extracorporeal thrombus formation during haemodialysis:* 1mg/kg (100IU/kg) introduced into the arterial line at the beginning of a dialysis session is sufficient for a 4-h session. In patients at high risk of haemorrhage: 5mg/kg for double vascular access or 0.75mg/kg for single vascular access.

2. *Common side effects*
   - The commonest are haemorrhagic complications (major haemorrhages in 4.2% of patients; somes cases can be fatal), local reactions at the injection site (irritation, pain, haematoma, ecchymosis, erythema, and skin necrosis), anaemia, and thrombocytopenia (type I, which usually is reversible during treatment). Injection site haematomas during the extended prophylaxis period after hip replacement surgery occurred in 9% of enoxaparin patients (compared to 1.8% of placebo patients). Bleeding can be reduced, but not completely reversed, by protamine (residual anti-Xa activity remains).
   - Others: nausea, oedema, reversible elevations of AST and ALT levels (>3 times ULN; 6%), allergic reactions (pruritus, rash, fever, cases of anaphylactoid reactions). Hypersensitivity reactions include vasculitis.
   - Hyperkalaemia occurs in patients with CKD or treated with potassium-sparing drugs. Alopecia and osteoporosis have also been reported following long-term therapy.
3. *Interactions*
   - Drugs that increase the risk of bleeding (anticoagulants, platelet inhibitors, thrombolytic agents, NSAIDs, dipyridamole, or sulfinpyrazone) should be discontinued prior to initiation of enoxaparin therapy. If they are co-administered, close clinical and laboratory monitoring is needed.
   - The pharmacokinetic properties of enoxaparin (and LMWHs) is not influenced by either CYP or P-gp inhibitors and/or inducers.
   - Avoid the combination with capecitabiline.
4. *Cautions/notes*
   - Enoxaparin should be used with caution in patients with a history of HIT with or without thrombosis. In patients receiving enoxaparin who experience platelet counts of 50,000–100,000/mm^3, the dose should be reduced to 2500IU daily until the platelet count recovers to ≥100,000/mm^3. In patients with platelet counts of <50,000/mm^3, enoxaparin should be discontinued until the platelet count recovers to above 50,000/mm^3.
   - Monitoring anticoagulant activity (anti-Xa levels) is not necessary, except in patients at an increased risk of bleeding (i.e. renal impairment, elderly, obesity, pregnancy, and extremes of weight) or actively bleeding.
   - Enoxaparin is given as a deep SC injection, not IM. It should not be mixed with other injections or infusions, unless specific compatibility data are available. For IV use (i.e. acute STEMI), enoxaparin can be mixed with normal saline solution (0.9%) or 5% glucose.
   - In obese patients LMWH dosing based on total body weight could cause supra-therapeutic anticoagulation. Monitoring anti-factor Xa levels is recommended in these patients.
   - In low-weight women (<45kg) or men (<57kg), an increase in enoxaparin exposure has been observed, which may lead to a higher risk of bleeding.

- LMWHs are not interchangeable, as they differ in their manufacturing process, molecular weights, specific anti-Xa activities, units, and dosage.
- When epidural/spinal anaesthesia or spinal puncture is employed, patients treated with enoxaparin are at risk of developing an epidural or spinal haematoma, which can result in long-term or permanent paralysis. The risk increased by the use of indwelling epidural catheters for the administration of analgesia, the concomitant use of drugs affecting haemostasis (e.g. NSAIDs, platelet inhibitors, other anticoagulants), or traumatic or repeated epidural or spinal puncture. Patients should be monitored frequently to detect any signs and symptoms of neurologic impairment (back pain, sensory or motor deficits, and bowel or bladder dysfunction). If signs or symptoms of spinal haematoma are suspected, urgent diagnosis and treatment may include spinal cord decompression.
- Elderly patients (especially ≥80 years) may be at an increased risk for bleeding complications within the therapeutic dosage ranges.
- There are no adequate studies in patients with prosthetic heart valves.

5. *Pregnancy and lactation*
   - Enoxaparin, as detected by anti-Xa activity, does not cross the placental barrier during the second trimester of pregnancy (Pregnancy category B). It is unknown whether enoxaparin is excreted in human breast milk.
6. *Contraindications*
   - Known allergies to LMWHs, heparin, sulfites, or benzyl alcohol.
   - Patients with active major bleeding and conditions with a high risk of uncontrolled haemorrhage, known haemorrhagic diathesis, serious coagulation disorders, acute bacterial endocarditis, injuries to and operations on the CNS, eyes, and ears.
   - Severe renal impairment.
   - History of HIT or HIT with thrombosis.
   - Undergoing epidural/neuraxial anaesthesia.
   - In patients receiving heparin for treatment, rather than prophylaxis, loco-regional anaesthesia in elective surgical procedures is contraindicated.

Eplerenone

Selective MRA (potassium-sparing diuretic).

CV indications

- In addition to standard therapy, including β-blockers, to reduce the risk of CV mortality and morbidity in stable patients with LVEF of ≤40% and clinical evidence of HF after recent MI.
- In addition to standard optimal therapy, to reduce the risk of CV mortality and morbidity in adult patients with NYHA class II (chronic) HF and LVEF of ≤30%.

Mechanism of action

Compared to spironolactone, eplerenone is 20–40 times less potent, but more selective (minimal binding to glucocorticoid, androgen, and progesterone receptors), than spironolactone.

Pharmacodynamics

In patients with acute MI complicated by LV dysfunction and HF (NYHA classes III–IV, LVEF ≤40%), eplerenone, added to standard therapy, reduces total mortality, CV mortality, and CV death or hospitalization for CV events, compared to placebo. It also reduces SCD.

Pharmacokinetics

Unlike spironolactone, eplerenone does not have an active metabolite. Steady-state C_{max} and AUC are increased with renal impairment, liver insufficiency, and HF and in the elderly, and reduced in blacks. (See Table 8.1.5.)

Practical points

1. *Doses*
   - Post-MI HF patients: 25mg od, titrated to a maintenance dose of 50mg od within 4 weeks. Eplerenone should usually be started within 3–14 days after an acute MI.
   - For patients with NYHA class II chronic HF: starting dose of 25mg od, titrated to 50mg od within 4 weeks. Reduce the doses when co-administered with ACEI/ARB.
   - When plasma K^+ levels are >5.5mmol/L or plasma creatinine levels >2.5mg/dL, the dose should be reduced (25mg/day) or discontinued. Avoid in patients with serum K^+ levels of >5mmol/L at baseline.
2. *Side effects*
   - Hyperkalaemia, increased creatinine concentration; hypotension, dizziness, headache, insomnia; diarrhoea, nausea, constipation, vomiting; rash, pruritus; muscle spasms, back pain, and asthenia.
3. *Interactions*
   - Co-administration with antihypertensives, vasodilatory drugs, alcohol, tricyclic antidepressants, neuroleptics, amifostine, and baclofen increases the risk of hypotension. It is recommended to monitor BP in these patients.
   - Concomitant use with drugs that raise serum K^+ levels (ACEIs, ARBs, other potassium-sparing diuretics, β-blockers, heparin, trimethoprim–sulfamethoxazole, NSAIDs, pentamidine, drospirenone, tolvaptan,

ciclosporin, tacrolimus, IV benzylpenicillin potassium, potassium salts or supplements) can precipitate serious hyperkalaemia, particularly in the elderly and patients with renal impairment. Monitor serum K^+ levels. Restrict dietary potassium and reduce/avoid potassium supplements without consulting the prescribing physician.

- Ciclosporin and tacrolimus may impair renal function and increase the risk of hyperkalaemia.
- NSAIDs reduce the antihypertensive effects of eplerenone and increase the risk of acute renal failure. Monitor plasma creatinine levels.
- Glucocorticoids reduce the antihypertensive effect of eplerenone.
- Use of eplerenone with strong CYP3A4 inhibitors is contraindicated due to potential enhanced effects (see Table 8.1.2). With mild to moderate CYP3A4 inhibitors, eplerenone should not be used at doses above 25mg.
- CYP3A4 inducers decrease eplerenone efficacy (see Table 8.1.2); this association is not recommended.
- Glucocorticoids and ACTH reduce the antihypertensive effects of eplerenone and increase the risk of hypokalaemia. Increase the dose of eplerenone, and monitor serum K^+ levels.
- Eplerenone reduces the renal clearance and increases the plasma levels of lithium. Re-adjust the dose of lithium, and monitor its plasma levels.
- There are no pharmacokinetic interactions when eplerenone is administered with digoxin, warfarin, midazolam, cisapride, ciclosporin, simvastatin, glyburide, or oral contraceptives (norethindrone/ethinylestradiol).

4. *Cautions/notes*
   - Serum K^+ levels should be monitored regularly to avoid hyperkalaemia, particularly in patients treated with RAAS inhibitors, in the elderly, and patients with renal and hepatic impairment.
   - Eplerenone should not be used concomitantly with potent CYP3A4 inhibitors/inducers (see Table 8.1.2), lithium, ciclosporin, or tacrolimus.
   - Eplerenone should not be used in patients with T2DM with hypertension and microalbuminuria, because of the risk of hyperkalaemia.
   - Tablets contain lactose and should not be administered in patients with galactose intolerance, Lapp lactase deficiency, or glucose–galactose malabsorption.
5. *Pregnancy and lactation*
   - Due to inadequate data, caution is required in pregnancy (Pregnancy category B). Balance of risks and benefits should be made in breastfeeding due to finding of the presence of eplerenone in rat breast milk.
6. *Contraindications*
   - Severe renal impairment (CrCl ≤30mL/min).
   - Hyperkalaemia (>5mEq/L) at initiation.
   - Severe (Child–Pugh score C) hepatic impairment.
   - Concomitant treatment with drugs that produce hyperkalaemia or potassium supplements and strong inhibitors of CYP3A4.
   - Hypersensitivity to the active substance or any of the excipients.

Epoprostenol

Synthetic PGI2 (or prostacyclin) indicated for continuous IV infusion.

CV indications

- Treatment of idiopathic or heritable PAH and PAH associated with connective tissue disease in patients with WHO functional class III–IV symptoms, to improve exercise capacity.
- In haemodialysis in emergency situations when the use of heparin carries a high risk of causing or exacerbating bleeding or when heparin is otherwise contraindicated.

Mechanism of action

Prostacyclin (PGI2) is produced predominantly by endothelial cells. PGI2 binds to IP receptors that are widely distributed, with higher expressions in the lungs, heart, and kidneys, activates adenylyl cyclase, and increases the cellular levels of cAMP, producing potent venous and arteriolar vasodilatation (reducing systemic and pulmonary vascular resistances). It also increases capillary density and reduces the increased vascular permeability caused by mediators such as serotonin or histamine in the microcirculation. PGI2 is the most potent endogenous inhibitor of platelet aggregation, stimulates endogenous fibrinolytic potential, and exerts cytoprotective and antiproliferative actions on vascular smooth muscle cells. IP expression and prostacyclin synthase activity are decreased in the pulmonary arteries of patients with PAH, resulting in a decrease in PGI2 and prostacyclin urinary metabolites.

Epoprostenol is a PGI2 analogue acting as a non-selective IP receptor agonist, as it can also activate other prostanoid receptors such as EP3 and EP4 receptors.

Pharmacodynamics

In idiopathic PAH (WHO functional classes III and IV) and PAH associated with scleroderma, IV epoprostenol improves functional class, symptoms, exercise capacity, and haemodynamics (increases cardiac index and stroke volume and decreases pulmonary vascular resistances, total pulmonary resistances, and mean systemic arterial pressure). It reduces total mortality by about 70%. Long-term persistence of efficacy has also been shown in idiopathic PAH, as well as in other associated PAH conditions and in non-operable CTEPH.

Pharmacokinetics

After continuous IV infusion, epoprostenol has an immediate effect and reaches steady-state levels within 15min. It is rapidly hydrolysed in plasma, which explains its poor tissue distribution (Vd 357mL/kg), is metabolized to two active metabolites, and presents a t½ of 3–5min. These active metabolites are eliminated in the urine (93%). The dose should be halved in patients with hepatic insufficiency.

Practical points

1. *Doses*
   - Starting dose: 2ng/kg/min IV under close observation in the ICU via a CVC coupled with a perfusion pump. The dose is further adjusted, based on adverse effects. Increase the dose by 2ng/kg/min every 15min until dose-limiting pharmacological effects are elicited. The optimal dose range for chronic therapy is 20–40ng/kg/min, and doses of >40ng/kg/min after 1 year of therapy are not uncommon.
   - *Renal dialysis*. Prior to dialysis: 4ng/kg/min IV for 15min; during dialysis: 4ng/kg/min into the arterial inlet of the dialyser. The infusion should be stopped at the end of dialysis.
   - Epoprostenol reconstituted solutions, prepared in real time, must not be administered over >12h when they are used at room temperature and must be protected from light. It is possible to refrigerate (2–8°C) epoprostenol reconstituted solutions without exceeding 40h of storage; in this case, the solutions should not be used over >8h when administered at room temperature. The reconstituted solution should be examined prior to administration. Its use is forbidden in the presence of discoloration or particles.
2. *Side effects*
   - Common: headache, flushing, hypotension, syncope, nausea, diarrhoea, skin rash, jaw and musculoskeletal pain, peripheral oedema, dizziness, paraesthesiae, tremor, rash, and urticaria. If excessive hypotension occurs, the dose should be reduced or the infusion discontinued.
   - Bradycardia, tachycardia (in response to direct vasodilatation and hypotension), lassitude, anxiety, agitation, insomnia, dry mouth, hyperglycaemia. Some patients with PAH have developed pulmonary oedema during dose-ranging, which may be associated with pulmonary veno-occlusive disease.
   - Chronic IV infusions are delivered using a small, portable infusion pump through a permanent indwelling CVC. Serious adverse events related to the delivery system include pump malfunction, local site infection, catheter obstruction, and sepsis. Local and systemic infections and infusion interruptions can be life-threatening. In controlled clinical trials of up to 12 weeks' duration, the local infection rate was about 18% and the rate for pain 11%. During long-term follow-up, sepsis was reported at a rate of 0.3 infections/patient per year. Guidelines for the prevention of CVC bloodstream infections have been proposed.
3. *Interactions*
   - Since PGI2 is a vasodilator, additive hypotensive effects are expected when co-administered with antihypertensive agents or vasodilating agents (riociguat). Dose adjustment might be required.
   - Epoprostenol inhibits platelet aggregation and may increase the risk of bleeding when co-administered with other anticoagulants, antiplatelet drugs, and NSAIDs in patients with other risk factors for bleeding. Careful monitoring is required.

4. *Cautions/notes*
    - Treatment should only be initiated and monitored by a physician experienced in the treatment of PAH and in experienced centres with adequate personnel and equipment for its administration and the systematic follow-up of patients.
    - Keep the vial in the outer carton in order to protect from light.
    - Patients must learn the techniques of sterile reconstitution and dilution of the medication to avoid infections, operation of the ambulatory infusion pump, and care of the CVC.
    - Abrupt interruption of epoprostenol infusion should be avoided, because in some patients, this may lead to PAH rebound, with symptomatic deterioration and even death.
    - Because of the high pH of the final infusion solutions, care should be taken to avoid extravasation due to the risk of tissue damage.
    - BP and heart rate should be monitored during treatment. Extreme caution is advised in patients with CAD.
    - Following establishment of a new chronic infusion rate, both standing and supine BP should be monitored for several hours.
    - Co-administer epoprostenol with anticoagulants, whenever possible, to reduce the risk of thromboembolism, but this combination may increase the risk of bleeding. Anticoagulant monitoring is required when given with UFH.
    - Chronic overdose sometimes results in high-output HF.
    - Caution in patients with impaired kidney or liver function.
    - Do not administer or dilute reconstituted solutions of epoprostenol with other parenteral solutions or medications. Use a multi-lumen catheter if other IV therapies are routinely administered.
    - This medicinal product contains sodium; this should be taken into consideration for patients on a controlled sodium diet.
5. *Pregnancy and lactation*
    - Fetal risk in animal studies (FDA category class B). It is not known whether treprostinil is excreted in breast milk. Thus, caution is advised when administered to nursing women.
6. *Contraindications*
    - Known hypersensitivity to the active substance or any of the excipients.
    - Decompensated HF.
    - Congenital or acquired valvular defects not related to PAH.
    - Patients who develop pulmonary oedema during dose-ranging.
    - SBP <85mmHg.
    - Severe CAD or UA; MI within the last 6 months.
    - Cerebrovascular events (e.g. TIA, stroke) within the last 3 months.
    - PAH due to veno-occlusive disease.
    - Conditions which increase the risk of bleeding.

Eptifibatide

Synthetic cyclic heptapeptide GPIIb/IIIa receptor antagonist (see ➔ Glycoprotein IIb/IIIa receptor antagonists, pp. 613–15).

CV indications

Eptifibatide is intended for use with ASA and UFH for the prevention of early MI in adults presenting with UA or non-Q-wave MI, with the last episode of chest pain occurring within 24h and with ECG changes and/or elevated cardiac enzymes. Patients most likely to benefit are those at high risk of developing MI within the first 3–4 days after the onset of acute angina symptoms, including, for instance, those who are likely to undergo early PTCA.

Mechanism of action

Eptifibatide reversibly inhibits platelet aggregation by preventing the binding of fibrinogen, von Willebrand factor, and other adhesive ligands to GPIIb/IIIa receptors. Platelet aggregation inhibition is reversible following cessation of eptifibatide infusion.

Pharmacokinetics

The effect of eptifibatide is observed immediately after administration of an IV bolus. It binds to plasma proteins (25%), and its Vd is 0.25L/kg. Platelet inhibition is readily reversed (>50% of platelet aggregation) 4h after stopping the continuous infusion. Renal clearance of eptifibatide and its metabolites accounts for approximately 50% of total body clearance. Plasma elimination t½ is 2–3h. In patients with CrCl of <50mL/min, the clearance of eptifibatide is reduced by approximately 50% and steady-state plasma levels are approximately doubled.

Practical points

1. *Doses*
   - *ACS*: 180mcg/kg IV bolus, followed by a continuous infusion of 2mcg/kg/min (1mcg/kg when CrCl <50mL/min) for up to 72h, until initiation of CABG surgery or until discharge from hospital, whichever comes first. In patients who undergo CABG surgery, the infusion should be discontinued prior to surgery. If PCI is performed during eptifibatide therapy, continue the infusion for 20–24h post-PCI (maximum duration of therapy 96h).

Eptifibatide should be given concomitantly with UFH, dosed to achieve a target aPTT of 50–70s and an ACT of 200–300s. Heparin infusion after PCI is strongly discouraged. Eptifibatide has no measurable effect on PT or aPTT.

2. *Side effects* (see ➔ Glycoprotein IIb/IIIa receptor antagonists, pp. 613–15)
   - Acute thrombocytopenia can develop as a result of naturally occurring drug-dependent antibodies or those induced by prior exposure to eptifibatide. Immune-mediated thrombocytopenia may be associated with hypotension and/or other signs of hypersensitivity.

3. *Interactions* (see ➔ Glycoprotein IIb/IIIa receptor antagonists, pp. 613–15)
4. *Cautions/notes* (see ➔ Glycoprotein IIb/IIIa receptor antagonists, pp. 613–15)
   - Decrease the dose in patients with moderate renal impairment.
   - Experience in patients with hepatic impairment is very limited. Administer with caution to patients in whom coagulation could be affected.
   - Patients requiring thrombolytic therapy should discontinue eptifibatide.
5. *Contraindications* (see ➔ Glycoprotein IIb/IIIa receptor antagonists, pp. 613–15)

Esmolol

IV ultrashort-acting β-blocker.

Indications

- For SVT (except for pre-excitation syndromes) and for rapid control of ventricular rate in patients with AF or atrial flutter in perioperative, post-operative, or other circumstances where short-term control of the ventricular rate with a short-acting agent is desirable.
- Treatment of tachycardia and hypertension occurring in the perioperative phase and non-compensatory sinus tachycardia where, in the physician's judgement, the rapid heart rate requires specific intervention.

Mechanism of action

Esmolol is a β1-selective adrenergic receptor blocking agent with a rapid onset and a very short duration of action.

Pharmacodynamics

(See ➲ Beta-adrenergic blocking agents, pp. 485–94.)

IV administration of esmolol rapidly reduces the heart rate at rest and during exercise, SBP/DBP, and MVO_2, prolongs the sinus node recovery time, and increases the antegrade Wenckebach cycle length. After termination of the infusion, full recovery from β-blockade is observed in 20–30min.

Because of its short t½, esmolol can be useful in situations in which on–off control of β-blockade is desired (i.e. SVT in the perioperative period, or sinus tachycardia or emergency hypertension in the perioperative period) or when there are relative contraindications or concerns about the use of a β-blocker (SVT, AF or atrial flutter, and associated COPD, UA and threatened MI when haemodynamic changes may call for the withdrawal of β-blockade, or LV dysfunction).

Pharmacokinetics

Following an initial IV bolus and infusion, onset of action occurs within 2min and 90% steady-state level within 5min. It is rapidly hydrolysed to inactive metabolites by esterases located in red blood cells, so that it has a t½ of approximately 9min. Total body clearance (20L/kg/h) is greater than the CO; thus, metabolism of esmolol is not limited by the rate of blood flow to metabolizing tissues, such as the liver, or affected by hepatic or renal blood flow. (See Tables 8.1.3 and 8.1.8.)

Practical points

1. *Doses*
   - *SVT.* IV loading dose (500mcg/kg over 1min), followed by an infusion of 50mcg/kg/min for 4min to maintain the desired heart rate and BP. If this fails, repeat the loading dose and increase the infusion to 100, 150, and 200mcg/kg/min (over 4min).
   - *Perioperative tachycardia and hypertension.* (1) For intraoperative treatment: bolus of 80mg (approximately 1mg/kg) over 15–30s, followed by a 150mcg/kg/min infusion (maximum dose 300mcg/kg/min), if needed; (2) upon awakening from anaesthesia: an infusion of 500mcg/kg/min for 4min, followed by a 300mcg/kg/min infusion.

- *For post-operative situations when time for titration is available*. Loading dose of 500mcg/kg/min over 1 min. Use titration steps of 50, 100, 150, 200, 250, and 300mcg/kg/min, given over 4min and stopping at the desired therapeutic effect.

2. *Side effects* (see ➔ Beta-adrenergic blocking agents, pp. 485–94)
   - The commonest are hypotension, nausea, dizziness, confusion, somnolence, headache, confusional state, diaphoresis, thrombophlebitis, and skin necrosis from extravasation, bradycardia, and bronchospasm. Local reactions at the injection site.
3. *Drug interactions*
   - Concomitant use of esmolol with drugs that decrease BP, heart rate, AV nodal conduction, or cardiac contractility increases the risk of hypotension, bradycardia, AVB, or cardiac dysfunction.
   - Co-administration with digoxin increases the risk of bradycardia and AVB.
   - Esmolol prolongs the duration of succinylcholine- and mivacuronium-induced neuromuscular blockade.
   - Esmolol increases the risk of clonidine, guanfacine, or moxonidine withdrawal rebound hypertension. In these patients, esmolol should be discontinued gradually.
   - In patients with depressed myocardial function, the combination of esmolol with diltiazem or verapamil can lead to bradycardia and AVB. Esmolol must not be administered within 48h of discontinuing verapamil.
   - Esmolol should not be administered to control tachycardia in patients receiving β-adrenergic agonists with positive inotropic and vasoconstrictive effects (adrenaline, noradrenaline, or dopamine).
4. *Cautions/notes*
   - Extravasation of the acid solution with risk of skin necrosis.
5. *Pregnancy and lactation*
   - There are limited data on the use of esmolol in pregnant women, and it is not known whether esmolol is excreted in human milk (Pregnancy category C).
6. *Contraindications* (see ➔ Beta-adrenergic blocking agents, pp. 485–94)
   - IV administration of verapamil or diltiazem.
   - Pulmonary hypertension.
   - Metabolic acidosis.
   - Hypersensitivity reactions, including anaphylaxis, to esmolol or any of the inactive ingredients of the product.

Evolocumab

Indications

- Adults with primary hypercholesterolaemia (heterozygous familial and non-familial) or mixed dyslipidaemia, as an adjunct to diet: (1) in combination with a statin or a statin with other lipid-lowering therapies in patients unable to reach LDL-C goals with the maximum tolerated dose of a statin; or (2) alone or in combination with other lipid-lowering therapies in patients who are statin-intolerant or for whom a statin is contraindicated.
- Adults with established atherosclerotic cardiovascular disease (MI, stroke, or PAD) to reduce cardiovascular risk by lowering LDL-C levels, as an adjunct to correction of other risk factors: (a) in combination with the maximum tolerated dose of a statin with or without other lipid-lowering therapies or (b) alone or in combination with other lipid-lowering therapies in patients who are statin-intolerant, or for whom a statin is contraindicated.
- In adults and adolescents aged 12 years and over with homozygous familial hypercholesterolaemia (HoFH), in combination with other lipid-lowering therapies.

Mechanism of action

(See ➔ Alirocumab, pp. 431–3.)

Pharmacodynamics

Evolocumab reduces LDL-C, non-HDL-C, Apo B, TGs, lipoprotein (a), VLDL-C, total-C/HDL-C, and Apo B/Apo A1 and increases HDL-C in patients with mixed dyslipidaemia. It significantly reduces TGs, Apo B, non-HDL-C, total-C/HDL-C, Apo B/Apo A1, and lipoprotein (a) from baseline to mean of weeks 10 and 12, compared to ezetimibe. Additionally, evolocumab reduces LDL-C by approximately 20–30% in patients with HoFH not on apheresis (approximately 15–25% in patients on apheresis).

In patients with atherosclerotic CV disease and already receiving statins, evolocumab reduces (15%) the risk of MI, stroke, CV death, coronary revascularization, and UA hospitalization, compared with placebo.

Pharmacokinetics

Evolocumab has limited tissue distribution and is degraded into small peptides and amino acids via catabolic pathways. As a monoclonal antibody, no renal excretion is anticipated due to its molecular size. (See Table 8.1.4.)

Practical points

1. *Doses*
   - *Primary hypercholesterolaemia and mixed dyslipidaemia in adults*: 140mg once every 2 weeks or 420mg once every 4 weeks; both doses are clinically equivalent.
   - *HoFH in adults and adolescents aged 12 years and over*: 420mg once every 4 weeks. After 12 weeks of treatment, the dose frequency can be uptitrated to 420mg once every 2 weeks, if required. Patients on apheresis: 420mg once every 4 weeks to correspond with their apheresis schedule.

No dose adjustment is necessary in patients with mild to moderate renal impairment, those with mild hepatic impairment, or in elderly patients. Patients with severe hepatic or renal impairment have not been studied.

The safety and efficacy of evolocumab in children <18 years have not been established in the indication for primary hypercholesterolaemia and mixed dyslipidaemia or in children aged <12 years for HoFH.

2. *Side effects*
   - Upper respiratory tract infections (influenza, nasopharyngitis), nausea, rash, urticaria, back pain, arthralgia, and injection site reactions.
3. *Drug interactions* (see ➔ Alirocumab, pp. 431–3)
4. *Cautions/notes*
   - Measure LDL-C levels 4–8 weeks after initiating, since response to therapy depends on the degree of LDL-R function.
   - The needle cover of the glass pre-filled syringe is made from dry natural rubber (a derivative of latex), which may cause allergic reactions.
5. *Pregnancy and lactation*
   - Human monoclonal antibodies in humans are unlikely to cross the placenta in the first trimester, but they are likely to cross the placenta in the second and third trimesters. It is uncertain whether evolocumab is excreted in human breast milk.
6. *Contraindications*
   - Hypersensitivity to the active substance or any of the excipients.

Ezetimibe

Oral antihyperlipidaemic agent acting as a cholesterol absorption inhibitor.

CV indications

- Primary (heterozygous familial and non-familial) hypercholesterolaemia: co-administration with a statin is indicated in patients who are not appropriately controlled with a statin alone or when statins are contraindicated or not tolerated.
- To reduce the risk of CV events in patients with CAD and a history of ACS when added to ongoing statin therapy or initiated concomitantly with a statin.
- HoFH: ezetimibe co-administered with a statin is indicated as adjunctive therapy to diet in these patients.
- Adjunctive therapy to diet and other treatments in patients with homozygous familial sitosterolaemia (phytosterolaemia).

Mechanism of action

Ezetimibe selectively binds to Niemann–Pick C1-Like 1 (NPC1L1) protein, which is responsible for the intestinal transport of cholesterol at the brush border membrane of the intestinal wall without affecting the absorption of vitamins A, D, and C. Thus, ezetimibe decreases the intestinal absorption of cholesterol and related plant sterols. This leads to an upregulation of LDL-Rs on the surface of hepatic cells and an increased LDL-C uptake into these cells, thus decreasing LDL-C plasma levels.

Pharmacodynamics

Ezetimibe inhibits intestinal cholesterol absorption by 54% and reduces LDL-C levels by 15–22% and increases HDL-C levels by 3.5% over 12 weeks. It also reduces elevated total-C, Apo B, TGs, and non-HDL-C levels. In combination with atorvastatin or simvastatin, ezetimibe is indicated for reducing elevated total-C and LDL-C levels in patients with HoFH.

Pharmacokinetics

Ezetimibe is extensively conjugated in the liver and small intestine to an active phenolic glucuronide (ezetimibe glucuronide) that also inhibits cholesterol absorption. In patients with moderate or severe hepatic impairment, the mean AUC values for ezetimibe increased approximately 3- to 4- and 5- to 6-fold, respectively. In patients with severe renal disease (CrCl ≤30mL/min/1.73m^2), mean drug exposure increased 1.5-fold. (See Table 8.1.4.)

Practical points

1. *Doses*
   - 10mg od, associated or not with a statin. No dosage adjustment is necessary in the elderly or in patients with mild hepatic impairment or with renal impairment. A combination of ezetimibe (10mg) with fenofibrate (160mg) can be used in patients with mixed hyperlipidaemia.

2. *Side effects*
   - GI (abdominal pain, diarrhoea, flatulence), headache, myalgia, arthralgia, upper respiratory tract infection, diarrhoea, and pain in extremities. Uncommon: hypersensitivity reactions (rash, urticaria, angio-oedema, and anaphylaxis), hepatitis; very rarely pancreatitis, cholelithiasis, thrombocytopenia, myopathy, and rhabdomyolysis. A higher percentage of patients had elevated levels (≥3 times ULN) of ALT and/or AST with ezetimibe and a statin together than with a statin alone.
3. *Interactions*
   - Colestyramine decreases the mean AUC of ezetimibe (55%) and the expected reduction in LDL-C levels. Administer ezetimibe either ≥2h before or ≥4h after the bile acid sequestrant.
   - Ezetimibe increases the plasma concentrations of ciclosporin (240%), fenofibrate (55%), and gemfibrozil (65–90%). Monitor ciclosporin plasma levels. With fenofibrate, it increases the risk of cholelithiasis and gall bladder disease.
   - There are post-marketing reports of increased INR in patients treated with ezetimibe and warfarin. Monitor the INR as appropriate.
   - No interactions with cimetidine, dapsone, dextromethorphan, digoxin, oral contraceptives (ethinylestradiol and levonorgestrel), glipizide, tolbutamide, statins, or midazolam.
4. *Cautions/notes*
   - Ezetimibe is not recommended in moderate to severe liver dysfunction.
   - In patients treated with statins and ezetimibe, elevations of transaminases (≥3 times ULN) have been observed. Thus, LFTs should be performed.
   - Patients on ezetimibe should be advised on the risk of myopathy and to report any unexplained muscle pain, tenderness, or weakness. If myopathy is suspected, based on muscle symptoms, or is confirmed by a CPK level of >10 times ULN, ezetimibe and/or statins should be immediately discontinued.
   - Avoid ezetimibe in patients with rare hereditary problems of galactose intolerance, Lapp lactase deficiency, or glucose–galactose malabsorption.
5. *Pregnancy and lactation*
   - No clinical data are available during pregnancy, and thus it should be given in pregnancy only if clearly necessary (Pregnancy category C). It is unknown if ezetimibe is excreted into human breast milk, and so it should not be used during lactation.
6. *Contraindications*
   - Hypersensitivity to the active substance or the excipients.
   - Co-administration with a statin is contraindicated during pregnancy and lactation.
   - Co-administration with a statin is contraindicated in patients with active liver disease or unexplained persistent elevations in serum transaminases.

Felodipine

Dihydropyridine L-type CCB (see also ➔ Calcium channel blockers, pp. 504–9).

CV indications

- Treatment of hypertension.
- Prophylaxis of chronic stable angina pectoris.

Pharmacodynamics

(See also ➔ Calcium channel blockers, pp. 504–9.)

Its antihypertensive effect appears within 2–5h and persists for 24h. In patients with CHF, felodipine added to standard therapy (including enalapril and diuretics) has no effect on mortality or hospitalization rates. Thus, it should be considered in patients with HFrEF when hypertension or angina persists despite standard treatment.

Pharmacokinetics

(See Table 8.1.6.)

Practical points

1. *Doses*
   - 5–10mg od (maximum 20mg od). Reduce the dose in the elderly and in patients with liver disease.
2. *Side effects* (see ➔ Calcium channel blockers, pp. 504–9)
3. *Interactions* (see ➔ Calcium channel blockers, pp. 504–9)
   - Felodipine does not interact with metoprolol, digoxin, indometacin, or spironolactone.
   - Cimetidine increases blood felodipine levels (reduce the dose).
4. *Cautions/notes* (see ➔ Calcium channel blockers, pp. 504–9)
   - Should be used with caution in severe LV dysfunction.
5. *Contraindications* (see ➔ Calcium channel blockers, pp. 504–9)

Fenofibrate

Oral PPAR-α receptor agonist (see also ➔ Fibrates, pp. 590–2).

CV indications

- Treatment of severe hypertriglyceridaemia with or without low HDL-C.
- Treatment of mixed hyperlipidaemia when a statin is contraindicated or not tolerated.
- Treatment of mixed hyperlipidaemia in patients at high CV risk, in addition to a statin, when TGs and HDL-C are not adequately controlled.

Mechanism of action

(See ➔ Fibrates, pp. 590–2.)

Pharmacodynamics

Fenofibrate reduces total-C (18–20%), LDL-C (20–31%), Apo B (25%), and TG (40–45%) levels, and increases HDL-C (11%) levels, when comparing 300mg fenofibrate daily to placebo over 6 months. Fenofibrate increases urinary excretion and reduces serum plasma uric acid levels, being the first-choice drug in hyperlipidaemic patients with hyperuricaemia. Fenofibrate reduces plasma levels of fibrinogen and lipoprotein (a). When statin–fibrate combination therapy is indicated, fenofibrate is preferred.

Pharmacokinetics

A high-fat meal increases (25%) drug exposure. Fenofibrate is a prodrug that is rapidly hydrolysed by esterases to the active metabolite fenofibric acid, which reaches peak plasma levels within 4–6h. Fenofibric acid binds to plasma proteins (99%) and is primarily glucoconjugated and then excreted in the urine (65%) and faeces (25%). Thus, neither compound undergoes oxidative CYP450 metabolism. In patients with severe renal impairment (eGFR <30mL/min/1.73m^2), fenofibrate exposure increases 2.7-fold. Thus, fenofibrate should be avoided in these patients and a dose reduction is required in patients having mild to moderate renal impairment. (See Table 8.1.4.)

Practical points

1. *Doses*
   - Doses varies with formulations. Capsules: 150mg od; tablets: 120–160mg od.
2. *Side effects* (see ➔ Fibrates, pp. 590–2)
   - Pancreatitis has been reported (especially in T2DM).
3. *Interactions* (see ➔ Fibrates, pp. 590–2)
   - Cases of myopathy, including rhabdomyolysis, have been reported when fenofibrate is co-administered with colchicine.
4. *Cautions/notes* (see ➔ Fibrates, pp. 590–2)
5. *Pregnancy and lactation* (see ➔ Fibrates, pp. 590–2)
6. *Contraindications* (see ➔ Fibrates, pp. 590–2)
   - Hypersensitivity to fenofibric acid or fenofibrate, known photoallergy or phototoxic reaction during treatment with ketoprofen.

Fibrates

(See also ➲ Bezafibrate, p. 495, ➲ Fenofibrate, p. 589, and ➲ Gemfibrozil, pp. 603–4.)

Fibrates are fibric acid derivative drugs used as hypolipidaemic agents.

CV indications

- They are indicated as adjunctive therapy to diet for the treatment of hyperlipidaemias of types IIa, IIb, III, IV, and V, especially in hypertriglyceridaemia or low HDL-C, when dietary measures alone have failed to produce an adequate response.
- Fibrates are the first-line therapy to reduce the risk for pancreatitis in patients with very high levels of plasma TGs; they can be useful with more modest TG elevations or when the prime problem is low HDL-C.

Mechanism of action

Fibrates bind specifically to, and activate, the hepatic isozyme PPARα, a nuclear transcription factor found mainly in the liver and skeletal muscle. PPARα modulates carbohydrate and fat metabolism and adipose tissue differentiation.

It is suggested that fibrates potentially alter lipoprotein levels via five mechanisms:

- Increase lipolysis of TG-rich remnant lipoproteins (TRLs) and VLDL due to an increase in lipoprotein lipase (LPL) activity or a reduction in Apo C-III (an inhibitor of LPL activity).
- Induce the hepatic β-oxidation pathway, with a concomitant decrease in fatty acid synthesis, which results in lower availability of fatty acids for TG production and VLDL synthesis.
- Fibrates result in the formation of LDL particles with a higher affinity for LDL-Rs, which are thus catabolized more rapidly.
- Reduce TG exchange between VLDL and HDL-C due to a reduction in plasma levels of TRLs.
- Increase the hepatic synthesis of Apo A1 and Apo AII, which may contribute to the increase in plasma HDL-C concentrations and more efficient reverse cholesterol transport.

Pharmacodynamics

Fibrates decrease fasting and postprandial TG levels and TRLs and slightly increase HDL-C levels, while they produce modest decreases in total-C and LDL-C levels. They modify the size and composition of LDLs from small, dense particles (more atherogenic due to their susceptibility to oxidation) to large particles that have a greater affinity for cholesterol receptors and are catabolized rapidly. Indeed, treatment of patients with elevated TGs due to type IV hyperlipoproteinaemia often results in a rise in LDL-C levels. In type IIb patients with elevations of both LDL-C and TG levels, fibrates minimally affected LDL-C levels. Fibrates increase HDL-C plasma levels (HDL2 and HDL3) and Apo A1 and Apo A2.

Pharmacokinetics

(See Table 8.1.4.)

Practical points

1. *Doses* (see ➔ Bezafibrate, p. 495, ➔ Fenofibrate, p. 589, and ➔ Gemfibrozil, pp. 603–4)
2. *Side effects*
   - Common: nausea, loss of appetite, vomiting, diarrhoea, constipation, dyspepsia, flatulence, abdominal discomfort, and cholelithiasis by increasing biliary secretion of cholesterol (more frequent in women, obese, and diabetics).
   - Increased liver transaminase, bilirubin, alkaline phosphatase, and CPK levels.
   - Musculoskeletal: myopathy (muscle pain with CPK elevations), myalgia, painful extremities. Isolated cases of rhabdomyolysis leading to renal failure have been described. Myopathy should be suspected in patients presenting with diffuse myalgia, myositis, muscular cramps and weakness, and/or marked increases in CPK levels, e.g. ≥5 times ULN. Risk increases with renal impairment, hypothyroidism, severe infection, trauma, surgery, or electrolyte imbalance and a high alcohol intake, in the elderly (>70 years), and patients with a personal or family history of hereditary muscular disorders or a previous history of muscle toxicity with another fibrate or statin.
   - CNS: dizziness, somnolence, paraesthesiae, depression, decreased libido, headache, blurred vision.
   - Others: impotence, anaemia, leucopenia, eosinophilia, rash, dermatitis, pruritus.
   - Fibrates increase serum creatinine and homocysteine levels. Changes are fully reversible after drug discontinuation. The fibrate-induced increase in homocysteine levels may blunt the increases in both HDL-C and Apo A1 levels and may promote thrombosis.
3. *Interactions*
   - Combination therapy with statins increases the risk of muscle toxicity. The risk is greater in patients with CKD but varies with different fibrates and statins.
   - Concomitant use with oral hypoglycaemics and/or insulin can produce hypoglycaemic reactions. Monitoring of plasma glucose levels is recommended.
   - Fibrates may potentiate the effects of warfarin and prolong the PT/INR. The dose of warfarin should be reduced (30–50%), and the INR should be monitored.
   - Isolated cases of reversible impairment of renal function have been reported when bezafibrate or fenofibrate are co-administered with ciclosporin and tacrolimus in organ transplant patients.
   - Bile acid-binding resins potentiate the lipid-lowering effects of fibrates but may reduce their oral bioavailability. To avoid the interaction, fibrates should be taken at least 1h before or 4–6h after resins.
   - Fibrates can displace other drugs (phenytoin, oral hypoglycaemic agents, thyroxine) from plasma proteins and increase their free plasma levels; doses of these drugs should be reduced, as needed.
   - Because fibrates are renally excreted, the risk/benefit ratio of the combination of fibrates and immunosuppressants (ciclosporin, tacrolimus) and other potentially nephrotoxic agents should be carefully and individually considered.

4. *Cautions/notes*
   - Periodic determination of serum lipids are necessary during treatment with fibrates. A paradoxical increase in total-C and LDL-C levels can occur in patients with hypertriglyceridaemia. If the response is insufficient after 3 months of therapy, treatment should be discontinued and an alternative treatment considered.
   - In some subjects with unsatisfactory responses to either statins or fibrates alone, the possible benefits of combined therapy do not outweigh the risks of severe myopathy, rhabdomyolysis, and acute renal failure. CPK levels should be measured before starting the combination in patients with risk factors for rhabdomyolysis.
   - Monitoring of LFTs is recommended prior to therapy, periodically after, and in patients who develop any signs or symptoms suggestive of liver injury. Consider to stop fibrates in cases of transaminase elevations to ≥3 times ULN or of ≥100IU. Patients who develop increased transaminase levels should be monitored until resolution.
   - Fibrates may also activate PPAR-γ, hence improving glucose utilization. Thus, monitoring of drug effects in diabetic patients is recommended.
   - Dose adjustment may be required in the elderly and in patients with renal dysfunction.
5. *Pregnancy and lactation*
   - Animal models suggest deleterious effects in pregnancy. In general, fibrates are not recommended in pregnant and breastfeeding women (Pregnancy category C).
6. *Contraindications*
   - Hypersensitivity to the fibrate or the excipients. Previous history of photoallergy or phototoxic reactions during treatment with fibrates.
   - Severe hepatic impairment (including biliary cirrhosis and unexplained persistent liver function abnormalities) and pre-existing gall bladder or biliary tract disease, with or without cholelithiasis.
   - Severe renal impairment (serum creatinine >135micromol/L or CrCl <60mL/min) or nephrotic syndrome (see ➔ Bezafibrate, p. 495, ➔ Fenofibrate, p. 589, and ➔ Gemfibrozil, pp. 603–4).
   - Chronic or acute pancreatitis (except acute pancreatitis due to severe hypertriglyceridaemia).
   - Combination with statins in patients with predisposing factors for myopathy.

Flecainide

Na^+ channel blocker with class 1C antiarrhythmic properties.

Indications

In patients without structural heart disease, it is indicated for the:

- Pharmacological cardioversion of recent-onset AF associated with disabling symptoms to sinus rhythm and maintenance of normal sinus rhythm following conversion by other means.
- Prevention of PSVT, including AVNRT, AVRT, and other SVTs in patients with disabling symptoms.
- Treatment of AV nodal reciprocating tachycardia; arrhythmias associated with WPW syndrome and similar conditions with accessory pathways, when other treatments have been ineffective.
- Treatment of severe symptomatic life-threatening paroxysmal ventricular arrhythmias not controlled by other drugs or when other treatments are not tolerated.
- Off-label: treatment of patients with LQTS3. Flecainide should be considered, in addition to β-blockers, in patients with CPVT who experience recurrent syncope or polymorphic/bidirectional VT while on β-blockers, when there are risks/contraindications for an ICD or an ICD is not available.

Mechanism of action

Flecainide and propafenone produce the most potent voltage- and frequency-dependent blockade of Na^+ channels. They slow intra-cardiac conduction velocity and decrease cardiac excitability; the depression of intra-cardiac conduction is more marked in the His–Purkinje system, widening the QRS complex. They do not modify the duration of the ventricular APD but prolong the effective refractory period by lenghthening the reactivation of the Na^+ channel and blocking several K^+ currents. Flecainide prolongs in a frequency-dependent manner the atrial APD, an effect that may facilitate the conversion of AF to sinus rhythm. They also prolong the PR, AH, HV, and QRS intervals of the ECG. Most of the QT prolongation is due to a widening of the QRS complex, so that the JT interval and the rate-corrected QT interval (QTc) remain almost unchanged. The marked depression of conduction velocity, together with a heterogenous prolongation of the APD, may explain the proarrhythmic effects of these drugs.

During chronic oral therapy, flecainide has minimal effects on BP or CO in patients with normal, or near-normal, ventricular function. However, it significantly reduces stroke volume index and LVEF and increases right atrial pressure and PCWP in patients with CAD, acute MI, or pre-existing LV dysfunction.

Pharmacodynamics

Flecainide should be considered, in addition to β-blockers, in patients with a diagnosis of CPVT who experience recurrent syncope or polymorphic/bidirectional VT while on β-blockers, when there are risks/contraindications for an ICD or an ICD is not available or is rejected by the patient.

Pharmacokinetics

Therapeutic plasma levels: 3–8mcg/mL. (See Table 8.1.3.)

Practical points

1. *Doses*
   - *PO*: 50mg bd (maximum 300mg/day) for SVT; 100–200mg bd (maximum 400mg/day) for ventricular arrhythmias. These high doses are associated with a higher risk of proarrhythmia and HF. Increase the dose every 4 days.
     —Chronic oral drug therapy to prevent AF recurrence: 150–300mg/day.
   - *IV*: bolus injection of 1–2mg/kg (maximum bolus dose 15mg) over no less than 10min or in divided doses, followed by 1.5mg/kg in the first hour, then 0.1–0.25mg/kg/h (maximum recommended dose over 24h: 600mg). ECG and plasma level monitoring is recommended.
   - In patients with renal impairment (GFR <35mL/min/1.73m^2), the initial dose should be 100mg daily (or 50mg bd).
2. *Common side effects*
   - (>10%): dizziness, visual disturbances, dyspnoea.
   - (1–10%): headache, nausea, fatigue, palpitation, chest pain, abdominal pain, constipation, tremor, oedema.
   - CV: sinus pause or arrest, AV dissociation, cardiac arrest, flushing, hot flushes, SVT, negative inotropism. Flecainide can convert AF to atrial flutter, which may conduct with a 1:1 AV ratio at a high ventricular rate. Proarrhythmic effects are related to non-uniform slowing of conduction and include monomorphic VT, aggravation of ventricular arrhythmias, and threat of sudden death. The risk of proarrhythmia increases in patients with prior MI, especially those with significant ventricular ectopy or pre-existing sinus node or AV conduction problems.
   - CNS: abnormal dreams, tremor, confusion, numbness, paraesthesiae, tinnitus, vertigo.
3. *Interactions*
   - Co-administration of flecainide with other class I AADs decreases further intra-cardiac conduction velocity and cardiac contractility, and is not recommended.
   - Co-administration with local anaesthetics and drugs which inhibit heart rate and/or myocardial contractility (e.g. β-blockers, tricyclic antidepressants) potentiates the cardiodepressant effects of flecainide.
   - Added negative inotropic and AV nodal depressant effects when co-administered with β-blockers, propafenone, verapamil, and diltiazem.
   - Plasma levels of flecainide and the risk of arrhythmia increase when combined with amiodarone (inhibits CYP2D6), cimetidine, antivirals (ritonavir, lopinavir, and indinavir), terfenadine, fluoxetine, paroxetine, tricyclic antidepresssants, and clozapine.
   - Flecainide increases plasma digoxin levels.

4. *Cautions/notes*
   - Flecainide should be started under careful clinical and ECG monitoring (assess QRS complex duration) and occasionally serum levels.
   - The risk of proarrhythmia increases in patients with structural heart disease and/or impaired LV function. In post-MI patients with asymptomatic non-sustained ventricular arrhythmias, flecainide increases mortality or non-fatal cardiac arrest among post-MI patients.
   - Flecainide is contraindicated in patients with structural heart disease (HF, CAD), Brugada syndrome, and acquired or congenital LQTS (other than LQTS3).
   - Use of flecainide in chronic AF has not been adequately studied and is not recommended.
   - Sinus node dysfunction and AVB, unless a pacemaker is present.
   - Flecainide increases endocardial pacing thresholds. It should be used with caution in patients with permanent pacemakers or temporary pacing electrodes; avoid its use in patients with existing poor thresholds or non-programmable pacemakers, unless suitable pacing rescue is available.
   - Prolonged parenteral administration over 24h is not recommended.
5. *Pregnancy and lactation*
   - Flecainide crosses the placenta (Pregnancy category C). It is also excreted in human breast milk, with levels reflecting maternal blood levels.
6. *Contraindications*
   - Structural heart disease (HF, CAD, MI, cardiogenic shock) or with abnormal LV function.
   - Asymptomatic ventricular extrasystoles or asymptomatic NSVT.
   - Patients with long-standing AF in whom there has been no attempt to convert to sinus rhythm.
   - Severe bradycardia, sinus node dysfunction, atrial conduction defects, second-degree or greater AVB, bundle branch block, or distal block (unless a pacemaker is available).
   - Severe hypotension.
   - Haemodynamically significant VHD.
   - In combination with class I AADs.
   - Brugada syndrome, inherited LQTS (other than LQTS3), concomitant treatments associated with QT interval prolongation.
   - Severe electrolyte imbalance (hypo-/hyperkalaemia).

Fluvastatin

Oral HMG CoA reductase inhibitor (see also Statins (3-hydroxy-3-methylglutaryl-coenzyme A reductase inhibitors), pp. 760–3).

CV indications

It is indicated as an adjunct to diet for the:

- Treatment of adults with primary hypercholesterolaemia or mixed dyslipidaemia when response to diet and other non-pharmacological treatments (e.g. exercise, weight reduction) is inadequate.
- Secondary prevention of CAD. Secondary prevention of major adverse cardiac events in adults with coronary heart disease after PCI.

Pharmacodynamics

At doses of 20–80mg/day, fluvastatin reduces LDL-C (22–35%), total-C (17–25%), and TG (12–19%) levels and increases HDL-C (3–6%) levels.

Pharmacokinetics

Administration of a high-fat meal delayed the absorption and increased the bioavailability by 50%. Drug pharmacokinetics are not affected by age; there are no pharmacokinetic data in the paediatric population. Fluvastatin AUC and C_{max} values increased approximately 2.5-fold in hepatic insufficiency. (See Table 8.1.4.)

Practical points

1. *Doses*
   - Dyslipidaemia: 20–80mg od (in the evening or at bedtime). No dose adjustments are needed in patients with mild to moderate renal impairment.
   - Secondary prevention in CAD after PCI: 80mg.
2. *Side effects* (see Statins (3-hydroxy-3-methylglutaryl-coenzyme A reductase inhibitors), pp. 760–3)
   - Transaminase elevations (>3 times ULN on two consecutive weekly measurements) occurred in 0.2%, 1.5%, and 2.7% of patients treated with 20, 40, and 80mg.
3. *Interactions* (see Statins (3-hydroxy-3-methylglutaryl-coenzyme A reductase inhibitors), pp. 760–3)
   - CYP2C9 inhibitors (see Table 8.1.2) increase plasma levels of fluvastatin; reduce the dose of fluvastatin. CYP2C9 inducers decrease plasma fluvastatin levels (see Table 8.1.2).
   - Fluvastatin increases the plasma levels of S-warfarin (monitor the INR).
   - Glibenclamide increases plasma fluvastatin levels; monitor drug effects.
   - Cimetidine/ranitidine/omeprazole reduce fluvastatin clearance and increase its plasma levels (43–70%).
   - Colestyramine reduces fluvastatin absorption and its plasma levels.
   - Not recommended with nelfinavir. Etravirine may increase the AUC of fluvastatin.
   - Plasma fluvastatin levels are not altered when co-administered with gemfibrozil, itraconazole, erythromycin, tolbutamide, or clopidogrel.
4. *Cautions and contraindications* (see Statins (3-hydroxy-3-methylglutaryl-coenzyme A reductase inhibitors), pp. 760–3)

Fondaparinux

A synthetic pentasaccharide (1728Da) structurally similar to the antithrombin-binding sequence found in heparin, acting as a selective inhibitor of activated factor X.

CV indications

- Prevention of VTE in: (1) adults undergoing major orthopaedic surgery of the lower limbs such as hip fracture, major knee surgery, or hip replacement surgery; (2) adults undergoing abdominal surgery who are judged to be at high risk of thromboembolic complications such as patients undergoing abdominal cancer surgery; and (3) adult medical patients who are judged to be at high risk for VTE and who are immobilized due to acute illness such as HF and/or acute respiratory disorders and/or acute infectious or inflammatory disease.
- Treatment of adults with: (1) acute symptomatic spontaneous superficial vein thrombosis of the lower limbs without concomitant DVT; (2) acute DVT and treatment of acute PE, except in haemodynamically unstable patients or patients who require thrombolysis or pulmonary embolectomy; (3) UA/NSTEMI for whom urgent (<120min) invasive management (PCI) is not indicated; (4) STEMI who are managed with thrombolytics or who initially are to receive no other form of reperfusion therapy; and (5) acute symptomatic spontaneous superficial vein thrombosis of the lower limbs without concomitant DVT.

Mechanism of action

Fondaparinux is a synthetic pentasaccharide that binds reversibly and non-covalently to antithrombin III (ATIII) with high affinity and potentiates (about 300 times) the innate neutralization of factor Xa by ATIII. Neutralization of factor Xa interrupts the blood coagulation cascade and thus inhibits thrombin formation and thrombus development. Fondaparinux does not inactivate thrombin (factor IIa), has no effect on platelet function, and does not bind significantly to other plasma proteins (including platelet factor 4) or affect fibrinolytic activity or bleeding time. The effect of fondaparinux can be quantified by anti-factor Xa activity.

Pharmacodynamics

The specific anti-Xa activity is approximately 7-fold higher than that of LMWHs. The main advantages of fondaparinux include a long t½ and a predictable, sustained anticoagulant effect which requires only a single daily SC administration; it causes less bleeding than heparin and does not cross-react with sera from patients with HIT. Fondaparinux does not affect routine coagulation tests such aPTT, PT, or INR in plasma nor bleeding time or fibrinolytic activity. Fondaparinux is superior to placebo, but not to UFH, in STEMI and is superior to LMWH in NSTEMI-ACS (lower bleeding and fewer deaths).

Pharmacokinetics

After SC injection, fondaparinux is rapidly and completely absorbed (bioavailability 100%), reaching peak plasma concentrations within 25min and steady state of plasma levels after 3–4 days. It is specifically bound to ATIII, but not to other plasma proteins. It is not metabolized, and up to 77% of the dose is eliminated unchanged in the urine in 72h. The specificity and selectivity of fondaparinux, combined with its long t½ and 100% bioavailability, allow once-daily anticoagulation, without the need for monitoring the ACT. (See Table 8.1.1.)

Plasma clearance is 1.3, 2, and 5 times lower in patients with mild (CrCl 50–80mL/min), moderate (CrCl 30–50mL/min), and severe (CrCl <30mL/min) renal impairment, respectively. The t½ increases to 29h in patients with moderate renal impairment and 72h in patients with severe renal impairment. Thus, fondaparinux is contraindicated in severe renal failure. Fondaparinux has not been studied in paediatric patients. No dose adjustment is required in patients with mild to moderate hepatic impairment.

Practical points

1. *Doses*

Fondaparinux is provided in a single-dose, pre-filled syringe, affixed to an automatic needle protection system. It should be administered SC (not IM) and needs no monitoring.

- *Patients undergoing major orthopaedic or abdominal surgery*: 2.5mg od by SC injection; the initial dose should be given 6h after surgery, provided haemostasis has been achieved. Treatment should be continued for 5–9 days. In patients undergoing hip fracture surgery, the risk of VTE continues beyond 9 days after surgery and the use of fondaparinux should be considered for up to an additional 24 days.
- *Medical patients who are at high risk for thromboembolic complications, based on an individual risk assessment*: 2.5mg od, administered by SC injection, for 6–14 days.
- *Treatment of superficial vein thrombosis*: 2.5mg od by SC injection for a minimum of 30 days, and up to a maximum of 45 days, in patients at high risk of thromboembolic complications. Patients with superficial vein thrombosis who are to undergo surgery or other invasive procedures: fondaparinux, where possible, should not be given during the 24h before surgery but may be restarted at least 6h post-operatively, provided haemostasis has been achieved.
- *UA/NSTEMI*: 2.5mg od as soon as possible following diagnosis and continued for up to a maximum of 8 days or until hospital discharge if this occurs earlier. If the patient undergoes PCI, the timing of restarting SC fondaparinux should be no earlier than 2h after sheath removal.
- *STEMI*: 2.5mg od. The first dose is administered IV, and subsequent doses are administered by SC injection. Treatment should be initiated as soon as possible following diagnosis and continued for up to a maximum of 8 days or until hospital discharge if this occurs earlier. If a patient is to undergo non-PPCI, treatment with fondaparinux should be restarted no earlier than 3h after sheath removal.
- *Patients undergoing CABG surgery*: fondaparinux should not be given during the 24h before surgery and may be restarted 48h post-operatively.
- *Treatment of adults with acute DVT and treatment of acute PE*: 7.5mg od SC (patients with body weight of ≥50 and ≤100kg). For patients

with body weight of <50kg, the recommended dose is 5mg; 10mg for patients with body weight of >100kg. Treatment should be continued for at least 5 days and until adequate oral anticoagulation is established (INR 2–3). Concomitant oral anticoagulation treatment should be initiated as soon as possible and usually within 72h. The average duration of administration is 7 days.

2. *Side effects*
   - Common: bleeding (GI, haematuria, haematoma, epistaxis, haemoptysis, utero-vaginal haemorrhage, haemarthrosis, ocular, bruises), purpura, anaemia, and thrombocytopenia. Epidural or spinal haematomas in patients given neuraxial anaesthesia or undergoing spinal punctures. The anticoagulant effect of fondaparinux may be reversed with recombinant factor VIIa.
   - Less common: GI disturbances (nausea, vomiting, dyspepsia), oedema, hepatic impairment, chest pain, dyspnoea, thrombocytopenia (but no HIT has been reported), rash, pruritus.
   - Rare: hypotension, flushing, cough, vertigo, dizziness, anxiety, drowsiness, confusion, headache, hypokalaemia, hyperbilirubinaemia, injection site reactions; also reported AF, tachycardia, and pyrexia.
   - Asymptomatic and reversible increases in AST/ALT levels of >3 times ULN are reported in up to 2.6% of patients.
3. *Interactions*
   - Concomitant use of oral anticoagulants, thrombolytics, heparins, and antiplatelets increases the risk of bleeding. If co-administration is essential, close monitoring is necessary.
   - Warfarin, platelet inhibitors (ASA), NSAIDs, and digoxin did not significantly affect the pharmacokinetics/pharmacodynamics of fondaparinux sodium.
4. *Cautions/notes*
   - Do not mix fondaparinux with other medications or solutions.
   - Fondaparinux should be used with caution in patients with an increased risk of haemorrhage: active GI ulcer disease; recent intracranial haemorrhage; brain, spinal, or ophthalmic surgery; spinal or epidural anaesthesia (risk of spinal haematoma); risk of catheter thrombus during PCI; low body weight; elderly patients; concomitant use of drugs that increase the risk of bleeding; hepatic impairment; renal impairment.
   - Fondaparinux should be used with caution in patients who have undergone recent surgery (<3 days) and only once surgical haemostasis has been established.
   - In patients receiving fondaparinux for treatment of VTE, rather than prophylaxis, spinal/epidural anaesthesia in cases of surgical procedures should not be used.
   - The risk of bleeding increases in patients with renal impairment. It is contraindicated in severe renal impairment.
   - Fondaparinux should be used with caution in patients with a history of HIT.
   - The needle shield of the pre-filled syringe contains dry natural latex rubber that has the potential to cause allergic reactions in latex-sensitive individuals.

- Fondaparinux can be used in patients with moderate hepatic impairment, although they present with a higher incidence of haemorrhage. Monitor for signs and symptoms of bleeding.
- The occurrence of major bleeding was doubled in patients with a body weight of <50kg.

5. *Pregnancy and lactation*
   - Animal studies have revealed harm to the fetus. However, there are no adequate studies in pregnant women (Pregnancy category B). It is not known whether this drug is excreted in human breast milk; caution should be exercised in nursing mothers.
6. *Contraindications*
   - Active clinically significant bleeding, impaired haemostasis.
   - Acute bacterial endocarditis.
   - Severe renal impairment (CrCl <30mL/min).
   - Patients with thrombocytopenia associated with a positive *in vitro* test for antiplatelet antibody in the presence of fondaparinux.
   - Hypersensitivity to the active substance or any of the excipients.

Furosemide

Loop diuretic (see ➔ Loop diuretics, pp. 645–50).

CV indications

- Furosemide is recommended when prompt diuresis is required, including oedema and/or ascites caused by cardiac or hepatic diseases, oedema caused by renal diseases (nephrotic syndrome), and pulmonary oedema (e.g. acute HF). It may be effective in patients unresponsive to thiazide diuretics.
- Acute pulmonary oedema/hypertensive crisis/increased intracranial pressure.
- Hyperkalaemia/hypermagnesaemia in advanced cardiac life support.

Mechanism of action

(See ➔ Loop diuretics, pp. 645–50.)

Pharmacodynamics

The onset of diuresis following PO administration is within 1.5h, with peak effects occurring within 1–2h. The duration of diuretic effects is 3–6h. By IV route, diuresis peak effects are observed within 15min.

Pharmacokinetics

Food reduces the absorption of furosemide; so it should be taken on an empty stomach. The elimination t½ is 0.5–2h (9h in ESRD). (See Table 8.1.5.)

Practical points

1. *Doses*
   - *Oedema*: 20–80mg PO od; not to exceed 600mg/day.
   - *HF*: 20–40mg, increased up to 40–240mg daily. In patients with new-onset acute HF or with chronic decompensated HF not receiving oral diuretics, the initial recommended dose is 20–40mg IV. For those on chronic diuretic therapy, the initial IV dose should be at least equivalent to the oral dose. Refractory CHF may necessitate larger doses.
   - *Hypertension*: 40–80mg bd. If the response is not satisfactory, add other antihypertensive agents.
   - *IV*: 20–40mg over 20min (increase in 20mg steps, if necessary, not less than every 2h; maximum dose 1.5g daily).
   - *Acute pulmonary oedema/hypertensive crisis/increased intracranial pressure*: 0.5–1mg/kg (or 40mg) IV over 1–2min; it may be increased to 80mg if there is no adequate response within 1h (not to exceed 160–200mg/dose).
   - *Hyperkalaemia in advanced cardiac life support*: 40–80mg IV.
   - *Hypermagnesaemia in advanced cardiac life support*: 20–40mg IV every 3–4h.
   - Dose selection for the elderly should be cautious, usually starting at low doses.

     —In patients with refractory HF and severe renal failure, furosemide (160–320mg) plus metolazone may be required to promote diuresis. When GFR is <20mL/min, high doses (up to 2g daily) may be needed because of reduced luminal excretion.

2. *Side effects* (see ➔ Loop diuretics, pp. 645–50)
   - Furosemide (like other sulfonamides) may precipitate photosensitive skin eruptions or may cause blood dyscrasias. A few patients on high-dose furosemide have developed severe hyperosmolar non-ketotic hyperglycaemic states.
3. *Interactions* (see ➔ Loop diuretics, pp. 645–50)
   - Furosemide may increase the ototoxicity of aminoglycoside antibiotics, especially in the presence of impaired renal function; avoid this combination.
   - In rheumatic patients treated with high doses of salicylates, furosemide may competitively inhibit the excretion of salicylates, increasing the risk of salicylate poisoning with tinnitus.
   - Phenytoin decreases intestinal absorption and interferes directly with the renal action of furosemide.
   - Methotrexate undergoes significant renal tubular secretion and may reduce the effect of furosemide.
   - Concomitant use of ciclosporin and furosemide decreases renal urate excretion and increases the risk of gouty arthritis.
4. *Cautions/notes* (see ➔ Loop diuretics, pp. 645–50)
5. *Pregnancy and lactation*
   - Furosemide crosses the placental barrier and is excreted in breast milk. Hence, it should be avoided in pregnancy and breastfeeding (Pregnancy category C).
6. *Contraindications* (see ➔ Loop diuretics, pp. 645–50)
   - Comatose or pre-comatose states associated with hepatic cirrhosis.

Gemfibrozil

Oral PPAR-α receptor agonist (see ➔ Fibrates, pp. 590–2).

CV indications

- Treatment of severe hypertriglyceridaemia with or without low HDL-C.
- Mixed hyperlipidaemia when statins are contraindicated or not tolerated.
- Primary hypercholesterolaemia when statins are contraindicated or not tolerated.
- Primary prevention: reduction of CV morbidity in males with increased non-HDL-C and at high risk for a first CV event when statins are contraindicated or not tolerated.

Pharmacodynamics

(See ➔ Fibrates, pp. 590–2.)

Gemfibrozil also inhibits synthesis of VLDL in the liver and increases the HDL2 and HDL3 sub-fractions, as well as Apo A1 and Apo A2.

Pharmacokinetics

Gemfibrozil undergoes conjugation to its acyl glucuronide, which is then oxidized via CYP2C8 to form successively hydroxymethyl and carboxyl metabolites (the main metabolite); approximately 70% of the dose is excreted in the urine, mainly as conjugates and its metabolites. (See Table 8.1.4.)

Practical points

1. *Doses*
   - 900–1200mg daily (30min before the evening meal). In patients with mild to moderate renal impairment (GFR >30mL/min/1.73m^2, respectively): starting dose of 900mg daily; assess renal function before increasing the dose. Contraindicated when GFR is <30mL/min.
2. *Side effects* (see ➔ Fibrates, pp. 590–2)
3. *Interactions* (see ➔ Fibrates, pp. 590–2)
   - Gemfibrozil inhibits CYP2C8, CYP2C9, CYP2C19, CYP1A2, UGTA1, and UGTA3, resulting in increased exposure of many medicinal products (see Table 8.1.2).
   - Gemfibrozil interferes with OATP1B1-mediated transport of statins into hepatocytes, which increases the plasma levels of statins. Gemfibrozil should be avoided in combination with lovastatin, pravastatin, and simvastatin, because it increases the risk of myopathy. Pitavastatin is unaffected by gemfibrozil.
   - Co-administration of gemfibrozil and colchicine may potentiate the development of myopathy, particularly in the elderly and in patients with renal impairment.
   - Combination with repaglinide increases the risk of hypoglycaemia and is contraindicated.
   - Gemfibrozil and its metabolite (gemfibrozil 1-*O*-β-glucuronide) are potent inhibitors of CYP2C8. This enzyme is important for the metabolism of dabrafenib, repaglinide, and dasabuvir; the combination of these drugs with gemfibrozil is contraindicated.

- Gemfibrozil increases exposure to rosiglitazone.
- Combination with bexarotene is not recommended, due to increases in plasma concentrations of bexarotene.
- Gemfibrozil potentiates VKA anticoagulants; monitor the INR.

4. *Cautions/notes*
   - Gemfibrozil should not be used in patients with type IIa hyperlipidaemia or with low HDL-C as their only lipid abnormality.
   - Hypoglycaemia has been reported with gemfibrozil, but not with bezafibrate and fenofibrate.
   - Patients with elevated TG levels should be closely monitored when treated with gemfibrozil, because it can produce a significant increase in LDL-C levels.
5. *Pregnancy and lactation* (see ➔ Fibrates, pp. 590–2)
6. *Contraindications* (see ➔ Fibrates, pp. 590–2)
   - Combination use of repaglinide or dasabuvir, repaglinide, or simvastatin.

Glucagon-like peptide 1 receptor agonists (GLP-1RAs)

Dulaglutide, exenatide, liraglutide, lixisenatide, semaglutide.

CV indications

- Adjunct to diet and exercise to improve glycaemic control in adults with T2DM: (a) as monotherapy, when metformin is considered inappropriate due to intolerance or contraindications, or (b) in addition to other medicinal products for the treatment of diabetes.
- Liraglutide to reduce the risk of major adverse cardiovascular events (cardiovascular death, non-fatal myocardial infarction, or non-fatal stroke) in adults with T2DM and established cardiovascular disease.
- Liraglutide as an adjunct to a reduced-calorie diet and increased physical activity for chronic weight management in adults with a BMI ≥30 (obesity) or adults with a BMI of ≥27 (overweight) who have at least one weight-related condition (e.g. hypertension, T2DM, dyslipidemia).

Mechanism of action

Native GLP-1 is a physiological hormone that binds to specific receptors (GLP-1R) expressed in pancreas, heart, vasculature, brain, immune system, and kidneys. However, GLP-1 has a half-life of 1.5–2min due to degradation by DPP-4.

Pharmacodynamics

GLP-1RAs selectively bind to and activate GLP-1 receptors (GLP-1R). In the presence of elevated glucose concentrations, GLP-1RAs increase intracellular cAMP in pancreatic beta cells, stimulate insulin secretion, and lower glucagon secretion decreasing hepatic glucose output, improve insulin sensitivity, and decrease HbA1C. They also delay gastric emptying in the early postprandial phase and reduce appetite, body weight, and body fat mass. GLP-1RAs have a beneficial effect on plasma lipids (decrease free fatty acid levels), reduce SBP, and in animal models slow the development of atherosclerosis by preventing aortic plaque progression and reducing inflammation in the plaque.

In cardiovascular outcome trials, liraglutide and semaglutide (but not exenatide or lixisenatide) reduced the relative risk of major cardiovascular events in patients with T2DM and increased cardiovascular risk. Liraglutide also reduced all-cause mortality in these patients.

Pharmacokinetics

These drugs are administered SC in abdomen, thigh, or upper arm; rotate injection site.

- Dulaglutide reaches peak plasma concentrations in 48h (bioavailability 65%) and steady-state plasma concentrations are achieved between 2 to 4 weeks of once-weekly administration. It presents a Vd of 0.25L/kg, is metabolized into its component amino acids by protein catabolism pathways, and presents a t½ of 4.6 days.

- Exenatide reaches peak plasma levels within 2h, presents a Vd of 0.4L/kg, and undergoes proteolytic degradation following glomerular filtration. Its t½ is 2.4h (immediate release) and 2 weeks (extended release).
- Liraglutide presents a bioavailability of 55% and reaches peak plasma levels within 8–12h. It binds to plasma proteins (>98%), presents a Vd of 0.07L/kg, and is metabolized by proteolytic degradation and eliminated in faeces and urine as inactive metabolites. It has a t½ of 13h.
- Lixisenatide reaches peak plasma levels after 1–3.5h. It binds to plasma proteins (55%), presents a Vd of 1.4L/kg, and is metabolized by proteolytic degradation. It has a t½ of 3h.
- Semaglutide presents a bioavailability of 89% and reaches peak plasma levels after 1–3 days. It binds to plasma proteins (>99%), presents a Vd of 12.5L/kg, and is metabolized by proteolytic cleavage of the peptide backbone and sequential beta-oxidation of the fatty acid side chain. It has a t½ of 1 week.

Practical points

1. *Doses*
   - Dulaglutide. Monotherapy: 0.75mg SC once weekly.
     Add-on-therapy: 1.5mg SC once weekly for inadequate glycaemic control. No dose adjustment required in the elderly or patients with hepatic or renal (eGFR < 90 to ≥ 15mL/min/1.73 m^2) impairment.
   - Exenatide (immediate release): 5mcg SC bd within 60min before morning and evening meals; after 1 month the dose can be increased to 10mcg SC bd based on clinical response. Severe renal impairment (CrCl <30mL/min) or ESRD: not recommended.
   - Exenatide QW: 2mg SC once weekly with or without meals.
   - Liraglutide: 0.6mg SC od for 1 week; then increase to 1.2mg od; if glycaemic control not acceptable, can increase dose to 1.8mg SC od. No dose adjustment is required for patients with mild, moderate, or severe renal impairment.
   - Lixisenatide: 10mcg SC od within 1h before the first meal of the day; on day 15 increase to 20mcg od. No dose adjustment is required for patients with mild or moderate renal impairment.
   - Semaglutide: 0.25mg SC once weekly for 4 weeks; then the dose can be increased to 0.5mg once weekly. After at least 4 weeks the dose can be increased to 1mg once weekly to further improve glycaemic control. No dose adjustment is required for patients with mild, moderate, or severe renal impairment.
2. *Adverse effects*
   - Very common: nausea, vomiting, diarrhoea, hypoglycaemia.
     Common: abdominal pain, dyspepsia, gastritis, eructation, flatulence, headache, acute event of gallbladder disease (cholelithiasis, cholecystitis), fatigue, decreased appetite, weight loss. Uncommon: injection-site reactions, sinus tachycardia, 1st degree AVB (dulaglutide).
   - Post-marketing reports: dehydration, pancreatitis (including fatal and non-fatal haemorrhagic or necrotizing pancreatitis), thyroid C-cell tumours (adenomas and/or carcinomas), serious hypersensitivity reactions (anaphylactic reactions and angioedema).

3. *Drug interactions*
   - The combination of GLP-1RAs with a sulfonylurea or insulin increases the risk of hypoglycaemia. Reduce the dose of sulfonylurea or insulin.
   - GLP-1RAs delay gastric emptying and have the potential to delay the absorption of concomitantly administered oral drugs (lisinopril, metoprolol). Oral medications that are particularly dependent on threshold concentrations for efficacy (antibiotics) or for which a delay in effect is undesirable (paracetamol) should be administered 1h before.
   - No drug interactions with atorvastatin, digoxin, lisinopril, metformin, oral contraceptives, paracetamol, or warfarin. In patients on warfarin or other coumarin derivatives, monitoring of INR is recommended.
4. *Cautions*
   - Not recommended as first-line therapy for patients inadequately controlled on diet and exercise.
   - Starting on lower doses and titrating slowly reduces the risk of nausea and other gastrointestinal effects. Correct volume depletion prior to treatment.
   - Some GLP-1RAs are supplied as single- or multi-dose pens; needle gauge requirements vary by product. Never share a pen between patients even if the needle is changed.
   - If pancreatitis is suspected, GLP-1RAs should be discontinued. If confirmed, they should not be restarted.
   - Patients with gastroparesis or severe gastroesophageal reflux disease because GLP-1RAs slow gastric emptying. Stop the treatment in patients with severe abdominal pain.
   - Patients treated with GLP-1RAs who experience gastrointestinal adverse reactions (nausea, vomiting, diarrhoea) can develop acute renal failure and worsening of chronic renal failure, which may sometimes require haemodialysis. Caution when initiating or escalating doses of GLP-1RAs in patients with renal impairment. Patients should be informed of the potential risk for worsening renal function.
   - Rapid improvement in glucose control has been associated with a temporary worsening of diabetic retinopathy in patients treated with semaglutide. Monitor patients with a history of diabetic retinopathy at baseline.
   - Inform patients of symptoms of thyroid tumours (e.g. a mass in the neck, dysphagia, dyspnoea, persistent hoarseness).
   - Because of the potentially immunogenic properties of protein and peptide pharmaceuticals, treated patients may develop anti-drug antibodies. With exenatide, if there is worsening glycaemic control or failure to achieve target glycaemic control, consider alternative antidiabetic therapy. A higher incidence of allergic reactions and injection site reactions occurred in antibody-positive patients.
5. *Pregnancy and lactation*
   - Limited data are available in pregnant women; no information regarding excretion in human milk. Use during pregnancy only if the potential benefit justifies the potential risk to the fetus.

6. *Contraindications*
    - Hypersensitivity to the active substance or any of the excipients.
    - History of anaphylaxis or angioedema to other GLP-1RAs.
    - Personal or family history of medullary thyroid carcinoma or multiple endocrine neoplasia syndrome type 2.
    - T1DM.
    - History of pancreatitis.
    - End-stage renal disease.

Glyceryl trinitrate (nitroglycerin, GTN)

Rapid and short-acting nitrate (see ➲ Nitrates, pp. 680–5).

CV indications

- Treatment and prophylaxis of angina pectoris and treatment of variant angina either alone or in combination with other anti-anginal therapy. Sublingual GTN is the standard to relieve angina pectoris.
- IV GTN for: (1) patients with unresponsive CHF, including that secondary to acute MI, provided there is no RV infarction; (2) patients with refractory unstable angina pectoris and coronary insufficiency, including Prinzmetal's angina; and (3) control of hypertensive episodes and/or myocardial ischaemia during and after cardiac surgery. For the induction of controlled hypotension for surgery.

Pharmacodynamics

(See ➲ Nitrates, pp. 680–5.)

Sublingual GTN can be used to prevent anginal attacks if taken a few minutes before activities known to possibly cause an attack (i.e. a meal, emotional stress, sexual activity, and in colder weather). An attack of angina that does not respond to short-acting GTN should be regarded as a possible MI.

IV GTN is the most appropriate preload-reducing agent, particularly in the early hours of acute MI when ischaemia may contribute to LV dysfunction. In acute pulmonary oedema, GTN relieves dyspnoea, reduces LV filling pressure, and increases CO. In ACS, IV GTN is very effective in the treatment of pain, but it should be continuously infused, under close haemodynamic monitoring to avoid a reduction of BP associated with tachycardia.

Pharmacokinetics

GTN is available for administration via sublingual, transdermal, PO, and IV routes. GTN is rapidly absorbed from mucous membranes, the skin, and the GI tract. When given orally, it undergoes extensive first-pass metabolism. It is metabolized in the liver by a reductase and largely by extrahepatic mechanisms (red blood cells and vascular wall) to 1,2- and 1,3-dinitroglycerols. Its Vd is 3L/kg, and its t½ is approximately 1–3min. Folllowing sublingual administration, its effects are usually present within 5–10min and persist for 20–30min; glyceryl trinitrate spray acts more rapidly. By IV route, the onset of action is 2–5min, with a duration of action of 5–10min.

Steady-state plasma concentrations of GTN are reached within about 2h after application of a patch and are maintained for the duration of wearing the system. Upon removal of the patch, the plasma concentration declines, with a t½ of 1h. (See Table 8.1.11.)

Practical points

1. *Doses*
   - *Sublingual*: 0.3–0.6mg (maximum dose 1.5mg). Peak levels at 2min and t½ of 7–10min. Take tablets in the sitting position (standing promotes light-headedness, especially just after rising from a recumbent or seated position) every 5min until the pain disappears (maximum 4–5 tablets). Sublingual GTN in repeated doses of 0.8–2.4mg every 5–10min can relieve dyspnoea within 15–20min, with a fall in LV filling pressure and a rise in CO.

Table 8.1.11 Pharmacokinetic properties of several anti-anginal drugs

Drug	F (%)	T_{max} (h)	PPB (%)	Vd (L/kg)	Metabolism	t½ (h)	Renal excretion* (%)
Glyceryl					Metabolized to 1,2 and 1,3-glyceryl		<1
trinitrate:	38	1–3min	60	3–3.3	dinitrate and glyceryl mononitrate	1–4min	
SL	70–85	10.5–1	60	3	via mitochondrial aldehyde	12–30	
PC	100	<1min	60	3	dehydrogenase-2	1–4min	
IV	–	2min	11–60	3			
Spray							
Isosorbide	20–25	1	0.7–2	–4	Metabolized to isosorbide	1–10	<1
dinitrate:	30–60		0.25–1		mononitrate glucuronide	30–50min	
Oral	33		–			–	
SL							
PC							
Isosorbide	90–100	1	<5	0.7	Metabolized to isosorbide	5.5–7	<5
mononitrate	77–80	1			mononitrate glucuronide		
ER							
Ivabradine	40	1	70	1.3	CYP3A4	Approximately 11	5
Nicorandil	Approximately 75	0.5–1	0.3–0.7	1	Hepatic denitration	1–1.7	<1
Ranolazine	30–50	2–5	62	2.3	CYP3A4	12 (6–22)	<5
Trimetazidine	100	2–3	20	4.8	Minimal	5–6.5	80

ER, extended release; F, oral bioavailability; h, hour; PC, percutaneous; PPB, protein plasma binding; t½, drug half-life; SL, sublingual; T_{max}, time to peak plasma levels; Vd, volume of distribution.

* Renal excretion without biotransformation.

- *Transdermal*: the onset of action of transdermal formulations is not sufficiently rapid to be useful in aborting an acute attack.
  —Patches: 0.1–0.8mg/h (patch on for 12h/off for 12h). Maximum dose 15mg in 24h.
  —Ointment: 2% cream, 15 × 15cm bd (6h intervals). Effects for 7h.
- Spray: one or two 400mcg/metered doses, sprayed under the tongue at the onset of angina or 2–3min before a provoking activity. Doses should be administered 5min apart and no more than three doses at once. Because of its rapid onset of action, it is indicated in patients with dry mouth.
- Buccal: 1–3mg tds (5mg in severe angina). Effects begin within minutes and last 3–5h.
- PO: 2.5–6.5mg bd/tds.
- IV: (1) unresponsive CHF: 10–200mcg/min under continuous monitoring of ECG, BP, heart rate, and CO. The infusion should be increased cautiously until the desired clinical response is achieved or up to 200mcg/min. (2) Management of severe hypertension: initial dose of 5mcg/min, which can be titrated to a maximum of 100mcg/min. (3) Refractory UA: an initial infusion rate of 10–15mcg/min; this may be increased cautiously in increments of 5–10mcg until relief of angina is achieved, headache prevents further increase in the dose, or the mean BP falls by >20mmHg.
- Use in surgery: initial infusion rate of 25mcg/min, which can be increased gradually until the desired systolic arterial pressure is attained. The usual dose is 25–200mcg/min.

2. *Side effects* (see ➲ Nitrates, pp. 680–5)
3. *Interactions* (see ➲ Nitrates, pp. 680–5)
   - GTN may slow the metabolism of morphine-like analgesics.
   - GTN activity decays when tablets are exposed to air, and opened containers should be discarded within 3 months; thus, GTN should be kept in airtight containers.
   - Patients should be carefully instructed about how to use short-acting sublingual GTN for acute relief of symptoms. When angina starts, the patient should rest sitting (standing promotes syncope; lying down enhances venous return and heart work) and take sublingual glyceryl trinitrate (0.3–0.6mg) every 5min until the pain goes or a maximum of 1.2mg has been taken within 15min. GTN should be placed under the tongue, but it should not be chewed or swallowed. Patients should be informed of the need to seek medical advice if chest pain persists after a total of three tablets in a 15-min period (or for 10–20min after resting) and/or is not relieved by sublingual nitrate. GTN spray acts more rapidly.
   - GTN may reduce the anticoagulant effect of heparin. The heparin dosage must be adjusted accordingly, while closely monitoring blood coagulation parameters. After discontinuation of GTN, it can be necessary to reduce the heparin dose.
   - In patients previously treated with organic nitrates, a higher dose of GTN may be necessary to achieve the desired haemodynamic effect.

4. *Cautions/notes* (see ➔ Nitrates, pp. 680–5)
   - Acute interruption of IV glyceryl trinitrate infusion in patients with UA is often associated with acute myocardial ischaemia. Transdermal GTN has been more clearly associated with rebound ischaemia than oral long-acting nitrate treatment.
   - The IV formulation contains propylene glycol that may react with heparin.
   - GTN can produce hypotension, accompanied by paradoxical bradycardia and increased angina pectoris. It should be used with caution in patients who may be volume-depleted or already hypotensive.
   - Because the hypotension associated with GTN overdose is due to venodilatation and hypovolaemia, therapy should be directed to increase central fluid volume.
   - Nitrate sprays are inflammable.
5. *Pregnancy and lactation* (see ➔ Nitrates, pp. 680–5)
6. *Contraindications* (see ➔ Nitrates, pp. 680–5)
   - Simultaneous administration of GTN with heparin.
   - Patients with possible increased intracranial pressure (e.g. cerebral haemorrhage or head trauma).

Glycoprotein IIb/IIIa receptor antagonists

(See ➔ Abciximab, pp. 416–17, ➔ Eptifibatide, pp. 580–1, and ➔ Tirofiban, p. 779.)

Indications

GPIIb/IIIa receptor antagonists, combined with aspirin and heparins (UFH/LMWH), are indicated in patients with ACS without ST-segment elevation at high risk of death or non-fatal MI, in whom intervention by PCI is likely or indicated.

Mechanism of action

GPIIb/IIIa receptor is a member of the integrin family of adhesion receptors and the major platelet surface receptor involved in platelet aggregation. On unstimulated platelets, GPIIb/IIIa is present in a closed conformation that prevents ligand binding. Upon platelet activation, the receptor undergoes conformational changes and several binding sites for fibrinogen and other ligands are exposed. Fibrinogen binding to activated GPIIb/IIIa mediates platelet aggregation by cross-linking adjacent platelets in response to multiple agonists. GPIIb/IIIa receptor antagonists bind to the intact GPIIb/IIIa receptor and inhibit the binding of fibrinogen to the GPIIb/IIIa (αIIbβ3) receptor on the surface of activated platelets. Antagonists of the platelet GPIIb/IIIa receptors have the advantage that they inhibit the final common pathway for platelet aggregation induced by thrombin, thromboxane A2, ADP, collagen, catecholamines, and shear stress.

Pharmacodynamics

In patients with UA/non-Q-wave MI, GPIIb/IIIa receptor antagonists significantly reduce the incidence of death from any cause or new MI within 30 days. Patients most likely to benefit from treatment are those at high risk of developing MI within the first 3–4 days after the onset of acute angina symptoms, including those who are likely to undergo early PCI. In patients undergoing non-urgent PCI with intracoronary stenting, GPIIb/IIIa receptor antagonists significantly reduced the incidence of primary endpoints (death, MI, urgent target vessel revascularization). They are not recommended in low- to moderate-risk patients or in those in whom a conservative approach is chosen.

Pharmacokinetics

(See ➔ Abciximab, pp. 416–17, ➔ Eptifibatide, pp. 580–1, and ➔ Tirofiban, p. 779.)

Practical points

1. *Common side effects*
   - Bleeding (major and minor bleeding, including femoral artery access, CABG-related, GI, genitourinary, retroperitoneal, intracranial, haematemesis, haematuria, oral/oropharyngeal, haemoglobin/haematocrit decreased, and other). The risk of bleeding increases in patients with severe renal disease; they should be more closely monitored. If serious uncontrolled bleeding occurs, GPIIb/IIIa receptor antagonists should be discontinued; in most patients,

bleeding time returns to normal within 12h. The majority of major bleeding reactions occurred at vascular access sites and increased as patient weight decreased. This relationship was most apparent for patients weighing <70kg. Anaemia.

- Thrombocytopenia (<100,000 cells/microlitre) is a potentially major side effect of GPIIb/IIIa receptor antagonists, associated with haemorrhagic complications, particularly in those with low initial platelet counts and in the elderly. Treatment involves close monitoring of platelets before and after drug administration and transfusion of platelets if significant decreases are observed.
- Hypotension, leg pain, puncture site pain, peripheral oedema, phlebitis, abdominal pain, nausea or vomiting, fever, headache, bradycardia, cardiac arrest, VT, VF, AF, AVB, and CHF. Allergic (anaphylactic) reactions.

2. *Cautions*
   - Increased risk of bleeding when co-administered with heparins, other anticoagulants, thrombolytics, antiplatelet agents, dextran solutions, prostacyclin, and NSAIDs.
   - Before infusion of GPIIb/IIIa receptor antagonists, the following laboratory tests should be performed to identify pre-existing haemostatic abnormalities: haematocrit or haemoglobin, platelet count, serum creatinine, and PT/aPTT. In patients undergoing PCI, the ACT should also be measured. Additional platelet counts should be taken 2–4h following the bolus dose and at 24h.
   - Unnecessary arterial and venous punctures, IM injections, routine use of urinary catheters, nasotracheal intubation, NG tubes, non-compressible sites (e.g. subclavian or jugular veins), and automatic BP cuffs should be avoided. Sodium chloride solution or heparin locks should be considered for blood-drawing. Vascular puncture sites should be documented and monitored.
   - If serious bleeding cannot be controlled by compression, GPIIb/IIIa receptor antagonists and heparin should be discontinued immediately.
   - In patients treated with prasugrel or ticagrelor, GPIIb/IIIa inhibitors should be limited to bailout situations or thrombotic complications during PCI.
   - Avoid GPIIb/IIIa inhibitors in patients in whom the coronary anatomy is not known.
3. *Pregnancy and lactation*
   - There are no adequate data in pregnant women, and it is not known whether GPIIb/IIIa receptor antagonists are excreted in breast milk. Thus, they should not be used during pregnancy or breastfeeding, unless clearly necessary (Pregnancy category C).
4. *Contraindications*
   - Hypersensitivity to the active substance or the excipients.
   - GI, genitourinary, or other active internal bleeding.
   - History of bleeding diathesis, pre-existing thrombocytopenia (<100,000 cells/mm^3).
   - History of CVA within 2 years or CVA with a significant residual neurological deficit.

- History of stroke within 30 days or any history of haemorrhagic stroke; known history of intracranial disease (neoplasm, arteriovenous malformation, aneurysm).
- Severe hypertension on antihypertensive therapy, hypertensive retinopathy.
- Recent intracranial or intraspinal surgery or severe trauma within past 2 months.
- History of vasculitis, acute pericarditis, and cirrhosis or other clinically significant liver disease.
- Use of IV dextran before PCI or intent to use it during an intervention.
- PT >3 times control or INR ≥1.5.
- Renal impairment (CrCl <30mL/min or <15mL/min for eptifibatide and tirofiban, respectively).
- Concomitant or planned administration of another parenteral GPIIb/IIIa inhibitor.

Heparin (unfractionated heparin, UFH)

UFH is a heterogenous mucopolysaccharide, generally used for acute anticoagulation.

CV indications

- Treatment of DVT, PE, UA, and acute peripheral arterial occlusion.
- Prophylaxis against DVT and PE.
- Prophylaxis of mural thrombosis following MI.
- Prevention of clotting in the extracorporeal circuit during haemodialysis.
- Maintain the patency of indwelling catheters/cannulae.

In the prophylaxis and treatment of DVT, SC heparin has been replaced by LMWH or fondaparinux.

Mechanism of action

UFH is a family of sulfated glucosaminoglycans (mucopolysaccharides) of 5–30kDa (mean 15kDa, approximately 45 monosaccharide chains). It binds to, and activates, ATIII through a high-affinity pentasaccharide, which is present on about one-third of heparin molecules. The heparin–ATIII complex inhibits a number of coagulation factors, including factors IIa (thrombin), Xa, IXa, XIa, and XIIa by binding to the active serine site. Heparin inhibits thrombin and factor Xa, but human thrombin is about 10-fold more sensitive to inhibition by the heparin–ATIII complex than factor Xa. To inhibit thrombin, UFH must bind to both ATIII via the pentasaccharide and to thrombin by its 13 additional saccharide units, but to inhibit factor Xa, it is sufficient that UFH binds to ATIII. Thus, molecules of heparin containing <18 saccharides do not bind simultaneously to thrombin and ATIII and are unable to catalyse thrombin inhibition. In contrast, very small heparin fragments containing the high-affinity pentasaccharide sequence catalyse the inhibition of factor Xa by ATIII. By inactivating thrombin, heparin prevents fibrin formation and inhibits thrombin-induced activation of factors V and VIII. UFH also prevents the formation of a stable fibrin clot by inhibiting the activation of the fibrin stabilizing factor.

UFH and LMWH also induce the secretion of the tissue factor pathway inhibitor by vascular endothelial cells and reduce the procoagulant activity of the tissue factor–factor VIIa complex, an effect that may contribute to their antithrombotic action.

UFH binds to platelets and endothelial cells, which may contribute to heparin-induced bleeding via a mechanism independent of its anticoagulant effect. Additionally, UFH inhibits the proliferation of vascular smooth muscle cells, suppresses osteoblast formation, and activates osteoclasts that promote bone loss.

Pharmacodynamics

UFH is an anticoagulant, with a rapid and short duration of action. The main advantages, as compared to LMWH, are that the anticoagulant effects rapidly disappear by stopping the IV infusion and can be reversed by protamine sulfate and it is safer in patients with renal failure.

Daily laboratory monitoring (ideally at the same time each day, starting 4–6h after initiation of treatment) is essential during full-dose heparin treatment. Doses should be adjusted to maintain an aPTT value of 1.5–2.5 times of the normal range or control value. In the cardiac catheterization laboratory, UFH is adjusted to maintain the ACT.

In acute MI, UFH is given together with thrombolysis or primary angioplasty. It should be used in the initial 24–48h to prevent further thrombin generation and reduce the risk of reocclusion. In patients with UA, dose-adjusted heparin added to aspirin helps to prevent MI.

Pharmacokinetics

UFH is not absorbed by oral administration and should be given by intermittent IV injection, IV infusion, or deep SC injection. Peak plasma levels are achieved immediately by IV route or after 2–4h following SC administration. UFH binds to a number of plasma proteins, endothelial cells, and macrophages, which reduces its anticoagulant activity at low concentrations; this explains the marked variability of the anticoagulant response to UFH among patients with thromboembolic disorders and the phenomenon of heparin resistance. Heparin clearance involves a rapid, saturable, dose-dependent mechanism (due to its binding to receptors on endothelial cells and macrophages where it is depolymerized) and a much slower first-order renal mechanism. At therapeutic doses, heparin is cleared predominantly through the rapid mechanism. As a result, the t½ of UFH increases from approximately 30min following an IV bolus of 25U/kg to 60min with a bolus of 100U/kg, and 150min with a bolus of 400U/kg. Thus, to obtain a rapid and persistent effect, UFH is given IV as a bolus, followed by a perfusion. The t½ increases in patients with renal or hepatic insufficiency. (See Table 8.1.1.)

Practical points

1. *Doses*
   - UFH is administered by continuous IV infusion in 5% glucose or 0.9% sodium chloride or by intermittent IV injection or by SC deep injection. Due to its short t½, administration by IV infusion is preferable to intermittent IV injections. A different site should be used for each injection to prevent the development of haematoma. The anticoagulant effect is delayed for approximately 1h, and peak plasma levels occur at approximately 3h.
   - *Prophylaxis of DVT and PE*: 5000U SC, followed by 5000U SC every 8–12h, for 7–10 days or until the patient is fully ambulant.
   - *Treatment of DVT, PE, UA, and acute peripheral arterial occlusion*: 60–70IU/kg IV bolus, up to 5000IU (10,000IU may be required in severe PE), followed by 12–15IU/kg/h by IV infusion (up to a maximum of 1000IU/h) or 5000–10,000IU every 4h by IV injection. Doses should be adjusted according to an aPTT of 1.5–2.5 times the control value. Higher aPTTs increase the risk of cerebral bleeding, without conferring any survival advantage. The infusion rate should be decreased by 50% if the aPTT is three times the control value. If the aPTT is <1.5 times the control value, the infusion should be increased by 25% to a maximum rate of 2500IU/h.
   - *Prophylaxis of mural thrombosis following MI*: 12,500IU 12-hourly SC for at least 10 days.
   - *NSTE-ACS*: in the PCI setting, UFH is given as an IV bolus either under ACT guidance (in the range of 250–350s, or 200–250s if a GPIIb/IIIa inhibitor is given) or in a weight-adjusted manner (usually 70–100IU/kg,

or 50–70IU/kg in combination with a GPIIb/IIIa inhibitor). UFH should be stopped after PCI, unless there is an established indication related to the procedure or patient's condition.

- *Haemodialysis and haemofiltration*: 1000–5000IU; then 1000–2000IU/h adjusted to maintain clotting time of >40min.
- *Cardiopulmonary bypass*: 300IU/kg IV, adjusted thereafter to maintain the ACT in the range of 400–500s.
- *To maintain the patency of indwelling IV lines*: 200IU should be administered into the catheter/cannula every 4–8h or as required.

2. *Side effects*
   - Haemorrhage is the main complication, and bleeding can occur at any site. When bleeding occurs, discontinuance of heparin and neutralization with protamine sulfate are advisable as a very slow infusion of a 1% solution (≤50mg in any 10-min period).
   - HIT and HITTS occur in 3–5% of patients treated with UFH for >5 days. There are two types of HIT: type I is an early-onset, mild, and reversible decline in platelet count due to the direct platelet-aggregating effect of heparin; type II occurs 2–5 days after the initial heparin exposure and is due to the formation of antibodies (of the IgG or IgM class) against heparin when it is bound to platelet factor 4, leading to irreversible aggregation of platelets. To reduce the risk of HIT, IV UFH should not be given for >48h and all patients receiving UFH should have platelet counts on day 1 and every 2 days during treatment. Thrombocytopenia can be accompanied by severe thromboembolic complications (skin necrosis, gangrene of the extremities that may lead to amputation, MI, PE, stroke, and possibly death). Patients with HIT should be treated with thrombin inhibitors (argatroban, bivalirudin, lepirudin), fondaparinux, or danaparoid and later with warfarin when the platelet count has recovered.
   - Injection site reactions: irritation, erythema, mild pain, haematoma, or ulceration may follow deep SC injection.
   - Rare: osteoporosis, skin necrosis, transient alopecia, rebound hyperlipaemia, priapism, and elevations of serum glutamic-oxaloacetic transaminase (SGOT) and serum glutamic-pyruvic transaminase (SGPT).
   - Heparin can suppress adrenal secretion of aldosterone, leading to hyperkalaemia, particularly in patients with diabetes mellitus, CKD, or pre-existing metabolic acidosis or those taking potassium-sparing drugs.
   - Heparin hypersensitivity reactions: fever, urticaria, rhinitis, angio-oedema, asthma, and anaphylactoid reactions; itching and burning, especially on the plantar side of the feet.
   - Heparin resistance, defined as an inadequate response to heparin at a standard dose, occurs in approximately 5–30% of patients. They may require much higher doses of heparin to achieve the desired effect. ATIII deficiency is very rare but can cause thrombophilia and heparin resistance.
3. *Interactions*
   - Increased risk of bleeding when co-administered with NSAIDs, dextrans, antiplatelet drugs, fibrinolytics, oral anticoagulants, thrombolytics, dipyridamole, alprostadil, iloprost, or any other drug

which may interfere with coagulation. These drugs should be co-administered under close clinical and laboratory monitoring.

- When heparin sodium is given with dicoumarol or warfarin sodium, a period of at least 5h after the last IV dose should elapse before blood is drawn to determine the PT.
- Some cephalosporins (cefaclor, cefixime, ceftriaxone) may increase the risk of haemorrhage when used concurrently with heparin.
- Increased risk of hyperkalaemia when combined with ACEIs, ARBs, or aliskiren.
- Epoetin, digitalis, tetracyclines, antihistamines, or IV glyceryl trinitrate may partially counteract the anticoagulant action of UFH; careful monitoring of the aPTT and adjustment of heparin dosage are recommended.
- Increased risk of hypoglycaemia when UFH is co-administered with sulfonylureas.
- UFH displaces benzodiazepines from plasma proteins and increases their effects (use lorazepam).
- The activity of UFH is reduced when combined with IV GTN infusion.
- Nicotine may partially counteract the anticoagulant effect of UFH. Increased heparin dosage may be required in smokers.

4. *Cautions/notes*
   - Periodic platelet counts, haematocrits, and tests for occult blood in stool are recommended during treatment with UFH. All patients receiving prolonged heparin of any sort should have platelet counts on day 1 and every 2–4 days.
   - The risk of bleeding increases with the dose, in the elderly, and in patients receiving other drugs that increase the risk of bleeding, those with hepatic or renal impairment, or sometimes with surgery, trauma, invasive procedures, or concomitant haemostatic defects.
   - The IM route should be avoided because of the frequent occurrence of haematoma at the injection site.
   - Heparin may prolong the PT, and when co-administered with an oral anticoagulant, a period of at least 5h after the last IV dose or 24h after the last SC dose should elapse before obtaining a valid blood sample to determine the PT. If a continuous IV heparin infusion is used, the PT can usually be measured at any time. To ensure continuous anticoagulation, full heparin therapy must continue for several days after the PT has reached the therapeutic range; heparin therapy may then be discontinued without tapering.
   - To reduce the risk of HIT, IV heparin should not be given for >48h. Thrombocytopenia should be monitored closely. If the count falls below 100,000/mm^3 or if recurrent thrombosis develops, heparin should be promptly discontinued and alternative anticoagulants considered, if needed.
   - Serum K^+ levels should be monitored before starting heparin therapy and regularly thereafter if treatment is prolonged beyond about 7 days.
   - When UFH is given after fibrinolytic therapy in patients with ACS, it should be discontinued immediately after PCI.

- UFH is incompatible with many injectable preparations, e.g. some antibiotics, reteplase, opioid analgesics, antihistamines, and 'many other drugs'. Dobutamine and UFH should not be mixed or infused through the same IV line, as this causes precipitation.
- Interference with diagnostic tests: UFH may be associated with pseudo-hypocalcaemia (in haemodialysis patients), artefactual increases in total thyroxine and triiodothyronine, and simulated metabolic acidosis and may interfere with the determination of aminoglycosides by immunoassays.

5. *Pregnancy and lactation*
   - UFH is used for the management of VTE during pregnancy because it does not cross the placenta (Pregnancy category C) and is not excreted in human milk. The high doses (20,000IU daily) needed to reduce the risk of thrombosed maternal valves may cause osteoporosis when used for >5 months. Alternatives are fondaparinux or LMWH (Pregnancy category B).
6. *Contraindications*
   - Patients who consume large amounts of alcohol, who are actively bleeding, and with haemophilia and other bleeding disorders.
   - Previous thrombocytopenia (including a history of HIT).
   - Severe hypertension.
   - Severe liver disease (including oesophageal varices).
   - During surgery of the brain, spinal cord, and eye, in procedures at sites where there is a risk of bleeding, in patients who have had recent surgery, and in patients undergoing lumbar puncture or regional anaesthetic block. After major trauma or recent surgery to the eye or nervous system.
   - Patients with an actual or potential bleeding site, e.g. hiatus hernia, peptic ulcer, neoplasm, bacterial endocarditis, retinopathy, bleeding haemorrhoids, suspected intracranial haemorrhage, cerebral thrombosis, or threatened abortion.
   - Hypersensitivity to heparin or LMWHs.
   - When blood coagulation tests cannot be performed at appropriate intervals.
   - The occurrence of skin necrosis in patients receiving heparin contraindicates further use of heparin because of the risk of thrombocytopenia.

Hydralazine

Direct peripheral vasodilator.

CV indications

- Treatment of moderate to severe hypertension (in conjunction with a β-blocker and a diuretic) and hypertensive crisis, particularly those associated with pre-eclampsia and toxaemia of pregnancy. Treatment of hypertension with renal complications.
- In patients with HF when hypertension persists despite treatment with a combination of an ACEI (or ARB), a β-blocker, an MRA, and a diuretic. In patients with high LV filling pressure, it is recommended to combine hydralazine with a nitrate (ISDN 20mg and hydralazine 37.5mg tds).

Mechanism of action

Hydralazine is a direct peripheral vasodilator, primarily of arteries and arterioles, as compared to veins. Its mechanism of action is uncertain, but it may be related to: (1) the inhibition of Ca^{2+} release from the SR of vascular smooth muscle cells induced by inositol triphosphate (IP3); (2) the opening of K^+ channels, which produces hyperpolarization of the membrane potential of vascular smooth muscle cells; and (3) the stimulation of NO release, leading to an increase in cellular cGMP levels. Hydralazine inhibits the generation of reactive oxygen species and may delay the appearance of nitrate tolerance.

Pharmacodynamics

Hydralazine decreases PVR and BP and induces a reflex sympathetic activation of the heart, increasing the heart rate, stroke volume, and CO. It also increases renin release and activates the RAAS, producing sodium and water retention. Hydralazine maintains or increases renal and cerebral blood flow. Hydralazine has been traditionally recommended as a treatment of choice in acute and severe hypertension in pregnancy, but is no longer the drug of choice as its use is associated with more perinatal adverse effects than other drugs.

Hydralazine and isosorbide dinitrate should be considered in self-identified black patients with LVEF ≤35% or with an LVEF <45% combined with a dilated LV in NYHA class III–IV despite treatment with an ACEI, a beta-blocker and an MRA to reduce the risk of HF hospitalization and death.

Hydralazine and isosorbide dinitrate may be considered in symptomatic patients with HFrEF who cannot tolerate either an ACEI or an ARB (or they are contraindicated) to reduce the risk of death. This recommendation is based on a study which recruited symptomatic HFrEF patients who received only digoxin and diuretics.

Pharmacokinetics

Oral hydralazine is rapidly and completely absorbed (bioavailability approximately 26–55%), reaching peak plasma levels after approximately 0.5–1.5h. It binds to plasma proteins (approximately 90%) and undergoes extensive hepatic metabolism, but it is subject to polymorphic acetylation, so that slow acetylators generally have higher drug plasma levels and require lower doses to control BP. Hydralazine is excreted mainly in the form of metabolites (90%) in the urine and also in bile. Plasma t½ is approximately 2–7h but increases up to 16h in severe renal failure and decreases to approximately 45min in rapid acetylators, which explains why they often respond inadequately, even to doses of 100mg.

Practical points

1. *Doses*
   - *Hypertension*: 25mg bd, titrated up to a dose of 200mg/day.
   - *HF*: treatment should always be initiated in hospital. Starting dose: 50mg bd; maintenance dose: 50mg four times daily.

Doses should not be increased beyond 100mg/day without checking the patient's acetylator status. In patients with reduced renal or hepatic function, the dose or interval of dosing should be adjusted, according to clinical response.

   - *IV*: 5–10mg by slow IV injection, to avoid precipitous decreases in BP with a critical reduction in cerebral or utero-placental perfusion; the dose can be repeated after 20–30min. A satisfactory response can be defined as a decrease in DBP to 90/100mmHg. Hydralazine may also be given by continuous IV infusion of 50–300mcg/min. Maintenance flow rates must be determined individually and are usually within the range of 50–150mcg/min.

2. *Side effects*
   - (>10%): tachycardia, palpitations, headache, anorexia, nausea, vomiting, diarrhoea.
   - Prolonged treatment (>6 months), especially where daily dose exceeds 100mg and in slow acetylators, may provoke an SLE-like syndrome acompanied by fever, urticaria, arthralgia, myalgia, and pericarditis that may be associated with an immune-complex glomerulonephritis.
   - CV: flushing, hypotension, angina symptoms, oedema. Neurological: dizziness, peripheral neuritis. Musculoskeletal: arthralgia, joint swelling, myalgia. Hypersensitivity: rash, urticaria, pruritus, vasculitis, eosinophilia, hepatitis.
3. *Interactions*
   - Hydralazine potentiates the effects of other antihypertensives, vasodilators, anaesthetics, tricyclic antidepressants, major tranquillizers, nitrates, and alcohol.
   - MAOIs should be used with caution in patients receiving hydralazine.
   - Propranolol may increase the bioavailability of hydralazine.
   - The hypotensive effect of hydralazine may be antagonized by oestrogens or NSAIDs.
   - Hydralazine decreases nitrate tolerance, probably via the inhibition of free radical formation.
4. *Cautions/notes*
   - Due to the possibility of causing a hyperdynamic state, hydralazine may precipitate/exacerbate angina and should be used with caution in patients with CAD; co-administration of a β-blocker should be considered. Patients with MI should not receive hydralazine until stabilization.

- Patients on hydralazine who undergo surgery may present hypotension; do not use adrenaline to correct hypotension because it enhances the cardiac-accelerating effects of hydralazine.
- Hydralazine should be gradually withdrawn.
- Dizziness is more frequent in elderly patients, can limit the ability to drive, and is increased by alcohol, exercise, and hot weather.
- Early detection and timely diagnosis of an SLE-like syndrome, with appropriate treatment, is of utmost importance to prevent more severe complications.

5. *Pregnancy and lactation*
   - It should be avoided before the third trimester but may be used in later pregnancy if there is no safer alternative or when the disease itself carries serious risks for mother or child (Pregnancy category C). It passes into breast milk, but there are no reports so far showing adverse effects on the infant.
6. *Contraindications*
   - Hypersensitivity to hydralazine or dihydralazine.
   - Idiopathic SLE and related diseases.
   - Severe tachycardia and high-output cardiac failure.
   - Isolated right HF secondary to pulmonary hypertension (cor pulmonale), CAD, and myocardial insufficiency due to mechanical obstruction (e.g. aortic or mitral stenosis or constructive pericarditis).
   - Dissecting aortic aneurysm.

Hydrochlorothiazide

Oral thiazide diuretic (see also ➔ Thiazide and related diuretics, pp. 768–73).

CV and other indications

- Treatment of all grades of essential hypertension.
- Treatment of oedema caused by HF, liver disease, CKD, corticosteroids, or nephrotic syndrome.

Pharmacodynamics

Hydrochlorothiazide (HCTZ) is the most widely used diuretic in the treatment of arterial hypertension.

Pharmacokinetics

Drug absorption is reduced in patients with CHF. Both plasma levels and the elimination t½ are prolonged in patients with CKD. (See Table 8.1.5.)

Practical points

1. *Doses*
   - *Hypertension*: 12.5–50mg od. At low doses (12.5mg), adverse metabolic and lipid effects are minimized or completely avoided. There are multiple preparations where HCTZ is combined with other antihypertensive drugs in fixed doses.
   - *Oedema*: 25–100mg daily. Many patients respond to administration on alternate days or on 3–5 days each week.
   - *HF*: 25mg od, increased up to 100–200mg/day.
2. *Side effects* (see ➔ Thiazide and related diuretics, pp. 768–73)
3. *Interactions* (see ➔ Thiazide and related diuretics, pp. 768–73)
4. *Cautions/notes* (see ➔ Thiazide and related diuretics, pp. 768–73)
5. *Pregnancy and lactation*
   - Pregnancy category C. HCTZ crosses the placenta and is excreted in breast milk.
6. *Contraindications* (see ➔ Thiazide and related diuretics, pp. 768–73)

Idarucizumab

Specific reversal agent for dabigatran.

Indications

In patients treated with dabigatran when reversal of the anticoagulant effects of dabigatran is needed:

- For emergency surgery/urgent procedures.
- In the event of life-threatening or uncontrolled bleeding.

Mechanism of action

Idarucizumab is a humanized monoclonal antibody fragment (Fab) that binds very rapidly and with a very high affinity to dabigatran (approximately 300-fold more potent than the binding affinity of dabigatran for thrombin) and its acyl glucuronide metabolites, neutralizing their anticoagulant effects.

Pharmacodynamics

The plasma concentrations of unbound dabigatran were reduced to below the lower limit of quantification immediately after the administration of 5g idarucizumab.

Pharmacokinetics

Following IV infusion, idarucizumab presents a limited extravascular distribution (Vd 0.12L/kg) and is degraded to small peptides or amino acids. It presents an initial t½ of 47min and a terminal t½ of 10.3h. Renal impairment decreases the total clearance and increases exposure to idarucizumab, but no dose adjustment is required in the elderly or in patients with hepatic or renal impairment.

Practical points

1. *Doses*
   - The recommended dose is 5g IV (2 × 2.5g/50mL). A second 5g dose may be considered in recurrence of clinically relevant bleeding, together with prolonged clotting times, if potential rebleeding would be life-threatening and prolonged clotting times are observed, or if patients require a second emergency surgery/urgent procedure and have elevated coagulation parameters. Dabigatran treatment can be reinitiated 24h after administration of idarucizumab, if the patient is stable and adequate haemostasis has been achieved.
2. *Side effects*
   - Hypokalaemia, constipation, delirium, pyrexia, pneumonia, and headache. Idarucizumab causes transient proteinuria as a physiological reaction to renal protein overflow after an IV bolus of 5g idarucizumab. The safety and effectiveness of repeat treatment with idarucizumab have not been established.
3. *Drug interactions*
   - No formal interaction clinical studies have been performed.

4. *Cautions*
   - Reversing dabigatran therapy exposes patients to the thrombotic risk of their underlying disease. To reduce this risk, resumption of anticoagulant therapy should be considered as soon as medically appropriate.
   - In a limited number of patients in the clinical programme, between 12 and 24h after administration of 5g idarucizumab, administration of an additional 5g dose may be considered.
   - If an anaphylactic reaction or other serious allergic reaction occurs, immediately discontinue drug administration.
   - Idarucizumab contains 4g sorbitol as an excipient. Administration of sorbitol in patients with hereditary fructose intolerance can cause serious adverse reactions, including hypoglycaemia, hypophosphataemia, metabolic acidosis, increase in uric acid levels, and acute liver failure.
5. *Pregnancy and lactation*
   - There are no data in pregnant women, and it is unknown whether idarucizumab is excreted in human milk.

Iloprost

A chemically stable prostacyclin analogue, available for IV, oral, or aerosol administration.

CV indications

Treatment of adult patients with primary PAH, classified as NYHA functional class III, to improve exercise capacity and symptoms.

Mechanism of action

(See ➔ Epoprostenol, pp. 577–9.)

Pharmacodynamics

Iloprost inhaled 6–9 times a day improves functional class and increases exercise capacity (mean of 36m), functional class, and symptoms. In patients already treated with bosentan, iloprost increases exercise capacity, as compared with placebo. Oral iloprost has not been assessed in PAH.

Pharmacokinetics

When administered via inhalation, it reaches peak plasma levels at the end of the inhalation session. It binds to plasma proteins (65%) and is extensively metabolized, so that no unchanged substance is eliminated. Drug concentrations decline rapidly (t½ of 10–30min), so that within 0.5–2h after the end of inhalation, iloprost is not detectable in the central compartment. Thus, it should be inhaled 6–9 times daily.

Practical points

1. *Doses*
   - Initial dose: 2.5–5mcg/inhalation 6–9 times per day (mean 30mg/day) delivered via the mouthpiece of a nebulizer, based on individual tolerability; reduce to 2.5mcg 6–9 times daily if higher doses are not tolerated. Iloprost elimination is reduced in patients with hepatic dysfunction (maximum 6 times per day). Patients with CrCL of ≤30mL/min were not investigated in clinical trials. The safety and efficacy in children aged up to 18 years have not been established.
2. *Side effects* (see ➔ Epoprostenol, pp. 577–9)
   - Other serious side effects: dyspnoea, rash, diarrhoea, vomiting, hypersensitivity. The nebulizer solution should not come into contact with the skin and eyes.
3. *Interactions* (see ➔ Epoprostenol, pp. 577–9)
4. *Cautions/notes*
   - Iloprost is not recommended in patients with unstable PAH and advanced HF.
   - Patients stabilized on one nebulizer should not switch to another nebulizer without supervision by the treating physician.
   - Monitor vital signs (BP) during initial treatment to decrease the risk for syncope; avoid eye and skin contact and oral ingestion.
   - Caution with hepatic impairment; initially 2.5mcg no more frequently than six times a day.
   - Iloprost contains small amounts of ethanol (<100mg per dose).

- Iloprost inhalation may cause bronchospasm, especially in patients with bronchial hyperactivity. Patients with acute pulmonary infections, COPD, and severe asthma should be carefully monitored.
- Following interruption of therapy, careful monitoring of the patient should be performed, because of the risk of rebound effect.

5. *Pregnancy and lactation*
   - Fetal risk has been revealed in studies in animals, but not established or not studied in humans; may be used if the benefits outweigh the risk to the fetus (Pregnancy category C).
6. *Contraindications* (see ➲ Epoprostenol, pp. 577–9)

Indapamide

Oral thiazide diuretic with direct vasodilator effects (see ➔ Thiazide and related diuretics, pp. 768–73).

CV and other indications

- Treatment of essential hypertension.

Mechanism of action

In addition to its diuretic effects, indapamide blocks L-type Ca^{2+} channels, increases the release of prostacyclin, and reduces vascular reactivity to noradrenaline; all these effects reduce PVR and BP. Regarding the regression of LVH, indapamide was better than enalapril.

Pharmacokinetics

(See Table 8.1.5.)

Practical points

1. *Doses*
   - For hypertension and HF: 1.25–2.5mg od increased to 2.5–5mg od.
2. *Side effects* (see ➔ Thiazide and related diuretics, pp. 768–73)
   - Indapamide appears to be more lipid-neutral than other thiazides, and the sustained-release preparation causes less hypokalaemia. Maculopapular rashes.
3. *Interactions* (see ➔ Thiazide and related diuretics, pp. 768–73)
   - The risk of hypokalaemia increases by mineralocorticoids and amphotericin.
   - Hypotensive effects may be increased by baclofen, imipramine-like antidepressants, and neuroleptics, and attenuated by corticosteroids.
   - Increased risk of lactic acidosis with metformin and of acute renal failure with iodinated contrast media.
4. *Cautions/notes* (see ➔ Thiazide and related diuretics, pp. 768–73)
   - Serum electrolytes should be monitored in the first week of treatment used with an ACEI.
   - Indapamide may give a positive reaction in doping tests.
5. *Pregnancy and lactation* (see ➔ Thiazide and related diuretics, pp. 768–73)
6. *Contraindications* (see ➔ Thiazide and related diuretics, pp. 768–73)
   - Known allergy to sulfonamides.
   - Severe hepatic failure, hepatic encephalopathy, or severe impairment of liver function.
   - Hypokalaemia.

Irbesartan

ARB (see ➲ Angiotensin II AT1 receptor blockers, pp. 456–8).

Indications

- Treatment of hypertension.
- Treatment of renal disease in hypertensive T2DM patients.

Pharmacodynamics

In hypertensive patients with T2DM, irbesartan slows the rate of progression of microalbuminuria to overt proteinuria and facilitates regression to normoalbuminuria, as compared with placebo. In hypertensive patients with established diabetic nephropathy, irbesartan significantly reduced the relative risk in the primary combined endpoint of doubling serum creatinine, ESRD, or all-cause mortality, compared with amlodipine or placebo.

Pharmacokinetics

(See Table 8.1.9.)

Practical points

1. *Doses*
   - 150–300mg od. A lower starting dose (75mg) should be considered in those >75 years or with volume depletion. No dosage adjustment is necessary in patients with impaired renal function or with mild to moderate hepatic impairment.
2. *Sidee effects* (see ➲ Angiotensin II AT1 receptor blockers, pp. 456–8)
3. *Interactions* (see ➲ Angiotensin II AT1 receptor blockers, pp. 456–8)
4. *Cautions/notes* (see ➲ Angiotensin II AT1 receptor blockers, pp. 456–8)
5. *Contraindications* (see ➲ Angiotensin II AT1 receptor blockers, pp. 456–8)
   - Irbesartan contains lactose. Avoid in patients with rare hereditary problems of galactose intolerance, Lapp lactase deficiency, or glucose–galactose malabsorption.

Isosorbide dinitrate

Long-acting nitrate (see also ➲ Nitrates, pp. 680–5).

CV indications

- Prophylaxis and treatment of angina pectoris.
- As an adjunctive treatment in the management of severe acute or chronic congestive cardiac failure.
- IV administration: (1) treatment of unresponsive LV failure, secondary to acute MI; (2) unresponsive LV failure of various aetiologies; (3) severe or unstable angina pectoris; and (4) to facilitate or prolong balloon inflation and to prevent or relieve coronary spasm during percutaneous transluminal coronary angioplasty.

Pharmacodynamics

ISDN (5mg sublingually) helps to abort anginal attacks for about 1h. The oral preparation is frequently given for the prophylaxis of angina. It increases exercise duration for 6–8h. In African-American patients with HF (NYHA classes III/IV), treament with ISDN and hydralazine (20mg and 37.5mg tds, respectively) reduces mortality (44%) and hospitalizations (39%), compared with placebo.

Pharmacokinetics

ISDN is available in several formulations (sublingual spray, immediate- and modified-release tablets, IV). Absorption of ISDN after PO administration is near complete, but bioavailability is highly variable (mean 25%) due to extensive first-pass metabolism. ISDN reaches peak plasma levels within 1h, presents a Vd of approximately 2–4L/kg, and is metabolized predominantly in the liver to two active metabolites isosorbide mononitrate (ISMN) (75–85%) and 2-nitrate; it also undergoes extrahepatic metabolism. Only traces of the unchanged drug are eliminated in the urine. It has a t½ of approximately 1h.

Practical points

1. *Doses*
    - *Sublingual*: 2.5–15mg. Because ISDN requires hepatic conversion to the mononitrate, the onset of its effect is slower than with GTN, but its anti-anginal effect persists for 1h or longer. Thus, ISDN should be used only if the patient is unresponsive or intolerant to GTN.
    - *PO*: 30–120mg tds (in divided doses); for angina, maximum dose 240mg/day. Extended-release formulation: eccentric 40mg bd (in the morning and 7h later) are often used to avoid tolerance. In CHF: 40–240mg daily in divided doses.
    - *IV*: start with 1mg/h, increase up to 10mg/h. Higher doses (up to 20mg/h) may be required in UA.
    - *Intracoronary administration*: 1mg given as a bolus injection prior to balloon inflation. Additional doses may be given, not exceeding 5mg over 30min.
    - *Spray*: 1.25mg/metered dose with 1–3 doses given under the tongue, 30s apart; onset of effects: 1–3min. It may also be administered as a chewable tablet as a single 5mg dose; effects last for up to 2.5h.
    - *Transdermal*: 100mg daily as an ointment.

2. *Side effects* (see ➔ Nitrates, pp. 680–5)
3. *Interactions* (see ➔ Nitrates, pp. 680–5)
4. *Cautions/notes* (see ➔ Nitrates, pp. 680–5)
5. *Contraindications* (see ➔ Nitrates, pp. 680–5)
   - In patients who are allergic to the drug or to the adhesives used in glyceryl trinitrate patches.
   - Treatment of cardiogenic shock with ISDN 0.1% should only be undertaken if means of maintaining an adequate DBP are available.

Isosorbide mononitrate

Long-acting nitrate (see also ➲ Nitrates, pp. 680–5).

CV indications

- Prophylactic treatment of angina pectoris.
- As adjunctive therapy in CHF not responding to cardiac glycosides or diuretics.

Pharmacokinetics

ISMN is completely absorbed after PO administration but does not undergo first-pass metabolism, and so it has predictable clinical effects, with minimal intra- and inter-individual variation in plasma levels. ISMN is <5% protein-bound and presents a Vd of approximately 0.6L/kg. Elimination is primarily by denitration and conjugation in the liver and excretion of metabolites mainly in the urine, and the elimination t½ is approximately 5h. Hepatic and renal impairment do not appear to significantly affect the pharmacokinetics of ISMN.

Practical points

1. *Doses*
   - *PO*: 10mg bd as initial starting dose (increasing to a maximum dose of 120mg/day in divided doses) in an eccentric dose (doses spaced by 7h: 8 a.m. and 3 p.m.). Prolonged-release formulation: 40–60mg od, titrated to 90–120mg od; efficacy up to 12–14h. Dose varies with the manufacturer.
   - *IV*: 1mg/h; increase up to 10mg/h.
2. *Side effects* (see ➲ Nitrates, pp. 680–5)
3. *Interactions* (see ➲ Nitrates, pp. 680–5)
4. *Cautions* (see ➲ Nitrates, pp. 680–5)
5. *Contraindications* (see ➲ Nitrates, pp. 680–5)

Ivabradine

Selectively inhibits the pacemaker hyperpolarization-activated current I_f

Indications

- Symptomatic treatment of chronic stable angina pectoris in adults with normal sinus rhythm and heart rate of ≥70bpm who are unable to tolerate, or with a contraindication to the use of, β-blockers or in combination with β-blockers in patients inadequately controlled with an optimal β-blocker dose.
- In chronic HFrEF (NYHA classes II–IV) in sinus rhythm with a resting heart rate of ≥75bpm, in combination with standard therapy including β-blocker therapy or β-blocker therapy is contraindicated or not tolerated.

Mechanism of action

The hyperpolarization-activated, cyclic nucleotide-gated non-selective cation (HCN) channels carry the pacemaker current I_f, a mixed Na^+–K^+ inward current modulated by the autonomic nervous system, which regulates the rate of the slow diastolic depolarization in the SA node. Ivabradine selectively inhibits I_f and reduces the heart rate in a dose- and frequency-dependent manner; this effect is greater at faster heart rates, which limits the risks of symptomatic bradycardia. Thus, it diminishes the symptoms of angina by reducing MVO_2 and increasing the diastolic time when coronary perfusion takes place.

Pharmacodynamics

Ivabradine reduces resting and exercise heart rate by approximately 10bpm, so there is less risk of severe SA node depression than with β-blockers. Its anti-anginal potency is similar to that of atenolol or amlodipine, However, ivabradine has no effect on BP, AV nodal conduction, PR, QRS and QTc intervals, cardiac conduction, and contractility or ventricular repolarization. There is no risk of rebound angina on cessation of therapy.

Pharmacokinetics

It is rapidly and almost completely absorbed after oral administration, but its bioavailability is approximately 40% due to first-pass effect in the gut and liver. Food increased drug exposure by 20–30%, so that it should be administered during meals. (See Table 8.1.11.)

Practical points

1. *Doses*
   - *Chronic stable angina*: 5mg bd (starting dose), which can be increased to 7.5mg bd. It is advisable to use a lower starting dose in the elderly. The dose should be downtitrated with a resting heart rate of <50bpm or if symptoms of bradycardia (dizziness, fatigue, hypotension) persist, or increased to 7.5mg bd if resting heart rate is persistently >60bpm.
   - A lower starting dose should be considered for elderly patients. No dose adjustment is required in patients with CrCl of >15mL/min or mild hepatic impairment.

2. *Common side effects*
   - (>10%): flashing lights (phosphenes) that could impair driving at night; usually disappear with continued use.
   - (1–10%): first-degree AVB, bradycardia, ventricular extrasystoles, AF. Nausea, headaches, dizziness, blurred vision, eosinophilia, and hyperuricaemia. The risk of severe sinus node depression is less with ivabradine than with β-blockers.
3. *Interactions*
   - Concomitant use of potent CYP3A4 inhibitors/inducers increases/decreases ivabradine plasma levels (see Table 8.1.2); these combinations should be avoided.
   - The risk of bradycardia increases when ivabradine is given in combination with β-blockers, verapamil, or diltiazem.
   - Concomitant use of QT-prolonging drugs with ivabradine should be avoided since QT prolongation may be exacerbated by heart rate reduction.
   - There are no interactions with PPIs (omeprazole, lansoprazole), ACEIs, ARBs, sildenafil, statins, dihydropyridine CCBs, digoxin, warfarin, and aspirin.
4. *Cautions/notes*
   - ECG monitoring should be considered before initiation of treatment and when titration should be considered.
   - Ivabradine is not recommended in patients with AF or arrhythmias that interfere with sinus node function.
   - Ivabradine should be administered with caution in patients with mild hepatic impairment and retinitis pigmentosa, and, due to limited amount of data, in patients with chronic HF (NYHA class IV).
   - Chronic HF patients with intraventricular conduction defects (RBBB or LBBB) and ventricular dyssynchrony should be monitored closely.
   - Tablets contain lactose; avoid ivabradine in patients with rare hereditary problems of galactose intolerance, Lapp lactase deficiency, or glucose–galactose malabsorption.
5. *Pregnancy and lactation*
   - Women of childbearing potential should use appropriate contraceptive measures during treatment (Pregnancy category C). In animal studies, ivabradine is excreted in milk; avoid during breastfeeding.
6. *Contraindications*
   - Resting heart rate <70bpm prior to treatment.
   - Sick sinus syndrome, SA block, third-degree and SA heart block; AF.
   - Acute MI, UA.
   - Unstable or acute HF.
   - Cardiogenic shock.
   - Severe hepatic impairment.
   - Severe hypotension (<90/50mmHg).
   - Combination with potent CYP3A4 inhibitors.
   - Women of childbearing potential not using appropriate contraceptive measures.

Labetalol

Labetalol combines both competitive α1-adrenergic and non-selective, competitive β1- and β2-adrenergic blocking activity (see also ➔ Beta-adrenergic blocking agents, pp. 485–94).

CV indications

- Severe hypertension, including hypertension in pregnancy, when rapid control of BP is needed.
- Anaesthesia when a hypotensive technique is indicated.
- Hypertensive episodes following acute MI.

Pharmacokinetics

Oral bioavailability increases with food. After a bolus injection, maximum effect usually occurs within 5min. Elimination appears reduced in the elderly. (See Table 8.1.8.)

Practical points

1. *Doses*
   - *PO*: initial dose 100mg bd; maintenance dose 200–400mg bd. Patients with severe hypertension may require from 1200 to 2400mg per day, with or without thiazide diuretics. A reduced initial dose (50mg bd) is recommended in the elderly.
   - *IV*: 50mg bolus; doses may be repeated at 5-min intervals until a satisfactory response occurs (maximum dose 200mg).
2. *Side effects* (see ➔ Beta-adrenergic blocking agents, pp. 485–94)
3. *Interactions* (see ➔ Beta-adrenergic blocking agents, pp. 485–94)
4. *Cautions/notes* (see ➔ Beta-adrenergic blocking agents, pp. 485–94)
5. *Pregnancy and lactation*
   - Labetalol crosses the placental barrier, and perinatal and neonatal distress (bradycardia, hypotension, respiratory depression, hypoglycaemia, hypothermia) has been rarely reported; sometimes these symptoms have developed a day or two after birth (Pregnancy category C). Labetalol is excreted in breast milk; breastfeeding is therefore not recommended.

4. *Contraindications*(see ➔ Beta-adrenergic blocking agents, pp. 485–94)

Lacidipine

Dihydropyridine L-type CCB (see ➲ Calcium channel blockers, pp. 504–9).

Indications

- Treatment of hypertension, alone or in combination with other antihypertensive agents, including β-adrenoceptor antagonists, diuretics, and ACEIs.

Mechanism of action

(See ➲ Calcium channel blockers, pp. 504–9).

Pharmacodynamics

Lacidipine was superior to atenolol in restraining carotid atherosclerosis and limiting the development of new MetS. In patients with a renal transplant, lacidipine prevents an acute decrease in renal plasma flow and GFR after administering oral ciclosporin.

Pharmacokinetics

(See Table 8.1.6.)

Practical points

1. *Doses*
   - 2–6mg daily. In patients with hepatic impairment, its oral bioavailability and hypotensive effects increase; monitor BP. No dose modification is needed in patients with kidney disease.
2. *Side effects* (see ➲ Calcium channel blockers, pp. 504–9)
3. *Interactions* (see ➲ Calcium channel blockers, pp. 504–9)
4. *Cautions/notes* (see ➲ Calcium channel blockers, pp. 504–9)
5. *Contraindications* (see ➲ Calcium channel blockers, pp. 504–9)

Lercanidipine

Dihydropyridine L-type CCB (see ➔ Calcium channel blockers, pp. 504–9).

CV indications

- Treatment of hypertension.

Pharmacokinetics

Its oral bioavailability increases 4-fold when ingested up to 2h after a high-fat meal and is reduced to one-third when administered under fasting conditions; accordingly, lercanidipine should be taken before meals. Despite its short pharmacokinetic plasma t½ (2–5h), the antihypertensive effect of lercanidipine lasts for 24h due to its high membrane partition coefficient. (See Table 8.1.6.)

Practical points

1. *Doses*
   - 10mg od at least 15min before meals. Dose titration to 20mg, if needed.
   - Mild to moderate renal or hepatic dysfunction: the dose of 20mg od should be approached with caution. Care should be exercised when initiating treatment in the elderly.
2. *Side effects* (see ➔ Calcium channel blockers, pp. 504–9)
3. *Interactions* (see ➔ Calcium channel blockers, pp. 504–9)
4. *Cautions/notes*
   - The tablet contains 30mg lactose; caution in patients with Lapp lactase insufficiency, galactosaemia, or glucose–galactose malabsorption syndrome.
5. *Contraindications* (see ➔ Calcium channel blockers, pp. 504–9)
   - Severe renal (GFR <30mL/min) or hepatic impairment.
   - Co-administration with strong CYP3A4 inhibitors or ciclosporin.

Levosimendan

Calcium sensitizer of cardiac contractile proteins.

Indications

- Treatment of hospitalized patients with acutely decompensated CHF.

Mechanism of action

Levosimendan binds to cardiac troponin C (TnC) in a Ca^{2+}-dependent manner, stabilizes the conformation of the Ca^{2+}–TnC complex, and increases the binding affinity of TnC for intracellular Ca^{2+}. Thus, levosimendan increases cardiac contractility without increasing $[Ca^{2+}]_i$ or impairing diastolic relaxation. Levosimendan also activates ATP-sensitive K^+ (K_{ATP}) channels in vascular smooth muscle cells and produces systemic and pulmonary vasodilatation, which may promote reflex tachycardia. The combined inotropic and vasodilatory actions increase CO and decreases preload and afterload. The opening of mitochondrial cardiac K_{ATP} channels causes a cardioprotective effect under ischaemic conditions.

Pharmacodynamics

Levosimendan dose-dependently increases CO, stroke volume, and heart rate and decreases PCWP, mean BP, mean PAP, mean right atrial pressure, and total PVR. There is no tolerance to its effects, even with a prolonged infusion of up to 48h. Its haemodynamic effects are maintained up to 7–9 days after stopping the infusion, due to the formation of the active metabolite OR-1896.

Phamacokinetics

IV levosimendan is completely metabolized, and only trace amounts of the unchanged drug are excreted in the urine and faeces. Two metabolites are detected in plasma—OR-1855 and OR-1896. OR-1896 exhibits haemodynamic and pharmacologic properties similar to those of levosimendan. The elimination t½ of levosimendan is approximately 1h, while the mean elimination t½ of OR-1896 is approximately 80h and its plasma protein binding is about 40%. Age, gender, or renal function have no effect on the pharmacokinetics of levosimendan. However, the elimination of OR-1896 is prolonged 1.5-fold in patients with severe renal impairment or undergoing haemodialysis and in patients with moderate hepatic impairment.

Practical points

1. *Doses*
   - IV bolus of 12mcg/kg over 10min (optional); then 0.1mcg/kg/min, which can be decreased to 0.05 or increased to 0.2mcg/kg/min. The drug is diluted with glucose 5% solution before infusion. Furosemide, digoxin, and GTN can be given simultaneously in connected IV lines.
2. *Side effects*
   - The commonest are: headache, hypotension, arrhythmias (AF, extrasystoles, atrial and ventricular tachycardia), insomnia, dizziness, myocardial ischaemia, hypokalaemia, nausea, diarrhoea, vomiting, and haemoglobin decrease.

3. *Interactions*
   - Levosimendan must be given with caution with other vasoactive drugs due to the risk of hypotension.
   - There are no interactions between levosimendan and digoxin, itraconazole, warfarin, captopril, ISMN, felodipine, carvedilol, or alcohol.
4. *Cautions*
   - Levosimendan is preferable over dobutamine to reverse the effect of β-blockade if β-blockade contributes to hypotension and subsequent hypoperfusion. Because levosimendan is a vasodilator, it is not suitable for patients with hypotension or cardiogenic shock, unless in combination with other inotropes or vasopressors.
5. *Pregnancy and lactation*
   - There is no experience of using levosimendan in pregnant women (Pregnancy Category C). In rats, levosimendan is excreted in breast milk.
6. *Contraindications*
   - Hypersensitivity to levosimendan or any of the excipients.
   - Severe renal impairment (CrCl <30mL/min), severe hepatic impairment.
   - Significant mechanical obstructions affecting ventricular filling and/or outflow.
   - Severe hypotension.
   - Tachycardia.
   - History of TdP.

Lidocaine

Na^+ channel blocker with class 1B antiarrhythmic properties.

Indications

- Acute management of haemodynamically compromising ventricular arrhythmias, particularly those associated with myocardial ischaemia, acute MI, cardiac surgery, cardiac catheterization, or general anaesthesia. IV lidocaine may be considered for the treatment of recurrent sustained VT or VF not responding to β-blockers or amiodarone or in the presence of contraindications to amiodarone.
- Ventricular arrhythmias induced by digitalis, phenothiazines, or tricyclic antidepressants.
- Other indications: local anaesthesia.

Mechanism of action

Lidocaine binds preferentially to the inactivated state of Na^+ channels, with rapid onset–offset kinetics, and therefore, it acts selectively on ischaemic depolarized tissues where it promotes conduction block and suppresses re-entry circuits. Lidocaine is more effective in the presence of hyperkalaemia; thus, hypokalaemia must be corrected for maximum efficacy. Lidocaine also reduces automaticity by decreasing the slope of phase 4, via a mechanism unrelated to its action on fast voltage-gated Na^+ channels.

Lidocaine also shortens the duration of the action potential (does not produce QT prolongation) and effective refractory period (ERP) in ventricular tissues, possibly through an inhibitory effect of the late Na^+ current. The shortening is more marked in the Purkinje fibres than in the ventricular muscle, so that lidocaine reduces the dispersion of ventricular refractoriness and the re-entry of cardiac impulses.

Pharmacodynamics

Lidocaine does not prolong ventricular depolarization (QRS complex) or repolarization (QT intervals), heart rate and contractility (even in patients with CHF), AV conduction, and BP. It does not offer a greater benefit than either procainamide or sotalol in teminating VT in the absence of MI. Prophylactic use of lidocaine reduces VF by one-third but may increase mortality by approximately the same percentage.

Pharmacokinetics

Following an IV loading dose, lidocaine is rapidly distributed to all body tissues, so that a subsequent infusion or repeated doses should be administered to maintain therapeutic blood levels. About 65% is bound to the α1-acid glycoprotein and crosses the blood–brain and placental barriers, and 80% of the dose is metabolized rapidly in the liver via CYP1A2 (and, to a minor extent, CYP3A4) to active metabolites (monoethyl glycinexylidide and glycinexylidide), so that <10% is found unchanged in the urine. Therapeutic plasma levels are 1.5–6mcg/mL. At higher doses, there is an increase in CNS adverse effects. (See Table 8.1.3.)

Practical points

1. *Doses*
   - Initial IV loading dose: 50–100mg IV bolus once over 2–3min under ECG monitoring; the dose can be repeated after 5min, if necessary (do not exceed 300mg in a 1-h period). Then 1–4mg/min continuous IV infusion. As soon as possible, patients should be changed to an oral antiarrhythmic agent for maintenance therapy.
2. *Common side effects*
   - CV: hypotension, CV collapse, bradycardia which may lead to cardiac arrest, and arrhythmias. SA arrest when co-administered with other drugs that potentially depress nodal function.
   - CNS: nausea, light-headedness, drowsiness, speech disturbances, dizziness, tremor, nervousness, euphoria, tinnitus, blurred or double vision, nystagmus, vomiting, numbness, twitching, tremors, paraesthesiae, convulsions, unconsciousness, respiratory depression and arrest. Severe reactions may be preceded by somnolence and paraesthesiae.
   - Hypersensitivity reactions (e.g. skin lesions, urticaria, oedema, anaphylactoid reactions). Local ischaemia, tissue injury, and ulceration.
3. *Interactions*
   - Propranolol, metoprolol, halothane, amiodarone, and cimetidine reduce the hepatic clearance of lidocaine, so that the dose should be reduced by 50%.
   - The cardiac depressant effects of lidocaine are additive to those of other AADs. The risk increases when combined with β-blockers that reduce liver blood flow.
   - Lidocaine prolongs the action of suxamethonium.
4. *Cautions/notes*
   - Hepatic clearance of lidocaine is slowed when the hepatic blood flow decreases, i.e. the elderly, patients with severe HF, cardiogenic shock, or severe hepatic disease, or those treated with non-selective β-blockers or cimetidine. Reduce the doses of lidocaine.
   - Constant ECG monitoring is necessary during IV administration. Resuscitative equipment should be immediately available for the management of severe adverse CV, respiratory, or CNS effects. Hypokalaemia, hypoxia, and disorders of acid–base balance should be corrected before treatment with lidocaine begins.
   - Discontinue infusion if signs of excessive cardiac depression occur (e.g. prolongation of PR interval and QRS complex, appearance or aggravation of arrhythmias).
   - Lidocaine should not be given prophylactically, only against serious ventricular arrhythmias.
   - Lidocaine should be used with caution in patients with epilepsy, liver disease, CHF, severe renal disease, marked hypoxia, severe respiratory depression, hypovolaemia, or shock.
   - With CYP inducers (phenytoin, rifampin/rifampicin), the dose of lidocaine needs to be increased.
   - Lidocaine has no value in treating supraventricular tachyarrhythmias.

5. *Pregnancy and lactation*
   - Safety has not been established in women during pregnancy (Pregnancy category B). Lidocaine is excreted in breast milk and may produce fetal acidosis, respiratory depression, apnoea, and bradycardia in children, and so it should be used with caution in breastfeeding.
6. *Contraindications*
   - Known hypersensitivity to local anaesthetics of the amide type or to other drugs.
   - Adams–Stokes syndrome, severe degrees of SA, AV, or intraventricular heart block (unless a functioning pacemaker is present).

Lisinopril

Orally active ACEI (see ➔ Angiotensin-converting enzyme inhibitors, pp. 459–64).

Indications

- Treatment of hypertension.
- Treatment of symptomatic HF.
- Short-term (6 weeks) treatment of haemodynamically stable patients within 24h of acute MI.
- Treatment of renal disease in hypertensive patients with T2DM and incipient nephropathy.

Pharmacokinetics

Oral bioavailability (approximately 25%) and reduced to 16% in HF, but it is not affected by food. Lisinopril is not a prodrug and can be removed by dialysis. Excretion is reduced in patients with severe renal impairment (CrCl <30mL/min) when there is a 4.5-fold increase in the AUC. (See Table 8.1.10.)

Practical points

1. *Doses*
    - *Hypertension*: 10mg initially (titrated to a maximum of 80mg od). For patients with renovascular hypertension, salt and/or volume depletion, or cardiac decompensation, reduce the starting dose to 2.5–5mg od.
    - *HF*: 2.5mg od (increased in intervals of ≤10mg/2 weeks to maximum of 35mg od, if tolerated).
    - *Acute MI*: start within 24h if SBP >120mmHg with 5mg od (day 1), 5g (day 2), and 10mg maintenance (day 3 onwards), as tolerated. Start at 2.5mg if SBP <120mmHg, and avoid if SBP <100mmHg.
    - *Diabetic nephropathy*: 2.5mg od initially to usual dose of 10–20mg od.
    - Starting doses should be reduced in patients with renal impairment: 5–10mg in those with CrCl of 30–80mL/h; 2.5–5mg with CrCl of <30mL/h; and 2.5mg with CrCl of <10mL/h (including patients on dialysis).
2. *Common side effects* (see ➔ Angiotensin-converting enzyme inhibitors, pp. 459–64)
3. *Interactions* (see ➔ Angiotensin-converting enzyme inhibitors, pp. 459–64)
4. *Cautions/notes* (see ➔ Angiotensin-converting enzyme inhibitors, pp. 459–64)
5. *Contraindications* (see ➔ Angiotensin-converting enzyme inhibitors, pp. 459–64)

Loop diuretics

(See Furosemide, pp. 601–2, Bumetanide, p. 503, and Torasemide, p. 782.)

CV indications

- Chronic HF: diuretics are recommended to improve symptoms and exercise capacity and reduce the risk of HF hospitalization in patients with signs and/or symptoms of congestion.
- Acute HF.
- Treatment of cardiac, pulmonary, hepatic, renal, and peripheral oedema.
- Treatment of mild to moderate hypertension.

Mechanism of action

Loop diuretics reach their luminal site of action after being actively secreted via an organic acid transport mechanism in the proximal tubule. They reversibly inhibit the Na^+-K^+-$2Cl^-$ co-transporter (NKCC1) in the apical membrane of epithelial cells of the thick ascending limb of the loop of Henle after combining with its chloride binding site. This transporter normally reabsorbs about 15–25% of the Na^+ load, which explains why they are the most powerful diuretics. This reduction in the reabsorption of sodium chloride increases the delivery of filtered Na^+ to the distal and collecting ducts, which stimulates the aldosterone-sensitive Na^+-K^+ exchange mechanism [e.g. inwardly rectifying K^+ (ROMK1) and Na^+ channels in the luminal membrane, coupled with basolateral Na^+-K^+ ATPases], facilitating the exchange of Na^+ by K^+ and H^+, which are lost to the urine. Thus, loop diuretics reduce the reabsorption of Na^+, Cl^-, K^+, Ca^{2+}, and Mg^{2+}, increase both natriuresis and diuresis, and produce hypokalaemia and metabolic alkalosis. Because Cl^-, but not bicarbonate (HCO_3^-), is lost in the urine, the plasma concentration of HCO_3^- increases as plasma volume is reduced. Loop diuretics also reduce the tonicity of the medullary interstitium by preventing the normal uptake of solute in the absence of water, limiting the kidney's ability to concentrate urine and may contribute to the development of hyponatraemia. Loop diuretics decrease the excretion of uric acid.

Loop diuretics interact with NKCC1 in vascular smooth muscle cells, hyperpolarize their membrane potential, reduce myogenic tone, and produce a vasodilatory effect. In patients with pulmonary oedema, IV administration of loop diuretics produces a venodilator effect and reduces venous return (preload) and right atrial pressure and PCWP, even before the onset of the diuretic effect, due to a decreased responsiveness to vasoconstrictors (noradrenaline, angiotensin II), renal release of prostaglandins (PGE2 in the medulla and PGI2 in the glomeruli), and opening of K^+ channels in resistance arteries. The release of renal prostaglandins can also increase cortical renal blood flow and GFR.

Pharmacodynamics

(See Furosemide, pp. 601–2, Bumetanide, p. 503, and Torasemide, p. 782.)

Loop diuretics are effective in patients with renal impairment (eGFR <30mL/min) that often accompanies severe HF, and in contrast to thiazides, they present a wide dose–response curve, so that increasing doses increases diuretic responses.

- *Antihypertensive effects.* Loop diuretics reduce blood volume, CO, and PVR. The best responses are observed in elderly and black hypertensives and in patients with HF and renal failure. However, loop diuretics increase the release of renin because they decrease intravascular volume and activate renal baroreceptors and β1-adrenoceptors, produce hyponatraemia, and upregulate renin gene expression in the kidney. Activation of the RAAS and sympathetic tone causes Na^+ and water retention and vasoconstriction, effects that partly counteract their antihypertensive effects. This explains why co-administration of a loop diuretic with an ACEI or an ARB increases the antihypertensive response. IV furosemide can be used in malignant hypertension when associated with CHF and fluid retention and in the treatment of hypercalcaemia and hyperkalaemia.
- *Oedema.* Loop diuretics (furosemide) decrease blood volume, venous pressure, and capillary hydrostatic pressure, which reduces net capillary fluid filtration and oedema associated with HF, CKD, nephrotic syndrome, and chronic liver disease and ascites.
- *HF.* In patients with HFrEF, loop diuretics, added to standard therapy, are recommended to improve signs and symptoms of pulmonary and systemic congestion (oedema, rales, pulmonary oedema, etc.), volume overload, and exercise capacity. Loop diuretics produce symptomatic benefits more rapidly than any other drug. IV loop diuretics exhibit a rapid and direct venodilator effect in patients with pulmonary oedema that reduces venous return (preload), right atrial pressure and PCWP, and pulmonary congestion. Venodilatation appears within 5–15min (even before diuresis) and is synergistic with the effect of glyceryl trinitrate and morphine. Long-term treatment may also produce systemic vasodilatation, which reduces LV afterload and improves LVEF. Because loop diuretics activate the RAAS, they should not be used alone but always be prescribed in combination with ACEIs (or ARBs), β-blockers, and aldosterone receptor antagonists. However, the effects of loop diuretics on mortality and morbidity remain uncertain.
- *Renal failure.* Loop diuretics must be filtered at the glomerulus to reach their site of action in the lumen of the tubules; thus, in patients with a decrease in GFR, higher doses of furosemide are needed to produce the same level of diuresis.

Pharmacokinetics

Loop diuretics are rapidly absorbed from the GI tract, are highly bound to plasma proteins, and do not pass directly to the glomerular filtrate but are secreted in the proximal tubule by the organic acid transport mechanism to reach their site of action. Drug absorption by the oral route is impaired in severe HF; under these circumstances, the IV route can be useful. In nephrotic syndrome, loop diuretics bind to albumin in the tubular fluid and so are less available to act on the Na^+-K^+-$2Cl^-$ symporter (diuretic resistance). (See Table 8.1.5.)

Practical points

1. *Doses* (see ➲ Furosemide, pp. 601–2, ➲ Bumetanide, p. 503, and ➲ Torasemide, p. 782)
   - Twice-daily doses should be given early in the morning and mid afternoon to avoid nocturia and to protect against volume depletion.
   - Loop diuretics produce a more intense, but shorter, diuresis than thiazides, so that a once-daily dose may be inadequate, and their combination with a longer-acting thiazide-type diuretic may be useful to treat resistant oedema or an insufficient response.
   - Loop diuretics can be given IV in urgent situations (e.g. acute pulmonary oedema) or when intestinal absorption is reduced (e.g. CHF and reduced intestinal perfusion). The initial IV dose should be at least equal to the pre-existing oral dose.
   - Combination of a loop diuretic with thiazide-type diuretics or spironolactone may be considered in patients with resistant oedema or insufficient response.
   - The dose must be adjusted to avoid the risk of dehydration and renal dysfunction and to prevent recurrence of volume overload. In selected asymptomatic euvolaemic/hypovolaemic patients, diuretics may be (temporarily) discontinued. Self-adjustment of the diuretic dose, based on daily weight measurements and other clinical signs of fluid retention, is recommended. In cases of a sudden, unexpected weight gain of >2kg in 3 days, patients should contact their clinician. Low doses may be sufficient in the elderly.
2. *Side effects*
   - Electrolyte disturbances: hypovolaemia (with risk of prerenal azotaemia), hypokalaemia, hypomagnesaemia, hyponatraemia, hypochloraemia, metabolic alkalosis, and hypocalcaemia. Reduction or discontinuation of the diuretic dose, Na^+ intake, and occasionally restriction of water intake can correct hyponatraemia. Hypokalaemia can be treated by concomitant use of potassium-sparing diuretics or potassium supplements. Hypokalaemia and hypomagnesaemia cause symptoms (fatigue, tremor, muscle cramps, constipation, and anorexia), ECG abnormalities, and cardiac arrhythmias. The risk of hypokalaemia increases in the elderly and in patients with renal impairment or HF. Urinary retention may by noted from vigorous diuresis in older adults.
   - CV: rapid mobilization of oedema, particularly in elderly patients, can lead to postural hypotension and renal dysfunction. Arrhythmias resulting from hypokalaemia/hypomagnesaemia.
   - GI: anorexia, nausea, gastric irritation, constipation.
   - Central: dizziness, vertigo, paraesthesiae, headache.
   - Metabolic: hyperuricaemia, hyperglycaemia, and new-onset diabetes, increase TG and LDL-C levels and decrease HDL-C plasma levels. Hyperuricaemia is due to increased absorption in the proximal tubule secondary to extracellular volume contraction and competition with uric acid for renal tubular secretion.
   - Others: muscle cramps, tinnitus, reversible or irreversible loss of hearing (after large doses, prolonged or parenteral administration, or renal impairment). Blood dyscrasias, marrow suppression, and pancreatitis are uncommon. Photosensitive skin eruptions (furosemide).

3. *Interactions*
   - The risk of hypotension increases when loop diuretics are co-administered with antihypertensive agents, nitrates, alcohol, MAOIs, opioids, phenothiazines, tricyclic antidepressants, or baclofen.
   - The diuretic effects of loop diuretics are antagonized by NSAIDs (inhibit the synthesis of renal prostaglandins).
   - Glucocorticoids, oestrogen-containing oral contraceptives, sucralfate, and bile acid sequestrants (colestyramine and colestipol) inhibit the diuretic and antihypertensive effects. The intake of loop diuretics and resins or sucralfate should be separated by at least 2h.
   - Because they inhibit Na^+ reabsorption at different tubular sites of the nephron, loop diuretics can be combined with thiazide diuretics and/or potassium-sparing diuretics. This *sequential nephron blockade* produces a synergistic diuretic effect and may be needed in patients with resistant peripheral oedema. This combination requires careful monitoring of the fluid status and serum electrolytes to avoid dehydration, electrolyte disturbances, hypovolaemia, or renal dysfunction.
   - Combination with potassium-sparing diuretics reduces the risk of hypokalaemia.
   - Hypokalaemia may enhance the arrhythmogenic effect of digoxin, antiarrhythmic agents, or QT-prolonging drugs. The risk of hypokalaemia increases when used with amphotericin, β-agonists, ACTH, corticosteroids, tacrolimus, thiazide and related diuretics, carbenoxolone, reboxetine, and theophylline.
   - Antiarrhythmics (including amiodarone, disopyramide, flecainide, and sotalol): increase the risk of cardiac toxicity (because of furosemide-induced hypokalaemia).
   - The risk of hyponatraemia increases with carbamazepine and amphotericin.
   - Loop diuretics displace warfarin from plasma proteins. A reduction in warfarin dose may be required in patients receiving both drugs.
   - Loop diuretics also increase the risk of nephrotoxicity when co-administered with other nephrotoxic drugs (i.e. NSAIDs, aminoglycoside antibiotics, amphotericin, some cephalosporins), especially in patients with impaired renal function.
   - Co-administration of cisplatin and loop diuretics increases the risk of ototoxic and nephrotoxic effects. Thus, the dose should be reduced and a positive fluid balance should be maintained to achieve forced diuresis during cisplatin treatment.
   - Loop diuretics reduce the renal clearance of lithium and increase the risk of lithium toxicity.
   - The combination with aminoglycosides, polymyxins, and vancomycin increases the risk of otoxicity.
   - Loop diuretics can enhance the skeletal muscle-relaxing effect of suxamethonium.
   - The combination of loop diuretics with β-blockers is not recommended in patients with diabetes or MetS due to the risk of new-onset diabetes.
   - Loop diuretics do not alter plasma digoxin levels and do not interact with warfarin.

4. *Cautions/notes*
- Urine output, electrolytes, blood urea, glucose, lipid and creatinine levels, full blood counts, and uric acid levels should be monitored during long-term treatment, particularly in patients with cardiac disease, diabetes, or renal or hepatic impairment, and in elderly patients.
- Excessively rapid mobilization of oedema, particularly in elderly patients, may lead to postural hypotension and circulatory collapse.
- Loop diuretics should be used with caution in patients receiving nephrotoxic, ototoxic, or QT-prolonging drugs (hypokalaemia. increases the risk of TdP).
- The dose should be carefully monitored to avoid excessive volume depletion that can reduce CO. In patients with pulmonary congestion and high PCWP presenting a depressed and flattened Frank–Starling curve, loop diuretics reduce the LV end-diastolic pressure (LVEDP) and pulmonary pressures (congestion symptoms) without changing the LV stroke volume. When LVEDP is <12mmHg, the stroke volume falls because the heart will now be operating on the ascending limb of the Frank–Starling curve.
- High doses of loop diuretics produce overdiuresis, volume depletion, fatigue and listlessness, hypotension, and urinary retention (mainly in the elderly) and reduces intravascular volume and LV filling pressure, so that the CO decreases and tissues become underperfused.
- In patients with acute HF and signs of hypoperfusion, diuretics should be avoided before adequate perfusion is attained.
- Patients with HF present with gut wall oedema that slows and decreases drug absorption, so that peak urinary concentrations of the diuretic after oral administration are reduced, resulting in a less powerful diuretic effect; under these circumstances, the IV route can be useful.
- Loop diuretics produce a diminished natriuretic response in patients with CKD or nephrotic syndrome due to reduced renal excretion of loop diuretics occurring in parallel with the decrease in GFR. In these patients, higher doses are needed to produce the same level of diuresis. In nephrotic syndrome, loop diuretics bind to albumin in the tubular fluid and are not available to act on the Na^+-K^+-$2Cl^-$ symporter (diuretic resistance).
- Doses of loop diuretics should be individually tailored, according to the renal/hepatic functional status, to avoid the risk of dehydration and renal insufficiency. The risk of electrolyte disturbances is markedly enhanced when two diuretics are used in combination.
- Patients with hypotension (SBP <90mmHg), severe hyponatraemia or acidosis are unlikely to respond to diuretic treatment.
- High doses of loop diuretics produce overdiuresis, volume depletion, and hyponatraemia. Hypovolaemia and hyponatraemia stimulate the activation of the RAAS and of the sympathetic tone, which may counteract the benefit in patients with HF. Under these circunstances, loop diuretics should be used only in combination with a RAAS inhibitor and a β-blocker.
- In men with prostate hyperplasia, there is a risk of urinary retention.
- Loop diuretics should also be avoided on the day of surgery because of potential adverse interaction with surgery-dependent fluid depletion.

5. *Pregnancy and lactation*
   - Furosemide and bumetanide cross the placental barrier and are excreted in breast milk; thus, they should be avoided in pregnancy and breastfeeding (Pregnancy category C). Torasemide is relatively safe in pregnancy (Pregnancy category B).
6. *Contraindications*
   - Anuria or renal failure.
   - Hypovolaemia and dehydration (with or without accompanying hypotension).
   - HF without fluid retention.
   - Severe hyponatraemia or hypokalaemia.
   - Severe hepatic impairment.
   - Hypotension.
   - Addison's disease.
   - Furosemide and bumetanide are contraindicated in patients allergic to sulfonamides, and torasemide in those allergic to sulfonylureas.
   - Digitalis intoxication.
   - Anuria or renal failure, renal failure as a result of poisoning by nephrotoxic agents.

Losartan

Angiotensin AT1 receptor blocker (see ➔ Angiotensin II AT1 receptor blockers, pp. 456–8).

Indications

- Treatment of hypertension.
- Treatment of renal disease in patients with hypertension and T2DM with proteinuria of ≥0.5g/day, as part of an antihypertensive treatment.
- Treatment of chronic HF in adult patients when treatment with ACEIs is not considered suitable due to incompatibility, especially cough, or contraindications. Patients with HF who have been stabilized with an ACEI should not be switched to losartan. The patients should have an LVEF of ≤40% and should be clinically stable and on an established treatment regimen for HF.
- Reduction in the risk of stroke in hypertensive patients with LVH evidenced by ECG.

Pharmacodynamics

The antihypertensive effect reaches steady state after 3–6 weeks and is potentiated by diuretic action or a low-salt diet more than by dose increase. In *diabetic nephropathy*, losartan reduces ESRD and proteinuria.

Pharmacokinetics

Losartan undergoes first-pass metabolism to form an active metabolite, more potent than losartan, and inactive metabolites. Food reduces the absorption (30–40%). Peak levels of losartan and the active metabolite occur at approximately 1 and 3–4h, respectively. Losartan and its metabolite bind to plasma proteins (99%) and present a Vd of approximately 0.6L/kg and a t½ of approximately 2h and 6–9h, respectively. Losartan levels increase in patients on dialysis. (See Table 8.1.9.)

Practical points

1. *Doses*
    - *Hypertension*: 50–100mg od. Maximal antihypertensive effect is attained 3–6 weeks after initiation of therapy. Some patients may receive an additional benefit by increasing the dose to 100mg od (in the morning). When there is volume depletion or liver disease, the starting dose should be 25mg.
    - *Hypertensive T2DM with proteinuria of ≥0.5g/day*: 50mg od increased to 100mg od.
    - *HF*: 50mg od (titrated up gradually to 150mg od if tolerated).
    - *Reduction in the risk of stroke in hypertensive patients with LVH evidenced by ECG*: 50mg up to 100mg od, based on BP response.

Lower doses should be considered in patients with hepatic impairment or intravascular volume depletion.

2. *Side effects* (see ➔ Angiotensin II AT1 receptor blockers, pp. 456–8)
3. *Interactions* (see ➔ Angiotensin II AT1 receptor blockers, pp. 456–8)

4. *Cautions/notes* (see ➔ Angiotensin II AT1 receptor blockers, pp. 456–8)
   - Losartan is a uricosuric compound that can be used in hypertensive patients with thiazide-induced hyperuricaemia in patients who are intolerant to allopurinol.
   - A lower dose should be considered in hepatic impairment.
5. *Pregnancy and lactation* (see ➔ Angiotensin II AT1 receptor blockers, pp. 456–8)
6. *Contraindications* (see ➔ Angiotensin II AT1 receptor blockers, pp. 456–8)
   - Severe hepatic impairment.

Lovastatin

Oral HMG CoA reductase inhibitor (see also ➔ Statins (3-hydroxy-3-methylglutaryl-coenzyme A reductase inhibitors), pp. 760–3).

CV indications

- Primary hypercholesterolaemia, heterozygous familial hypercholesterolaemia (types IIa and IIb), or mixed dyslipidaemia to reduce elevated total-C and LDL-C levels when response to non-pharmacological treatments is inadequate.
- In adolescent patients (at least 1 year post-menarche, 10–17 years of age) with heterozygous familial hypercholesterolaemia to reduce total-C, LDL-C, and Apo B levels if after diet therapy, the following findings are present: (1) LDL-C levels remain ≥190mg/dL; or (2) LDL-C levels remain ≥160mg/dL and there is a positive family history of premature CV disease or two or more other CV risk factors are present in the adolescent patient.
- Primary prevention of CAD, in individuals without symptomatic CV disease, average to moderately elevated total-C and LDL-C levels, and below-average HDL-C levels, to reduce the risk of MI, UA, and coronary revascularization procedures.
- To slow the progression of coronary atherosclerosis in patients with CAD, as part of a treatment strategy to lower total-C and LDL-C to target levels.

Mechanism of action

(See ➔ Statins (3-hydroxy-3-methylglutaryl-coenzyme A reductase inhibitors), pp. 760–3.)

Pharmacodynamics

Primary hypercholesterolaemia: at doses of between 10 and 80mg, it reduces elevated LDL-C (21–40%), total-C (16–29%), and TGs (10–19%) levels, and increases HDL-C (5–9.5%) levels. Lovastatin, alone or in combination with colestipol and nicotinic acid, slows the progression of coronary lesions, increases the frequency of regression, and reduces the incidence of CV events.

Pharmacokinetics

Oral bioavailability decreases by approximately 50% when given without food. (See Table 8.1.4.)

Practical points

1. *Doses*
   - Initial dose: 20mg od with the evening meal; maximum dose 80mg od (60mg od for the extended-release formulation). Elderly patients may require a lower dose. In severe renal insufficiency (CrCl <30mL/min), doses of above 20mg/day should be carefully considered.
   - Adolescents (10–17 years) with heterozygous familial hypercholesterolaemia: 10–40mg/day.

2. *Side effects* (see ➔ Statins (3-hydroxy-3-methylglutaryl-coenzyme A reductase inhibitors), pp. 760–3)
3. *Interactions* (see ➔ Statins (3-hydroxy-3-methylglutaryl-coenzyme A reductase inhibitors), pp. 760–3)
   - Concomitant administration with strong CYP3A4 inhibitors (see Table 8.1.2) increases drug exposure and the risk of myopathy. For patients taking potent CYP3A4 inhibitors, the dose of lovastatin should not exceed 20mg od. A 20-mg dose of lovastatin should not be exceeded in patients taking danazol, diltiazem, or verapamil; the 40-mg dose should not be exceeded with amiodarone.
   - Myopathy, including rhabdomyolysis, has been reported when co-administered with colchicine.
   - The risk of myopathy may also increase when combined with ranolazine.
   - No interactions between lovastatin and propranolol, glipizide, or digoxin.
   - Avoid the combination of lovastatin with boceprevir or telaprevir.
4. *Cautions/notes* (see ➔ Statins (3-hydroxy-3-methylglutaryl-coenzyme A reductase inhibitors), pp. 760–3)
5. *Contraindications* (see ➔ Statins (3-hydroxy-3-methylglutaryl-coenzyme A reductase inhibitors), pp. 760–3)

Macitentan

Orally active potent dual endothelin receptor antagonist (see ➔ Bosentan, pp. 500–2).

Indications

- As monotherapy or in combination for the long-term treatment of PAH in adult patients with WHO functional classes II–III. Efficacy has been shown in patients with idiopathic and heritable PAH, PAH associated with connective tissue disorders, and PAH associated with corrected simple congenital heart disease.

Mechanism of action

Macitentan is a potent dual endothelin receptor antagonist, with approximately 100-fold increased selectivity for ETA, as compared with ETB, receptors. Macitentan displays high affinity and sustained occupancy of ET1 receptors in human pulmonary arterial smooth muscle cells and presents a much slower dissociation rate. This slow dissociation could contribute to an enhanced pharmacological activity of macitentan, as compared to bosentan or ambrisentan.

Pharmacodynamics

Macitentan significantly reduced the time from initiation of treatment to first occurrence of a composite endpoint of death, atrial septostomy, lung transplantation, initiation of treatment with IV or SC prostanoids, or worsening of PAH in patients with PAH and also increased exercise capacity. Benefits were shown both for patients who had not received treatment previously and for those receiving additional therapy for PAH.

Pharmacokinetics

Macitentan is well absorbed, orally reaching peak plasma concentrations approximately 8h after oral dosing in humans. It is metabolized via CYP3A4 (with minor contributions of CYP2C8, CYP2C9, and CYP2C19) into ACT-132577, an active depropylated metabolite. Macitentan and its active metabolite are highly bound to plasma proteins (>99%) and present a Vd of 50L and 40L, respectively. The t½ of macitentan is approximately 16h, while ACT-132577 has a t½ of approximately 48h. Excretion involves both renal (50%) and faecal routes.

Practical points

1. *Doses*
    - 10mg od with or without food. The film-coated tablets are not breakable and are to be swallowed whole with water. Treatment should only be initiated and monitored by a physician experienced in the treatment of PAH. No dose adjustments are necessary in the elderly or in patients with moderate or severe hepatic impairment. There is no clinical experience in PAH patients with severe renal impairment.

2. *Side effects*
   - The commonest side effects are anaemia (decreases blood haemoglobin to ≤8g/dL), headache, oedema, fluid retention, hypotension, upper respiratory tract infections (nasopharyngitis/pharyngitis/bronchitis), and urinary tract infections. Other side effects: elevations of liver transaminases, rash, pruritus, decreased spermatogenesis.
3. *Interactions*
   - Macitentan and its active metabolite are not inhibitors of hepatic or renal uptake transporters, including the organic anion transporting polypeptides (OATP1B1 and OATP1B3); they are not relevant substrates of OATP1B1 and OATP1B3, and are not inhibitors of hepatic or renal efflux pumps, including the multidrug resistance protein (P-gp, MDR-1) and multidrug and toxin extrusion transporters (MATE1 and MATE2-K), the bile salt export pump (BSEP) and the sodium-dependent taurocholate co-transporting polypeptide (NTCP).
   - Caution should be exercised when macitentan is administered concomitantly with strong CYP3A4 inhibitors/inducers (see Table 8.1.2). Avoid this combination, if possible.
   - Macitentan does not interact with warfarin or sildenafil, ciclosporin, and oral contraceptives.
4. *Cautions/notes*
   - The safety and efficacy of macitentan in children have not been established.
   - If signs of pulmonary oedema occur during treatment, the possibility of pulmonary veno-occlusive disease should be considered.
5. *Pregnancy and lactation*
   - Macitentan is contraindicated in pregnancy (Pregnancy category X). Treatment should only be initiated in women of childbearing potential when the absence of pregnancy has been verified, appropriate advice on contraception provided, and reliable contraception is practised.
6. *Contraindications*
   - Pregnancy, women of childbearing potential who are not using reliable contraception, and breastfeeding.
   - Patients with severe hepatic impairment (with or without cirrhosis).
   - Baseline values of hepatic transaminases (ALT, AST) >3 times ULN.
   - Tablets contain lactose and lecithin derived from soya. Patients with rare hereditary problems of galactose intolerance, Lapp lactase deficiency or glucose–galactose malabsorption or hypersensitivity to soya should not take the drug.

Methyldopa

Central antihypertensive drug.

Specific indications

Treatment of hypertensive disorders during pregnancy.

Mechanism of action

The antihypertensive effect of methyldopa is probably due to its metabolism to α-methylnoradrenaline, an agonist of CNS presynaptic α2-adrenergic receptors. Activation of these receptors in the brainstem inhibits sympathetic nervous system output, lowers BP, and reduces plasma renin activity. Methyldopa is also a competitive inhibitor of DOPA decarboxylase, which converts L-DOPA into dopamine; this inhibition results in reduced dopaminergic and adrenergic neurotransmission in the peripheral nervous system.

Pharmacodynamics

Methyldopa reduces BP, with infrequent symptomatic postural hypotension, but has no direct effect on cardiac (although, in some patients, the heart rate is slowed) or renal function. BP returns to baseline values within 4h following drug discontinuation.

Pharmacokinetics

Absorption of oral methyldopa is variable and incomplete (bioavailability 25%), reaching peak concentrations within 2–3h. Renal excretion accounts for about two-thirds of drug clearance from plasma. Plasma t½ is 1.8–2h.

Practical points

1. *Doses*
   - Initial dosage: usually 250mg bd or tds for 2 days (125–250mg bd in the elderly). The dose can be increased at intervals of not less than 2 days (maximal daily dosage 3g). Patients with impaired renal function may respond to smaller doses. Many patients experience sedation at the begining of treatment or when the dose is increased; thus, it may be desirable to increase the evening dose first.
2. *Side effects*
   - Methyldopa produces many side effects: central (parkinsonism, nightmares, depression, headache, sedation, asthenia or weakness, dizziness, light-headedness, paraesthesiae), hepatic (hepatitis, jaundice, abnormal LFTs), CV (hypotension, bradycardia, oedema, aggravation of angina pectoris, CHF), GI (diarrhoea, nausea, flatus), hyperprolactinaemia, arthralgia, myalgia, anaemia, bone marrow depression, pericarditis, vasculitis, fever, rash, amenorrhoea, gynaecomastia, lactation, impotence, or decreased libido.
3. *Interactions*
   - When methyldopa and lithium are given concomitantly, monitor for lithium toxicity.
   - Methyldopa potentiates the effects of antihypertensive and vasodilator drugs.

- The antihypertensive effect of methyldopa may be diminished by sympathomimetics, phenothiazines, tricyclic antidepressants, and MAOIs.
- Ferrous sulfate or ferrous gluconate decrease the oral bioavailability of methyldopa.

4. *Cautions/notes*
   - A positive Coombs' test, haemolytic anaemia, and liver disorders may occur during methyldopa therapy. Blood counts and LFTs should be performed in the first 6–12 weeks or when fever occurs. A positive direct Coombs' test occurs in 10–20% of patients and is dose-related, with the lowest incidence occurring in patients receiving ≥1g of methyldopa daily.
   - Methyldopa can also interfere with measurement of urinary uric acid, serum creatinine, AST, catecholamines (but it does not interfere with the measurements of vanillyl mandelic acid), antinuclear antibodies, and rheumatoid factor, depending on the method used.
   - It should be used with extreme caution in patients or patients' near relatives with hepatic porphyria.
   - Since methyldopa is largely excreted by the kidneys, patients with impaired renal function may respond to comparatively low doses.
   - Methyldopa is not recommended for treatment of hypertension associated with phaeochromocytoma.
   - A thiazide may be added to methyldopa if effective control of BP cannot be maintained on 2g of methyldopa daily.
5. *Pregnancy and lactation*
   - Methyldopa crosses the placental barrier and appears in cord blood and breast milk, although no obvious teratogenic effects have been reported. Oral and IV methyldopa has been assigned to Pregnancy category B and C, respectively.
6. *Contraindications*
   - Active hepatic disease (acute hepatitis and active cirrhosis).
   - Hypersensitivity to the active substance.
   - Depression; treatment with MAOIs.
   - Catecholamine-secreting tumours (phaeochromocytoma or paraganglioma).
   - Porphyria.

Metolazone

Metolazone is a substituted quinazolinone thiazide-like diuretic, (see ➲ Thiazide and related diuretics, pp. 768–73).

CV and other indications

- Treatment of hypertension.
- Treatment of oedema.

Mechanism of action

(See ➲ Thiazide and related diuretics, pp. 768–73.)

Pharmacodynamics

Diuresis begin within 1h and persist for 24h, particularly at the higher recommended dosages. Metolazone is around ten times as potent as HCTZ, and in contrast to other thiazides, it remains effective in renal impairment, but at risk of excessive diuresis. In combination with furosemide, it produces profound diuresis, with a risk of hypovolaemia and hypokalaemia. Metolazone is often used in addition to a prior combination with a loop diuretic, a thiazide, and an aldosterone inhibitor in patients with CHF and resistant peripheral oedema.

Pharmacokinetics

(See Table 8.1.5.)

Practical points

1. *Doses*
   - *Hypertension*: 2.5–5mg od initially; may be increased to 20mg.
   - *HF*: 2.5mg od, increased to 10mg od.
   - *Oedema*: 2.5–10mg od to a maximum of 80mg, if required.

Given its potency, it is advisable to start metolazone at doses lower than those recommended, especially when given in combination with a loop diuretic.

2. *Side* effects (see ➲ Thiazide and related diuretics, pp. 768–73)
3. *Interactions* (see ➲ Thiazide and related diuretics, pp. 768–73)
4. *Cautions*/notes (see ➲ Thiazide and related diuretics, pp. 768–73)
5. Contraindications (see ➲ Thiazide and related diuretics, pp. 768–73)
   - Anuria, hepatic coma or pre-coma, and documented hypersensitivity to metolazone or sulfonamides.

Metoprolol

Cardioselective β1-adrenergic receptor antagonist, with high lipid solubility and membrane-stabilizing activity (see also ➔ Beta-adrenergic blocking agents, pp. 485–94).

CV indications

- Hypertension.
- Angina pectoris.
- Tachycardias, particularly SVT.
- Prevention of cardiac death and reinfarction after the acute phase of MI.
- Prophylaxis of migraine.

Pharmacokinetics

Metoprolol tartrate (immediate-release formulation) is almost completely absorbed, but its bioavailability is approximately 40–50% due to hepatic first-pass metabolism. Peak plasma concentrations occur 1.5–2h after dosing. Metoprolol undergoes extensive oxidative metabolism in the liver, primarily via CYP2D6. Its oxidative metabolism is under genetic control. Poor metabolizers have higher plasma levels; there are marked ethnic differences in the prevalence of the poor metabolizer phenotype (87% of Caucasians and <1% of Asians). Its t½ is approximately 3–5h (7.5h in poor metabolizers and 2.8h in extensive metabolizers), but the effects persists for 12h. The pharmacokinetic properties of metoprolol are unaltered in patients with renal failure. The biological t½ of metoprolol exceeds the plasma t½ considerably, so that twice-daily dosages of standard metoprolol are effective, even in angina pectoris.

Metoprolol succinate [controlled-release (CR)/extended-release (XL) formulations] has lower bioavailability (approximately 70%, compared with the immediate-release formulation) and is characterized by lower C_{max}, longer time to peak plasma levels (to approximately 8h), and lower peak-to-trough variation. (See Table 8.1.8.)

Practical points

1. *Doses*
   - *Hypertension*: 50mg bd or 100mg od; then 100–200mg in single or divided doses.
   - *Angina pectoris*: start with 50mg bd; then 50–100mg bd.
   - *HF* (metoprolol CR/XL): 12.5–25mg od, increased up to 200mg od.
   - *Cardiac arrhythmias*: 100–150mg/day, increased if needed.
   - *Prevention of cardiac death and reinfarction after IV treatment of acute MI*: start once the patient is haemodynamically stable with 50mg PO bd.
   - *Prophylaxis after MI*: maintenance dose 100mg bd.
   - *Prophylaxis of migraine*: 50–100mg bd.
   - Dose adjustment is not usually required in hepatic impairment, except with severe dysfunction.
2. *Side effects* (see ➔ Beta-adrenergic blocking agents, pp. 485–94)
3. *Interactions* (see ➔ Beta-adrenergic blocking agents, pp. 485–94)
   - CYP2D6 inhibitors/inducers may increase/decrease plasma concentrations of metoprolol (see Table 8.1.2).

4. *Cautions/notes* (see ➲ Beta-adrenergic blocking agents, pp. 485–94)
5. *Pregnancy and lactation*
   - Metoprolol crosses the placenta and is found in breast milk. Its use is not recommended in pregnancy and breastfeeding (Pregnancy category C).
6. *Contraindications* (see ➲ Beta-adrenergic blocking agents, pp. 485–94)

Mexiletine

Class IB AAD (see ➲ Lidocaine, pp. 641–3).

CV indications

- Treatment of life-threatening ventricular arrhythmias (sustained VT).
- Off-label: treatment of patients with LQTS3.

Mechanism of action

(See ➲ Lidocaine, pp. 641–3.)

Pharmacokinetics

Administration with food or antacid is recommended. Therapeutic range: 0.5–2mg/L. (See Table 8.1.3.)

Practical points

1. *Doses*
   - Initial: 200mg PO every 8h; may load with 400mg, followed by 200mg PO every 8h, if necessary, for rapid control of ventricular arrhythmia. A minimum of 2–3 days between dose adjustments is recommended. Maximum dose: 1200mg/day. Reduce the dose in patients with CrCl of <10mL/min (50–75% of normal dose) or hepatic impairment or CHF (25–30% of normal dose).
2. *Side effects* (see ➲ Lidocaine, pp. 641–3)
   - Common (>10%): nausea, vomiting, heartburn, ataxia, dizziness, light-headedness, tremor, coordination difficulties. Less common (2–8%): palpitations, hypotension, headache, insomnia, confusion, depression, visual disturbances, paraesthesiae, changes in sleep habits, rash, and arrhythmias.
   - ALTs have been reported in the first weeks of therapy in patients with CHF or ischaemia.
3. *Interactions*
   - Mexiletine is metabolized via CYP2D6 and CYP1A2 enzymes. Inhibition or induction of either of these enzymes would be expected to increase or decrease, respectively, plasma mexiletine concentrations (see Table 8.1.2).
   - Cimetidine can increase, decrease, or leave unchanged plasma mexiletine levels.
   - Mexiletine may increase plasma theophylline levels. Proper adjustment of the theophylline dose should be considered.
4. *Cautions/notes*
   - Clinical and ECG evaluations are needed to determine whether the desired antiarrhythmic effect has been obtained and to guide titration and dose adjustment.
   - Use with caution in CHF, hypotension, and a history of seizures.
   - Because of its proarrhythmic effects, its use in patients with asymptomatic VPBs or conduction disturbances is not recommended.
   - Prior to use, electrolyte imbalances (especially hypokalaemia and hypomagnesaemia) must be corrected.
   - Mexiletine should be used with caution in patients with hypotension and severe CHF because of the potential for aggravating these conditions.

5. *Pregnancy and lactation*
   - Pregnancy category C. Mexiletine is present in breast milk, reaching concentrations comparable to those in maternal plasma.
6. *Contraindications*
   - Hypersensitivity to mexiletine.
   - Cardiogenic shock, pre-existing second-/third-degree AVB if no pacemaker is present.

Milrinone

Selective inhibitor of cAMP PDE-3 in cardiac and vascular muscle cells.

Indications

- Short-term (up to 35h) IV treatment of patients with acute decompensated HF unresponsive to conventional therapy, including low-output states following cardiac surgery.
- Short-term treatment (up to 35h) of severe CHF unresponsive to conventional maintenance therapy (glycosides, diuretics, vasodilators, and/or ACEIs).

Mechanism of action

(See ➔ Positive inotropic agents, pp. 700–1.)

Milrinone increases cAMP levels by blocking PDE-3, the enzyme that breaks down cAMP in cardiac and vascular smooth muscle cells. This leads to an increase in intracellular cAMP levels that increases intracellular free Ca^{2+} levels, myocardial contractility, and MVO_2, while producing peripheral arterial and venous vasodilatation, i.e. milrinone acts as an inovasodilator drug. The increased levels of myocardial cAMP predispose to atrial and ventricular arrhythmias.

Pharmacodynamics

Milrinone increases CO and decreases PCWP and PVR. These effects are accompanied by mild to moderate increases in heart rate or MVO_2. In most patients, improvement in haemodynamic function occurs within 5–15min of initiation of therapy. Milrinone has a favourable inotropic effect in fully digitalized patients, without causing signs of glycoside toxicity. Combined with low doses of dobutamine, milrinone increases cardiac contractility and decreases LV filling pressures. When the BP is low, milrinone can be combined with high-dose dopamine.

Pharmacokinetics

Following IV injections of 12.5mcg/kg, milrinone binds to plasma proteins by 70% and presents a Vd of 0.38–0.45L/kg and a mean terminal t½ of 2.3h. The primary route of excretion is via the urine (83% as milrinone; 12% as its *O*-glucuronide metabolite).

Practical points

1. *Doses*
   - Loading dose of 25–50mcg/kg over 10min, followed by a continuous infusion of 0.35–0.75mcg/kg/min; maximum daily dose 1.13mg/kg. The initial load can be omitted to avoid hypotensive effects. Reduce the dose according to the CrCl (CrCl 40mL/min/1.73m^2: 0.38mcg/kg/min; CrCl 20mL/min/1.73m^2: 0.28mcg/kg/min).
2. *Side effects*
   - Common: headaches, supraventricular and ventricular arrhythmias, ventricular ectopic activity, non-sustained or sustained VT, hypotension, hypokalaemia, tremor, thrombocytopenia, and infusion site reactions. Long-term oral use increased ventricular arrhythmias and mortality in patients with HF.
   - Others: thrombocytopenia, angina/chest pain.

3. *Interactions*
   - There are no interactions with digitalis, lidocaine, quinidine, nitrates, hydralazine, prazosin, chlortalidone, furosemide, HCTZ, spironolactone, captopril, heparin, warfarin, diazepam, insulin, and potassium supplements.
   - There is an immediate chemical interaction, with the formation of a precipitate, when furosemide is injected into an IV line of an infusion of milrinone.
4. *Cautions/notes*
   - Patients should be closely monitored (ECG, electrolytes, renal function, BP), including the facility for immediate treatment of potential cardiac events (including life-threatening ventricular arrhythmias).
   - In patients with AF/atrial flutter, milrinone can increase the ventricular rate response by improving AV nodal conduction. Digoxin can avoid this increase in ventricular rate.
   - Milrinone should not be diluted in sodium bicarbonate IV infusion.
5. *Pregnancy and lactation*
   - There are no adequate and well-controlled studies in pregnant women (Pregnancy category C). It is unknown whether it is excreted in human milk.
6. *Contraindications*
   - Hypersensitivity to milrinone or any of the excipients, severe hypovolaemia.

Morphine

Competitive agonist at μ opiate receptors, which are responsible for many other actions, including respiratory depression, euphoria, inhibition of gut motility, and physical dependence.

Indications

- Symptomatic relief of severe pain; relief of dyspnoea of LV failure and pulmonary oedema; preoperative use.

Mechanism of action

Morphine sulfate is an opioid agonist. It is relatively selective for the μ receptor, although it can interact with other opioid receptors at higher doses.

Pharmacodynamics

Morphine combines a potent analgesic effect with haemodynamic actions, including a venodilator action that reduces ventricular preload, a mild arterial vasodilator action that reduces afterload, and bradycardia. These effects reduce the MVO_2 demands and may result in orthostatic hypotension. Morphine also decreases sympathetic outflow and releases histamine. It also helps to relieve anxiety and insomnia which may be associated with severe pain.

Pharmacokinetics

Variably absorbed after oral administration; rapidly absorbed after SC or IM administration. After an oral dose, peak plasma levels are reached after 15–60min, and within 10–20min after an IM or IV dose. Morphine is bound to plasma proteins (35%) and is widely distributed (Vd 2–3L/kg), but it does not readily cross the placenta. Morphine is extensively metabolized by the liver, and the metabolites are excreted mainly via the renal route (10% of the dose is excreted unchanged in the urine) and 7–10% in the faeces. The terminal t½ is 2h.

Practical points

1. *Doses*
   - Sulfate may be given by the SC, IM, or IV route. The SC route is not suitable for oedematous patients. SC/IM: 10mg every 4h (5–20mg). If pain persists or if the patient is agitated or pulmonary congestion is present: 4–8mg by slow IV push, followed by 2–8mg at 5–15min intervals. PO: 60mg/day, up to 90–120mg/day. A reduction in dosage should be considered in hepatic and renal impairment.
2. *Side effects*
   - The commonest are: GI (nausea, dyspepsia, paralytic ileus, abdominal pain, anorexia, biliary spasm), CV (bradycardia, tachycardia, palpitations, hypotension, syncope, facial flushing, oedema), and respiratory depression (potentially increasing the need for invasive ventilation).
   - Others: psychiatric disorders (restlessness, mood changes, hallucinations, delirium, disorientation, excitation, sleep disturbance), nervous system disorders (headache, vertigo, euphoria, dysphoria, dizziness, taste disturbances, seizures, paraesthesiae), visual (nystagmus,

miosis), musculoskeletal (muscle fasciculation, myoclonus, muscle rigidity), urinary disorders (ureteric spasm, urinary retention), rashes, urticaria, pruritus, dry mouth, sweating, hypothermia, malaise, asthenia, pain and irritation at the injection site, impotence, decreased libido.

3. *Interactions*
   - The CNS depressant effects of morphine are increased by other CNS depressants, including alcohol, anaesthetics, muscle relaxants, hypnotics, sedatives, tricyclics, neuroleptics, and phenothiazines. Such combinations should be used with extreme caution.
   - Combined with alcohol, antidepressants, and antipsychotics, the hypotensive effect of morphine may be enhanced. Alcohol can increase plasma morphine levels, leading to a potentially fatal overdose of morphine.
   - Concomitant use of MAOIs with morphine results in CNS excitation or depression with hyper- or hypotensive crises and is contraindicated.
   - Morphine may reduce the efficacy of diuretics by inducing the release of ADH.
   - The combination of morphine with anticholinergics may enhance constipation and urinary retention.
   - Co-administration with antidiarrhoeal and antiperistaltic agents may increase the risk of severe constipation.
   - Cimetidine and ranitidine interfere with the metabolism of morphine and can potentiate morphine-induced respiratory depression.
   - Metoclopramide and domperidone may antagonize morphine's GI effects; metoclopramide enhances its sedative effect.
   - Ritonavir can increase the metabolism of morphine and reduce its analgesic effects.
   - Morphine may enhance the action of skeletal muscle relaxants and produce an increased degree of respiratory depression.
4. *Cautions/notes*
   - Assess each patient's risk for opioid abuse/misuse prior to prescribing morphine.
   - Serious, life-threatening, or fatal respiratory depression can occur at any time. Monitor patients with significant COPD or cor pulmonale and patients having a substantially decreased respiratory reserve, hypoxia, hypercapnia, or pre-existing respiratory depression.
   - Monitor patients for signs of sedation and respiratory depression, and consider using a lower dose of the concomitant CNS depressant.
   - Morphine may cause severe hypotension. Monitor these patients for signs of hypotension. In patients with circulatory shock, it may cause vasodilatation that can further reduce CO and BP.
   - In the presence of hypovolaemia, morphine may cause profound hypotension.
   - Morphine should be avoided in patients with biliary disorders or given with an antispasmodic.
   - Monitor patients with head injury or increased intracranial pressure.
   - Morphine may aggravate convulsions in patients with convulsive disorders.
   - Do not abruptly discontinue morphine, but gradually taper the dose.

5. *Pregnacy and lactation*
   - Morphine is not recommended for use in pregnancy (Pregnancy category C). Administration during labour may cause respiratory depression in the newborn infant. Morphine has been shown to suppress lactation, is secreted in breast milk, and may cause respiratory depression in the infant.
6. *Contraindications*
   - Hypersensitivity to morphine or other opioid preparations.
   - Acute respiratory depression; acute or severe bronchial asthma; HF secondary to chronic lung disease.
   - Head injury; raised intracranial pressure.
   - Paralytic ileus; biliary and renal tract spasm.
   - Phaeochromocytoma (due to the risk of pressor response to histamine release).

Moxonidine

Oral centrally acting imidazoline-selective receptor subtype 1 (I_1) agonist.

Indications

- Adults (>18 years) with moderate hypertension.

Mechanism of action

Moxonidine selectively interacts with I_1-imidazoline receptors within the brainstem (in the rostral ventrolateral medulla) and reduces sympathetic nervous activity. Indeed, it reduces plasma levels of adrenaline and noradrenaline. Moxonidine also promotes Na^+ excretion.

Pharmacodynamics

Moxonidine reduces PVR and BP and increases Na^+ excretion, while heart rate, CO, stroke volume, and PAPs are not affected. LVH has been found to regress after 6 months' treatment with moxonidine. In patients with HFrEF (NYHA classes II–IV), moxonidine sustained-release (1.5mg bd) increases mortality hospitalization for HF, acute MI, and adverse events, as compared to placebo.

Pharmacokinetics

Oral moxonidine is well absorbed (bioavailability approximately 90%), reaching peak plasma levels in 1h. It is approximately 7% bound to plasma proteins, and its Vd is approximately 2.5L/kg. Moxonidine is mostly excreted unchanged in the urine (75%); only 1% is eliminated via the faeces. The mean elimination t½ is 2.5h, which is prolonged by renal insufficiency. However, the antihypertensive effect lasts longer than would be expected from its t½, as moxonidine is suitable for once-daily administration.

Practical points

1. *Doses*
   - Initial dose of 0.2mg in the morning (up to a maximum of 0.6mg in divided doses). In moderate renal dysfunction (GFR >30 to <60mL/min), the starting dose should not exceed 0.2mg and the daily dose 0.4mg.
2. *Side effects*
   - (>1%): dry mouth, headache, fatigue, asthenia, dizziness, anorexia, nausea, sleep disturbances (insomnia, somnolence), facial flush, oedema, and hypotension.
   - Others: sedation (<1%), skin reactions (rash/itching), bradycardia, inability to get or maintain an erection, isolated cases of angio-oedema.

The frequency and intensity of these symptoms often decrease in the course of treatment.

3. *Interactions*
   - The risk of hypotension increases when co-administered with other antihypertensives or vasodilators. Moxonidine potentiate the vasodilator effect of benzodiazepines, antidepressants, hypnotics, and alcohol. Monitor BP.

4. *Cautions/notes*
   - If treatment with a β-blocker has to be stopped, the β-blocker should be discontinued first, then moxonidine after a few days.
   - Where necessary, moxonidine should be withdrawn gradually over 2 weeks.
   - Moxonidine is not recommended in patients with HFrEF.
   - Patients should not drive or operate machinery if they feel dizzy or drowsy, while taking moxonidine.
5. *Pregnancy and lactation*
   - There are not adequate data in pregnant women (Pregnancy category B). It is excreted in breast milk. Due to limited therapeutic evidence, it should not be used in breastfeeding mothers.
6. *Contraindications*
   - Hypersensitivity to the active substance or any of the excipients.
   - Severe hepatic or renal (GFR <30mL/min) disease.
   - History of angioneurotic oedema.
   - Sick sinus syndrome, SA block, second- or third-degree AVB, bradycardia, malignant arrhythmias.
   - Severe HF, severe CAD, or UA.
   - Intermittent claudication, depression, glaucoma, Raynaud's syndrome, and Parkinson's disease.

Nadolol

Non-selective β-adrenergic blocker (see ➲ Beta-adrenergic blocking agents, pp. 485–94).

CV indications

- Long-term treatment of hypertension.
- Long-term treatment of angina pectoris.
- Treatment of cardiac arrhythmias.
- Prophylactic management of migraine headache.
- Relief of symptoms of hyperthyroidism and preoperative preparation of patients for surgery.

Mechanism of action

(See ➲ Beta-adrenergic blocking agents, pp. 485–94.)

Pharmacodynamics

(See ➲ Beta-adrenergic blocking agents, pp. 485–94.)

Pharmacokinetics

(See Table 8.1.8.)

Practical points

1. *Doses*
   - *Hypertension*: 40–320mg daily.
   - *Angina pectoris*: initial 40mg/day od, increased gradually every 3–7 days. Doses of up to 160–240mg/day may be needed. No dose adjustment in hepatic impairment. Renal impairment: CrCl 31–50mL/min, give the dose every 24–36h; CrCl 10–30mL/min: every 24–48h; CrCl <10mL/min: every 40–60h.
   - *Cardiac arrhythmias*: 40–160mg od.
   - *Migraine*: 40mg od, up to 160mg od. If a satisfactory response is not obtained after 4–6 weeks at the maximum dose, nadolol should be withdrawn gradually.
   - *Thyrotoxicosis*: 80–160mg od.
2. *Side effects* (see ➲ Beta-adrenergic blocking agents, pp. 485–94)
3. *Interactions* (see ➲ Beta-adrenergic blocking agents, pp. 485–94)
4. *Cautions/notes* (see ➲ Beta-adrenergic blocking agents, pp. 485–94)
5. *Contraindications* (see ➲ Beta-adrenergic blocking agents, pp. 485–94)

Naftidrofuryl oxalate

5-HT2 receptor antagonist in vascular smooth muscle cells.

Indications

- Peripheral vascular disorders (intermittent claudication, night cramps, rest pain, incipient gangrene, trophic ulcers, Raynaud's syndrome, diabetic arteriopathy, and acrocyanosis).

Mechanism of action

Naftidrofuryl oxalate increases cellular oxidative capacity and ATP levels and decreases lactic acid levels in ischaemic conditions. Furthermore, it is a powerful antispasmodic agent.

Pharmacodynamics

Naftidrofuryl oxalate is a powerful peripheral and cerebral vasodilator agent. In a Cochrane meta-analysis, an improvement in time to initial pain on treadmill walking over a 3- to 6-month period was noted.

Pharmacokinetics

Naftidrofuryl presents an oral bioavailability of 24% and reaches peak plasma levels within 0.5–0.75h. It binds to plasma proteins (80%), is widely distributed (reaching the brain), is metabolized in the liver, and is excreted principally via the urine as metabolites. The plasma t½ is approximately 1h.

Practical points

1. *Doses*
   - 100–200mg tds. The capsules should be administered with a sufficient amount of water (one glass) during or after food.
2. *Side effects*
   - Diarrhoea, nausea, vomiting, and epigastric pain; skin rash, dizziness, headache; calcium oxalate kidney stones. Rarely, hepatitis and liver failure have been reported.
3. *Cautions/notes*
   - Administration of naftidrofuryl without liquid before going to bed may cause local oesophagitis; thus, it should always be taken with a sufficient amount of water.
   - Naftidrofuryl may modify the composition of the urine, promoting the formation of calcium oxalate kidney stones.
4. *Pregnancy and lactation*
   - There are no clinical data.
5. *Contraindications*
   - Patients with a history of hyperoxaluria or recurrent calcium-containing stones.
   - Hypersensitivity to the active substance or any of the excipients.

Nebivolol

β1-adrenergic receptor blocking agent (see ➔ Beta-adrenergic blocking agents, pp. 485–94).

Indications

- Treatment of hypertension, alone or in combination with other antihypertensives.
- Treatment of stable mild and moderate chronic HF, in addition to standard therapies, in elderly patients aged ≥70 years.
- Control of ventricular rate in AF.

Mechanism of action

(See ➔ Beta-adrenergic blocking agents, pp. 485–94.)

Nebivolol is a highly cardioselective β1-blocker, with direct vasodilating properties mediated by the release of NO.

Pharmacodynamics

In hypertensive patients, nebivolol improves the lipid profile, increases insulin sensitivity, and reverses endothelial dysfunction, which may explain the improvement of erectile dysfunction. In extensive CYP2D6 metabolizers (most of the population) and at doses of ≤10mg, nebivolol is preferentially a β1-selective blocker. In poor metabolizers and at higher doses, nebivolol blocks both β1- and β2-adrenoceptors.

Pharmacokinetics

Oral bioavailability of nebivolol is 12% in extensive metabolizers, and 96% in poor metabolizers. Nebivolol has a terminal t½ of approximately 10h in extensive metabolizers, and 32h in poor metabolizers.

Metabolites probably account for the vasodilatation and long biological t½. Drug clearance is greatly reduced in patients with significant renal impairment. Due to its extensive hepatic metabolism, peak plasma concentrations increase 3-fold, exposure (AUC) increases 10-fold, and the apparent clearance decreases by 86% in patients with moderate hepatic impairment (Child–Pugh class B). Drug clearance is reduced by 50% in patients with severe renal impairment (CrCl <30mL/min). (See Table 8.1.8.)

Practical points

1. *Doses*
   - *Hypertension*: the starting dose is 5mg od; the dose can be increased at 2-week intervals up to 40mg. In patients with severe renal impairment (CrCl <30mL/min) or moderate hepatic impairment, the recommended initial dose is 2.5mg od. The drug has not been studied in patients with severe hepatic impairment. No dose adjustments are necessary in the elderly or in CYP2D6 poor metabolizers.
   - *HF*: the starting dose is 1.25mg od; it can be increased up to 10mg od.
   - *Control of ventricular rate in AF*: 20–80mg/day.
2. *Side effects* (see ➔ Beta-adrenergic blocking agents, pp. 485–94)
   - Nevibolol increases BUN, uric acid, TG levels, and decreases HDL-C levels and platelet count.

3. *Interactions* (see ➔ Beta-adrenergic blocking agents, pp. 485–94)
   - Drugs that inhibit CYP2D6 may increase plasma levels of nebivolol (see Table 8.1.2).
4. *Cautions/notes* (see ➔ Beta-adrenergic blocking agents, pp. 485–94)
5. *Pregnancy and lactation* (see ➔ Beta-adrenergic blocking agents, pp. 485–94)
   - Well-controlled studies in pregnant women have failed to demonstrate a risk to the fetus (Pregnancy category B).
6. *Contraindications* (see ➔ Beta-adrenergic blocking agents, pp. 485–94)

Nicardipine

L-type CCB (see ➲ Calcium channel blockers, pp. 504–9).

Indications

- Prophylaxis of patients with chronic stable angina.
- Treatment of hypertension: IV nicardipine can be used in malignant arterial hypertension/hypertensive encephalopathy, aortic dissection (when short-acting β-blockers are not suitable or in combination with β-blockers when β-blockers alone are not effective), severe pre-eclampsia, when other IV antihypertensives are not recommended or are contraindicated, or post-operative hypertension.

Pharmacokinetics

Because nicardipine is extensively metabolized by the liver, plasma drug levels increase in patients with severe liver disease (hepatic cirrhosis); in these patients, the t½ of nicardipine is prolonged from 8.6 to 19h. (See Table 8.1.6.)

Practical points

1. *Doses*
   - *Prophylaxis of chronic stable angina*. Starting dose: 20mg every 8h, titrating up to 30mg every 8h, as required (60–120mg/day).
   - *Hypertension*. Starting dose: 20mg every 8h, titrating up to 30mg every 8h. In the elderly, titrate upwards with care. IV nicardipine (10mg) should only be administered by specialists in well-controlled environments, with continuous monitoring of BP.
2. *Interactions* (see ➲ Calcium channel blockers, pp. 504–9)
   - Severe hypotension has been reported when combined with other antihypertensives or during fentanyl anaesthesia.
3. *Side effects* (see ➲ Calcium channel blockers, pp. 504–9)
4. *Interactions* (see ➲ Calcium channel blockers, pp. 504–9)
5. *Cautions/notes* (see ➲ Calcium channel blockers, pp. 504–9)
6. *Contraindications* (see ➲ Calcium channel blockers, pp. 504–9)

Nicorandil

Nitrate derivative of nicotinamide, which activates ATP-dependent K^+ channels.

CV indications

- Treatment of adults with stable angina pectoris who are inadequately controlled or have a contraindication or intolerance to first-line anti-anginal therapies (such as β-blockers and/or CCBs).

Mechanism of action

Nicorandil exerts a dual mode of action, leading to the relaxation of peripheral and coronary vascular smooth muscle cells. It is an organic nitrate, acting as an NO donor that activates guanylyl cyclase, increases cGMP cellular levels, and predominantly relaxes vascular smooth muscle in veins and causes epicardial coronary vasodilatation. In addition, it selectively activates ATP-dependent K^+ channels at the sarcolemmal and mitrochondrial level in ischaemic cardiomyocytes, which results in membrane hyperpolarization, inhibition of Ca^{2+} entry via L-type Ca^{2+} channels, and arteriolar dilatation. Unlike nitrates, there is no drug tolerance with prolonged use of nicorandil.

Pharmacodynamics

Nicorandil reduces the frequency of angina as effectively as other anti-anginal drugs. In patients with stable angina, nicorandil reduced major coronary events (CAD death, ACS, non-fatal MI, or unplanned hospital admission for cardiac chest pain). Long-term use of oral nicorandil may stabilize coronary plaque in patients with stable angina.

Pharmacokinetics

The pharmacokinetics remain unaltered in elderly persons and in patients with renal or hepatic impairment. (See Table 8.1.11.)

Practical points

1. *Doses*
   - 10mg bd (maximum dose 40mg bd). Gradual titration from 5mg bd may reduce the likelihood of headaches. No dose adjustment is needed in renal or hepatic impairment.
2. *Side effects*
   - Headaches appear to be dose-dependent and resolve despite continued treatment, but they may contribute to drug withdrawal. Dizziness, nausea, vomiting, flushing, palpitations, weakness, hypotension, myalgia, rash, and pruritus. Occasional reports of oral, intestinal, and perianal mucosal ulcerations, which resolved on discontinuation of nicorandil.
3. *Interactions*
   - Risk of hypotension when nicorandil is taken with other antihypertensives and vasodilators (tricyclic antidepressants, MAOI antidepressants, dipyridamole, PDE-5 inhibitors, riociguat, alcohol).
   - No interactions with β-blockers, CCBs, digoxin, or furosemide.
   - Increased risk of GI ulceration if co-administered with corticosteroids.
   - Metformin has the potential to close ATP-dependent K^+ channels and may antagonize the effects and benefits of nicorandil.

4. *Pregnancy and lactation*
   - Well-controlled studies in pregnant women have failed to demonstrate a risk to the fetus (Pregnancy category B).
5. *Contraindications*
   - Hypersensitivity to nicorandil or any of the excipients.
   - Cardiogenic shock, acute pulmonary oedema, or acute MI with LV failure and low filling pressures.
   - Severe hypotension, hypovolaemia.
   - Aortic stenosis.
   - Co-administration with PDE-5 inhibitors or riociguat due to the risk of hypotension.
   - Acute pulmonary oedema.

Nifedipine

Dihydropyridine derivative L-type CCB (see ➔ Calcium channel blockers, pp. 504–9).

CV indications

- Treatment of hypertension.
- Prophylaxis of chronic stable angina pectoris, either as monotherapy or in combination.
- Treatment of Raynaud's phenomenon.

Pharmacokinetics

The pharmacokinetics varies widely between preparations and brands (see Table 8.1.6).

- *Standard preparation*: after oral administration, nifedipine is rapidly absorbed, but it undergoes a significant first-pass effect, so that its availability is approximately 45–56%, reaching peak plasma concentrations after 1–2h. Nifedipine is extensively metabolized in the liver by CYP3A4 and is excreted predominantly via the urine, but also in the faeces (approximately 5–15%). The terminal elimination t½ is 1.6–3.5h.
- *Extended-release preparations*: they have longer onsets and durations of action, as well as lower peak-to-trough fluctuations in concentrations, so that the risk of large BP variations and reflex tachycardia is reduced. Simultaneous food intake leads to delayed absorption but does not reduce total absorption. It presents a terminal t½ of approximately 6–11h.

Practical points

1. *Doses*
   - The different formulations of nifedipine are not directly interchangeable. Clinical effects vary considerably between them, due to differences in pharmacokinetics. Consequently, brands and formulations should be specified when nifedipine is prescribed.
   - *Unmodified immediate-release preparations*: 5mg tds (increased to a maximum of 20mg tds, as required) for Raynaud's phenomenon.
   - *Extended-release preparations*: 30mg, increased to 90mg (either od or bd, depending on the formulation). Modified-release nifedipine is also available in preparations containing other antihypertensive drugs.
2. *Side effects* (see ➔ Calcium channel blockers, pp. 504–9)
3. *Interactions* (see ➔ Calcium channel blockers, pp. 504–9)
   - Nifedipine decreases the plasma levels of quinidine but increases the plasma levels of digoxin and tacrolimus; dose reductions are possibly required.
   - Limit the dose of simvastatin to 20mg.
   - Cimetidine (inhibits CYP3A4) and liver disease increase nifedipine plasma levels.
   - Volatile anaesthetics and nifedipine exhibit additive cardiac inhibitory effects.

4. *Cautions/notes*
   - Nifedipine should be used with caution in patients with LV dysfunction, as worsening HF has occasionally been observed when used in high doses in the management of CAD and particularly post-MI.
   - Extended-release formulations (i.e. Adalat® LA, GITS, Procardia® XL) should not be broken or chewed, and the tablet may appear in the faeces. They should be given with caution in patients with obstructive symptoms, inflammatory bowel disease or Crohn's disease, or a history of oesophageal and GI obstruction.
   - Short-acting preparations of nifedipine produce rapid arteriolar dilatation and cause a rapid drop in BP, reflex tachycardia, and neurohumoral activation, that may lead to myocardial ischaemia and worsening of patients with ACS. Therefore, they are not recommended for the treatment of hypertension or angina.
   - Nifedipine XR contains 30mg lactose. Avoid in patients with Lapp lactase insufficiency, galactosaemia, or glucose–galactose malabsorption syndrome.
5. *Pregnancy and lactation* (see ➔ Calcium channel blockers, pp. 504–9)
6. *Contraindications* (see ➔ Calcium channel blockers, pp. 504–9)

Nitrates

(See ➔ Glyceryl trinitrate (nitroglycerin, GTN), pp. 609–12, ➔ Isosorbide dinitrate, pp. 631–2, and ➔ Isosorbide mononitrate, p. 633.)

CV indications

- Prophylaxis and treatment of effort, vasospastic, and microvascular angina. Nitrates should also be considered when angina persists despite treatment with a β-blocker or in patients unable to tolerate a β-blocker, to relieve angina. Short-acting nitrates provide acute symptomatic relief.
- Acute and chronic HF.
- IV GTN is very effective in the treatment of pain in patients with recurrent angina and ACS and in the management of severe hypertension. IV nitrates are more effective than sublingual nitrates with regard to symptom relief in NSTE-ACS.

Mechanism of action

Endothelial NO has several important functions, including relaxation of vascular smooth muscle cells (vasodilatation) via the activation of soluble guanylyl cyclase and the formation of cGMP that reduces intracellular Ca^{2+} concentrations and inhibits platelet aggregation (antithrombotic) and leucocyte–endothelial interactions (anti-inflammatory). Under physiological conditions, the endothelium releases NO that acts as an endogenous nitrate, producing coronary vasodilatation. In patients with IHD, in whom the coronary endothelium is damaged, nitrates induce the formation of NO in smooth muscle cells, i.e. nitrates act as nitrovasodilators when the endogenous production of NO is impaired.

Organic nitrates (GTN, ISDN, and ISMN) produce non-specific and direct smooth muscle relaxation that is independent of a known receptor and the presence or absence of a functional endothelium. They present in their molecule nitrate groups (R-NO2) that are chemically reduced to release NO or interact with enzymes and intracellular sulfhydryl groups that reduce the nitrate groups to S-nitrosothiols, which are then reduced to NO in the smooth muscle cell. NO can react directly with the heme moiety of soluble guanylyl cyclase (sGC) and stimulates the NO–sGC–cGMP pathway. cGMP reduces intracellular Ca^{2+} concentrations and stimulate a cGMP-dependent protein kinase (PKG) which: (1) activates the sarcolemmal Ca^{2+} efflux and increases K^{+} efflux, leading to membrane hyperpolarization that inhibits voltage-gated L-type Ca^{2+} channels; and (2) activates myosin light chain (MLC) phosphatase, the enzyme that dephosphorylates myosin light chains, which regulate the contractile state in smooth muscle. Overall, the result is vascular smooth muscle relaxaion. Like NO, nitrates inhibit platelet aggregation.

Pharmacodynamics

1. *Angina*. Organic nitrates are used extensively to treat effort and resting angina. At *therapeutic doses*, nitrates cause venous and coronary dilatation. Venodilatation promotes pooling of blood in the splanchnic and mesenteric veins and decreases venous return to the heart, thereby reducing LV end-diastolic volume and pressure and PCWP.

The preload reduction improves the signs of pulmonary congestion and decreases myocardial wall tension and ventricular size, which, in turn, reduces MVO_2. Nitrates directly vasodilate large epicardial arteries and arterioles with a diameter of >100 microns, producing a redistribution of coronary blood flow from epicardial to endocardial regions (i.e. improves subendocardial perfusion), and reduce coronary vascular tone, suppressing coronary vasospasm, especially at epicardial sites. The selective vasodilatation of large arteries in the coronary circulation increases myocardial blood flow to deeper ischaemic regions where resistance vessels are already maximally dilated by adenosine-mediated autoregulation. Additionally, the reduction of intraventricular pressure and volume indirectly decreases the mechanical compression of subendocardial vessels and increases subendocardial blood flow and the subendocardial:epicardial blood flow ratio. Nitrates also have been shown to dilate coronary collateral vessels and reverse vasoconstriction of small coronary arteries distal to a coronary obstruction.

Intracoronary GTN is often used to minimize ischaemia caused by coronary spasm.

Nitrates improve the oxygen supply:demand ratio, relieve anginal pain, and prolong exercise tolerance, time to onset of symptoms, and time to ST-depression during exercise testing both in patients with exercise and in those with resting angina. However, it is unknown whether nitrates improve survival in patients with chronic stable angina. Nitrates are highly effective in acute coronary vasospasms. In most patients, the combination of long-acting nitrates and high doses of calcium antagonists will improve the symptoms. Nitrates failed to reduce mortality in patients with ACS (UA, NSTEMI, or STEMI). Therefore, the goal of nitrate therapy in acute MI is pain relief in patients with recurrent or ongoing angina or ischaemia.

Nitrates also reduce platelet aggregation in patients with stable angina, an effect most likely mediated by the release of NO. Although the contribution of inhibition of platelet aggregation to the therapeutic efficacy of nitrates is controversial, it might have potential for preventing thrombus formation in UA.

At higher doses, nitrates produce arterial vasodilatation, reduce PVR (afterload) and BP, and increases CO, counteracting the possible decrease of CO caused by the reduction in preload. The reduction in ventricular preload and afterload improves haemodynamics without compromising stroke volume or increasing MVO_2. However, at these high doses, nitrate use is also associated with arterial hypotension and an adrenergic-mediated reflex tachycardia that can overcome the decrease in MVO_2 worsening of myocardial ischaemia.

2. *HF*. Because they reduce both pre- and afterload, nitrates are used in acute and severe chronic HF, particularly in patients with ACS. Venous dilatation reduces LVEDP and PCWP, signs of pulmonary congestion (without compromising stroke volume or increasing MVO_2), and exercise tolerance and relieves pulmonary congestion when nitrates are added to standard therapy. Arterial dilatation reduces LV afterload on the failing ventricle and leads to an increase in stroke volume and ejection fraction. Reduction in both afterload and preload improves

mechanical efficiency of the heart and reduces wall stress and MVO_2 on the failing heart. The overall effect on CO depends on the LVEDP. When LVEDP is high, nitrates can increase CO; when LVEDP is normal, nitrates do not modify, or can even decrease, CO when the LVEDP decreases below 12mmHg. Nitrates should not be administered to patients with acute inferior MI with RV involvement, because the decrease in preload may aggravate hypotension. IV administration of GTN or ISDN may be considered in patients with pulmonary congestion/oedema and an SBP of >110mmHg, who do not have severe mitral or aortic stenosis, to reduce PCWP and PVR.

Hydralazine and isosorbide dinitrate should be considered in self-identified black patients with LVEF ≤35% or with an LVEF <45% combined with a dilated LV in NYHA class III–IV despite treatment with an ACEI, a beta-blocker and an MRA to reduce the risk of HF hospitalization and death.

Hydralazine and isosorbide dinitrate may be considered in symptomatic patients with HFrEF who cannot tolerate either an ACEI or an ARB (or they are contraindicated) to reduce the risk of death. This recommendation is based on a study which recruited symptomatic HFrEF patients who received only digoxin and diuretics.

Pharmacokinetics

Nitrates are rapidly absorbed from the skin, mucous membranes, or GI tract and undergo enzymatic denitration to release NO. (See Table 8.1.11.)

Practical points

1. *Doses* (see ➲ Glyceryl trinitrate (nitroglycerin, GTN), pp. 609–12, ➲ Isosorbide dinitrate, pp. 631–2, and ➲ Isosorbide mononitrate, p. 633)
   - Rapidly acting formulations of GTN or ISDN provide rapid and effective symptom relief, being the drugs of choice to treat acute anginal attacks. The effect of GTN is almost immediate, while the onset effect of sublingual ISDN is slower, so that it should be prescribed in patients unresponsive or intolerant to sublingual administration of GTN. Both drugs are useful to prevent anginal attacks if taken a few minutes before activities known to possibly cause an attack ('situational prophylaxis'). An anginal attack that does not respond to GTN should be regarded as a possible MI.
2. *Common side effects*
   - (≥10%): headaches that necessitate either a dose reduction or cessation of treatment (25–50%) and flushing. Headaches disappear or decrease in intensity after prolonged usage (1–2 weeks). Aspirin relieves headaches, improves drug compliance, and protects from coronary events.
   - (0.1–10%): dizziness, facial flushing, nausea, vomiting; hypotension, tachycardia, bradycardia (in patients with acute MI), vertigo, nervousness, dizziness, light-headedness, cold sweats, syncope. Overdosing may cause postural hypotension and reflex cardiac sympathetic activation with tachycardia, leading to 'paradoxical' angina. Hypotension is more frequent in volume-depleted or already

hypotensive patients and, on some occasions, can lead to syncope. When GTN results in bradycardia and hypotension, discontinuation of the drug, leg elevation, rapid fluid administration, and atropine are appropriate. In patients with cor pulmonale, the vasodilator effect of nitrates may also produce venous mixture and aggravate hypoxaemia by increasing V/Q mismatch.

- Others: postprandial hypotension, blurred vision, halitosis (sublingual formulations). Methaemoglobinaemia with prolonged high doses (very rarely); give IV methylene blue (1–2mg/kg).
- Cutaneous rash or exfoliative dermatitis are observed with topical preparations (ointment, patch). To avoid irritation, it is advisable to rotate the site of application.
- The safety and effectiveness in paediatric patients have not been established.

3. *Interactions*
    - The vasodilator effect of nitrates can be potentiated by β-blockers, CCBs, ACEIs, ARBs, diuretics, alcohol, neuroleptics, and tricyclic antidepressants.
    - Nitrates, β-blockers, and CCBs are combined in many patients with angina pectoris. These three group of drugs decrease MVO_2; nitrates and CCBs also increase coronary blood flow, and β-blockers suppress the tachycardia induced by nitrates.
    - Life-threatening hypotension and myocardial ischaemia appear when nitrates are co-administered with PDE-5 inhibitors (e.g. sildenafil, tadalafil, vardenafil) in patients with erectile dysfunction or PAH. Nitrates may be started 24h after sildenafil or vardenafil and 48h after taladafil. In cases of inadvertent PDE-5–nitrate combinations, emergency α-adrenergic agonists (noradrenaline) may be needed.
    - In men with prostatic problems taking tamsulosin, nitrates can be prescribed.
4. *Cautions/notes*
    - Only short-acting nitrates (but not long-acting nitrates with slow onset of action) should be used in the management of acute angina attacks. Sublingual GTN can be used 5–10min to prevent chest pain before physical activity.
    - Symptoms and haemodynamics should be monitored frequently during administration of IV nitrates. Because the hypotension associated with GTN overdose is due to venodilatation and hypovolaemia, therapy should be directed to increase central fluid volume.
    - The hypotensive effects of nitrates are potentiated by concurrent administration of PDE-5 inhibitors used for the treatment of erectile dysfunction or PAH, which markedly increase the fall in BP, leading to severe side effects (e.g. syncopes, paradoxical myocardial ischaemia). This combination is contraindicated.
    - It is useful to warn the patient of the need to protect against potential hypotension by sitting on the first number of occasions when taking sublingual nitrate and also of other possible side effects, particularly headache.

5. *Nitrate tolerance*

A limitation of nitrates is a reduction in the intensity and duration of their effects when they are taken over a prolonged period without a nitrate-free or nitrate-low interval of about 8–10h (tolerance). Nitrate tolerance appears with all nitrates, and there is cross-tolerance between formulations, which explains the poor protection against angina attacks and resistance to the pain-relieving effects of short-acting GTN in patients treated with long-acting nitrates. Tolerance appears within 8–24h of administration of preparations that allow for maintenance of stable plasma nitrate levels (IV patch), but the vasodilator response recovered quickly after a short (8–24h) 'nitrate-free interval'. Thus, patients treated with transdermal GTN patches should remove them during part of the day or at night to achieve the nitrate-free interval.

Nitrate tolerance has been attributed to:

- Impaired bioactivation of nitrates, leading to a decrease in the release of NO, due to inhibition of mitochondrial aldehyde dehydrogenase (GTN) or cytochrome P450 reductase (ISMN, ISDN). Tolerance to GTN is associated with an impairment to its conversion to glyceryl-1,2-dinitrate, and tolerance to ISDN with its denitration to 2-mononitrate (15–25%) and 5-mononitrate (75–85%). Inhibition of both enzymes is associated with an increase in the production of free radicals. GTN can potently and rapidly inactivate aldehyde dehydrogenase, including aldehyde dehydrogenase 2.
- Increased endothelial and vascular smooth muscle formation of free radicals (peroxynitrite, superoxide) from nicotinamide adenine dinucleotide phosphate (NADPH) oxidase activation by protein kinase C, leading to endothelial dysfunction. This can lead to:
    - Direct inhibition of nitric oxide synthase (NOS) activation and NO availability.
    - Increased clearance of NO.
    - Uncoupling of endothelial NOS caused by limited BH4 availability, resulting from peroxynitrite-induced oxidation of BH4 and reduced expression of GTP-cyclohydrolase I (GTPCH-I).
    - Increased inactivation of cGMP by PDEs.
    - Inhibition of smooth muscle sGC by superoxide and peroxynitrite, leading to a decrease in the intracellular levels of cGMP.
- Increased release of vasoconstrictors (angiotensin II, catecholamines, endothelin) that counteract the vasodilator effect of nitrates.

Tolerance can be avoided by intermittent dosing, leaving at least a 10-h dose-free interval every day or using eccentric dosage schedules with 8–12h nitrate-free intervals. Patients should remove the patches during part of the day or at night to achieve the nitrate-free interval. Hydralazine can overcome tolerance, and sulfhydryl donors (i.e. acetylcysteine, hydralazine, ACEIs, carvedilol, nebivolol, atorvastatin) can potentiate the effects of nitrates, although it is unclear whether these drugs can prevent tolerance.

6. *Pregnancy and lactation*
    - Safety of nitrates in pregnancy and breastfeeding have not been established (Pregnancy category C). Nitrates should be given to a pregnant woman only if clearly needed.

7. *Contraindications*
   - Hypertrophic obstructive cardiomyopathy (nitrates may exaggerate outflow obstruction), constrictive pericarditis, mitral/aortic stenosis, cardiac tamponade.
   - Hypotension (SBP <90mmHg), hypovolaemia.
   - Severe cerebrovascular insufficiency, head trauma, cerebral haemorrhage.
   - Acute inferior MI with RV involvement, because they may aggravate hypotension.
   - Treatment with PDE-5 inhibitors (e.g. sildenafil, tadalafil, vardenafil).
   - Marked anaemia.
   - Closed-angle glaucoma.
   - Acute circulatory failure (shock, circulatory collapse), hypotensive shock.
   - Cardiogenic shock, unless intra-aortic counterpulsation or positively inotropic drugs ensure an adequately high LVEDP.
   - Hypersensitivity to nitrates.

Noradrenaline

Sympathetic neurotransmitter.

Indications

- For restoration of BP in cases of acute hypotension. Noradrenaline may be considered in patients with cardiogenic shock, despite treatment with another inotrope, to increase BP and vital organ perfusion. It should be used when a shock-like state is accompanied by peripheral vasodilatation ('*warm shock*').

Mechanism of action

Sympathomimetic drug with prominent β1- and α-effects and less β2-stimulation.

Pharmacodynamics

Noradrenaline produces simultaneous stimulation of α- and β-adrenergic receptors in the heart and vessels. Noradrenaline is a peripheral vasoconstrictor (α-adrenergic action) that increases PVR and BP. Vasoconstriction may result in decreased blood flow in the kidneys, liver, skin, and smooth muscles; the increase in BP may cause a reflex decrease in heart rate. It is also a coronary vasodilator and a positive inotropic agent (β-adrenergic action). Local vasoconstriction may cause haemostasis and/or necrosis.

Pharmacokinetics

Noradrenaline is rapidly degraded and should be administered by the IV route. The effect on BP disappears 1–3min after stopping the infusion.

Practical points

1. *Doses*
   - Initial rate of infusion of 0.05–0.8mg/h of noradrenaline base (0.2–1.0mcg/kg/min). Once an infusion of noradrenaline is established, the dose should be titrated in steps of 0.05–0.1mcg/kg/min of noradrenaline base, according to the pressor effect observed. Noradrenaline should be continued for as long as vasoactive drug support is indicated. The aim should be to establish a low normal SBP (100–120mmHg) or to achieve an adequate mean arterial BP (>65–80mmHg—depending on the patient's condition). Administer as a diluted solution via a CVC. The infusion should be at a controlled rate, using either a syringe pump or an infusion pump or a drip counter.
2. *Side effects*
   - Headache, tachycardia, bradycardia, hypertension, arrhythmias, hypoxia, anxiety, respiratory difficulty. Severe peripheral vasoconstriction. Extravasation necrosis at the injection site. Prolonged administration of any potent vasopressor may result in plasma volume depletion, which should be continuously corrected by appropriate fluid and electrolyte replacement therapy. If noradrenaline is continuously administered to maintain BP in the absence of blood volume replacement, severe peripheral and visceral vasoconstriction, decreased renal perfusion and urine output, poor systemic blood flow despite 'normal' BP, tissue hypoxia, and lactic acidosis may occur.

3. *Interactions*
   - Cyclopropane and halothane anaesthetics sensitize the myocardium to the effect of noradrenaline. Avoid this combination because of the risk of VT/VF.
   - Noradrenaline should be administered with extreme caution in patients receiving MAOIs, tricyclic antidepressants, or adrenergic-serotoninergic drugs, because severe, prolonged hypertension may result.
4. *Cautions/notes*
   - Noradrenaline should only be administered by healthcare professionals who are familiar with its use and in conjunction with appropriate volume replacement.
   - Noradrenaline can cause sinus tachycardia and may induce myocardial ischaemia and arrhythmias; thus, ECG monitoring is required.
   - Special caution in patients with coronary, mesenteric, or peripheral vascular thrombosis, because noradrenaline may increase the ischaemia and extend the area of infarction. Similar caution in patients with hypotension following MI and in patients with variant angina, diabetes mellitus, hypertension, or hyperthyroidism.
   - The risk of cardiac arrhythmias increases in patients with profound hypoxia or hypercarbia.
   - Extravasation of the solution may cause local tissue necrosis. If extravasation occurs, the infusion should be stopped and the area should be infiltrated with phentolamine without delay.
5. *Pregnancy and lactation*
   - Noradrenaline may impair placental perfusion and induce fetal bradycardia (Pregnancy category C). It may also exert a contractile effect on the uterus and lead to fetal asphyxia in late pregnancy.
6. *Contraindications*
   - Hypotension from blood volume deficits, except as an emergency measure to maintain coronary and cerebral artery perfusion until blood volume replacement can be completed.
   - Mesenteric or peripheral vascular thrombosis.
   - Cyclopropane and halothane anaesthetics.
   - Profound hypoxia or hypercarbia.
   - Late pregnancy and pre-existing excess vasoconstriction.

Olmesartan medoxomil

Selective angiotensin AT1 receptor antagonist (see ➲ Angiotensin II AT1 receptor blockers, pp. 456–8).

Indications

- Treatment of hypertension.

Pharmacodynamics

Olmesartan (40mg/day) delays the onset of microalbuminuria in patients with T2DM and normoalbuminuria.

Pharmacokinetics

Olmesartan medoxomil is a prodrug that is converted to the pharmacologically active metabolite olmesartan by esterases from the GI tract. Food does not affect its oral bioavailability. The AUC and C_{max} increase in patients with moderate hepatic impairment. The AUC also increases in patients with severe renal impairment (CrCl <20mL/min). (See Table 8.1.9.)

Practical points

1. *Doses*
   - *Starting dose*: 10mg od in patients who are not volume-contracted. The dose can be increased to 40mg. No dosage adjustment is required in the elderly or in patients with mild hepatic impairment. The maximum dose in patients with CrCl of 20–60mL/min is 20mg od, and in patients with moderate hepatic impairment, it should not exceed 20mg od.
2. *Side effects* (see ➲ Angiotensin II AT1 receptor blockers, pp. 456–8)
   - The commonest side effects are: headache, dizziness, back pain, bronchitis, rhinitis, increase in blood CPK, diarrhoea, dyspepsia, gastroenteritis, hyperglycaemia, hypertriglyceridaemia, influenza-like symptoms, and rash,
3. *Interactions*
   - No significant drug interactions were reported with antacids, digoxin, warfarin, or CYP450 inducers/inhibitors.
   - In elderly people and in patients who are volume-depleted or with impaired renal function, co-administration of NSAIDs with olmesartan medoxomil may result in deterioration of renal function. Monitor the renal function in these patients.
   - Colesevelam reduces systemic exposure and peak plasma concentrations of olmesartan. To avoid possible interactions, olmesartan should be administered at least 4h before colesevelam.
4. *Cautions* (see ➲ Angiotensin II AT1 receptor blockers, pp. 456–8)
   - The antihypertensive effect of olmesartan may be attenuated by NSAIDs.
   - Olmesartan increases serum lithium concentrations and lithium toxicity. Monitor serum lithium levels during concomitant use.
5. *Pregnancy and lactation* (see ➲ Angiotensin II AT1 receptor blockers, pp. 456–8)
6. *Contraindications* (see ➲ Angiotensin II AT1 receptor blockers, pp. 456–8)

Omega-3-fatty acids (ethyl esters)

The omega-3 series of polyunsaturated fatty acids contain eicosapentaenoic acid (EPA) and docosahexaenoic acid (DHA). Both are essential fatty acids.

CV indications

- Adjuvant treatment in secondary prevention after MI, in addition to other standard therapy (e.g. statins, antiplatelet medicinal products, β-blockers, ACEIs).
- Endogenous hypertriglyceridaemia as a supplement to diet when dietary measures alone are insufficient to produce an adequate response: (1) type IV in monotherapy; and (2) type IIb/III in combination with statins, when control of TGs is insufficient. However, it is not indicated in exogenous hypertriglyceridaemia (type 1 hyperchylomicronaemia).

Mechanism of action

Omega-3-fatty acids reduce the hepatic synthesis of TGs, leading to a decrease in serum TG levels up to 45% by several mechanisms: (1) reduce substrate availability, as EPA and DHA are poor substrates for the enzymes responsible for TG synthesis; (2) decrease the activity of TG-synthesizing enzymes (diacylglycerol acyltranferase, phosphatidic acid phosphohydrolase, and hormone-sensitive lipase; and (3) increase peroxisomal β-oxidation of fatty acids in the liver and stimulate Apo B degradation. All these effects reduce the quantity of free fatty acids available for the synthesis of TGs and the hepatic release of VLDL-C. Their effects on other lipoproteins are trivial, although LDL-C can increase in some patients.

Omega-3-fatty acids also decrease thromboxane A2 and inhibit platelet aggregation and produce vasodilatation and antiarrhythmic and anti-inflammatory effects.

Pharmacodynamics

Diets leading to high consumption of long-chain omega-3 fatty acids are associated with a low prevalence of CAD in epidemiological studies. Some studies found that omega-3 fish oils reduce the combined endpoint of all-cause and CV deaths and non-fatal MI, but with no reduction in non-fatal CV events or fatal and non-fatal strokes.

In patients with severe hypertriglyceridaemia, Omacor® (one capsule contains approximately 465mg of EPA and 380mg of DHA) significantly reduces mean TG (45%), total-C (15%), VLDL-C (32%), and LDL-C (31%) levels, and increases HDL-C (13%) levels. The effect of Omacor® on the risk of pancreatitis in patients with very high TG levels has not been evaluated.

Pharmacokinetics

Omega-3 fatty acids are absorbed when administered as ethyl esters orally and induce an increase in serum phospholipid EPA content (increases in DHA content are less marked). Omega-3 fatty acids can be: (1) transported to the liver where they are incorporated into various lipoproteins and then channelled to the peripheral lipid stores; (2) incorporated in cell membrane phospholipids and can then act as precursors for various eicosanoids; and (3) oxidized to meet energy requirements.

Practical points

1. *Doses*
   - *Post-MI*: one capsule daily.
   - *Hypertriglyceridaemia*: two capsules daily; the dose may be increased to four capsules daily.
3. *Side effects*
   - Common: GI disorders (abdominal distension, abdominal pain, constipation, diarrhoea, dyspepsia, flatulence, eructation, gastro-oesophageal reflux disease, nausea, or vomiting).
   - Uncommon: epistaxis, hyperglycaemia, gout, dizziness, dysgeusia, headache, hypotension, rash, epistaxis, and GI haemorrhage.
   - Rare: increase in transaminases, skin rash, urticaria.
   - Their antithrombotic effects may increase the propensity to bleeding, especially when given in addition to aspirin/clopidogrel.
4. *Interactions*
   - High doses (4g daily) of omega-3 fatty acids prolong bleeding time, so that patients receiving anticoagulant therapy should be monitored periodically. Monitor the PT when combined with warfarin.
   - Monitoring of hepatic function is required in hepatic impairment, especially with high doses.
5. *Cautions/notes*
   - The capsules may be taken with food to avoid GI disturbances.
6. *Pregnancy and lactation*
   - Potential risk unknown (Pregnancy category C). Should not be used during pregnancy and lactation, unless clearly necessary.
7. *Contraindications*
   - Hypersensitivity to the active substance, soya, or any of the excipients.

Patiromer

The active ingredient is patiromer sorbitex calcium, which consists of the active moiety patiromer, a non-absorbed cation exchange polymer, and a calcium-sorbitol counterion.

Indications

It is indicated for the treatment of hyperkalaemia.

Mechanism of action

Patiromer binds potassium in the lumen of the GI tract, particularly in the colon, and increases its faecal excretion, leading to a reduction of serum K^+ levels. It also binds magnesium in the colon, leading to hypomagnesaemia.

Pharmacokinetics

Patiromer is not absorbed systemically following oral administration and is excreted in the faeces. No differences in effectiveness were observed between young and elderly (≥75 years), and no dose adjustments are needed for patients with CKD. Drug efficacy and safety have not been analysed in paediatric patients.

Practical points

1. *Doses*
   - The recommended starting dose is 8.4g PO od. The dose can be uptitrated, based on serum K^+ levels at 1-week or longer intervals, in increments of 8.4g, up to a maximum dose of 25.2g od. No dose adjustments are needed in renal impairment. The oral suspension should be prepared and the mixture taken immediately after preparation with food.
2. *Side effects*
   - The commonest side effects are: constipation, hypomagnesaemia, diarrhoea, nausea, abdominal discomfort, and flatulence. Older patients reported more GI adverse reactions. Approximately 4.7% of patients developed hypokalaemia (<3.5mEq/L) and approximately 9% hypomagnesaemia (<1.4mg/dL).
   - Patiromer binds many orally administered medications, which could decrease their GI absorption and reduce their efficacy.
3. *Interactions*
   - In healthy volunteers, patiromer does not alter the systemic exposure of amlodipine, cinacalcet, clopidogrel, furosemide, lithium, metoprolol, trimethoprim, verapamil, or warfarin. However, patiromer decreases the exposure of ciprofloxacin, levothyroxine, and metformin; no interaction when patiromer and these drugs were taken 3h apart.
4. *Cautions/notes*
   - Severe constipation, bowel obstruction, or impaction, including abnormal post-operative bowel motility disorders, because patiromer may be ineffective and may worsen GI conditions.

- To avoid possible interactions, other oral medications should be administered at least 3h before or after patiromer. Monitor for clinical response when possible.
- Patiromer can produce hypomagnesaemia; consider magnesium supplementation.

5. *Pregnancy and lactation*
   - Patiromer is not absorbed systemically following oral administration; thus, it is not expected to be harmful during pregnancy or lactation.
6. *Contraindications*
   - Patients with hypersensitivity to patiromer or any of its components.

Pentoxifylline

Xanthine derivative.

Indications

- Treatment of peripheral vascular disease, including intermittent claudication and rest pain.

Mechanism of action

Pentoxifylline is a competitive, non-selective PDE inhibitor, which activates cAMP–PKA signalling, inhibits TNF-α and leucotriene synthesis, and reduces inflammation.

Pharmacodynamics

Pentoxifylline improves blood flow by decreasing blood viscosity and increasing red blood cell flexibility. In a comparative trial, cilostazol, but not pentoxifylline, improved both functional status and the walking impairment questionnaire. Thus, benefits of pentoxifylline are marginal and not well established.

Pharmacokinetics

After oral administration, pentoxifylline bioavailability is 10–30%, reaching peak plasma levels within 1h. It is extensively metabolized in the liver, and several metabolites reach plasma levels 5–8 times greater than pentoxifylline. The t½ of pentoxifylline is 0.4–0.8h, and that of its metabolites 1–1.6h. Drug excretion is mainly urinary, with 50–80% as metabolites (<5% is recovered in the faeces).

Practical points

1. Doses
   - 400mg tds. Renal impairment (CrCl <30mL/min): decrease the dose to 400mg/day.
2. *Side effects*
   - Nausea, vomiting, dizziness, easy bruising/bleeding, allergic reactions.
3. *Interactions*
   - Pentoxifylline increases the anticoagulant activity of VKAs, exerts an additive effect with platelet aggregation inhibitors and antihypertensive agents, and can intensify the hypoglycaemic action of insulin and oral hypoglycaemic agents.
4. *Cautions/notes*
   - Careful monitoring is required in patients with risk factors for haemorrhage or impaired renal function.
   - Pentoxifylline may increase theophylline plasma levels in some patients.
5. *Pregnancy and lactation*
   - There are no controlled data in human pregnancy (Pregnancy category C). Pentoxifylline and its metabolites are excreted into human milk.
6. *Contraindications*
   - Hypersensitivity to pentoxifylline or xanthine derivatives.
   - Recent retinal or cerebral haemorrhage.

Perindopril

Orally active ACEI (see ➲ Angiotensin-converting enzyme inhibitors, pp. 459–64).

Indications

- Treatment of hypertension.
- Treatment of symptomatic HFrEF.
- Reduction of risk of cardiac events in patients with a history of MI and/or revascularization.

Pharmacokinetics

About 25% of administered perindopril reaches the bloodstream as the active metabolite perindoprilat, which reaches peak concentrations within 3–4h. Ingestion of food decreases the conversion to perindoprilat, and hence its bioavailability; thus, perindopril should be administered orally in the morning before a meal. Elimination of perindoprilat is decreased in the elderly and in patients with heart or renal failure. In patients with cirrhosis, hepatic clearance of the parent molecule is reduced by half. (See Table 8.1.10.)

Practical points

1. *Doses*
   - *Hypertension, diabetes, and CV risk*: 2–4mg od in the morning (2mg in the elderly), titrated to a maximum of 8mg, if required.
   - *HF*: 2mg od. This dose may be increased after 2 weeks to 4mg od, if tolerated.

   Doses should be reduced in patients with renal impairment, as follows:

CrCl	Maximum dose
>60mL/min	4mg/day
30–60mL/min	2mg/day
15–30mL/min	2mg on alternate days
Haemodialysis	2mg on day of dialysis

2. *Side effects* (see ➲ Angiotensin-converting enzyme inhibitors, pp. 459–64)
3. *Interactions* (see ➲ Angiotensin-converting enzyme inhibitors, pp. 459–64)
4. *Cautions/notes* (see ➲ Angiotensin-converting enzyme inhibitors, pp. 459–64)
5. *Contraindications* (see ➲ Angiotensin-converting enzyme inhibitors, pp. 459–64)

Perhexiline

Anti-anginal drug with a narrow therapeutic index and high inter- and intra-individual pharmacokinetic variability.

Indications

- Anti-anginal drug for patients who have contraindications or do not respond to other anti-anginal drugs.

Mechanism of action

Perhexiline inhibits mitochondrial carnitine palmitoyl transferase 1 (and 2) and shifts the myocardial substrate of utilization from free fatty acids to glucose oxidation, resulting in increased glucose and lactate utilization. This results in increased ATP production for the same oxygen consumption and increases myocardial efficiency during myocardial ischaemia. Perhexiline also potentiates platelet responsiveness to NO.

Pharmacodynamics

Perhexiline relieves symptoms of angina, improves exercise tolerance, and increases the workload needed to induce ischaemia when used as monotherapy. Perhexiline is used as short-term therapy (<3 months' duration) in patients with severe ischaemia awaiting coronary revascularization and as long-term therapy in patients with ischaemic symptoms refractory to other therapeutic measures.

Pharmacokinetics

Perhexiline is well absorbed (>80%) from the GI tract. It is highly protein-bound (>90%) and is extensively metabolized by CYP2D6, and only 0.1% of a dose is eliminated as unchanged drug in the urine. Its t½ is long and variable, and ranges from 1 to 2 days in extensive metabolizers to up to 30–40 days in poor metabolizers.

Practical points

1. *Doses*
   - *Starting dose*: 100mg PO daily; the dose can be increased at 2- 4-weekly intervals, based on the results of plasma level monitoring, up to a maximum dose of 300mg/day.
2. *Side effects*
   - The most commonly reported side effects are headache, dizziness, nausea and vomiting, hypoglycaemia in diabetic patients, hypertriglyceridaemia, and weight loss. Rare cases of TdP. At plasma concentrations of >0.6mg/L, perhexiline can cause muscle weakness, ataxia, peripheral neuropathy (sometimes not reversible), and hepatitis/cirrhosis (potentially fatal hepatotoxicity). These serious side effects are associated with CYP2D6 polymorphisms. Serum liver enzymes [SGPT, SGOT, alkaline phosphatase, lactate dehydrogenase (LDH)] should be assessed prior to treatment and at least every month thereafter.

3. *Interactions*
    - Perhexiline can increase doxorubicin toxicity.
    - CYP2D6 inhibitors or substrates can increase perhexiline exposure (see Table 8.1.2); monitor perhexiline blood levels, and dose adjustment may be required.
4. *Cautions/notes*
    - Plasma perhexiline concentrations should be maintained between 0.15 and 0.60mcg/mL.
    - Perhexiline is not recommended in patients with hepatic or renal impairment.
    - The safety and efficacy of perhexiline following MI have not been established.
    - Perhexiline can aggravate ventricular conduction disturbances.
    - Perhexiline increases the risk of hypoglycaemia in diabetic patients receiving insulin or sulfonylureas over the first 3 days of therapy. Monitor blood glucose levels.
5. *Pregnancy and lactation*
    - It is not known whether it enters breast milk or crosses the placenta (Pregnancy category B).
6. *Contraindications*
    - History of porphyria.
    - Impaired hepatic or renal function.
    - Known hypersensitivity to perhexiline maleate or any of the ingredients.

Phenoxybenzamine

Non-selective, non-competitive, long-acting, α-adrenergic receptor antagonist.

CV indications

- Hypertensive episodes associated with phaeochromocytoma.

Mechanism of action

It is a non-selective, irreversible α-adrenergic receptor antagonist, preventing adrenaline and noradrenaline from binding.

Pharmacodynamics

Block of α-adrenoceptors produces vasodilatation and decreases PVR and BP. Concomitant β-adrenergic blockade may be necessary to control tachycardia and arrhythmias when tumours of the adrenal gland secrete an appreciable amount of adrenaline and/or noradrenaline.

Pharmacokinetics

Approximately 20–30% of the oral dose is absorbed. Onset of action is gradual over several hours, and the effects persist for 3–4 days after a single oral dose, possibly due, in part, to its stable covalent bonding. Phenoxybenzamine is extensively metabolized in the liver and excreted in the urine and bile. The t½ is approximately 24h.

Practical points

1. *Doses*
   - *PO*: 10mg od. This may be increased by 10mg daily until control of hypertensive episodes is achieved or postural hypotension occurs. Concomitant β-adrenergic blockade may be necessary to control tachycardia and arrhythmias.
2. *Side effects*
   - Postural hypotension, dizziness, and compensatory tachycardia. Inhibition of ejaculation, nasal congestion, GI disturbances, drowsiness, and weakness. A sudden and drastic fall in BP can occur after administering the first dose. Post-operative hypotension can be avoided by discontinuing the drug several days before an operation.
3. *Interactions*
   - Risk of hypotension when combined with antihypertensive or vasodilator drugs.
4. *Cautions/notes*
   - Use with caution in patients in whom a BP fall or tachycardia is undesirable (e.g. elderly, HF, CV disease, renal disease). Tachycardia which can be controlled with a cardioselective β-blocker. In patients with a phaeochromocytoma, β-blockers must never be used prior to adequate α-blockade (for 1 week) to avoid a hypertensive crisis.
   - In patients treated with drugs that stimulate both α- and β-adrenergic receptors (i.e. adrenaline), phenoxybenzamine can produce hypotension and tachycardia.

- Administer with caution in patients with marked cerebral or coronary arteriosclerosis or renal damage.
- Avoid intake of alcohol or other sedating medications to prevent excessive drowsiness and dizziness.

5. *Pregnancy and lactation*
   - There is no evidence of safety in pregnancy, and so it should not be used in pregnancy unless essential (Pregnancy category B). It is also excreted in breast milk and can cause hypotension in the newborn; avoid during breastfeeding.
6. *Contraindication*
   - Any conditions in which a fall in BP is undesirable.
   - CVA; during the recovery period (usually 3–4 weeks) post-MI.
   - Hypersensitivity to the drug or its components

Pitavastatin

HMG CoA reductase inhibitor (see ➲ Statins (3-hydroxy-3-methylglutaryl-coenzyme A reductase inhibitors), pp. 760–3).

Indications

It is indicated as an adjunctive therapy in adult patients with primary hyperlipidaemia or mixed dyslipidaemia to reduce elevated total-C, LDL-C, Apo B, and TG levels and to increase HDL-C levels.

Pharmacodynamics

Depending on the dose, pitavastatin can be expected to reduce LDL-C (31–45%) and TG (13–22%) levels and increase HDL-C levels by 1–8%.

Pharmacokinetics

A high-fat meal decreases the C_{max} of pitavastatin by 43% but does not reduce the AUC. The C_{max} and AUC are higher in women. Pitavastatin is metabolized by hepatic uridine 5′-diphosphate glucuronosyltransferases (UGT1A3 and UGT2B7) but is marginally metabolized via CYP2C9 (and CYP2C8). Age, race, and gender have no effect on drug pharmacokinetics. Its t½ increases with moderate hepatic impairment. (See Table 8.1.4.)

Practical points

1. *Doses*
   - 1–4mg od at any time of the day, with or without food. Doses of >4mg od are associated with an increased risk for severe myopathy and should be avoided. In patients with moderate to severe renal impairment or in haemodialysis, the starting dose is 1mg od and the maximum dose 2mg od.
2. *Side effects* (see ➲ Statins (3-hydroxy-3-methylglutaryl-coenzyme A reductase inhibitors), pp. 760–3)
3. *Interactions* (see ➲ Statins (3-hydroxy-3-methylglutaryl-coenzyme A reductase inhibitors), pp. 760–3)
   - Pitavastatin is unlikely to interact with CYP3A4 inhibitors/inducers and does not interact with antiretrovirals.
   - Ciclosporin, erythromycin, and rifampicin reduce the clearance of pitavastatin and increase the C_{max} of pitavastatin 6.6-, 3.6-, and 2-fold, respectively. With erythromycin, the maximal dose of pitavastatin is 1mg od, and in patients taking rifampicin 2mg od. Co-administration of ciclosporin is contraindicated.
   - Metabolism of pitavastatin via CYP2C9 is unaffected by gemfibrozil.
4. *Cautions/notes* (see ➲ Statins (3-hydroxy-3-methylglutaryl-coenzyme A reductase inhibitors), pp. 760–3)
   - In patients with moderate to severe renal impairment, the C_{max} of pitavastatin increases by 60% and 40%, respectively.
   - The C_{max} of pitavastatin increases 2.7-fold in patients with moderate hepatic impairment (Child–Pugh B disease).
5. *Pregnancy and lactation* (see ➲ Statins (3-hydroxy-3-methylglutaryl-coenzyme A reductase inhibitors), pp. 760–3)
6. *Contraindications* (see ➲ Statins (3-hydroxy-3-methylglutaryl-coenzyme A reductase inhibitors), pp. 760–3)
   - Hypersensitivity to any component of this product.
   - Co-administration with ciclosporin.

Positive inotropic agents

Digoxin, dobutamine, dopamine, levosimendan, and PDE-3 inhibitors (milrinone).

Indications

In patients with acute HF:

- Short-term IV infusion of inotropic agents may be reserved for patients with systolic HF, hypotension (SBP <90mmHg), and/or signs/symptoms of hypoperfusion despite adequate filling status, to increase cardiac contractility and CO, to reduce LV filling pressures, to increase BP, to improve peripheral perfusion, and to maintain end-organ function. They should be used with caution, starting from rather low doses and uptitrating, with close monitoring.

An IV infusion of levosimendan or a PDE-3 inhibitor may be considered to reverse the effect of β-blockers if they are thought to be contributing to hypotension with subsequent hypoperfusion.

Mechanism of action

(See ➔ Digoxin, pp. 542–6, ➔ Dobutamine, pp. 555–8, ➔ Dopamine, pp. 559–61, ➔ Levosimendan, pp. 639–40, and ➔ Milrinone, pp. 664–5).

Sympathomimetics (dopamine, dobutamine) increase extracelular Ca^{2+} entry through L-type channels, Ca^{2+} transients, and cardiac contractility by increasing cellular levels of 3′,5′-cAMP in cardiac myocytes, leading to the activation of cAMP-dependent PKA. PKA produces the phosphorylation of: (1) L-type Ca^{2+} channels, increasing extracellular Ca^{2+} entry during the plateau phase of the cardiac action potential; (2) ryanodine receptors (RyR2) located in the SR, which induces further release of Ca^{2+} at this level via a Ca^{2+}-induced Ca^{2+} release mechanism—as a result of both mechanisms, the $[Ca^{2+}]i$ and the contractile force increase; (3) phospholamban, so that its ability to inhibit Ca^{2+} transport via SERCA2a is lost, enhancing Ca^{2+} uptake by the SR; and (4) troponin I, which decreases Ca^{2+} affinity of the contactile proteins. These two latter effects result in an acceleration of cardiac relaxation. Thus, inotropic agents that increase cAMP levels produce both inotropic and lusitropic effects.

Pharmacodynamics

When needed, inotropic agents should be administered as early as possible and withdrawn as soon as adequate organ perfusion is restored and/or congestion reduced. Although inotropes may acutely improve signs, symptoms, and haemodynamics in patients with acute HF, they may promote and accelerate the progression of HF, causing further myocardial injury. Indeed, dopamine, dobutamine, milrinone, noradrenaline, and adrenaline increase in-hospital mortality, as compared with patients treated solely with diuretics and vasodilators.

In some patients with cardiogenic shock, inotropic agents may stabilize patients at risk of progressive haemodynamic collapse or serve as a life-sustaining bridge to mechanical circulatory support, ventricular assist devices, or cardiac transplantation.

Practical points

1. *Cautions*
   - Use of an inotrope should be reserved for patients with a severe reduction in CO resulting in compromised vital organ perfusion, which occurs most often in hypotensive acute HF.
   - It is recommended to monitor ECG and BP when using inotropic agents, as they can cause sinus tachycardia and ventricular arrhythmias and increase myocardial ischaemia. Effects of dopamine on BP vary according to the dose used; levosimendan and PDE-3 inhibitors also cause hypotension.
   - Inotropic agents are not recommended in cases of hypotensive acute HF where the underlying cause is hypovolaemia or other potentially correctable factors, before elimination of these causes.
   - Inotropic agents should be prescribed in hospitalized patients under close monitoring.

Prasugrel

Inhibitor of platelet activation and aggregation through the irreversible binding of its active metabolite to the P2Y12 class of ADP receptors on platelets.

Indications

- Co-administered with ASA, is indicated for the prevention of atherothrombotic events in adult patients with ACS (i.e. UA/NSTEMI or STEMI) undergoing primary or delayed PCI.

Mechanism of action

Prasugrel inhibits platelet activation and aggregation through the irreversible binding of its active metabolite to the P2Y12 class of ADP receptors on platelets.

Pharmacodynamics

Following a 60mg loading dose, prasugrel produces 50% inhibition of ADP-induced platelet aggregation by 1h. Mean maximum steady-state inhibition (approximately 70–80%) of platelet aggregation can be reached after 3–5 days of dosing at 10mg daily after a 60mg loading dose. Platelet aggregation gradually returns to baseline values over 5–9 days after discontinuation of prasugrel; this time course reflects new platelet production, rather than the pharmacokinetics of prasugrel. Prasugrel-mediated inhibition of platelet aggregation is approximately 5–9 times more potent than that of clopidogrel. The effect in patients ≥75 years of age is somewhat smaller, and bleeding risk is higher in these individuals. Prasugrel given as early as possible after an ACS may be superior to clopidogrel, particularly in patients with diabetes mellitus. Prasugrel should be considered in patients with stent thrombosis despite compliance with clopidogrel therapy. Prasugrel has several pharmacological advantages over clopidogrel—it is more effectively converted into its active metabolite and displays a faster onset of action and a greater degree of platelet inhibition, with less variability in response.

Pharmacokinetics

Prasugrel is rapidly absorbed but is not detected in plasma because it is rapidly hydrolysed in the intestine to a thiolactone, which is then converted to the active metabolite primarily by CYP3A4 and CYP2B6 and, to a lesser extent, by CYP2C9 and CYP2C19. The active metabolite reaches peak plasma levels approximately 30min after dosing, is highly bound to plasma albumin (98%), presents a Vd of 1.25L/kg, is metabolized to two inactive compounds, and presents an elimination t½ of approximately 7 (2–15) h. Prasugrel is excreted in the urine (68%) and faeces (27%) as inactive metabolites. (See Table 8.1.7.)

Practical points

1. *Doses*
   - *Starting dose*: 60mg oral loading dose, and then 10mg PO od for up to 12 months recommended in patients who are proceeding to PCI if no contraindication. Patients taking prasugrel should also take aspirin (75–325mg) daily.

- In patients with stable CAD, mean platelet inhibition in subjects <60kg taking 5mg prasugrel was similar to that in subjects ≥60kg taking 10mg prasugrel. Thus, the maintenance dose should be lowered to 5mg in patients <60kg. No dose adjustment is necessary for patients with mild to moderate impaired hepatic function or with ESRD, but it must not be used in patients with severe hepatic impairment.

2. *Side effects*
   - Haemorrhagic events, including epistaxis, ecchymosis, haemoptysis, GI, pericardial, subcutaneous haematoma, post-procedural haemorrhage, retroperitoneal haemorrhage, pericardial effusion/haemorrhage/tamponade, puncture site haematoma/haemorrhage.
   - Non-haemorrhagic: anaemia, thrombocytopenia, thrombotic thrombocytopenic purpura, abnormal hepatic function, allergic reactions, and angio-oedema.
3. *Interactions*
   - The risk of bleeding increases when prasugrel is co-administered with heparins, warfarin, aspirin, or NSAIDs (used chronically), although these drugs did not alter prasugrel-mediated inhibition of platelet aggregation.
   - Administration of a prasugrel loading dose without concomitant use of PPIs may provide the most rapid onset of action.
4. *Cautions*
   - Prasugrel should be used with caution in patients ≥75 years due to the potential risk of bleeding in this population.
   - In patients with ACS who are managed with PCI, premature discontinuation of prasugrel could result in an increased risk of thrombosis, MI, or death due to the patient's underlying disease. A treatment of up to 12 months is recommended, unless contraindicated.
   - In patients undergoing elective non-cardiac surgery, prasugrel should be discontinued 7 days before surgery, unless the patient is at high risk of stent thrombosis.
   - Some PPIs widely used in patients with ACS inhibit CYP2C19, decreasing the formation of the active metabolite of clopidogrel. This interaction is not present with prasugrel.
   - There are no drug interactions with ranitidine or lansoprazole, atorvastatin, digoxin, or potent P450 inhibitors or inducers.
5. *Pregnancy and lactation*
   - Prasugrel is only recommended for use during pregnancy when benefit outweighs risk (Pregnancy category B). Because there are no data, caution is recommended if used in nursing women.
6. *Contraindications*
   - Hypersensitivity to prasugrel or any component of the product.
   - Active pathological bleeding.
   - Prior stroke or TIA.
   - Severe hepatic impairment (Child–Pugh class C).

Pravastatin

HMG CoA reductase inhibitor (see ➲ Statins (3-hydroxy-3-methylglutaryl-coenzyme A reductase inhibitors), pp. 760–3).

CV indications

- Treatment of primary hypercholesterolaemia or mixed dyslipidaemia, when response to diet and other non-pharmacological treatments (e.g. exercise, weight reduction) is inadequate.
- *Primary prevention*: reduction in CV mortality and morbidity in patients with moderate or severe hypercholesterolaemia and at high risk of a first CV event, as an adjunct to diet.
- *Secondary prevention*: reduction in CV mortality and morbidity in patients with a history of MI or UA and with either normal or increased cholesterol levels, as an adjunct to correction of other risk factors. It is indicated to reduce total mortality by reducing coronary deaths and to reduce recurrent MI, revascularization, and stroke or TIA.
- Reduction of post-transplantation hyperlipidaemia in patients receiving immunosuppressive therapy following solid organ transplantation.

Pharmacodynamics

Primary hypercholesterolaemia: at doses between 10 and 40mg/day, it reduces elevated LDL-C (19–34%), total-C (14–25%), and TG (14–24%) levels and increases HDL-C (2–11.5%) levels.

Pharmacokinetics

Pravastatin does not undergo metabolism through the CYP system but is metabolized by sulfation and conjugation. The major degradation product of pravastatin is the 3-α-hydroxy isomeric metabolite, which has one-tenth to 1/40th of HMG CoA reductase inhibitor activity of the parent compound. Peak plasma levels markedly increased in cirrhotic patients. (See Table 8.1.4.)

Practical points

1. *Doses*
   - Hypercholesterolaemia: 10–40mg od.
   - CV prevention: the starting and maintenance dose is 40mg daily.
   - Dosage after transplantation: starting dose of 20mg od in patients receiving ciclosporin, with or without other immunosuppressive therapy (up to 40mg under close supervision).
   - The recommended dose is 20mg in children aged 8–13 years, and 40mg in adolescents aged 14–18 years.
2. *Side effects* (see ➲ Statins (3-hydroxy-3-methylglutaryl-coenzyme A reductase inhibitors), pp. 760–3)
3. *Interactions* (see ➲ Statins (3-hydroxy-3-methylglutaryl-coenzyme A reductase inhibitors), pp. 760–3)
   - Co-administration of pravastatin with ciclosporin, fibrates, niacin (nicotinic acid), colchicine, clarithromycin, and erythromycin increases the risk of myopathy/rhabdomyolysis and should be avoided. The maximum daily dose of pravastatin should be 20mg if co-administered with ciclosporin, and 40mg if co-administered with clarithromycin.

- Darunavir increases the AUC of pravastatin.
- There is no interaction with cimetidine, digoxin, erythromycin, ketoconazole, or warfarin.

4. *Cautions/notes* (see ➔ Statins (3-hydroxy-3-methylglutaryl-coenzyme A reductase inhibitors), pp. 760–3)
   - Moderate to severe renal or significant hepatic impairment: starting dose 10mg daily.
   - Combination with fibrates is not recommended.
5. *Contraindications* (see ➔ Statins (3-hydroxy-3-methylglutaryl-coenzyme A reductase inhibitors), pp. 760–3)

Prazosin

Selective post-synaptic competitive α1-adrenoreceptor blocker.

CV indications

- Treatment of hypertension.
- Treatment of CHF added to the standard therapy in patients who are resistant or refractory to conventional therapy.
- Raynaud's phenomenon and Raynaud's disease.
- Benign prostatic hyperplasia.

Pharmacodynamics

Prazosin reduces PVR through selective inhibition of post-synaptic α1-adrenoreceptors in vascular smooth muscle cells. It does not produce adverse changes in the serum lipid profile or rebound elevation of BP following abrupt cessation of therapy. In patients with HF, prazosin reduces LV filling pressure and increases CO. It does not cause reflex tachycardia or hypotension in normotensive patients with HF. However, prazosin is ineffective in prolonging survival in patients with HF.

Prazosin reduces the severity of the signs, symptoms, frequency, and duration of attacks in patients with Raynaud's disease.

Pharmacokinetics

Oral prazosin presents a bioavailability of 60%, reaching peak plasma concentrations within 2–3h. It binds to plasma proteins (97%), is extensively metabolized in the liver (by demethylation and conjugation), is excreted mainly via bile and faeces (<10% in urine), and presents a t½ of approximately 7h. Prazosin can be used safely in patients with renal impairment.

Practical points

1. *Doses*
   - *Hypertension*: 0.5–5mg od, administered in the evening (maximum dose 20mg in divided doses).
   - *HF*: 0.5mg 2–4 times daily (maximum dose 4–20mg/day in divided doses).
   - *Raynaud's phenomenon and Raynaud's disease*: starting dosage is 0.5mg bd for 7 days; maintenance dosage: 1–2mg bd.
   - *Benign prostatic hyperplasia*: 0.5mg bd for 3–7 days; maintenance dose: 2mg bd.
   - *Starting dose*: 0.5mg in patients with renal and hepatic impairment.
2. *Common side effects*
   - Depression, nervousness, vertigo; palpitations, nasal congestion, oedema, orthostatic hypotension, dyspnoea, syncope; blurred vision; constipation, diarrhoea, dry mouth, vomiting; oedema, weakness, rash. During cataract surgery, an intraoperative floppy iris syndrome (IFIS) has been reported in patients on α1-blocker therapy.
3. *Interactions*
   - Use with other antihypertensives or vasodilators (PDE-5 inhibitors) may produce a substantial fall in BP. This can be minimized by reducing the dose (1–2mg tds).

4. *Cautions/notes*
   - Monitor BP and fluid balance in patients treated with antihypertensives or vasodilators. Post-operative hypotension can be avoided by discontinuing the drug several days before surgery.
   - Clinical efficacy may decline with time on treatment (tachyphylaxis).
   - Prazosin may produce false positives in some tests for phaeochromocytoma.
5. *Pregnancy and lactation*
   - Safety in pregnancy is uncertain (Pregnancy category C). Prazosin is excreted in breast milk. Thus, caution should be used in either pregnancy or breastfeeding.
6. *Contraindications*
   - Patients with sensitivity to quinazolines, prazosin, or any other excipient.

Procainamide

IV Na^+ channel blocker with class IA antiarrhythmic properties.

CV indications

- Treatment of symptomatic or sustained VT. Because of the risk of proarrhythmia and serious haematological disorders (0.5%), it is not recommended with lesser arrhythmias.

Mechanism of action

(See ➲ Quinidine, pp. 716–19.)

Pharmacodynamics

Compared with other class I AADs, procainamide produces less depression of cardiac contractility. It exhibits a weak anticholinergic effect, most prominent in the SA and AV nodes. At high doses, procainamide can produce peripheral vasodilatation.

Pharmacokinetics

Procainamide is metabolized in the liver to the active metabolite *N*-acetylprocainamide (NAPA), 16–21% of an administered dose in 'slow acetylators' and 24–33% in 'fast-acetylators'. It is predominantly (60%) excreted unchanged in the urine (6–50% as NAPA) by active tubular secretion, as well as by glomerular filtration. Therapeutic plasma levels: 3–8mcg/mL. Its elimination t½ increases in the elderly and in patients with renal and hepatic impairment. (See Table 8.1.3.)

Practical points

1. *Doses*
   - They should be adjusted for the individual patient, based on the degree of underlying myocardial disease, patient's age, and hepatic or renal function.
   - IV. Loading dose (15–18mg/kg over 30 min) or 100mg at a rate lower than 50mg/min, repeated every 5min as needed to a total dose of 1g. Maintenance dose: 1–4mg/min.
2. *Common side effects*
   - Anorexia, nausea, diarrhoea, myalgia, blood dyscrasias (leucopenia or agranulocytosis, sometimes fatal). Elevations of transaminases, with and without elevations of alkaline phosphatase and bilirubin.
   - CV (see ➲ Quinidine, pp. 716–19).
   - A lupus erythematosus-like syndrome with arthralgia, pleural or abdominal pain, arthritis, pleural effusion, pericarditis, fever, and myalgia.
3. *Interactions*
   - Risk of bradycardia, intra-cardiac blockade, and proarrhythmia when given with class I and III AADs. Risk of TdP when given with QT-prolonging drugs.
   - Amiodarone increases the plasma levels of procainamide.
   - Patients treated with procainamide require lower doses of suxamethonium.

- Its combination with captopril can cause neutropenia and/or SJS.
- Co-administration with anticholinergic agents exerts additive antivagal effects on the sinus rate and AV conduction.

4. *Cautions/notes*
   - Monitor ECG and BP during treatment. If hypotension or excessive widening of QRS or bradycardia occur, the drug should be discontinued.
   - Caution in patients with HF, ACS, cardiogenic shock, or cardiomyopathy due to the risk of reduced myocardial contractility.
   - Procainamide may worsen symptoms of asthma and myasthenia gravis by reducing acetylcholine release.
5. *Pregnancy and lactation*
   - Procainamide crosses the placenta, and its safety has not been established in pregnancy (Pregnancy category C). It is excreted in breast milk; avoid during breastfeeding.
6. *Contraindications* (see ➔ Quinidine, pp. 716–19)
   - Brugada syndrome.
   - Severe renal failure.
   - Hypersensitivity: in patients sensitive to procaine or other ester-type local anaesthetics.
   - SLE.

Propafenone

Na^+ channel blocker with class 1C antiarrhythmic properties (see ➲ Flecainide, pp. 593–5).

Indications

In patients without structural heart disease, it is indicated for the:

- Treatment of AV nodal reciprocating tachycardia, arrhythmias associated with WPW syndrome, and similar conditions with accessory pathways.
- Pharmacological cardioversion of recent-onset AF associated with disabling symptoms to sinus rhythm and maintenance of normal sinus rhythm following conversion by other means.
- Treatment of severe symptomatic life-threatening paroxysmal ventricular arrhythmias not controlled by other drugs or when other treatments are not tolerated.

Mechanism of action

(See ➲ Flecainide, pp. 593–5.)

Pharmacodynamics

(See ➲ Flecainide, pp. 593–5.)

Propafenone has moderate L-type Ca^{2+} channel antagonistic activity and β-blocking properties, especially when the dose exceeds 450mg daily. A clinically relevant reduction of LV function is to be expected only in patients with pre-existing poor ventricular function. There appears to be a close relationship between plasma concentrations and AV conduction times.

Pharmacokinetics

It is metabolized in the liver into two main active metabolites, which have antiarrhythmic activity, comparable with propafenone. Therapeutic plasma levels: 0.2–3mcg/mL. More than 90% of patients rapidly and extensively metabolizing the drug (by CYP2D6, 3A4, and 1A2). In <10% of whites, CYP2D6 is genetically absent, so that its metabolism is slower and the elimination t½ is approximately 10–32h. (See Table 8.1.3.)

Practical points

1. *Doses*
    - *Supraventricular arrhythmias*: 50mg bd (increasing at a minimum of 3-day intervals to 300mg bd). *Ventricular arrhythmias*: 100mg bd (maximum dose 400mg daily).
    - IV: 2mg/kg, followed by an infusion of 2mg/min.
    - *Cardioversion and prevention of recurrences of AF*: 1.5–2mg/kg IV over 10–20min. PO: 400–600mg/day.
    - *Liver dysfunction*: a reduction in the recommended dose may be necessary.
    - *Renal dysfunction*: 50mg bd or 100mg od.

Therapy should be initiated under hospital conditions, and the dose should be determined under ECG monitoring and BP control. The elderly may respond to a lower dose.

2. *Common side effects*
   - (>10%): dizziness, nausea and vomiting, unusual taste.
   - (1–10%): ventricular proarrhythmia (monomorphic VT, occasional TdP), HF, reduced LVEF, weakness, intraventricular conduction delay, fatigue, dyspnoea, headache, ataxia, tremor, rash, blurred vision, constipation, dyspepsia, joint pain. AVB, sinus bradycardia, sinus node dysfunction, negative inotropism. Propafenone can convert AF in atrial flutter, resulting in 1:1 AV conduction and increased ventricular rate that can be prevented with AV nodal blocking agents (β-blockers, diltiazem, verapamil).
3. *Interactions* (see ➲ Flecainide, pp. 593–5)
   - Propafenone can produce conduction abnormalities and potential arrhythmias when used with amiodarone and increases the risk of lidocaine-related CNS side effects.
   - QT-prolonging drugs can increase the risk of serious proarrhythmia.
   - SA and AV node depression when combined with verapamil or diltiazem. Conduction defects may increase when combined with class IA antiarrhythmics.
   - Propafenone enhances the effects of oral anticoagulants; reduce the dose of warfarin, and monitor the INR.
   - Propafenone increases the plasma levels of digoxin, propranolol, metoprolol, ciclosporin, theophylline, and desipramine. Doses of these drugs should be reduced.
   - Drugs that inhibit CYP2D6, CYP1A2, and CYP3A4 (see Table 8.1.2) increase the plasma levels of propafenone. Patients should be monitored closely and doses adjusted accordingly when propafenone is administered with such drugs.
   - The effects of propafenone may also be increased by concomitant use of cimetidine, paroxetine, or fluoxetine and decreased by rifampicin.
   - Propafenone should not be used in combination with ritonavir.
   - CYP3A4 inducers (see Table 8.1.2) reduce the efficacy of propafenone, so that the response to propafenone should be monitored.
4. *Cautions/notes*
   - Patients with structural heart disease are predisposed to serious side effects.
   - Monitor the patients (clinically and by ECG) prior to and during therapy.
   - Care should be exercised in the treatment of patients with obstructive airways disease or asthma (due to its β-blocking effect).
   - The weak negative inotropic effect of propafenone may predispose to LV failure.
   - Due to altered sensitivity and thresholds, appropriate adjustments may be required for pacemakers.
   - Blurred vision, dizziness, fatigue, and postural hypotension may affect the patient's speed of reaction and impair the individual's ability to operate machinery or motor vehicles.
   - Propafenone increases endocardial pacing thresholds and should be used with caution in patients with permanent pacemakers or

temporary pacing electrodes; avoid its use in patients with existing poor thresholds or non-programmable pacemakers, unless suitable pacing rescue is available.

5. *Pregnancy and lactation*
   - Propafenone should not be used during pregnancy and lactation (Pregnancy category C).
6. *Contraindications* (see ➔ Flecainide, pp. 593–5)
   - Severe COPD, asthma or marked hypotension.
   - Myasthenia gravis (may be worsened).

Propranolol

Non-selective β-adrenergic receptor blocking drug (see also ➲ Beta-adrenergic blocking agents, pp. 485–94).

Indications

- Treament of arterial hypertension.
- Treatment of chronic stable angina pectoris.
- Long-term prophylaxis against reinfarction after recovery from acute MI.
- Treament of hypertrophic obstructive cardiomyopathy.
- Treatment of supraventricular and ventricular arrhythmias.
- Control of ventricular rate in patients with AF/atrial flutter.
- Treatment of phaeochromocytoma perioperatively (with an α-blocker).
- Treament of essential tremor.
- Relief of situational anxiety and generalized anxiety symptoms.
- Adjunctive management of hyperthyroidism and thyrotoxicosis.
- Prophylaxis of common migraine headache, probably by inducing vasoconstriction.
- Prophylaxis of upper GI bleeding in patients with portal hypertension and oesophageal varices.

Mechanism of action

(See ➲ Beta-adrenergic blocking agents, pp. 485–94.)

Pharmacodynamics

(See ➲ Beta-adrenergic blocking agents, pp. 485–94.)

In patients with hypertrophic obstructive cardiomyopathy, propranolol (200–400mg/day) slows the heart rate, prolongs the diastolic filling period, relieves symptoms (dyspnoea, fatigue, angina), and improves NYHA functional class.

Propranolol is used in patients with hyperthyroidism and thyrotoxicosis to control symptoms (tachycardia, palpitations, tremor, and nervousness) and reduce the vascularity of the thyroid gland, thereby facilitating surgery.

Pharmacokinetics

Propranolol is almost completely absorbed but undergoes an extensive first-pass effect, so that oral bioavailability is 25%. Propranolol crosses the blood–brain barrier and the placenta and is distributed into breast milk. The plasma t½ is 3–4h (longer after chronic administration). The biological t½ of propranolol exceeds the plasma t½ considerably, so that twice-daily dosages of standard propranolol are effective, even in angina pectoris. Oral bioavailability, steady-state plasma levels, and the t½ of propranolol increase in patients with hepatic impairment, so that the initial dose should not exceed 20mg tds. Plasma levels of propranolol may increase in patients with significant renal impairment and haemodialysis. (See Tables 8.1.3 and 8.1.8.)

Practical points

1. *Doses*
   - *Hypertension*: starting dose is 80mg bd, which may be increased at weekly intervals up to 160–320mg/daily. Propranolol sustained-release: 80–320mg/day.

- *Angina, migraine, and essential tremor*: initially 40mg bd or tds, increasing up to 160mg daily (migraine, essential tremor) or 120–240mg daily (angina). Angina: Propranolol sustained-release 80–320mg/day.
- *Arrhythmias, anxiety tachycardia, hypertrophic obstructive cardiomyopathy, and thyrotoxicosis*: 10–40mg tds or four times daily.
- *Situational and generalized anxiety*: 40mg bd or tds.
- *Post-MI*: treatment should be initiated between days 5–21 after MI, with an initial dose of 40mg four times daily for 2–3 days, then 80mg bd.
- *Phaeochromocytoma* (preoperatively) 60mg daily for 3 days. Non-operable malignant cases: 30mg daily.
- *Portal hypertension*: begin with 40mg bd, up to 160mg bd, depending on heart rate response.
- *Arrhythmias*: 0.25–0.5mg/kg 3–4 times daily, as required.
- *Thyrotoxicosis*: IV propranolol (1mg/min, up to a total of 5mg at a time) can be given if LV function is normal.

2. *Common side effects* (see ➲ Beta-adrenergic blocking agents, pp. 485–94)
3. *Interactions* (see ➲ Beta-adrenergic blocking agents, pp. 485–94)
   - Blood levels and/or side effects of propranolol increase by co-administration with substrates or inhibitors of CYP2D6, CYP1A2, or CYP2C19 (see Table 8.1.2).
   - Blood levels of propranolol decrease by co-administration with CYP inducers such as rifampicin, ethanol, phenytoin, and phenobarbital (see Table 8.1.2).
   - Propranolol inhibits the metabolism and reduces the clearance of lidocaine; decrease the dose of lidocaine to avoid its adverse side effects.
   - The effects of propranolol can be antagonized by dobutamine or isoprenaline, and propranolol may reduce sensitivity to dobutamine stress echocardiography.
   - Severe hypertension and bradycardia in patients treated with propranolol and adrenaline.
   - Propranolol increases (100%) the AUC of propafenone.
   - The metabolism of propranolol is reduced by quinidine, leading to a 2- to 3-fold increase in plasma propranolol levels.
   - Nisoldipine and nicardipine increase the C_{max} and UAC of propranolol.
   - Propranolol increases the C_{max} and AUC of nifedipine.
   - Propranolol decreases the oral clearance of theophylline.
   - Propranolol increases the plasma levels of diazepam, while the pharmacokinetics of oxazepam, triazolam, lorazepam, and alprazolam are not affected.
   - Propranolol increases the plasma levels of thioridazine.
   - Co-administration of chlorpromazine with propranolol increases the plasma levels of both drugs and the risk of hypotension and bradycardia.
   - Co-administration of propranolol and haloperidol increases the risk of hypotension and cardiac arrest.

- MAOIs reduce the antihypertensive effect of propranolol and lead to hypertensive reactions.
- NSAIDs can inhibit the antihypertensive effect of propranolol.
- Fluvoxamine increases the plasma levels of propranolol, leading to severe bradycardia.
- Cimetidine increases, while aluminum hydroxide gel decreases, the plasma levels of propranolol.
- Colestyramine and colestipol decrease (50%) the plasma concentrations of propranolol.
- Propranolol increases warfarin bioavailability. Monitor the PT/INR.
- Tobacco smoking can reduce the beneficial effects of propranolol on heart rate and BP.
- Methoxyflurane may depress myocardial contractility when administered with propranolol.
- Administration of ergotamine and propranolol can produce vasospastic reactions.

4. *Cautions/notes*
   - Propranolol interfere with the estimation of serum bilirubin by the diazo method and with the determination of catecholamines by methods using fluorescence.
   - Propranolol should be used with great caution in patients with Raynaud's disease/syndrome or intermittent claudication.
   - Propranolol may enhance an anaphylactic reaction and may cause a more severe reaction to a variety of allergens in patients with a history of severe anaphylactic reactions. These patients may be unresponsive to the doses of adrenaline used to treat allergic reactions.
   - After chronic therapy with propranolol, administration of adrenaline may develop uncontrolled hypertension due to α-receptor stimulation.
5. *Pregnancy and lactation* (see ➔ Beta-adrenergic blocking agents, pp. 485–94)
6. *Contraindications* (see ➔ Beta-adrenergic blocking agents, pp. 485–94)
   - Known hypersensitivity to propranolol hydrochloride.

Quinidine

CV indications

- Conversion of AF/atrial flutter.
- Mantainance of sinus rhythm after cardioversion of AF.
- Suppression of recurrent ventricular arrhythmias. However, it is not recommended for the treatment of asymptomatic VPBs.
- Patients with a diagnosis of SQTS who present a contraindication to ICD or refuse it; in asymptomatic patients with a diagnosis of SQTS and a family history of SCD.
- Patients with Brugada syndrome to treat electrical storms. Quinidine should be considered in patients who qualify for an ICD but present a contraindication or refuse it and in patients who require treatment for supraventricular arrhythmias.

Mechanism of action

Class I AADs bind to the α-subunit of voltage-gated Na^+ channels and inhibit Na^+ entry, decrease the amplitude of the fast cardiac action potentials generated in non-nodal cardiomyocytes (widening the QRS complex), and reduce cardiac excitability and slow intra-cardiac conduction. These effects may convert unidirectional into bidirectional conduction block, suppressing re-entrant arrhythmias, but sometimes they may favour the appearance of such re-entrant arrhythmias (i.e. proarrhythmia). Class IA AADs present a high affinity for the activated and/or inactivated state of the channel (the latter predominates in ischaemic–depolarized cardiac tissues) and prolong the reactivation of the channel, which determines the shortest time between two cardiac beats (cardiac effective refractory period) independently of the changes in the APD. The effects of class IA AADs increase at fast driving rates (increase the time that the channel spends in the active activated/inactive inactivated state) and in depolarized (ischaemic) cardiac tissues, because depolarization of the resting membrane potential inactivated the Na^+ channels. Thus, they produce a frequency (use)- and voltage-dependent Na^+ channel block.

Pharmacodynamics

Class IA AADs slow the heart rate, prolong the QRS, PR, and QT intervals on the ECG, and exert an anticholinergic effect, most prominent in the SA and AV nodes. They exert a negative inotropic effect. Class IA AADs have other mechanisms of action not associated with their effects on Na^+ channels. Thus, they can reduce the automaticity of the SA node, as well as the automaticity of the His–Purkinje system, by decreasing the slope of phase 4 and shifting the threshold potential to less negative values. Both effects suppress the automaticity of cardiac ectopic pacemakers. Class IA AADs also block several outward-repolarizing K^+ currents, including the rapid component of the delayed rectifier potassium current (I_{Kr}). Therefore, they prolong the APD (QT interval) and the effective refractory period, due to prolongation of the reactivation of the I_{Na} and the blockade of several outward-repolarizing K^+ currents. The inhomogenous prolongation of the QT interval facilitates re-entry, and prolongation of the APD can lead to the development of early after-depolarizations and polymorphic VT, including

TdP. They can also block the L-type Ca^{2+} current, leading to a decrease in cardiac contractility (negative inotropic effect), more evident in patients with previous LV dysfunction or HF. Class IA AADs increased mortality among patients with previous MI. In patients treated for sustained VT, these agents may provoke more frequent, and often more difficult to cardiovert, episodes of sustained VT.

They also exert anticholinergic effects, most prominent in the SA and AV nodes, due to their extensive vagal innervation. This vagolytic activity may cause sinus tachycardia and facilitate AV conduction, i.e. effects just opposite to the direct depressant effects of these drugs on the SA and AV nodes. This anticholinergic effect can produce a sudden increase in the ventricular rate in patients with atrial flutter or AF. To avoid this increase, class IA AADs should be administered with AV-blocking drugs.

Pharmacokinetics

(See Table 8.1.3.)

Practical points

1. *Doses*
   - Oral:
     —AF (quinidine sulfate): 300–400mg every 8h.
     —PSVT (quinidine sulfate/gluconate): 400–600mg every 2–3h until paroxysm is terminated.
     —Atrial/ventricular premature contractions (quinidine sulfate): 200–300mg every 6–8h.
     —Maintenance: (1) quinidine sulfate: 200–400mg every 6–8h or 600mg of sustained-release every 8–12h; (2) quinidine gluconate: 648mg bd or 324–660mg tds. No more than 3–4g/day.
   - IV (quinidine gluconate): usual <5mg/kg (up to 10mg/kg) at 0.25mg/kg/min.
2. *Common side effects*
   - Diarrhoea, nausea, headache, dizziness, light-headedness, auditory and visual disturbances, fatigue, and vomiting.
   - CV: bradycardia, intra-cardiac conduction abnormalities (AVB and bundle branch block), palpitations, tachyarrhythmias (VT/VF, TdP), hypotension, and HF. Proarrhythmia increases in patients with hypokalaemia or structural heart disease. Because of its negative inotropic effect, episodes of HF, or even cardiogenic shock, have also been described in patients with structural heart disease.
   - Anticholinergic effects: urinary retention, blurred vision, dry mouth, abdominal pain.
   - Autoimmune and inflammatory syndromes, including pneumonitis, fever, urticaria, flushing, exfoliative rash, bronchospasm, pruritus, haemolytic anaemia, vasculitis, agranulocytosis, arthralgia, myalgia, and a disorder resembling SLE.
3. *Interactions*
   - Quinidine inhibits CYP2D6 and increases the plasma concentrations of tricyclic antidepressants, metoprolol, procainamide, and antipsychotics (haloperidol). Quinidine decreases the efficacy of codeine.

- Amiodarone, diltiazem, verapamil, and cimetidine increase, while nifedipine decreases, plasma quinidine levels.
- Co-administration of quinidine with β-blockers, diltiazem, or verapamil increases the risk of bradycardia, AVB, and hypotension and decreases cardiac contractility. Propranolol increases peak serum levels and decreases the Vd and total clearance of quinidine.
- Drugs that alkalinize the urine (carbonic anhydrase inhibitors, sodium bicarbonate, thiazide diuretics) reduce the renal elimination of quinidine.
- Plasma quinidine levels increase when co-administered with CYP3A4 inhibitors but decrease when co-administered with CYP3A4 inducers (see Table 8.1.2). Avoid these combinations.
- Quinidine inhibits P-gp and increases serum digoxin levels. Reduce the dose of digoxin.
- Quinidine potentiates the anticoagulant effect of warfarin; reduce the dose of warfarin, and monitor the INR.
- Quinidine's anticholinergic, vasodilating, and negative inotropic actions may be additive to those of other drugs with these effects.
- Quinidine potentiates the actions of depolarizing (suxamethonium) and non-depolarizing (pancuronium) neuromuscular blocking agents.
- Combinations with other AADs should be avoided.

4. *Cautions/notes*
   - The proarrhythmic and non-cardiac side effects of quinidine, together with its potential for drug interactions, are key limitations for its use.
   - Periodic monitoring of the QRS and QTc intervals of the ECG are recommended. The dose should be reduced or therapy discontinued if the QRS widens by 30%, QRS duration >140ms, or QTc >500ms, or if the patient develops tachycardia, symptomatic bradycardia, or hypotension.
   - Treatment of acute quinidine toxicity includes stopping quinidine, reducing plasma K^+ levels if elevated, and acidifying the urine to increase renal excretion of the drug.
   - Due to its anticholinergic effects, quinidine shortens the refractoriness of the AVN and can produce a paradoxical increase in the ventricular rate in patients with atrial flutter/AF. The risk can be reduced by giving AV nodal drugs (digoxin, diltiazem, verapamil, β-blockers) prior to quinidine therapy.
   - Drugs that induce hypokalaemia potentiate the risk of proarrhythmia.
   - Atropine and other anticholinergic drugs potentiate the atropine-like effect of disopyramide and quinidine; pyridostigmine (90–180mg tds) reduces these anticholinergic effects.
5. *Pregnancy and lactation*
   - There are no adequate and well-controlled studies in pregnant women (Pregnancy category C). Quinidine is present in human milk at levels slightly lower than those in maternal serum, so that its administration should be avoided in breastfeeding.
6. *Contraindications*
   - Patients allergic to the drug or who have developed thrombocytopenic purpura during prior therapy with quinidine or quinine.

- Severe sinus node disease or second- or third-degree AVB (unless a pacemaker is present); severe intraventricular conduction disturbances.
- Ventricular tachyarrhythmias associated with, or caused by, inherited or acquired QT prolongation or when QT-prolonging drugs are prescribed. In combination with other AADs, likely to provoke ventricular proarrhythmia.
- Severe hepatic impairment.
- Cardiogenic shock, hypotension.
- Severe HF, reduced LVEF (unless due to arrhythmia), CAD, previous MI.
- Myasthenia gravis.

Ramipril

Orally active ACEI (see ➔ Angiotensin-converting enzyme inhibitors, pp. 459–64).

Indications

- Treatment of hypertension.
- Treatment of symptomatic HF.
- CV prevention: reduction of CV morbidity and mortality in patients with: (1) manifest atherothrombotic CV disease (history of CAD or stroke or peripheral vascular disease); or (2) diabetes with at least one CV risk factor.
- Treatment of renal disease: (1) incipient glomerular diabetic nephropathy, as defined by the presence of microalbuminuria; (2) manifest glomerular diabetic nephropathy, as defined by macroproteinuria in patients with at least one CV risk factor; and (3) manifest glomerular non-diabetic nephropathy, as defined by macroproteinuria of ≥3g/day.
- Secondary prevention after acute MI: reduction in mortality from the acute MI in patients with clinical signs of HF when started >48h following acute MI.

Pharmacokinetics

(See Table 8.1.10.)

Practical points

1. *Doses*
   - *Hypertension and CV risk*: 1.25–2.5mg od (titrated to maximum of 10mg od). The full effect is potentiated by thiazides and loop diuretics or a low-salt diet more than by dose increase. In hypertensives in whom the diuretic is not discontinued, ramipril should be initiated at a dose of 1.25mg od.
   - *HF*: 1.25mg od. Double the dose every 1–2 weeks to a maximum dose of 10mg.
   - *Secondary prevention after acute MI and HF*: after 48h following MI in a clinically and haemodynamically stable patient, the starting dose is 1.25–2.5mg bd for 3 days; after 2 days, 2.5–5mg bd. If the dose cannot be increased to 2.5mg bd, the treatment should be withdrawn.
   - *Diabetic nephropathy and patients with diabetes and at least one CV risk*: 1.25mg od initially to the usual dose of 10mg od.
   - *CV prevention*: the initial dose is 2.5mg od, titrated up to 10mg od.
   - *Non-diabetic nephropathy*: the initial dose is 1.25mg od, titrated to 5mg od.
   - Doses should be reduced in patients with renal impairment. In those with CrCl of 30–60mL/min, it is not necessary to adjust the initial dose (2.5mg/day), but the maximum daily dose will be 5mg od. If CrCl is 10–30mL/min: initial dose 1.25mg/day, maximum dose 5mg/day. In haemodialysed hypertensives, the initial dose is 1.25mg/day and the maximum daily dose is 5mg; the drug should be administered a few hours after haemodialysis.

- In patients with hepatic impairment, ramipril must be initiated only under close medical supervision, and the maximum daily dose is 2.5mg.
- In the *elderly*, the initial dose should be 1.25mg od and subsequent dose titration should be more gradual because of the risk of side effects.
- Doses should be reduced in the elderly. In hepatic impairment, treatment with ramipril must be initiated only under close medical supervision and the maximum daily dose is 2.5mg. An initial dose of 1.25mg should be considered for those who may be sodium- or fluid-depleted, in whom hypotension is a particular risk.

2. *Common side effects* (see ➔ Angiotensin-converting enzyme inhibitors, pp. 459–64)
   - Common: dizziness, vertigo; fatigue; hypotension; hyperkalaemia, rise in urea and creatinine levels.
   - Others: nausea, vomiting; chest infection; headache; angio-oedema has been reported with some ARBs.
3. *Interactions* (see ➔ Angiotensin-converting enzyme inhibitors, pp. 459–64)
4. *Cautions/notes* (see ➔ Angiotensin-converting enzyme inhibitors, pp. 459–64)
5. *Contraindications* (see ➔ Angiotensin-converting enzyme inhibitors, pp. 459–64)

Ranolazine

Selective late Na^+ current (I_{NaL}) inhibitor.

CV indications

- As an add-on therapy for the symptomatic treatment of patients with stable angina pectoris who are inadequately controlled or intolerant to first-line anti-anginal therapies (such as β-blockers and/or calcium antagonists).

Mechanism of action

Most cardiac Na^+ channels open transiently, within milliseconds, but then rapidly inactivate following depolarization. However, a small percentage of Na^+ channels either fail to inactivate properly (i.e. fail to close) or close and then reopen during the plateau phase, carrying the so-called persistent or late Na^+ current (I_{NaL}) that facilitates the entry of Na^+ during the plateau phase of the action potential.

During myocardial ischaemia, the amplitude of the I_{NaL} and intracellular Na^+ levels increase, which, in turn, activate the reverse mode of the Na^+–Ca^{2+} exchanger and increases the intracellular Ca^{2+} levels. The increase in intracellular Na^+ and Ca^{2+} levels results in contractile (increased diastolic tension, reduced contractility and coronary blood supply), metabolic (decreased ATP formation), and electrophysiologic disturbances (arrhythmias). Under these conditions, ranolazine selectively inhibits the I_{NaL}.

Pharmacodynamics

In patients with chronic stable angina, ranolazine significantly reduces the frequency of angina and increases exercise duration, time to onset of angina, and time to 1-mm ST-segment depression at trough (12h after dose) and peak in patients treated with other anti-anginal drugs. However, ranolazine does not modifiy the mean heart rate, BP, or the RR, PR, and QRS intervals on the ECG. In patients with recent NSTE-ACS, ranolazine does not modify the composite endpoint of CV death, MI, or recurrent ischaemia, but in patients with prior chronic angina, it reduces the risk of recurrent ischaemia. In these patients, ranolazine decreases the incidence of arrhythmias, as assessed by Holter monitoring performed for the first 7 days after randomization.

In diabetic patients with chronic stable angina or NSTE-ACS, ranolazine significantly reduces HbA1c and recurrent ischaemia. In patients with T2DM and chronic stable angina receiving one or two anti-anginal drugs, ranolazine reduces the episodes of angina and the use of sublingual glyceryl trinitrate; the benefits appeared more prominent in patients with higher, rather than lower, HbA1c levels.

Ranolazine (off-label) is effective to maintain sinus rhythm in patients with recurrent AF, facilitates electrical cardioversion of AF, prevents post-operative AF, and at high doses (2g PO) produces the conversion of recent-onset AF (<48h duration). The combination of ranolazine (750mg bd) and dronedarone (225mg bd) reduces AF burden vs placebo in patients with paroxysmal AF. In LQT3 patients IV ranolazine shortens the QTc interval without changes in PR and QRS intervals, AV conduction or blood pressure, and improves diastolic dysfunction.

Pharmacokinetics

The pharmacokinetics of ranolazine are unaffected by age, gender, or food, but drug clearance is reduced by renal and hepatic impairment. Plasma levels increase (40–50%) in patients with mild, moderate, or severe renal impairment and those with mild to moderate hepatic impairment. (See Table 8.1.11.)

Practical points

1. *Doses*
   - Initial dose: 375mg bd, which can be increased to 750mg bd.
   - Careful dose titration is recommended in renal and hepatic impairment, in the elderly, and when used concomitantly with CYP3A4 and P-gp inhibitors (see Table 8.1.2).
2. *Side effects*
   - Dizziness, constipation, nausea, headache; asthenia.
   - Bradycardia, hypotension, palpitations, QTc prolongation.
   - Others: peripheral oedema, abdominal pain, dry mouth, dyspepsia, anorexia, vomiting, tinnitus, vertigo, blurred vision, confusional state, hyperhidrosis.
   - The incidence of adverse events is higher in the elderly.
3. *Interactions*
   - Ranolazine is a substrate of cytochrome CYP3A4. Potent CYP3A inhibitors increase exposure to ranolazine (see Table 8.1.2). This combination should be avoided. The dose of ranolazine should be limited to 500mg bd in patients treated with moderate CYP3A inhibitors.
   - Dose adjustment of CYP3A4 substrates (atorvastatin, lovastatin, simvastatin, ciclosporin, tacrolimus, sirolimus, everolimus) are required when co-administered with ranolazine.
   - CYP3A inducers decrease plasma ranolazine levels (see Table 8.1.2). This combination should be avoided.
   - Ranolazine is a substrate for P-gp. P-gp inhibitors (e.g. ciclosporin, verapamil) increase the plasma levels of ranolazine; careful dose titration of ranolazine is recommended in patients treated with P-gp inhibitors (see Table 8.1.2).
   - Ranolazine is a mild inhibitor of CYP2D6, and CYP2D6 inhibitors may increase the plasma concentrations of ranolazine (see Table 8.1.2).
   - The risk of ventricular arrhythmia may be increased when used concomitantly with QT-prolonging drugs: class IA and III (sotalol) antiarrhythmic agents, antipsychotics (thioridazine, ziprasidone), antidepressants (e.g. imipramine, amitriptyline), erythromycin, and antihistamines (terfenadine, mizolastine). However, ranolazine shortens the QT interval in patients with LQTS due to blockade of the I_{NaL}.
   - Ranolazine increases the plasma levels of digoxin. Thus, digoxin levels should be monitored, following initiation and termination of ranolazine therapy.
   - Plasma exposure of metformin increases when co-administered with ranolazine. Thus, the dose of metformin should not exceed 1700mg/day.
   - There are no interactions with warfarin, atenolol, or amlodipine.

4. *Cautions/notes*
   - Ranolazine should be used with caution in patients with known QT prolongation (e.g. congenital LQTS other than LQTS3), those taking QT-prolonging drugs, and those with a previous history of VT.
   - Careful dose titration is recommended in patients treated with moderate CYP3A4 inhibitors or P-gp inhibitors (see Table 8.1.2), in patients with mild to moderate renal impairment (CrCl 30–80mL/min) and with mild hepatic impairment and CHF (NYHA classes III–IV).
   - Avoid the combination of ranolazine with class I/III (except amiodarone) AADs.
   - Swallow tablets whole; do not crush, chew, or split.
   - Ranolazine contains lactose. Avoid in patients with rare hereditary problems of galactose intolerance, the Lapp lactase deficiency, or glucose-galactose malabsorption.
5. *Pregnancy and lactation*
   - The potential effects of ranolazine on fetal development and lactation have not been adequately studied (Pregnancy category C).
6. *Contraindications*
   - Hypersensitivity to the active substance or any of the excipients.
   - Pre-existing QT prolongation, co-administration of QT-prolonging drugs.
   - Severe renal impairment (CrCl <30mL/min).
   - Severe or moderate hepatic impairment.
   - Co-administration of potent CYP3A inhibitors.
   - Concomitant use with class I or III (except amiodarone) antiarrhythmics.

Reteplase

This thrombolytic drug is a recombinant non-glycosylated form of tPA, produced by recombinant DNA technology in *Escherichia coli*. It contains the kringle 2 and protease domains of human tPA and 355 of the 527 amino acids of native tPA (amino acids 1–3 and 176–527) (see ➜ Thrombolytic agents, pp. 774–6).

Indications

- For the thrombolytic treatment of suspected MI with persistent ST-elevation or recent LBBB within 12h after the onset of acute MI symptoms.

Pharmacodynamics

(See ➜ Thrombolytic agents, pp. 774–6.)

Reteplase catalyses the cleavage of plasminogen to generate plasmin, which degrades the fibrin matrix of the thrombus, thereby exerting its thrombolytic action. Reteplase decreases fibrinogen levels, which return to baseline values after 48h. In patients treated within 6–12h of the onset of symptoms, reteplase increases coronary artery perfusion through the infarct-related artery, the percentage of patients with partial or complete flow [Thrombolysis in Myocardial Infarction (TIMI) grade 2 or 3] and complete flow (TIMI grade 3), and ventricular function. Patients with known cerebrovascular disease or other bleeding risks and those with a SBP of >200mmHg or a DBP of >100mmHg were excluded from clinical studies.

Pharmacokinetics

Based on the measurement of thrombolytic activity, reteplase is cleared very rapidly from plasma by the liver and kidney, with an effective t½ of 13–16min.

Practical points

1. *Doses*
   - IV reteplase is administered as a 10 + 10U double-bolus injection (each bolus 2min). The second bolus is given 30min after initiation of the first injection. No other medication should be added to the injection solution containing reteplase.
2. *Side effects* (see ➜ Thrombolytic agents, pp. 774–6)
   - More patients treated with retaplase experienced haemorrhagic strokes than patients treated with streptokinase.
3. *Interactions* (see ➜ Thrombolytic agents, pp. 774–6)
   - Heparin and aspirin are given concomitantly with and following the administration of reteplase in patients with acute MI.
   - Co-administration with heparins, VKAs, aspirin, dipyridamole, and abciximab may increase the risk of bleeding. Careful monitoring for bleeding is advised.
4. *Cautions/notes* (see ➜ Thrombolytic agents, pp. 774–6)
   - Each bolus injection should be given via an IV line in which no other medication is being simultaneously injected or infused. UFH and reteplase are incompatible when combined in solution.

- Reteplase lyses fibrin of the haemostatic plug formed at needle puncture sites. Therefore, reteplase therapy requires careful attention to potential bleeding sites (e.g. catheter insertion sites, arterial puncture sites).
- Careful monitoring for bleeding is required, especially at arterial puncture sites.
- Reteplase may decrease plasminogen and fibrinogen and can degrade fibrinogen in blood samples for analysis.

5. *Pregnancy and lactation*
   - There are no controlled data in human pregnancy (Pregnancy category C) and should only be used during pregnancy when benefit outweighs risk. There are no data on the excretion of reteplase into human milk.
6. *Contraindications* (see ➔ Thrombolytic agents, pp. 774–6)

Riociguat

Stimulator of sGC.

Indications

- Treatment of adults with WHO functional classes II–III with inoperable CTEPH or persistent or recurrent CTEPH after surgical treatment or persistent or recurrent CTEPH after surgical treatment, to improve exercise capacity.
- As monotherapy or in combination with ERAs for the treatment of adult patients with PAH with WHO functional classes II–III, to improve exercise capacity. Efficacy has been shown in idiopathic or heritable PAH or PAH associated with connective tissue diseases.

Mechanism of action

PAH is associated with endothelial dysfunction, impaired synthesis of NO, and insufficient stimulation of the NO–sGC–cGMP pathway. Intracellular cGMP plays an important role in regulating processes that influence vascular tone, proliferation, fibrosis, and inflammation. Riociguat has a dual mode of action. It sensitizes sGC to endogenous NO by stabilizing the NO–sGC complex and also directly stimulates sGC via a different binding site, independently of NO. As a consequence, it restores the NO–sGC–cGMP pathway and leads to increased generation of cGMP, which produces vasodilatation, antiproliferative, antifibrotic, and anti-inflammatory properties.

Pharmacodynamics

Riociguat improves WHO functional class, haemodynamics (systemic and pulmonary vascular resistance, SBP, and CO), and time to clinical worsening, compared with placebo, and increases exercise ability (improves 6MWT). It also significantly reduces plasma NT-pro-BNP levels. There is a direct relationship between the plasma concentration of riociguat and haemodynamic parameters such as systemic and pulmonary vascular resistances, SBP, and CO.

Pharmacokinetics

Oral bioavailability of riociguat is approximately 94%, and C_{max} is reached within 1.5h after drug intake. Food does not affect bioavailability. Riociguat is highly bound to plasma proteins (95%), presents a Vd of 0.42L/kg, and is metabolized mainly via CYP1A1, CYP3A, CYP2C8, and CYP2J2. The active metabolite (M1) of riociguat is one-third to one-tenth as potent as riociguat. The drug is excreted in the urine (53%) and faeces, and its terminal t½ is 12h in PAH patients. Riociguat is a substrate of P-gp and breast cancer resistance protein (BCRP).

Practical points

1. *Doses*
   - The recommended starting dosage is 1mg tds (6–8h apart) for 2 weeks. If SBP is >95mmHg and the patient has no signs or symptoms of hypotension, uptitrate the dose by 0.5mg tds up to 2.5mg tds. If at any time, the patient has symptoms of hypotension, decrease the dosage by 0.5mg tds. Smokers may need dosages

higher than 2.5mg tds, if tolerated; a dose decrease may be required in patients who stop smoking. No dose adjustment is warranted, based on age, sex, weight, or race/ethnicity. Patients with severe hepatic impairment (Child–Pugh class C) have not been studied; patients with moderate hepatic impairment (Child–Pugh class B) showed higher drug exposure, and care should be exercised. Data in patients with severe renal impairment (CrCl <30mL/min) are limited.

2. *Side effects*
   - The commonest are: dizziness, headache, hypotension, peripheral oedema, flushing, and GI (vomiting, dyspepsia, gastritis, nausea, diarrhoea). Common: gastroenteritis, hypotension, palpitations, bleeding (epistaxis), anaemia, gastro-oesophageal reflux disease, abdominal pain, constipation.
   - In pulmonary hypertension patients, there is an increased likelihood for respiratory tract bleeding (serious haemoptysis), particularly among patients receiving anticoagulation therapy.
3. *Interactions*
   - Co-administration with nitrates, nicorandil, or NO donors produces profound systemic hypotension and is contraindicated.
   - Co-administration with specific PDE-5 inhibitors (sildenafil, tadalafil, or vardenafil) and non-specific PDE inhibitors (i.e. dipyridamole or theophylline) produces an additive hypotensive response; this combination is contraindicated.
   - Riociguat produces additive BP-lowering effects with other antihypertensives and vasodilator drugs. Consider whether patients on antihypertensive therapy or with resting hypotension, hypovolaemia, severe LV outflow obstruction, or autonomic dysfunction could be adversely affected by riociguat.
   - Plasma concentrations of riociguat are reduced (50–60%) in smokers, as compared to non-smokers. Thus, a dose reduction should be considered in patients who stop smoking.
   - Co-administration of riociguat with strong CYP1A1 inhibitors (erlotinib, gefitinib) and strong P-gp/BCRP inhibitors (ciclosporin, ketoconazole, itraconazole) or HIV PIs (ritonavir) increases riociguat exposure and may result in hypotension. Monitor BP, and consider a starting dose of 0.5mg tds.
   - Strong inducers of CYP3A reduce plasma levels of riociguat (see Table 8.1.2).
   - Bosentan decreases steady-state plasma concentrations of riociguat by 27%.
   - Co-administration of riociguat and warfarin does not alter the PT.
   - Co-administration with aspirin does not affect bleeding time or platelet aggregation.
   - Riociguat did not affect the pharmacokinetics of sildenafil.
   - Antacids containing aluminum hydroxide/magnesium hydroxide decrease riociguat absorption and should not be taken within 1h of taking riociguat.
4. *Cautions/notes*

- Pulmonary vasodilators may worsen the CV status of patients with pulmonary veno-occlusive disease. Discontinue riociguat in these patients.
- The risk of serious and fatal respiratory tract bleeding may be further increased by riociguat, especially in the presence of risk factors.
- Riociguat should be avoided in patients with a history of serious haemoptysis or who have previously undergone bronchial arterial embolization.

5. *Pregnancy and lactation*
   - Riociguat may cause fetal harm and is contraindicated in pregnant women. Pregnancy tests should be performed prior to initiation and monthly during treatment (Pregnancy category X).
6. *Contraindications*
   - Pregnancy.
   - Co-administration with nitrates, NO donors, specific PDE-5 inhibitors (sildenafil, tadalafil, or vardenafil), or non-specific PDE inhibitors (dipyridamole, theophylline).
   - Severe hepatic impairment (Child–Pugh class C).
   - Hypersensitivity to the active substance or any of the excipients.
   - Baseline SBP <95mmHg.
   - Patients with PAH associated with idiopathic interstitial pneumonia.

Rivaroxaban

Rivaroxaban is an orally active, direct, specific, and selective inhibitor of factor Xa that does not require ATIII as cofactor for activity (see ➲ Apixaban, pp. 465–8).

CV indications

- Prevention of stroke and systemic embolism in adult patients with NVAF with one or more risk factors such as CHF, hypertension, age ≥75 years, diabetes mellitus, and prior stroke or TIA.
- Treatment of DVT and PE, and prevention of recurrent DVT and PE in adults.

Mechanism of action

(See ➲ Apixaban, pp. 465–8.)

Pharmacodynamics

Maximum inhibition of factor Xa occurred within 1–4h after administration and ranged from 20% to 61% for the 5–80mg doses.

Pharmacokinetics

Drug elimination decreases with advancing age, renal insufficiency (most trials excluded patients with CrCl of <30mL/min), and hepatic impairment (Child–Pugh class A or B) and in the presence of strong CYP3A4 inhibitors (see Table 8.1.2). A moderate hepatic impairment results in a 2.3-fold increase in AUC for rivaroxaban. Simulations in virtual patient populations with AF showed that rivaroxaban (15mg od) in patients with CrCl of 30–49mL/min would achieve AUC and C_{max} values similar to those observed with 20mg od in patients with normal renal function. It has a terminal t½ of 5–13h in healthy individuals (11–13h in the elderly), but factor Xa is inhibited for up to 24h, allowing once-daily dosage. (See Table 8.1.1.)

Practical points

1. *Doses*
   - *Prevention of stroke and systemic embolism*: 20mg od, with food, continued long term; reduce to 15mg daily in those with moderate to severe renal impairment (CrCl 15–50mL/min).
   - *Treatment of DVT and PE, and prevention of recurrent DVT and PE*: initial dose is 15mg bd for the first 3 weeks; then 20mg od for continued treatment. The duration of therapy should be individualized after careful assessment of the treatment benefit against the risk for bleeding.
   - *Prophylaxis of VTE following knee replacement surgery in adult over 18 years*: 10mg od for 2 weeks, starting 6–10h after surgery, provided that haemostasis has been established.
   - *Prophylaxis of VTE following hip replacement surgery in adult over 18 years*: 10mg od for 5 weeks, starting 6–10h after surgery, provided that haemostasis has been established.
   - *Converting from VKAs to rivaroxaban*: discontinue warfarin, and start rivaroxaban when the INR is ≤3.0. For patients treated for DVT and PE and prevention of recurrence, rivaroxaban should be initiated once the INR is ≤2.5. When converting patients from VKAs to rivaroxaban, INR values will be falsely elevated after the intake of rivaroxaban.

- *Converting from rivaroxaban to VKA*: VKA should be given concurrently until the INR is ≥2.0. For the first 2 days of the conversion period, standard initial dosing of the VKA should be used, followed by VKA dosing as guided by INR testing. While patients are on both rivaroxaban and VKA, the INR should not be tested earlier than 24h after the previous dose, but prior to the next dose of rivaroxaban. Once rivaroxaban is discontinued, INR testing may be done reliably at least 24h after the last dose.
- *Converting from parenteral anticoagulants to rivaroxaban*: discontinue the parenteral anticoagulant, and start rivaroxaban 0–2h before the time that the next scheduled administration of the parenteral drug (i.e. LMWH) would be due or at the time of discontinuation of a continuously administered parenteral drug (IV UFH).
- *Converting from rivaroxaban to parenteral anticoagulants*: give the first dose of the parenteral anticoagulant at the time of the next rivaroxaban dose.
- *Patients undergoing cardioversion*: rivaroxaban should be started at least 4h before cardioversion to ensure adequate anticoagulation. Decisions on initiation and duration of treatment should take established guideline recommendations.
- *Discontinuation for surgery and other interventions*: if anticoagulation must be discontinued to reduce the risk of bleeding with surgery or other procedures, rivaroxaban should be stopped at least 24h before the procedure. Rivaroxaban should be restarted after surgery or other procedures as soon as adequate haemostasis has been established, noting that the time to onset of therapeutic effect is short.

2. *Side effects*
   - Common: haemorrhage, headache, dizziness, post-procedural haemorrhage (including post-operative anaemia and wound haemorrhage), thrombocytopenia, GI (nausea, constipation, diarrhoea, dyspepsia, dry mouth, vomiting), hypotension, and tachycardia. Pruritus, rash, ecchymosis, cutaneous and subcutaneous haemorrhage, pain in extremities. Increase in transaminases.
   - Others: oedema, thrombocythaemia, syncope, dizziness, renal impairment, pain in extremities or back, pruritus, and rash.
   - Less common: asthenia, fatigue, hypotension, oedema, urinary tract infection, increased bilirubin and plasma alkaline phosphatase, insomnia, muscular spasm, oropharyngeal pain, agranulocytosis.
3. *Interactions* (see ➔ Apixaban, pp. 465–8)
   - As with other anticoagulants, patients need to be carefully observed for signs of bleeding, and caution is recommended under conditions with an increased risk of haemorrhage.
   - The risk of bleeding increases when rivaroxaban is co-administered with other anticoagulants, platelet anti-aggregants, heparins, and NSAIDs.
   - Rivaroxaban is a substrate of CYP3A4 and P-gp. Avoid the concomitant use of rivaroxaban with strong inhibitors of both CYP3A4 and P-gp inhibitors abiraterone, aprepitant, crizotinib, dronedarone, enzalutamide, HIV-1 protease inhibitors, idelalisib, imatinib, itraconazole, ketoconazole, posoconazole, and voriconazole.

- Reduce the dose of rivaroxaban (15mg od) when combined with amiodarone, clarithromycin, ciclosporin, erythromycin, fluconazole, lapatinib, nilotinib, paclitaxel, pazopanib, prednisone, quinidine, sirolimus, tacrolimus, tamoxifen, temserolimus.
- Strong dual inducers of CYP3A4 and P-gp (dexamethasone, doxorubicin, rifampicin, St John's wort, sunitinib, vandetanib, vermurafenib, vinblastine) decrease the exposure to rivaroxaban and its anticoagulant activity. Avoid the combination.
- No interactions have been described between rivaroxaban and ranitidine, the antacid aluminum hydroxide/magnesium hydroxide, atorvastatin, digoxin, midazolam, or omeprazole.

4. *Cautions/notes* (see ➔ Apixaban, pp. 465–8)
   - Carefully monitor for bleeding in patients who require chronic treatment with low-dose aspirin and/or NSAIDs.
   - In patients with severe renal impairment (CrCl <30mL/min), plasma rivaroxaban levels increases 1.6-fold, which may lead to an increased bleeding risk. Use with caution in patients with CrCl of 15–29mL/min; not recommended with CrCl of <15mL/min. No dose adjustment is required in patients with mild hepatic impairment; avoid rivaroxaban in patients with moderate-severe hepatic impairment (Child–Pugh B–C).
   - For patients who are unable to swallow whole tablets, they may be crushed and mixed with food immediately prior to use and administered PO.
   - Andexanet alfa is the antidote of the anticoagulant effects of rivaroxaban in patients with life-threatening or uncontrolled bleeding.
5. *Pregnancy and lactation*
   - Rivaroxaban passes through the placenta, and in animal models, it produces reproductive toxicity. Thus, it is contraindicated in pregnant woman (Pregnancy category C). No data are available in breastfeeding women.
6. *Contraindications* (see ➔ Apixaban, pp. 465–8)
   - Strong inhibitors of both CYP3A4 and P-gp.
   - Rivaroxaban contains lactose; avoid in patients with rare hereditary problems of galactose intolerance, Lapp lactase deficiency, or glucose–galactose malabsorption.
   - Moderate–severe hepatic impairment (Child–Pugh B–C).
   - Severe renal impaiment (CrCl<15mL/min).

Rosuvastatin

Oral HMG CoA reductase inhibitor (see ➔ Statins (3-hydroxy-3-methylglutaryl-coenzyme A reductase inhibitors), pp. 760–3).

CV indications

- Treatment of hypercholesterolaemia in: (1) adults, adolescents, and children aged 6 years or older with primary hypercholesterolaemia (type IIa, including heterozygous familial hypercholesterolaemia) or mixed dyslipidaemia (type IIb), as an adjunct to diet when response to diet and other non-pharmacological treatments (e.g. exercise, weight reduction) is inadequate; (2) HoFH to reduce LDL-C, total-C, and Apo B levels, as an adjunct to other lipid-lowering treatments or if such treatments are not appropriate.
- Patients with hypertriglyceridaemia or with primary dysbetalipoproteinaemia (type III hyperlipoproteinaemia).
- Slows the progression of atherosclerosis, as part of a treatment strategy to lower total-C and LDL-C to target levels.
- Primary prevention of CV disease: in patients without clinically evident CAD, but with an increased risk of CV disease [≥50 years old in men and ≥60 years old in women, high-sensitivity C-reactive protein (hsCRP) ≥2mg/L, and presence of at least one additional CV disease risk factor such as hypertension, low HDL-C, smoking, or family history of premature CAD] to reduce the risk of MI, stroke, and arterial revascularization procedures.

Mechanism of action

(See ➔ Statins (3-hydroxy-3-methylglutaryl-coenzyme A reductase inhibitors), pp. 760–3.)

Pharmacodynamics

At doses between 10 and 40mg/day, rosuvastatin reduces serum levels of LDL-C (43–63%), total-C (31–46%), TGs (23–30%), and Apo B (7%) and increases HDL-C (10–14%) and Apo AI (36–54%) levels.

Pharmacokinetics

(See Table 8.1.4.)

Practical points

1. *Doses*
   - Starting dose: 5–10mg daily at any time of the day, with or without food; maximum dose 40mg od. Dose adjustments can be made after 4 weeks. Because of the increased risk of side effects, a dose of 40mg should be considered only in patients with severe hypercholesterolaemia at high CV risk who do not achieve their treatment goal on 20mg. For elderly patients, the recommended starting dose is 5mg od.
   - The recommended start dose is 5mg in patients with CrCl of <60mL/min.
   - In patients with hepatic impairment (Child–Pugh class B), the C_{max} and AUC of rosuvastatin increase; it is contraindicated in patients with active liver disease.

- Increased exposure to rosuvastatin is observed in Asian subjects. The recommended start dose is 5mg, and a 40mg dose is contraindicated.
- Patients with predisposing factors to myopathy and the elderly: the recommended starting dose is 5mg, and a 40mg dose is contraindicated.

2. *Side effects* (see ➔ Statins (3-hydroxy-3-methylglutaryl-coenzyme A reductase inhibitors), pp. 760–3)
   - Proteinuria with microscopic haematuria, mostly tubular in origin, has been observed in patients treated with high doses. In most cases, it was transient or intermittent and has not been shown to be predictive of acute or progressive renal disease.
3. *Interactions* (see ➔ Statins (3-hydroxy-3-methylglutaryl-coenzyme A reductase inhibitors), pp. 760–3)
   - Rosuvastatin is neither an inhibitor nor an inducer of cytochrome P450 isoenzymes. In addition, rosuvastatin is a poor substrate for these isoenzymes.
   - Concomitant use of aluminium/magnesium antacids reduces plasma levels of rosuvastatin (50%); administer the antacid 2h after rosuvastatin.
   - Gemfibrozil increased rosuvastatin exposure and the risk of myopathy/rhabdomyolysis; this interaction is not expected with fenofibrate. In combination with gemfibrozil, rosuvastatin should be limited to 5mg od.
   - Myopathy and rhabdomyolysis have been reported when co-administered with colchicine or niacin (≥1g/day).
   - Ciclosporin and gemfibrozil reduce rosuvastatin clearance; reduce the dose of rosuvastatin.
   - Co-administration with certain PIs (simeprevir, combinations of atazanavir/ritonavir or lopinavir/ritonavir) increases rosuvastatin exposure up to 5-fold. Therefore, in HIV patients receiving PIs, rosuvastatin is not recommended. The dose should be limited to 10mg od with atazanavir, with or without ritonavir, or lopinavir with ritonavir.
   - Erythromycin decreases (20–30%) rosuvastatin exposure, possibly due to an increase in gut motility.
   - Ciclosporin increases rosuvastatin exposure 7-fold, but the combination did not increase the plasma levels of ciclosporin. Avoid the combination.
   - Rosuvastatin increases the AUC of oral contraceptives (ethinylestradiol and norgestrel AUC increases by 26% and 34%, respectively).
   - No relevant interactions with digoxin or inhibitors/inducers of CYP3A4 or 2A6 are expected.
4. *Cautions/notes* (see ➔ Statins (3-hydroxy-3-methylglutaryl-coenzyme A reductase inhibitors), pp. 760–3)
5. *Pregnancy and lactation* (see ➔ Statins (3-hydroxy-3-methylglutaryl-coenzyme A reductase inhibitors), pp. 760–3)
6. *Contraindications* (see ➔ Statins (3-hydroxy-3-methylglutaryl-coenzyme A reductase inhibitors), pp. 760–3)
   - Severe renal impairment (CrCl <30mL/min).
   - Patients treated with ciclosporin.
   - A 40mg dose is contraindicated in patients with predisposing factors for myopathy/rhabdomyolysis.

Sacubitril/valsartan

This medicine combines the moieties of valsartan, an AT1 receptor antagonist, and sacubitril, a neprilysin (neutral endopeptidase) inhibitor.

Indications

- Treatment of symptomatic chronic HFrEF to reduce the risk of CV death and hospitalization. Entresto® is usually administered in the place of an ACEI (or an ARB).

Mechanism of action

Sacubitril/valsartan contains valsartan and sacubitril, which is then metabolized to the neprilysin inhibitor LBQ657. The CV and renal effects of sacubitril/valsartan are attributed to the increased levels of natriuretic peptides that are degraded by neprilysin and the simultaneous inhibition of the deleterious effects of angiotensin II mediated via the stimulation of AT1 receptors by valsartan. Natriuretic peptides exert their effects by activating membrane-bound guanylyl cyclase-coupled receptors (types A and B), resulting in increased concentrations of cGMP, which produces vasodilatation, natriuresis and diuresis, increased GFR and renal blood flow, inhibition of renin and aldosterone release, reduction in sympathetic activity, and antihypertrophic and antifibrotic effects. Stimulation of AT1 receptors produces vasoconstriction, hypertrophy, fibrosis, adverse remodelling, and sodium and water retention, increases oxidative stress and sympathetic tone, and inhibits angiotensin II-dependent aldosterone release.

Pharmacodynamics

In hypertensive patients, sacubitril/valsartan reduces PVR and SBP/DBP. In patients with HFrEF, sacubitril/valsartan increases natriuresis, urine atrial natriuretic peptide (ANP) and cGMP, and plasma cGMP and mid-regional pro-atrial natriuretic peptide (MR-proANP) and NT-pro-BNP, compared to valsartan. The risk of CV and all-cause mortality and HF hospitalizations was reduced by 20% in sacubitril/valsartan-treated patients, compared to enalapril-treated patients. Similar reduction was observed in sudden death and pump failure. Risk reduction was consistently observed across subgroups, including gender, age, race, NYHA class (II/III), LVEF, renal function, history of diabetes or hypertension, prior HF therapy, and AF.

Pharmacokinetics

Sacubitril/valsartan is well absorbed (oral bioavailability of sacubitril and valsartan is >60% and 23%, respectively) but is rapidly converted by esterases into valsartan and sacubitril, which is further metabolized to LBQ657. Peak plasma concentrations of sacubitril, LBQ657, and valsartan are reached in 0.5, 2, and 1.5h, respectively, and steady-state levels are reached in 3 days. In sacubitril/valsartan, 26, 51, and 103mg of valsartan are equivalent to 40, 80, and 160mg of valsartan in other marketed tablet formulations, respectively. Sacubitril, LBQ657, and valsartan are highly bound to plasma proteins (94–97%), and the Vd of valsartan and sacubitril are 75L and 103L, respectively. LBQ657 is not further metabolized, and valsartan is minimally metabolized (20%). Sacubitril (50–68%) and valsartan (approximately 13%) are excreted in the urine; 37–48% of sacubitril and

86% of valsartan are excreted in faeces. The t½ of sacubitril, LBQ657, and valsartan are 1.4, 11.5, and 9.9h, respectively. Exposure of valsartan was similar in patients with moderate and severe renal impairment, compared to patients with mild renal impairment, while exposure of patients with moderate and severe renal impairment to LBQ657 was 1.4-fold and 2.2-fold higher, compared to patients with mild renal impairment. Because LBQ657 and valsartan are highly bound to plasma protein, they are unlikely to be effectively removed by dialysis. (See Table 8.1.9.)

Practical points

1. *Doses*
   - The starting dose is 49/51mg bd (24/26mg bd in patients not currently taking an ACEI or an ARB); the dose can be doubled after 2–4 weeks to 97/103mg bd. A starting dose of 24/26mg bd is recommended for patients with moderate renal impairment (eGFR <30mL/min/1.73m^2). Treatment should not be initiated in patients with serum K^+ levels of >5.4mmol/L or with SBP of <100mmHg. No starting dose adjustment is needed for mild hepatic impairment; limited clinical experience in patients with moderate to severe hepatic impairment (Child–Pugh classes B and C) or severe renal impairment (eGFR <30mL/min/1.73m^2).
2. *Side effects*
   - The commonest are hypotension, hyperkalaemia, cough, nausea, diarrhoea, gastritis, fatigue, asthenia, dizziness, headache, decreases in haemoglobin/haematocrit, renal impairment, and angio-oedema. In the PARADIGM-HF trial, the incidence of angio-oedema was higher in patients treated with sacubitril/valsartan than enalapril (0.5% and 0.2%, respectively).
3. *Interactions* (see ➲ Valsartan, p. 791)
   - Co-administration of sacubitril/valsartan with drugs that induce/inhibit CYP450 enzymes is not expected to affect the pharmacokinetics of the drug.
   - Combination of sacubitril/valsartan with an ACEI increases the risk of angio-oedema and is contraindicated. Avoid the use of sacubitril/valsartan with any other ARB, because it contains valsartan.
   - The combination of sacubitril/valsartan with aliskiren is associated with hypotension, hyperkalaemia, and decreased renal function. This combination is contraindicated in patients with diabetes or renal impairment (eGFR <60mL/min/1.73m^2).
   - Co-administration of sacubitril/valsartan with potassium-sparing diuretics (e.g. spironolactone, triamterene, amiloride), potassium supplements, or heparin may increase serum K^+ and creatinine levels. Monitor serum K^+ levels.
   - Co-administration with PDE-5 inhibitors (i.e. sildenafil) produces a greater reduction in BP.
   - LBQ657 and valsartan are OATP1B1, OATP1B3, OAT1, and OAT3 substrates; valsartan is also an MRP2 substrate. Co-administration of sacubitril/valsartan with inhibitors of OATP1B1, OATP1B3, OAT3 (e.g. rifampicin, ciclosporin), OAT1 (e.g. tenofovir, cidofovir), or MRP2 (e.g. ritonavir) may increase the systemic exposure of LBQ657 or valsartan.

- No drug interactions with amlodipine, atorvastatin, carvedilol, digoxin, furosemide, HCTZ, levonorgestrel/ethinylestradiol, omeprazole, or warfarin.

4. *Cautions/notes*
   - Co-administration with NSAIDs in elderly patients, volume-depleted patients (treated with diuretics), or those with compromised renal function may increase the risk of worsening of renal function. Renal function should be monitored periodically.
   - Co-administration of sacubitril/valsartan with an ACEI (or ARBs) is contraindicated. Sacubitril/valsartan must not be administered until 36h after discontinuing ACEI therapy.
5. *Pregnancy and lactation*
   - There are no controlled data in human pregnancy or during lactation, but the limitations of valsartan can be applied (see ➔ Angiotensin II AT1 receptor blockers, pp. 456–8).
6. *Contraindications*
   - Hypersensitivity to the active substances or any of the excipients.
   - Concomitant use with ACEIs (or ARBs).
   - Known history of angio-oedema related to previous ACEI or ARB therapy. Hereditary or idiopathic angio-oedema.
   - Concomitant use with aliskiren-containing medicinal products in patients with diabetes mellitus.
   - Renal impairment (eGFR <60mL/min/1.73m^2).
   - SBP <90mmHg.
   - Severe hepatic impairment, biliary cirrhosis, and cholestasis.
   - Second and third trimester of pregnancy.

Selexipag

Oral non-prostanoid selective IP prostacyclin receptor agonist, distinct from prostacyclin and its analogues. A clear advantage of selexipag is its oral administration.

Indications

- Treatment of PAH in adult patients with WHO functional classes II–III, either as combination therapy in patients insufficiently controlled with an ERA and/or a PDE-5 inhibitor or as monotherapy in patients who are not candidates for these therapies.

Mechanism of action

Selexipag and its active metabolite, which is approximately 37-fold as potent as selexipag, are potent selective agonists of the prostacyclin IP receptor versus other prostanoid receptors (EP1-4, DP, FP, and TP). Activation of the IP receptor expressed in vascular smooth muscle cells and platelets stimulates adenylyl cyclase and increases cAMP levels, leading to vasodilatation, antiproliferative, and antifibrotic effects and inhibition of platelet aggregation. This selectivity for the IP receptor can minimize the frequent GI side effects (nausea, vomiting) resulting from activation of other prostanoid receptors.

Pharmacodynamics

Selexipag has been studied in patients with idiopathic and heritable PAH, PAH associated with connective tissue disorders, and PAH associated with corrected congenital heart disease with repaired shunts. In patients receiving ERAs and/or PDE-5 inhibitors, selexipag reduces (40%) a composite endpoint (including all-cause death, hospitalization for worsening of PAH, worsening of PAH resulting in the need for lung transplantation or atrial septostomy, initiation of parenteral prostanoids or chronic oxygen for worsening of PAH, and disease progression).

Pharmacokinetics

Selexipag is rapidly absorbed after oral administration (bioavailability 49%). It binds to plasma proteins (97–99%), present a Vd of 11.7L, and is biotransformed by hepatic carboxylesterase 1 to its metabolite ACT-333679, which is present at 3- to 4-fold higher plasma concentrations than the parent drug. Peak plasma concentrations of selexipag and its active metabolite are reached within 1–3h and 3–4h, respectively. Selexipag and its active metabolite undergo oxidative metabolism by CYP2C8 and CYP3A4; glucuronidation of the active metabolite is catalysed by UGT1A3 and UGT2B7. Selexipag is eliminated in the faeces (93%) and presents a t½ of 0.8–2.5h; the t½ of the active metabolite is 6.2–13.5h. No clinically relevant effects of sex, race, age, or body weight on the pharmacokinetics of selexipag have been observed in PAH patients.

Drug exposure increases 1.4- to 1.7-fold in patients with severe renal impairment (eGFR <30mL/min/1.73m^2) and 4-fold (and that of the metabolite 2-fold) in patients with moderate to severe hepatic impairment.

Practical points

1. *Doses*
   - Starting dose: 200mcg PO bd. Increase the dose by increments of 200mcg bd, usually at weekly intervals, to the highest tolerated dose (1600mcg bd). No dosage adjustment is required in the elderly and in patients with renal impairment or mild hepatic impairment. In mild hepatic impairment (Child–Pugh class B), the starting dose is 200mcg od; increase by increments of 200mcg/day at weekly intervals, as tolerated. Avoid the drug in patients with severe hepatic impairment. No change in the starting dose is required in patients with severe renal impairment (eGFR <30mL/min/1.73m^2). The tablets should not be split, crushed, or chewed and are to be swallowed with water.
2. *Side effects*
   - Very common: headache, diarrhoea, nausea, vomiting, jaw pain, pain in extremities, myalgia, flushing, arthralgia, anorexia, nasopharyngitis, and rash.
   - Common: anaemia, haemoglobin decrease, hyperthyroidism, anorexia, weight decrease, hypotension, abdominal pain, rash, urticaria, erythema.
3. *Interactions*
   - Selexipag and its active metabolite do not inhibit cytochrome P450 enzymes.
   - Lopinavir/ritonavir, a strong CYP3A4 inhibitor, increases exposure to selexipag 2-fold, whereas exposure to the active metabolite of selexipag did not change. Given the 37-fold higher potency of the active metabolite, this effect is not clinically relevant.
   - Use of selexipag in combination with both an ERA and a PDE-5 inhibitor resulted in 30% lower exposure of the active metabolite.
   - Selexipag inhibits platelet aggregation *in vitro* but does not increase the risk of bleeding when co-administered with anticoagulants or inhibitors of platelet aggregation. The pharmacokinetics of selexipag and its active metabolite are not affected by warfarin.
4. *Cautions/notes*
   - Treatment should only be initiated and monitored by a physician experienced in the treatment of PAH.
   - Selexipag can lower BP, particularly in patients on antihypertensive therapy or with hypotension, hypovolaemia, severe LV outflow obstruction, or autonomic dysfunction.
   - Selexipag can produce hyperthyroidism. Montor thyroid function tests.
   - Pulmonary oedema have been reported with prostacyclins when used in patients with pulmonary veno-occlusive disease. If pulmonary oedema occurs, treatment with selexipag should be discontinued.
   - Experience in the elderly (≥65 years) is limited.
   - Exposure to selexipag and its active metabolite increases in subjects with moderate hepatic impairment (Child–Pugh class B); it should be dosed once daily.
   - In patients with severe renal impairment (eGFR <30mL/min/1.73m^2), caution should be exercised during dose titration.

5. *Pregnancy and lactation*
   - No adequate and well-controlled studies with selexipag exist in pregnant women, and it is unknown whether it is excreted in human breast milk (Pegnancy category C). Thus, it is recommended to discontinue nursing or to discontinue selexipag.
6. *Contraindications*
   - Hypersensitivity to the active substance or any of the excipients.
   - Severe CAD, UA, and MI within the last 6 months.
   - Decompensated HF.
   - Severe arrhythmia.
   - Cerebrovascular events (e.g. TIA, stroke) within the last 3 months.
   - Congenital or acquired valvular defects with clinically relevant myocardial function disorders not related to pulmonary hypertension.
   - Co-administration with strong CYP2C inhibitors (abiraterone, clopidogrel, and gemfibrozil).

Sildenafil

Orally active, potent, and selective PDE-5 inhibitor.

CV indications

- Treatment of adult patients with PAH classified as WHO functional classes II and III, to improve exercise capacity. Efficacy has been shown in primary PAH and PAH associated with connective tissue disease.
- Treatment of paediatric patients aged 1–17 years with PAH. Efficacy has been shown in primary PAH and PAH associated with congenital heart disease.
- Other indications: treatment of erectile dysfunction.

Mechanism of action

PAH is associated with impaired release of NO because of reduced expression of NO synthase in the vascular endothelium of pulmonary arteries and an upregulation of PDE-5 activity in the pulmonary vasculature, which rapidly degrades cGMP. Inhibition of PDE-5 increases intracellular cGMP levels, which mediates the antiproliferative and vasodilating effects of endogenous NO in the pulmonary vasculature and in the corpus cavernosum of the penis.

Sildenafil inhibits PDE-5, the enzyme responsible for the degradation of cGMP, and activates the NO–guanylyl cyclase–cGMP pathway. Thus, it produces pulmonary and systemic vasodilatation, increase cardiac contractility (i.e. it acts as an inodilator), and exerts antiproliferative effects.

Pharmacodynamics

Studies with sildenafil have been performed in forms of PAH related to primary (idiopathic), connective tissue disease associated, or congenital heart disease associated forms of PAH. Sildenafil reduces mean right arterial pressure and pulmonary and systemic vascular resistances, and improves functional class, symptoms, exercise capacity (6MWT), haemodynamics, and time to clinical worsening. Addition of sildenafil to epoprostenol produces an improvement after 12 weeks in 6MWT and time to clinical worsening.

Pharmacokinetics

Oral absorption is rapid (bioavailability 40%), reaching peak plasma levels within 30–120min. Drug absorption is reduced and delayed when taken with a high-fat meal. Protein-binding is 96%, and the Vd is large (1.3L/kg). It is hepatically metabolized by CYP450 3A4 (2C9 is a minor route) and is excreted as active and inactive metabolites in the faeces (80% of the administered oral dose) and in the urine (13%). The terminal t½ is 3–5h.

Practical points

1. *Doses*
   - 10mg tds (for symptomatic treatment of PAH). Age >65 and hepatic and renal impairment (CrCl <30mL/min) decreased clearance of sildenafil. Reduce the dose to 20mg bd in such patients, if recommended doses are not tolerated.
   - Based on pharmacokinetics data, an IV formulation of sildenafil has been proposed as a bridge for PAH patients on long-term oral treatment who are temporarily unable to ingest tablets.

- Initial dose adjustments are not required in patients with severe renal (CrCl <30mL/min) or moderate hepatic impairment (Child–Pugh classes A and B).
- 10mg bd when sildenafil is co-administered with CYP3A4 inhibitors such as erythromycin or saquinavir; 10mg od when co-administered with potent CYP3A4 inhibitors (see Table 8.1.2).

2. *Side effects*
   - Very common: headache, flushing, epistaxis, dyspepsia, diarrhoea, pain in extremities.
   - Common: GI (vomiting, gastritis, gastro-oesophageal reflux disease, abdominal pain, dry mouth), dizziness, insomnia, skin rashes, hypotension, myalgia, back pain, alopecia, erythema, epistaxis, cough, nasal congestion, reduced visual acuity, and diplopia.
   - Potency of sildenafil for PDE-6 (which is found within the retina and involved in the phototransduction pathyway) is about one-tenth. Thus, patients may experience visual disturbances, including photophobia, blurred vision, and increased sensitivity to light and blue/green tingeing at higher doses.
   - Rare: sudden vision loss caused by non-arteritic anterior ischaemic optic neuropathy (NAION), priapism, severe hypotension, MI, increased intraocular pressure, and sudden hearing loss.
   - In males with erectile dysfunction, serious CV events, including UA, MI, SCD, ventricular arrhythmia, cerebrovascular haemorrhage, TIA, hypertension, and hypotension, have been reported in temporal association with the use of sildenafil.
3. *Interactions*
   - Concomitant use of antihypertensives and vasodilator drugs (nitrates, nicorandil) increases the risk of hypotension. Combination with α1-blockers may lead to low BP; this effect does not occur if they are taken at least 4h apart.
   - Co-administration of bosentan (125mg bd) with sildenafil (80mg tds) resulted in a 63% decrease in the sildenafil AUC and a 50% increase in the bosentan AUC. Caution is recommended in the case of co-administration. Bosentan reduces tadalafil (40mg od) systemic exposure by 42% and C_{max} by 27%; tadalafil does not affect the exposure (AUC and C_{max}) of bosentan or its metabolites.
   - Co-administration with powerful CYP450, 3A4, and 2C9 inhibitors (see Table 8.1.2) increases plasma levels, even when dose adjustments may not be required.
   - Co-administration of sildenafil with guanylyl cyclase stimulators (riociguat) may potentially lead to symptomatic hypotension and is contraindicated.
   - CYP3A4 inducers (see Table 8.1.2) may significantly lower sildenafil levels.
   - Sildenafil can increase the plasma levels of atorvastatin and simvastatin, and these drugs can increase the levels of sildenafil.
   - There may be potential for an increased risk of bleeding when sildenafil is initiated in patients already using a VKA, particularly in patients with PAH secondary to connective tissue disease.
   - Ritonavir and saquinavir (potent P450 inhibitors) markedly increase the plasma levels of oral sildenafil; this combination is contraindicated.

4. *Cautions/notes*
   - Assess CV status before use; caution with LV outflow obstruction or in conditions aggravated by hypotension.
   - Sildenafil has not been studed in clinically or haemodynamically unstable patients or in those with severe PAH (functional class IV) or with WHO functional class I PAH.
   - The safety of sildenafil has not been studied in patients with retinitis pigmentosa.
   - Sildenafil should be used with caution in patients with anatomical deformation of the penis or conditions which may predispose them to priapism (such as sickle-cell anaemia, multiple myeloma, or leukaemia).
   - The use of sildenafil is contraindicated in patients with severe hepatic impairment, a recent history of stroke or MI, or severe hypotension (BP <90/50mmHg) at initiation.
   - Sildenafil should not be used in patients with pulmonary hypertension secondary to sickle-cell anaemia. because of the risk of vaso-occlusive crises requiring hospitalization.
5. *Pregnancy and lactation*
   - Sildenafil is safe in pregnancy (Pregnancy category B). Avoid in pregnant women, unless strictly necessary.
6. *Contraindications*
   - Hypersensitivity to the active substance or any of the excipients.
   - Concurrent or intermittent use of NO donors or organic nitrates in any form.
   - Co-administration with guanylyl cyclase stimulators or potent 3A4 inhibitors (see Table 8.1.2).
   - Visual loss due to NAION.
   - Severe hepatic impairment; recent stroke or MI; severe hypotension (BP <90/50mmHg).
   - Lactose monohydrate is present in the tablet film coat. Patients with rare hereditary problems of galactose intolerance, Lapp lactase deficiency, or glucose–galactose malabsorption should not take this medicine.

Simvastatin

Oral HMG CoA reductase inhibitor (see also ➔ Statins (3-hydroxy-3-methylglutaryl-coenzyme A reductase inhibitors), pp. 760–3).

CV indications

It is indicated as an adjunct to diet.

- Hypercholesterolaemia: (1) treatment of primary hypercholesterolaemia or mixed dyslipidaemia when response to diet and other non-pharmacological treatments (e.g. exercise, weight reduction) is inadequate; and (2) treatment of HoFH, as an adjunct to other lipid-lowering treatments (e.g. LDL apheresis) or if such treatments are not appropriate.
- CV prevention: reduction in CV mortality and morbidity in patients with manifest atherosclerotic CV disease or diabetes mellitus, with either normal or increased cholesterol levels, as an adjunct to correction of other risk factors and other cardioprotective therapy.

Pharmacodynamics

At doses between 10 and 40mg/day, simvastatin reduces serum levels of LDL-C (18–41%), total-C (20–45%), TGs (10–18%), and Apo B and increases HDL-C (up to 12%) levels.

Pharmacokinetics

Simvastatin is an inactive lactone, which is readily hydrolysed in the liver to the corresponding β-hydroxy acid, a potent inhibitor of HMG CoA reductase. The major metabolites of simvastatin present in human plasma are β-hydroxy acid and four additional active metabolites. (See Table 8.1.4.)

Practical points

1. *Doses*
   - The dosage range is 5–80mg daily (in the evening). The 80mg dose is only recommended in patients with severe hypercholesterolaemia and at high risk for CV complications.
   - *Hypercholesterolaemia*: starting dose is 10–20mg daily. Patients who require a large reduction in LDL-C levels may be started at 20–40mg/day.
   - *HoFH*: 40mg in the evening, as an adjunct to other lipid-lowering treatments.
   - *CV prevention*: 20–40mg in the evening in patients at high risk of coronary heart disease (with or without hyperlipidaemia).
   - Simvastatin is also available in combination with ezetimibe (10mg of ezetimibe with 20, 40, or 80mg of simvastatin).
2. *Side effects* (see ➔ Statins (3-hydroxy-3-methylglutaryl-coenzyme A reductase inhibitors), pp. 760–3)
   - Persistent increases (>3 times ULN) in serum transaminases occurred in 1% of patients.

3. *Interactions* (see ➔ Statins (3-hydroxy-3-methylglutaryl-coenzyme A reductase inhibitors), pp. 760–3)
   - Simvastatin modestly potentiates coumarin anticoagulants. Monitor the INR.
   - Simvastatin is a substrate of CYP3A4 and of the transport protein OATP1B1. The risk of myopathy and rhabdomyolysis significantly increased when combined with potent CYP3A4 inhibitors (see Table 8.1.2).
   - Avoid the combination of doses higher than 20mg in patients taking amiodarone, verapamil, and diltiazem.
4. *Cautions/notes* (see ➔ Statins (3-hydroxy-3-methylglutaryl-coenzyme A reductase inhibitors), pp. 760–3)
   - Patients titrated to the 80mg dose should receive additional LFTs prior to titration, 3 months after titration to the 80mg dose, and periodically for the first year. Dosages above 10mg/day should be carefully considered in severe renal insufficiency (CrCl <30mL/min).
5. *Contraindications* (see ➔ Statins (3-hydroxy-3-methylglutaryl-coenzyme A reductase inhibitors), pp. 760–3)
   - Concomitant administration of gemfibrozil, ciclosporin, danazol, or potent CYP3A4 inhibitors (see Table 8.1.2).

Sodium–glucose co-transporter 2 inhibitors (SGLT2Is)

Canaglifozin, dapagliflozin, empagliflozin, ertugliflozin, sotagliflozin.

CV indications

- As an adjunct to diet and exercise to improve glycaemic control in patients with T2DM as: monotherapy, when metformin is considered inappropriate due to intolerance, and/or in addition to other medicinal products, including insulin, when they do not provide adequate glycaemic control.
- Canagliflozin: to reduce the risk of major adverse cardiovascular events (cardiovascular death, non-fatal MI, and stroke) in adults with T2DM and established cardiovascular disease.
- Empagliflozin: to reduce the risk of cardiovascular death in adults with T2DM and cardiovascular disease.

Mechanism of action

SGLT2 is selectively expressed in the proximal renal tubules and is responsible for the majority (90%) of the reabsorption of filtered glucose from the tubular lumen. SGLT2Is selectively inhibit SGLT2, reduce the tubular reabsorption of filtered glucose, and thereby increase urinary glucose excretion, lowering elevated plasma glucose concentrations by this insulin-independent mechanism in patients with T2DM. Because glucose is exchanged by Na^+, SGLT2Is also produce an osmotic diuresis, which may reduce intravascular volume and decrease blood pressure.

In cardiovascular outcome trials performed in T2DM patients, empagliflozin reduced major cardiovascular events (MACE: cardiovascular death, non-fatal MI, or non-fatal stroke), CV mortality, all-cause mortality, and hospitalization for HF); canagliflozin reduced MACE and all-cause mortality, and hospitalization for HF, but not CV mortality; and dapagliflozin did not result in a higher or lower rate of MACE than placebo but did result in a lower rate of CV death or hospitalization for HF. Empagliflozin, canagliflozin, and dapagliflozin also reduced the progression of renal disease. These cardiac and renal protective effects were observed regardless of the presence of atherosclerotic CVD or HF at baseline.

Pharmacodynamics

SGLT2Is decrease plasma glucose concentrations and HbA1c levels, plasma volume, blood pressure, and arterial stiffness. Urinary glucose excretion (70g/day) is associated with an osmotic diuresis and transient natriuresis, caloric loss (280kcal/day) and reduction in body weight and visceral adiposity. SGLT2 inhibitors also increase haemoglobin and haematocrit and produce a uricosuric effect.

It has been proposed that the cardiorenal protective effects of SGLT2 inhibitors can be related to a metabolic shift in cardiorenal metabolism from conventional fatty acids and glucose oxidation to ketone bodies and to a reduction in intracellular sodium ($[Na^+]_i$) by inhibiting the sarcolemmal Na^+-H^+ exchanger (NHE1 and 3).

Pharmacokinetics

- Canagliflozin presents an oral bioavailability of 65% and reaches peak plasma levels within 1–2h. It binds to plasma proteins (99%), presents a Vd of 1.7L/kg, and is metabolized via UGT1A9 and UGT2B4 to inactive metabolites (7% by CYP3A4). It is eliminated in faeces (41.5%) and urine (33%; <15% unchanged). Its t½ is 10–13h.
- Dapagliflozin is rapidly absorbed (bioavailability 78%) and reaches peak plasma levels within 2h. It binds to plasma proteins (91%), presents a Vd of 1.7L/kg, and is metabolized through UGT1A9-mediated O-glucuronidation to inactive metabolites. It is eliminated in faeces (21%) and urine (55%). Its t½ is 12–13h.
- Empagliflozin presents an oral bioavailability of 65% and reaches peak plasma levels within 1.5h. It binds to plasma proteins (88%), presents a Vd of 0.97L/kg, and is metabolized by uridine 5'-diphospho-glucuronosyltransferases to inactive metabolites. It is eliminated in faeces (41.5%) and urine (54%) and has a t½ of 12.4h.
- Ertugliflozin is rapidly and completely absorbed (oral bioavailability 100%) and reaches peak plasma levels after 1h. It binds to plasma proteins (93.5%), presents a Vd of 1.2L/kg, and is metabolized by UGT1A9 and UGT2B7. It is eliminated in faeces (41%) and urine (50%; 1.5% unchanged). Its t½ is 16.6h.

Practical points

1. *Doses*
   - Canagliflozin: 100mg PO od taken before the first meal of the day. The dose can be increased to 300mg/day in patients who have eGFR ≥60mL/min/1.73m^2 and require additional glycaemic control. eGFR <60mL/min/1.73m^2: do not exceed 100mg/day. eGFR <45mL/min/1.73m^2: do not initiate canagliflozin.
   - Dapagliflozin: 10mg od. No dose adjustment is recommended in the elderly or in hepatic impairment. It should be discontinued when eGFR <60mL/min/1.73m^2.
   - Empagliflozin: 10mg od. In tolerant patients who have an eGFR ≥60ml/min/1.73m^2 and need tighter glycaemic control, the dose can be increased to 25mg od. It should be discontinued when eGFR is <45mL/min/1.73m^2.
   - Ertugliflozin: 5mg od, taken in the morning. The dose can be increased to 15mg od if additional glycaemic control is needed. eGFR 30–60mL/min/1.73m^2: not recommended.
2. *Side effects*
   - Common: genital mycotic infections, volume depletion, hypotension, polyuria, thirst, hypoglycaemia (when used with sulphonylurea or insulin), haematocrit increased, urinary tract infections (including life-threatening urosepsis and pyelonephritis), weight loss, increase in LDL-C levels and renal adverse effects (increase in plasma creatinine and urea levels, decrease in eGFR).
   - Uncommon: symptomatic hypotension.
   - Rare: euglycaemic ketoacidosis (including life-threatening and fatal cases), worsening renal function and acute kidney failure (mainly if volume depletion), necrotizing fasciitis of the perineum (Fournier gangrene).

- Canagliflozin increases the risk of lower-limb amputations (mainly of the toe) and bone fractures. Before treatment consider factors in the patient history that may increase the risk for amputation. It is unknown whether this constitutes a class effect.

3. *Interactions*
   - Hypoglycaemia risk increases with insulin and insulin secretagogues (e.g. sulfonylureas); use a lower dose of insulin or insulin secretagogue to reduce the risk of hypoglycaemia.
   - Co-administration with thiazide and loop diuretics and may increase the risk of dehydration and hypotension.
   - No interaction with ciclosporin, gemfibrozil, glimepiride, hydrochlorothiazide, linagliptin, metformin, oral contraceptives (ethinylestradiol and levonorgestrel), pioglitazone, ramipril, simvastatin, sitagliptin, torasemide, verapamil, warfarin.
   - Colestyramine may potentially reduce canagliflozin exposure. Administer canagliflozin at least 1h before or 4–6h after colestyramine.
   - Rifampicin decreases canagliflozin exposure and may reduce its efficacy.
   - Patients taking digitalis or dabigatran should be monitored appropriately if combined with canagliflozin.
4. *Cautions*
   - Symptomatic hypotension may occur, particularly in patients with renal impairment, low SBD, on diuretics, or in the elderly. Correct volume status and monitor renal function before initiating and periodically during treatment.
   - Risk of genital mycotic infections increase in patients with history of genital mycotic infections and in uncircumcised males.
   - Acute kidney injury increases in patients with hypovolaemia, HF, and CKD, or treated with diuretics, ACE inhibitors, NSAIDs, or angiotensin receptor blockers.
   - Assess patients who present with signs and symptoms of metabolic acidosis for ketoacidosis, regardless of blood glucose level. In clinical situations that may predispose to ketoacidosis a temporary discontinuation of therapy is required.
   - Before initiating the treatment consider the presence of factors that may predispose for amputation, such as a history of prior amputation, peripheral vascular disease, neuropathy, and diabetic foot ulcers. Counsel patients about the importance of routine preventative foot care. Monitor patients for signs and symptoms of infection (including osteomyelitis), new pain, or tenderness, sores, or ulcers involving the lower limbs, and discontinue if these complications occur.
   - Necrotizing fasciitis of the perineum (Fournier gangrene): if suspected, discontinue SGLT2Is and start treatment immediately with broad-spectrum antibiotics and surgical debridement if necessary.
   - Monitoring glycemic control with 1,5-AG assay is not recommended in patients taking SGLT2Is. Use alternative methods to monitor glycaemic control. Monitoring glycaemic control with urine glucose tests is not recommended as SGLT2Is increase urinary glucose excretion and will lead to positive urine glucose tests.

5. *Pregnancy and lactation*
   - Limited data are available in pregnant women; no information regarding excretion in human milk. Use during pregnancy only if the potential benefit justifies the potential risk to the fetus. SGLT2Is are not recommended while breastfeeding.
6. *Contraindications*
   - Serious hypersensitivity reaction to SGLT2Is or any of excipients.
   - T1DM.
   - Any type of acute metabolic acidosis.
   - eGFR <30mL/min/1.73m^2 (ertugliflozin), <45mL/min/1.73m^2 (canagliflozin, empagliflozin), or <60ml/min/1.73m^2 (dapagliflozin).
   - Acute conditions with the potential to alter renal function such as: dehydration, severe infection, shock.

Sodium nitroprusside

IV direct NO donor.

CV indications

- Immediate reduction of BP in patients with hypertensive crisis. It should be administered with other long-acting antihypertensives to minimize the duration of treatment.
- Treatment of acute CHF. IV sodium nitroprusside is the vasodilator of choice for severe low-output left-sided HF, because it acts rapidly and has a balanced effect on afterload and preload.
- Controlled hypotension in anaesthesia to reduce bleeding during surgery.
- In patients with pulmonary oedema secondary to severe acute or chronic mitral or aortic regurgitation, IV sodium nitroprusside is probably the agent of choice.

Mechanism of action

Sodium nitroprusside is a non-organic nitrate that acts as a direct NO donor. Endothelial NO relaxes vascular smooth muscle (vasodilatation) through the activation of sGC and the formation of cAMP. NO also inhibits platelet aggregation (antithrombotic) and leucocyte–endothelial interactions (anti-inflammatory) and exhibits antiproliferative properties. By mimicking the actions of endogenous NO, sodium nitroprusside causes dilatation of peripheral arteries and veins. Venodilatation decreases venous return to the heart, thereby reducing LVEDP (preload) and PCWP. Arteriolar relaxation reduces PVR (afterload) and BP and increases the heart rate, with variable effects on CO. In hypertensive patients, sodium nitroprusside induces renal vasodilatation, without changes in renal blood flow or GFR.

Pharmacodynamics

After IV administration, sodium nitroprusside produces a rapid and potent relaxation of vascular smooth muscle cells, producing a more marked venous than arterial dilatation and a decrease in BP. Its vasodilator effect appears immediately, but changes in BP dissipates rapidly after the infusion is discontinued. Due to its potency and rapid onset of action, its use in severe hypertension can lead to compensatory mechanisms that may cause reflex tachycardia, volume expansion, and increases in plasma renin activity. Sodium nitroprusside also produces coronary arterial vasodilatation, although a significant reduction in regional blood flow (coronary steal) can occur in patients with CAD. The hypotensive effect of sodium nitroprusside is associated with reduced blood loss in a variety of major surgical procedures.

In patients with acute HF and increased PVR (associated to hypertension), with mitral or aortic regugitation, or with severe HF complicating an acute MI, after cardiac surgery, or in patients with acute exacerbation of chronic HF, sodium nitroprusside reduces PVR and LV filling pressure and increases CO.

Pharmacokinetics

IV infusion of sodium nitroprusside produces an almost immediate reduction in BP, but BP begins to rise immediately when the infusion is slowed or stopped and returns to pre-treatment levels within 1–10min. It is distributed to the extracellular space and is cleared by an intra-erythrocyte reaction with haemoglobin to form cyanomethaemoglobin and cyanide ions, so that its t½ is approximately 2–3min. Cyanide ions then reacts with thiosulfate to produce thiocyanate, which is excreted in the urine (t½ 2.7–7 days; longer in patients with decreased renal function and hyponatraemia), and some cyanide is removed as expired hydrogen cyanide. Cyanide ions not removed by these pathways are enzymatically converted to thiocyanate by the hepatic mitochondrial enzyme thiosulfate-cyanide sulfur transferase and may cause toxicity through inhibition of oxidative phosphorylation.

Practical points

1. *Doses*
   - Dosage varies between individuals. The solutions should be made in saline (avoid alkaline solutions) and used as soon as possible, under continuous BP monitoring to avoid excessive hypotension. Discolored solutions or solutions with visible particulate matter should not be used. If properly protected from light with aluminum foil or opaque materials, the freshly diluted solution is stable for 24h.
   - *Hypertensive crises*: initial dose of approximately 0.3mcg/kg/min (uptitrated to 0.5–10mcg/kg/min). The infusion dose should never last for >10min to avoid the danger of cyanide toxicity. In hypertensive patients, receiving concomitant antihypertensive medication, smaller doses might be required.
   - *Acute HF*: initial dose of 0.3mcg/kg/min, and increase up to 5mcg/kg/min. Sometimes it is permissible to use low-dose nitroprusside for up to 3 days when using this agent as a bridge to a mechanical assist device or to cardiac transplantation.
   - Due to an increased risk of cyanide poisoning, doses of sodium nitroprusside should be reduced in renal impairment. Risk of toxicity may also be reduced by not exceeding a dose equivalent to 2mcg/kg/min (over a maximum of 48h). Toxic cyanide can reach potentially lethal levels.
2. *Side effects*
   - The commonest side effects are: hypotension, headache, dizziness, drowsiness, fatigue, disorientation, palpitations, tachycardia, bradycardia, nausea, vomiting, abdominal pain, apprehension, and diaphoresis. Retrosternal discomfort have been noted when the reduction in BP is too rapid. Sodium nitroprusside may cause a coronary steal syndrome and myocardial ischaemia and increase intracranial pressure. These symptoms disappear when the rate of infusion is decreased or the infusion is temporarily discontinued and do not reappear with a continued slower rate of administration.
   - Pulmonary hypoxia may result from increased V/Q mismatch with pulmonary vasodilatation.

- Others: rash, hypothyroidism (thiocyanate interferes with iodine uptake by the thyroid), decreased platelet aggregation, flushing, venous streaking, irritation at the infusion site, cyanide toxicity (changed mental status, convulsions, lactic acidosis, and venous hyperoxaemia with bright red venous blood), and thiocyanate toxicity (tinnitus, miosis, hyperreflexia at serum levels of 1mmol/L). To maintain steady-state thiocyanate levels of <1 mmol/L, a prolonged infusion of sodium nitroprusside should not exceed a dose of 3mcg/kg/min (1mcg/kg/min in anuric patients).
- Cyanide toxicity is treated with sodium nitrite, available in a 3% solution (0.2mL/kg over 2–5min), followed by an infusion of sodium thiosulfate (12.5g in 50mL of 5% glucose over 10min). Repeat, if needed, at half these doses.
- At high doses, nitroprusside can lead to methaemoglobin formation through dissociation of cyanmethaemoglobin and by direct oxidation of haemoglobin by the released nitroso group. Treatment of methaemoglobinaemia is 1–2mg/kg of methylthioninium chloride.

3. *Interactions*
   - The vasodilator and hypotensive effects of sodium nitroprusside increase when co-administered with other vasodilators or antihypertensives and some anaesthetic agents.
4. *Cautions/notes*
   - Sodium nitroprusside should be administered by IV infusion via a controlled infusion pump that allows precise measurement of flow rates, under careful continuous monitoring, and it should be protected from light to minimize degradation.
   - Nitroprusside treatment should not be abruptly withdrawn because of the danger of rebound hypertension. Extravasation must be avoided.
   - Infusions may be continued for several days (normally should not exceed 3 days), but care must be taken to ensure that serum cyanide concentrations do not exceed 100mcg/100mL and blood thiocyanate concentrations 100mcg/mL. Risk of toxicity is increased in renal impairment.
   - Elderly patients appear to be more sensitive to the hypotensive effects of the drug, and it should be administered with caution in this age group.
   - Progressive tachyphylaxis to the hypotensive effects of sodium nitroprusside has been described, but the mechanism remains unknown.
   - In patients with acute HF, monitor the haemodynamic response and urine output, but improvements in CO and LV filling pressure must not be reached at the price of undue hypotension and tissue hypoperfusion.
5. *Pregnancy and lactation*
   - Sodium nitroprusside crosses the placental barrier, with fetal cyanide levels dose-related to maternal levels of nitroprusside. It is not known whether sodium nitroprusside can cause fetal harm when administered to a pregnant woman (Pregnancy category C). It is not known if sodium nitroprusside is excreted in breast milk. Therefore, it should be used with caution in breastfeeding mothers.

6. *Contraindications*
   - Hypotension (SBP <90mmHg). Compensatory hypertension (arteriovenous shunt or aortic coarctation).
   - Acute HF associated with reduced PVRs (i.e. high-output HF observed in endotoxic sepsis).
   - Inadequate cerebral circulation and compensatory hypertension.
   - Severe vitamin B12 deficiency, hepatic and renal insufficiency, and Leber's optic atrophy (due to the metabolites cyanide and thiocyanide).
   - Acute MI is not a contraindication, provided that excess hypotension is avoided.

Sotalol

Non-selective β1-adrenergic receptor antagonist with high lipid solubility (see ➔ Beta-adrenergic blocking agents, pp. 485–94). Mixed class II and III antiarrhythmic agent.

CV indications

- Treatment of life-threatening sustained and non-sustained ventricular tachyarrhythmias. Because of the proarrhythmic risks, sotalol is not recommended in patients with less severe arrhythmias, even if symptomatic.
- Maintenance of sinus rhythm following cardioversion of atrial flutter or AF and to control ventricular rate. Sotalol can be given to patients with structural heart disease and without an additional agent to slow AV nodal conduction. Sotalol is not effective in converting recent-onset or persistent AF.
- Prophylaxis of paroxysmal AT, paroxysmal AVRT and paroxysmal AVNRT using accessory pathways, and paroxysmal SVT after cardiac surgery.
- Sotalol may be considered in patients with a diagnosis of SQTS who qualify for an ICD but present a contraindication to the ICD or refuse it and in asymptomatic patients with a diagnosis of SQTS and a family history of SCD.

Mechanism of action

In addition to acting as a β-blocker with related class II antiarrhythmic activity, sotalol also exerts additional class III antiarrhythmic activity through the blockade of the rapid component of the delayed rectifier K^+ current (IKr) responsible for phase 3 of the cardiac action potential. This results in a dose-dependent prolongation of the QT interval and an effective refractory period.

Pharmacodynamics

(See ➔ Beta-adrenergic blocking agents, pp. 485–94.)

Sotalol is a racemic mixture of dextro- and levo-isomers; the l-isomer is responsible for its β-blocking effects and class II antiarrhythmic activity. Its β-blocking effects occur with oral doses as low as 25mg, but class III effects are seen at higher doses (>160mg/day).

Sotalol slows the heart rate, decreases AV nodal conduction, increases AV nodal refractoriness, and prolongs the APD and refractoriness in all cardiac tissues. Furthermore, sotalol inhibits conduction along any bypass tract in both directions. It produces a dose-dependent increase in the QTc, RR, and PR intervals but does not modify the QRS interval. The APD prolongation can explain why the negative inotropic effect is less than expected but may cause early after-depolarizations, triggering TdP.

In hypertensive patients, sotalol reduces both SBP/DBP. Sotalol is usually well tolerated haemodynamically, but caution should be exercised in patients with reduced LVEF and VT. d-sotalol increased mortality in post-MI patients with a low LVEF.

Sotalol reduces dose-dependently VPBs and NSVT. In patients with sustained ventricular arrhythmias and ICD, sotalol significantly reduced the incidence of recurrences of sustained ventricular tachyarrhythmias, but it did not improve survival. Sotalol can be considered for acute conversion of haemodynamically stable monomorphic sustained VT. In patients with previous MI, sotalol did not increase survival. Sotalol can be used safely in patients with CAD, unless they have HF.

Pharmacokinetics

(See Tables 8.1.3 and 8.1.8.)

Practical points

1. *Doses*
   - The recommended initial dose is 80mg bd. In patients with ventricular arrhythmias, the dose may be increased in increments of 80mg/day every 3 days, provided the QTc is <500ms, up to a total daily dose of 160–320mg/day in two doses. Oral doses as high as 480–640mg/day have been utilized in patients with refractory life-threatening arrhythmias.
   - Prevention of recurrence of AF/atrial flutter: 120mg bd.
   - Doses should be reduced in renal impairment (half dose with CrCl of 30–60mL/min, quarter dose with CrCl of 10–30mL/min), in elderly patients, or when there are risk factors for proarrhythmia. Another alternative is to prolong the dosing interval up to 24h and 36–48h in patients with CrCl of 30–59mL/min and 10–29mL/min, respectively. In patients with CrCl of <10mL/min or QTc >450, sotalol is contraindicated.
2. *Side effects* (see ➔ Beta-adrenergic blocking agents, pp. 485–94)
   - The most important side effects are TdP and other serious new ventricular arrhythmias occurring in a dose-dependent manner (0.3% at 320mg/day, but goes up to 4% at the highest doses). Avoid daily doses of ≥320mg.
   - Bradycardia, fatigue, dyspnoea, chest pain, palpitations, oedema, hypotension, proarrhythmia, syncope, HF, presyncope, asthenia, and dizziness.
3. *Interactions* (see ➔ Beta-adrenergic blocking agents, pp. 485–94)
   - Sotalol should be administered with caution with QT-prolonging drugs.
   - Additive effects are expected if sotalol is co-administered with other β-blockers.
   - Co-administration with digoxin can increase the risk of bradycardia and AVB.
   - Sotalol should be administered with caution with diltiazem or verapamil, because they may exert additive effects, leading to hypotension, bradycardia, or AVB.
   - The dosage of insulin or antidiabetic drugs may require adjustment because of the risk of hyperglycaemia. Additionally, sotalol masked the symptoms of hypoglycaemia.
   - β2-receptor agonists should be administered at increased dosages in patients treated with sotalol.
   - Administration of sotalol within 2h of antacids containing aluminum oxide and magnesium hydroxide reduces sotalol exposure.

4. *Cautions/notes* (see ➔ Beta-adrenergic blocking agents, pp. 485–94)
   - Renal function, safety (heart rate, BP, QT interval), and ECG must be closely monitored.
   - The risk of TdP increases in females, at high doses (>320mg/day), in the presence of bradycardia, when the baseline QT interval is >450ms, in severe LV failure, and in patients treated with QT-prolonging drugs. Electrolyte disturbances (hypokalaemia and hypomagnesaemia) should be corrected.
   - For the initial treatment in patients with recurrent AF or flutter, the patient should be monitored for 3 days while the dose is increased.
   - Sotalol may precipitate bronchospasm.
5. *Pregnancy and lactation* (see ➔ Beta-adrenergic blocking agents, pp. 485–94)
   - There are no well-controlled studies in pregnant women, but sotalol crosses the placenta and may depress fetal vital functions, and is present in breast milk (Pregnancy category B).
6. *Contraindications* (see ➔ Beta-adrenergic blocking agents, pp. 485–94)
   - Hypersensitivity to any of the components of the formulation.
   - Renal failure (CrCl <10mL/min).
   - Asthma. In bronchospastic disease with caution (sotalol is a non-selective β-blocker).
   - Sinus bradycardia, sick sinus syndrome, or second- and third-degree AVB (unless a functioning pacemaker is present).
   - Congenital or acquired LQTS.
   - Cardiogenic shock or decompensated HF.
   - Prinzmetal's angina.
   - Raynaud's phenomenon and severe peripheral circulatory disturbances.

Spironolactone

Competitive MRA (potassium-sparing diuretic).

CV indications

- HFrEF (NYHA classes III–IV) to increase survival and to reduce hospitalizations for HF when used in addition to standard therapy.
- Arterial hypertension, particularly in patients with resistant hypertension.
- Diagnosis and treatment of primary aldosteronism.
- Oedema associated with hyperaldosteronism (hepatic cirrhosis with ascites, nephrotic syndrome, vasculorenal hypertension).
- Prophylaxis and treatment of hypokalaemia.

Mechanism of action

Aldosterone is a mineralocorticoid released by the glomerulosa cells of the adrenal cortex that plays an important role in the regulation of Na^+ and K^+ homeostasis, extracellular fluid volume, and BP. Aldosterone binds to mineralocorticoid receptors in both epithelial (e.g. kidney) and non-epithelial (e.g. heart, blood vessels, and brain) tissues. In the kidney, it binds to mineralocorticoid receptors in cells of the collecting duct, activates specific amiloride-sensitive ENaCs, and increases the number and action of Na^+/K^+-ATPase pumps. Reabsorbed Na^+ is pumped out of the cell by the Na^+/K^+-ATPase pump in the basolateral (peritubular) membrane. Thus, aldosterone is responsible for the reabsorption of about 2% of filtered Na^+ in the kidneys and the excretion of K^+. In addition, aldosterone can cause endothelial dysfunction (increases NADPH and decreases NOS activity), increases both sympathetic tone and the vasoconstrictor response to angiotensin II, and produces CV fibrosis and hypertrophy and may lead to cardiac arrhythmias. Additionally, aldosterone also exerts mineralocorticoid receptor-independent effects, and in both mineralocorticoid receptor-dependent and independent effects, genomic and non-genomic effects are described.

Spironolactone is a potent non-specific antagonist of aldosterone that prevents aldosterone-dependent synthesis of ENaCs, and consequently Na^+-K^+ exchange in the renal distal convoluted tubule. Thus, it promotes excretion of Na^+, Cl^-, and water and the retention of K^+ and H^+. Spironolactone exhibits poor selectivity for the mineralocorticoid receptor and presents progestogenic and anti-androgenic activities responsible for sexual side effects.

Pharmacodynamics

In patients with mild to moderate hypertension, spironolactone has a gradual onset and a prolonged action. It is indicated in hypertensive patients with CHF, post-MI, and in primary and secondary hyperaldosteronism. Added to thiazides or loop diuretics, it increases diuresis and serum K^+ remains within the normal range.

Spironolactone is indicated in HF patients with: (1) recent or current symptoms despite ACEIs (or ARBs), diuretics, digoxin, and β-blockers; (2) chronic, severe systolic HF; and (3) systolic HF after MI. It reduces mortality and reduce the rates of sudden death in patients with HF who are already receiving ACEIs and β-blocker therapy.

Pharmacokinetics

Spironolactone is extensively metabolized to active metabolites, including thiomethylspironolactone and canrenone; their t½ are 9–12h and 10–35h, respectively. This explains why the renal action of spironolactone persists for at least 24h. These metabolites are eliminated in the urine and via biliary excretion in the faeces. (See Table 8.1.5.)

Practical points

1. *Doses*
   - *Hyperaldosteronism*: 25–200mg od (to a maximum of 400mg od) in preparation for surgery or when used as a diagnostic agent. Select the lowest dose in each patient.
   - *Hypertension*: 25–100mg PO in 1–2 doses; adjust to patient response.
   - *For HF*: starting dose of 12.5–25mg od, up to 50mg od. If 25mg/day is not tolerated, reduce to 25mg every other day. Monitor serum K^+ levels within 1 week; if <5mEq/L: 25mg od. If K^+ reaches 5.5mEq/L, the drug should be discontinued.
   - *Liver cirrhosis with oedema and/or ascites; nephrotic syndrome*: 25–200mg od or bd for 5 days; if no clinical response, add a second diuretic with a different mechanism of action.
   - *Diagnosis/treatment of primary aldosteronism*: 400mg daily for 3–4 weeks. For patients unsuitable for surgery, spironolactone may be employed for long-term maintenance therapy at the lowest effective dosage.
   - Hypokalaemia: 25–100mg PO od.
2. *Side effects*
   - Gynaecomastia, painful breasts, hyperkalaemia, GI upset (diarrhoea, nausea, vomiting). If the patient develops gynaecomastia, triamterene or amiloride can replace spironolactone.
   - Others: headache, rash, hyponatraemia, leg cramps, metabolic acidosis, leucopenia, thrombocytopenia, loss of libido, impotence, menstrual irregularities, testicular atrophy.
3. *Interactions*
   - Antihypertensives, vasodilatory drugs, alcohol, tricyclic antidepressants, and neuroleptics increase the risk of hypotension when co-administered with an MRA. Monitor BP in these patients.
   - Concomitant use with drugs known to cause hyperkalaemia (ACEIs, ARBs, other potassium-sparing diuretics, β-blockers, heparin, trimethoprim–sulfamethoxazole, NSAIDs, pentamidine, drospirenone, tolvaptan, ciclosporin, tacrolimus, IV benzylpenicillin potassium, potassium salts or supplements) can precipitate serious hyperkalaemia, particularly in the elderly and in patients with renal impairment. Monitor serum K^+ levels, restrict dietary potassium, and reduce/avoid potassium supplements.
   - Spironolactone decreases the renal excretion of digoxin and increases its plasma concentrations. Reduce the dose of digoxin, and monitor plasma levels of digoxin.
   - Spironolactone reduces the renal clearance of lithium. Readjust the dose of lithium, and monitor its plasma levels to avoid the risk of toxicity.

- NSAIDs reduce the antihypertensive effects of spironolactone; monitor BP levels. Indometacin combined with spironolactone may precipitate acute renal failure; monitor plasma creatinine levels.
- Co-administration with thiazides and/or loop diuretics increases diuresis and reduces renal K^+ and Mg^{2+} excretion. Monitor BP and serum K^+ levels.

4. *Cautions/notes*
   - Plasma creatinine and electrolytes should be closely monitored, particularly in the elderly and those with renal and hepatic impairment.
   - Monitor renal function.
5. *Pregnancy and lactation*
   - Avoid in pregnancy due to the risk of feminization of the fetus (observed in animal studies) (Pregnancy category C). Metabolites are present in breast milk; an alternative method of infant feeding should be instituted.
6. *Contraindications*
   - Anuria; deteriorating or severely impaired renal function.
   - Hyperkalaemia (>5.5mEq/L), concurrent treatment with other potassium-sparing diuretics or potassium supplements.
   - Addison's disease.
   - Hypersensitivity to spironolactone or any of the excipients.

Statins (3-hydroxy-3-methylglutaryl-coenzyme A reductase inhibitors)

Statins are HMG CoA reductase inhibitors, e.g. atorvastatin, fluvastatin, lovastatin, pitavastatin, pravastatin, rosuvastatin, and simvastatin.

CV indications

(See ➲ Atorvastatin, pp. 480–1, ➲ Fluvastatin, p. 596, ➲ Lovastatin, pp. 653–4, ➲ Pitavastatin, p. 699, ➲ Pravastatin, pp. 704–5, ➲ Rosuvastatin, pp. 733–4, and ➲ Simvastatin, pp. 744–5.)

- Primary hypercholesterolaemia or mixed dyslipidaemia, as an adjunct to diet, when response to non-pharmacological treatments is inadequate, to reduce elevated plasma levels of total-C and LDL-C.
- Primary and/or secondary prevention in patients at high risk of CV events.
- To slow the progression of atherosclerosis in adult patients, as part of a treatment strategy to lower total-C and LDL-C to target levels.

Mechanism of action

Hepatic HMG CoA reductase is the rate-limiting enzyme that converts 3-hydroxy-3-methylglutaryl coenzyme A to mevalonate, a precursor for cholesterol. Statins are selective and competitive inhibitors of HMG CoA reductase and reduce the hepatic synthesis of cholesterol. This reduction in intracellular cholesterol concentration results in an increase in the expression of LDL-Rs on the surface of hepatocytes and the uptake of LDL-C from blood, reducing the plasma levels of LDL-C. At present, it is uncertain whether a variety of pleiotropic effects associated with statins (including effects on endothelial function; reduction in the fibrinogen and inflammatory process; antioxidant, antiproliferative, and immunodepressant properties; inhibition of platelet activation and coagulation, with decreased thrombus formation) may also contribute to the therapeutic effects of statins in CV disease.

Pharmacodynamics

In patients with primary hypercholesterolaemia, statins reduce in a dose-dependent manner the plasma levels of total-C, LDL-C, Apo B, and TGs, and produce variable increases in HDL-C levels. The magnitude of the response on LDL-C, TGs, and HDL-C varies significantly with different statins. The LDL-C-lowering effects of statins are proportional to pre-treatment levels. Consistent with epidemiological data, each 1mmol/L (40mg/dL) reduction in LDL-C concentration by statin therapy is associated with a fall (20%) in major CV events (MI, coronary death, coronary revascularization, or stroke) and in all-cause mortality rate (12%). These benefits are broadly similar across a wide range of levels of baseline CV risk. Statin treatment significantly reduces CV risk more in diabetic than in non-diabetic patients in both primary and secondary prevention.

Large-scale trials have demonstrated that statins substantially reduce CV morbidity and mortality in both primary and secondary prevention, in both genders and in all age groups. In patients with CAD, intensive lipid-lowering treatment with statins slowed the progression, or even promoted the regression, of coronary atherosclerosis.

Pharmacokinetics

Statins differ in their pharmacokinetic properties. Lovastatin and simvastatin are prodrugs, while other statins are administered in their active form. Systemic bioavailability is generally low. Atorvastatin, lovastatin, and simvastatin undergo CYP34 metabolism, fluvastatin, pitavastatin, and rosuvastatin CYP2C9 metabolism, and pravastatin is the only statin that does not undergo CYP450 metabolism. (See Table 8.1.4.)

Practical points

1. *Doses* (see ➲ Atorvastatin, pp. 480–1, ➲ Fluvastatin, p. 596, ➲ Lovastatin, pp. 653–4, ➲ Pitavastatin, p. 699, ➲ Pravastatin, pp. 704–5, ➲ Rosuvastatin, pp. 733–4, and ➲ Simvastatin, pp. 744–5)
   - Statins are more effective when given with the evening meal, as cholesterol synthesis occurs mainly at night. This recommendation can be avoided for statins with a long t½ or with metabolites with a prolonged t½.
2. *Side effects*
   - Common: abdominal pain, dyspepsia, nausea, flatulence, constipation, diarrhoea, insomnia, headache, dizziness, asthenia, allergic reactions, rash. An increase in proteinuria has been reported for all statins, due to reduced tubular reabsorption, and not to glomerular dysfunction.
   - Other side effects vary between individual drugs but are largely dose-related:

     —A dose-dependent increase in serum ALT levels (>3 times the ULN on two consecutive weekly measurements) occurred in 0.2–2.7%. Progression to liver failure is exceedingly rare. Therefore, routine monitoring of ALT during statin treatment is no longer recommended. Stopping or reducing the dose of statins should be considered in transamInase elevations to ≥3 times the ULN or ≥100IU. Following dose reduction, drug interruption, or discontinuation, transaminase levels return to, or near, pre-treatment levels without sequelae. If liver injury with clinical symptoms and/or hyperbilirubinaemia or jaundice occurs, treatment should be discontinued inmmediately. Statins should be used with caution in patients who consume substantial quantities of alcohol and/or with a history of liver disease. In patients with mild ALT elevation due to steatosis, there is no indication that statins cause any worsening of liver disease.

     —Statins can produce muscle pain, tenderness, or weakness (myalgia). Myopathy is defined as unexplained muscle symptoms, such as pain or tenderness, muscle weakness, or muscle cramps, plus an increase in CPK levels; the actual frequency of this side effect is unclear. Very rarely, cases of rhabdomyolysis, characterized by severe muscular pain, muscle necrosis, CPK levels at least ten times the ULN, and myoglobinuria potentially leading to renal failure and death, have been reported (approximately 1 per 100,000 patient-years).

     —Statins increased the development of new-onset T2DM and increases HbA1c and fasting plasma glucose levels. The absolute risk is higher with the more potent statins in high doses. However, the absolute reduction in the risk of CV disease in high-risk patients outweighs the possible side effects of a small increase in the incidence of diabetes.

There are post-marketing reports about potential non-serious and reversible *cognitive side effects* (memory loss, confusion, etc.).

3. *Interactions*
   - The risk of dose-related side effects, including myopathy, increases when co-administered with:
     —Strong inhibitors of CYP3A4 (see Table 8.1.2) that increase the plasma concentration of atorvastatin, lovastatin, and simvastatin and the risk of side effects.
     —Colchicine, ciclosporin, ezetimibe, everolimus, gemfibrozil (replace by fenofibrate), sirolimus, and tacrolimus.
     —Alternative therapies, dose reduction, or temporary suspension of statin therapy should be considered with co-administration of these medications.
   - Concomitant administration with CYP3A4 inducers reduces the plasma levels of atorvastatin, lovastatin, and simvastatin (see Table 8.1.2).
   - Combinations of statins with fibrates increase the risk for myopathy. This risk is highest for gemfibrozil, but the risk decreases when combining a statin and a fibrate that are metabolized by non-competing pathways—fluvastatin or rosuvastatin with fenofibrate.
   - The lowering effects on total-C and LDL-C levels increased when statins are combined with resins (colestyramine, colestipol), but they reduce the absorption of statins. Statins should be given either 1h before or at least 4h after the resin.
   - Reduce the dose when given in patients taking amiodarone or verapamil.
   - The INR should be monitored following the initiation of a statin or a change in statin dose. The impact on the INR appears lowest for fluvastatin, pitavastatin, and rosuvastatin.
4. *Cautions/notes*
   - Prior to therapy, patients should be on a cholesterol-lowering diet and a lipid profile performed to assess total-C, LDL-C, HDL-C, and TG levels; causes of hypercholesterolaemia should be excluded/treated.
   - Dose adjustment may be required in moderate to severe renal and hepatic dysfunction (see ➲ Atorvastatin, pp. 480–1, ➲ Fluvastatin, p. 596, ➲ Lovastatin, pp. 653–4, ➲ Pitavastatin, p. 699, ➲ Pravastatin, pp. 704–5, ➲ Rosuvastatin, pp. 733–4, and ➲ Simvastatin, pp. 744–5).
   - Monitoring of LFTs is recommended prior to therapy and in patients who develop any signs or symptoms suggestive of liver injury, i.e. fatigue, anorexia, right upper abdominal discomfort, dark urine, or jaundice.
     —Stop or reduce the dose of statins when transaminase levels increase to ≥3 times the ULN or ≥100IU. Patients with increased transaminase levels should be monitored until resolution.
   - Monitoring for muscular disorders:
     —Myopathy must be considered in cases of unexplained muscle symptoms (pain or tenderness, muscle weakness, or muscle cramps), and CPK levels should be measured. CPK levels should not be measured following strenuous exercise or in the presence of any plausible alternative cause of CPK increase. If CPK levels are >5 times the ULN, statins should be discontinued and levels remeasured within 5–7 days to confirm the results.

—Renal impairment and concomitant use of higher doses of statins increase the risk of myopathy/rhabdomyolysis.

—Statins should be prescribed with caution, temporarily withheld, or discontinued in patients with predisposing factors for rhabdomyolysis (renal impairment, hypothyroidism, personal or family history of hereditary muscular disorders, previous history of muscular toxicity with a statin or fibrates, previous history of liver disease, and/or high alcohol consumption; age >70 years; severe acute infection, hypotension, major surgery, trauma, severe metabolic, endocrine, and electrolyte disorders, and uncontrolled seizures).

- Statins do not modify the plasma levels of testosterone and do not impair adrenal reserve. Caution should also be exercised when statins are administered to patients also receiving drugs (e.g. spironolactone, cimetidine) that may decrease the levels/activity of endogenous steroid hormones.
- Avoid atorvastatin, lovastatin, pitavastatin, and simvastatin in combination with ciclosporin, everolimus, sirolimus, or tacrolimus. The maximum daily doses of fluvastatin, pravastatin, or rosuvastatin should be limited to 40, 20, and 5mg daily, respectively.
- A non-CYP3A4-metabolized statin is preferred in combination with diltiazem or verapamil.

5. *Pregnancy and lactation*
   - Statins may cause fetal harm and are contraindicated in women who are pregnant or may become pregnant (Pregnancy category X). Up to 6 months should be allowed from stopping treatment to planned conception. Discontinuation of statin therapy during pregnancy has little impact on the outcome of long-term therapy of primary hypercholesterolaemia. Statins are secreted into breast milk and have the potential to cause serious adverse reactions in nursing infants.
6. *Contraindications*
   - Active liver disease or unexplained persistently elevated serum transaminases.
   - Pregnancy (or women who are planning to become pregnant) and breastfeeding.
   - Rare hereditary problems of galactose intolerance, Lapp lactose deficiency, or glucose–galactose malabsorption.
   - Concomitant administration of certain medications (see ➔ Atorvastatin, pp. 480–1, ➔ Fluvastatin, p. 596, ➔ Lovastatin, pp. 653–4, ➔ Pitavastatin, p. 699, ➔ Pravastatin, pp. 704–5, ➔ Rosuvastatin, pp. 733–4, and ➔ Simvastatin, pp. 744–5).
   - Hypersensitivity to any component of this medication.

Streptokinase

Thrombolytic agent (47kDa) produced by group C (β-haemolytic) streptococci (see also ➔ Thrombolytic agents, pp. 774–6).

CV indications

- Acute massive PE.
- Acute, subacute, or chronic (not older than 6 weeks) occlusion of peripheral arteries.
- Extensive DVT.
- Central retinal venous or arterial thrombosis (arterial occlusions not older than 8h, venous occlusions not older than 10 days).

Mechanism of action

Streptokinase (SK) binds to plasminogen to form a 1:1 complex that becomes an active enzyme that converts plasminogen to plasmin, which degrades fibrin clots, fibrinogen, and other plasma proteins. Thus, IV infusion of SK is followed by increased fibrinolytic activity, which decreases plasma fibrinogen levels for 24–36h, blood viscosity, and red blood cell aggregation and increases the amount of circulating fibrinogen degradation products. This hyperfibrinolytic effect disappears a few hours after discontinuation. The TT and aPTT usually diminish within 3–4h following the administration of SK; values return to normal by 24h. IV administration of SK reduces PVRs and BP.

Pharmacodynamics

SK administered via the intracoronary route has resulted in thrombolysis, usually within 1h, and results in improvement of cardiac function and reduction in mortality. LVEF increased in patients treated with intracoronary SK, when compared to patients treated with conventional therapy.

Pharmacokinetics

IV infusion of SK is followed by increased fibrinolytic activity, which decreases plasma fibrinogen levels for 24–36h. This effect disappears within a few hours after discontinuation, but a prolonged TT may persist for up to 24h. The drug is cleared primarily by the liver (>5% in the urine), and its t½ is approximately 23min. The complex plasminogen–SK is inactivated, in part, by antistreptococcal antibodies present in individuals with recent streptococcal infections or following the administration of SK.

Practical points

1. *Doses*
   - *MI*: administer SK as soon as possible after onset of symptoms. IV infusion: 1.5 million IU within 60min. Intracoronary infusion: 20,000IU by bolus, followed by 2000IU/min for 60min.
   - *PE*: an initial dose of 250,000IU during 30min, followed by a maintenance IV infusion: 100,000IU/h over 12–24h (72h if concurrent DVT is suspected). As an alternative: 1,500,000IU infused into a peripheral vein, preferably over a short time of 1–2h.
   - *DVT*: an IV bolus of 250,000IU should be infused into a peripheral vein over 30min, followed by a maintenance drip at 100,000IU/h for up to 3 days.

- *Occlusive peripheral arterial diseases*: (1) gradual infusion: 1000–2500IU at an interval of 3–5min for a maximum of 10h (maximum dose 250,000IU); (2) prolonged continuous low-dose infusion (using an infusion pump): 5000–10,000IU/h for up to a maximum of 5 days. For difficult arterial access or multiple occlusions: initial dose of 250,000IU infused over 30min and a maintenance infusion of 100,000IU/h for a maximum of 5 days.
- *Central retinal vessel occlusion*: initial dose of 250,000IU infused into a peripheral vein over 30min; maintenance infusion of 100,000IU/h for 12h.
- *Arteriovenous cannula occlusion*: slowly instil 250,000IU into each occluded limb of the cannula. Clamp off the cannula limb(s) for 2h, and then aspirate the contents of the cannula limb(s), flush with saline, and reconnect the cannula.

2. *Common side effects* (see ➔ Thrombolytic agents, pp. 774–6)
   - Serious haemorrhage calls for discontinuation of SK, followed by administration of clotting factors or a proteinase inhibitor (aprotinin: 200,000–1 million KIU, followed by 50,000KIU/h IV until bleeding stops).
   - Hypotension and bradycardia, due to the formation of plasmin that generates kinins.
   - Allergic reactions: minor breathing difficulty to bronchospasm, periorbital swelling or angioneurotic oedema, urticaria, flushing, headache, or nausea. Anaphylactic shock is very rare (≤0.1%). tPA is indicated in patients allergic to SK and in those having SK within a period of 12 months.
   - Fever and shivering, transient elevations of serum transaminases.
   - Others: cholesterol embolism, chest pain, non-cardiogenic pulmonary oedema, polyneurophaty, PE.
3. *Interactions* (see ➔ Thrombolytic agents, pp. 774–6)
   - In patients with acute MI, addition of aspirin to SK causes a minimal increase in the incidence of major bleeding. Thus, the use of aspirin is recommended, unless contraindicated, while the use of anticoagulants should be carefully decided.
   - Continuous IV infusion of heparin, without a loading dose, has been recommended following termination of SK.
4. *Cautions/notes* (see ➔ Thrombolytic agents, pp. 774–6)
   - In patients previously treated with coumarin derivatives, the INR should be below 1.3 before starting therapy with SK.
   - The effect of SK is blocked by antibodies, which appear a few days after the initial dose. At least 1 year must elapse before SK is used again.
   - If uncontrollable bleeding occurs, SK infusion should be terminated immediately and aminocaproic acid may be considered in an emergency situation.
   - If the TT or any other parameter of lysis after 4h of therapy is not significantly different from baseline, discontinue SK because excessive resistance is present.
5. *Pregnancy and lactation* (see ➔ Thrombolytic agents, pp. 774–6)
6. *Contraindications* (see ➔ Thrombolytic agents, pp. 774–6)
   - Major recent streptococcal infection (it causes SK resistance).
   - Previous treatment with SK, because the antibodies diminish efficacy and increase the risk of allergy.

Telmisartan

Angiotensin AT1 receptor blocker (see ➔ Angiotensin II AT1 receptor blockers, pp. 456–8).

Indications

- Treatment of essential hypertension in adults.
- CV prevention: reduction in CV morbidity in adults with manifest atherothrombotic CV disease (history of CAD, stroke, or peripheral arterial disease) or T2DM with documented target organ damage.

Mechanism of action

(See ➔ Angiotensin II AT1 receptor blockers, pp. 456–8.)

Telmisartan has dual AT1 blocker/PPARγ agonist activity. This latter effect might account for the superior reduction in microalbuminuria versus valsartan at equivalent BP levels.

Pharmacokinetics

(See Table 8.1.9.)

Practical points

1. *Doses*
   - *Hypertension*: 20–40mg od (titrated to a maximum of 80mg/daily).
   - *CV prevention*: 80mg od. When initiating telmisartan therapy for reduction in CV morbidity, close monitoring of BP is recommended.

No dose adjustment is required for the elderly or patients with mild to moderate renal impairment. A starting dose of 20mg is recommended in severe renal impairment or dialysis. In patients with mild to moderate hepatic impairment, the posology should not exceed 40mg. Telmisartan is contraindicated in patients with severe hepatic impairment.

2. *Side effects* (see ➔ Angiotensin II AT1 receptor blockers, pp. 456–8)
3. *Interactions* (see ➔ Angiotensin II AT1 receptor blockers, pp. 456–8)
   - Telmisartan increases the plasma levels of digoxin (20–40%).
   - Avoid use of aliskiren with telmisartan in patients with diabetes mellitus or renal impairment (GFR <60mL/min/1.73m^2).
4. *Cautions/notes* (see ➔ Angiotensin II AT1 receptor blockers, pp. 456–8)
5. *Pregnancy and lactation* (see ➔ Angiotensin II AT1 receptor blockers, pp. 456–8)
6. *Contraindications* (see ➔ Angiotensin II AT1 receptor blockers, pp. 456–8)
   - Severe hepatic impairment; biliary obstructive disorders.

Tenecteplase

Tenecteplase (70kDa, 527 amino acids) is a recombinant fibrin-specific plasminogen activator, derived from native tPA with amino acid substitutions at three sites (Thr103Asn and Asn117Gln within the kringle 1 domain; Lys296-His297–Arg298-Arg299 to Ala in the protease domain) (see also ➲ Thrombolytic agents, pp. 774–6).

CV indications

- Thrombolytic treatment of suspected MI with persistent ST-elevation or recent LBBB within 6h after the onset of acute MI symptoms.

Mechanism of action

Tenecteplase binds to the fibrin component of the thrombus and selectively converts thrombus-bound plasminogen to plasmin, which degrades the fibrin matrix of the thrombus. Tenecteplase has a higher fibrin specificity, a longer plasma t½ (so that it can be given as a single bolus injection), and greater resistance to inactivation by its endogenous inhibitor (PAI-1), compared to native tPA.

Pharmacodynamics

In patients with acute MI of <6h duration, tenecteplase was therapeutically equivalent to alteplase in reducing mortality at 30 days. Rates of intracranial bleeding were similar, but tenecteplase is associated with a significantly lower incidence of non-intracranial major bleeding.

Pharmacokinetics

After administration as a single IV bolus, tenecteplase distribution approximates plasma volume and exhibits a biphasic disposition, with an initial t½ of 20–24min and a terminal t½ of 90–130min. Hepatic metabolism is the main clearance mechanism of the drug. No clinically relevant antibody formation was detected at 30 days.

Practical points

1. *Doses*
    - Tenecteplase should be administered IV, based on the body weight. Maximum dose of 6000U (30mg) in patients of <60kg, and 10,000U (50mg) in patients of ≥90kg. It is not necessary to adjust the tenecteplase dose in patients with hepatic and severe renal insufficiency.
2. *Side effects* (see ➲ Thrombolytic agents, pp. 774–6)
3. *Interactions* (see ➲ Thrombolytic agents, pp. 774–6)
4. *Cautions/notes* (see ➲ Thrombolytic agents, pp. 774–6)
5. *Contraindications* (see ➲ Thrombolytic agents, pp. 774–6)

Thiazide and related diuretics

They include standard thiazides (bendroflumethiazide, HCTZ, metolazone) and thiazide-like diuretics such as chlortalidone and indapamide (see ➲ Diuretics, pp. 553–4).

CV indications

(See ➲ Bendroflumethiazide, p. 484, ➲ Hydrochlorothiazide, p. 624, ➲ Metolazone, p. 659, ➲ Chlortalidone, p. 519, and ➲ Indapamide, p. 629.)

They are indicated in the treatment of:

- Hypertension.
- Oedema associated with CHF, hepatic cirrhosis, various forms of renal dysfunction (nephrotic syndrome, acute glomerulonephritis, and CKD), and corticosteroid and oestrogen therapy.
- Severe resistant oedema (in combination with loop diuretics).
- Other indications: treatment of Dent's disease, prevention of recurrent stone formation in idiopathic hypercalciuria (to decrease the formation of renal stones), and nephrogenic diabetes insipidus (decrease 'free water' clearance).

Mechanism of action

Thiazide diuretics are actively secreted via a renal organic anion transporter (rOAT1) in the proximal tubule, and they bind to the Cl^- site of the electroneutral Na^+-Cl^- co-transporter (NCCT), located in the apical membrane of the early segment of the distal convoluted tubules where approximately 5–10% of the filtered Na^+ is normally absorbed. They inhibit NCCT, causing natriuresis and diuresis. As a result of an increased delivery of Na^+ to the distal segment of the distal tubule, K^+, Mg^{2+}, and H^+ loss is increased due partly to stimulation of the aldosterone-sensitive Na^+ pump and partly due to activation of the RAAS caused by natriuresis and a fall in BP. Consequently, thiazides can cause hypokalaemia with hypochloraemic alkalosis. At high doses, some thiazides also inhibit a membrane-bound form of carbonic anhydrase in the proximal convoluted tubule and increases HCO_3^- and phosphate excretion.

Thiazides also increase Ca^{2+} reabsorption in the proximal tubule and decrease urinary Ca^{2+} excretion, and hypercalcaemia can be observed in patients with pre-existing hyperparathyroidism or vitamin D-treated hypoparathyroidism. Therefore, thiazides are useful in preventing calcium-containing kidney stones. They also stimulate osteoblast differentiation and increase bone mineral formation and density, independently of their renal actions. This effect is associated with a positive Ca^{2+} balance and an increase in bone mineral density and a decrease in the incidence of hip fractures attributable to osteoporosis.

Thiazide diuretics reduce free water clearance and impair the ability of the kidneys to excrete dilute urine during water diuresis, as they: (1) decrease the extracellular fluid volume and the eGFR, which triggers a compensatory increase in proximal Na^+ reabsorption and reduces the delivery of fluid to the distal dilutes sites and the amount of water for excretion; (2) stimulate vasopressin release, which increases water reabsorption in the collecting ducts; and possibly (3) exert a direct effect on water flow in the collecting duct. These effects predispose to the development of dilutional hyponatraemia if patients ingest large quantities of water.

Pharmacodynamics

Hypertension. Low-dose thiazides are the first-choice drugs, especially in low-renin groups, such as older adults, females, black patients, and patients with HF, but are less effective in younger white patients. If a diuretic is not the first choice, a thiazide can be added to produce an additive decrease in BP because they exert a different, but complementary, effect on PVR and can counteract the increase in Na^+ and water retention produced by other antihypertensives. Compared with placebo, low doses of thiazides reduce the risk of stroke and CAD and reduce mortality in patients with mild to moderate hypertension. However, thiazides increase the risk of new-onset diabetes and the risk increases if combined with a β-blocker. Thus, thiazides are not recommended as initial therapy in patients prone to diabetes or with MetS. There are no outcome studies with standard thiazides, but with thiazide-like agents (chlortalidone and indapamide).

The mechanism of the antihypertensive effect is unknown but involves a decrease in BP, a negative Na^+ balance, and direct arteriolar vasodilatation. This vasodilatation is the result of: (1) a reduction in vascular reactivity to angiotensin II, noradrenaline, and thromboxane A2; (2) the opening of large-conductance Ca^{2+}-activated K^+ (BK) channels, which hyperpolarizes vascular smooth muscle cells, reduces the activation of voltage-dependent L-type Ca^{2+} channels, and decreases $[Ca^{2+}]i$; (3) an endothelium-dependent mechanism involving the release of NO; (4) the release of endogenous vasodilators, including prostaglandins E2 and F2α; and (4) inhibition of voltage-dependent L-type Ca^{2+} channels, an effect exerted by indapamide, but not by other thiazide diuretics.

The initial BP lowering is related to the inhibition of the NCC1, which increases diuresis and natriuresis, decreases extracellular and plasma volume, and reduces venous return and CO. This reduction in CO induces an increase in PVR due to an increase in sympathetic tone and activation of the RAAS that partly counteract the BP reduction. In fact, co-administration of a thiazide with an ACEI or ARB inhibits the increase in PVR and increases the antihypertensive response. Combination of a thiazide with a potassium-sparing diuretic reduces the risk of hypokalaemia. In hypertension, standard doses of diuretics should not be combined, if possible, with other drugs with unfavourable effects on blood lipids, such as β-blockers, but rather with ACEIs, ARBs, or CCBs, which are lipid-neutral.

Paradoxically, thiazides reduce the urine volume in patients with diabetes insipidus by interfering with the production of hypotonic fluid in the distal tubule, and thus, they reduce free water clearance.

HF. In mild to moderate HF with modest fluid retention, thiazides can be used, alone or in combination with loop diuretics, to achieve and maintain euvolaemia with the lowest achievable dose. In patients with HFrEF, thiazides are recommended to improve symptoms and exercise capacity in patients with signs and/or symptoms of congestion, and they should be considered to reduce the risk of HF hospitalization in these patients. However, their effects on mortality and morbidity have not been studied in

RCTs. In patients with chronic HF, the effect of thiazide diuretics may be inhibited by poor renal perfusion and Na^+ excretion that stimulate the release of renin. Thus, an ACEI (or ARB) should be administered with the diuretic.

The dose of the diuretic must be adjusted according to individual needs over time, and in selected asymptomatic euvolaemic/hypovolaemic patients, diuretics might be (temporarily) discontinued. Patients can be trained to self-adjust their diuretic dose, based on monitoring of symptoms/signs of congestion and daily weight measurements.

Pharmacokinetics

(See Table 8.1.5.)

Practical points

1. *Doses*
   - Thiazide diuretics present a flat dose–response curve, so that higher doses are no more effective to lower BP but significantly increase the risk of hydroelectrolytic and metabolic side effects. Thus, if low doses of thiazide-like diuretics are insufficient to reduce BP, rather than increasing the dose, a second antihypertensive drug, such as an ACEI or an ARB, which exerts a synergistic reduction in BP and reduces the hypokalaemia, should be added. At the recommended low doses used in monotherapy, or in combination with other antihypertensives, the side effects of thiazides are mild and transient.
2. *Common side effects*

The most frequent side effects produced by thiazides are:

- Hydroelectrolyte disturbances: dehydration, hypovolaemia, hypokalaemia, hypomagnesaemia, hyponatraemia; hypercalcaemia; hypochloraemic alkalosis. Excessive diuresis can cause fatigue and listlessness. Thiazides increases proximal tubular reabsorption of Ca^{2+}.
- CV: hypovolaemia and postural hypotension, particularly in the elderly, and hypokalaemia-induced arrhythmias. Hyponatraemia occurs especially in older patients in whom free water excretion is impaired, leading to fatigue and nausea, confusion, seizures, coma, and death. Hypokalaemia (and hypomagnesaemia) causes symptoms (fatigue, muscle cramps, constipation, anorexia) and ECG abnormalities and supraventricular/ventricular arrhythmias. The order of potency to reduce serum K^+ levels by 0.4mmol/L is: bendroflumethiazide > chlortalidone > HCTZ. The risk of hypokalaemia (<3.5mmol/L) increases with the dose, particularly in the elderly and polymedicated patients, as well as in patients with CHF.
- GI: anorexia, nausea, gastric irritation, constipation.
- Central: dizziness, vertigo, paraesthesiae, headache.
- Metabolic: thiazide diuretics dose-dependently impair glucose tolerance and increase new-onset diabetes, plasma levels of total-C, LDL-C, and TGs, and the ratio of Apo B to Apo A1; HDL-C levels can decrease. Lipid abnormalities are more evident in blacks, males, diabetics, and non-responders treated with higher doses of thiazides. The diuretic-induced dyslipidaemia has been related to worsened insulin sensitivity and/or reflex activation of the sympathetic tone and RAAS in response to volume depletion. During chronic

thiazide therapy, a lipid-lowering diet should be recommended. Thiazide diuretics increase renin levels, and ACEIs or ARBs decrease the metabolic side effects of thiazides. Diuretic-induced glucose intolerance is likely related to hypokalaemia or to total body K^+ depletion. Hypokalaemia can be avoided by the use of a low-dose thiazide with a potassium-retaining drug (amiloride, triamterene, spironolactone, or eplerenone). Concurrent ACEI or ARB therapy also also counters hypokalaemia.

- Thiazide diuretics increase urate reabsorption in the renal proximal tubule and compete with uric acid for tubular secretion into the proximal tubule through rOAT1. Thus, they decrease urate excretion and increase blood uric acid levels (up to 35%). Co-administration of losartan lessens the rise in uric acid levels.
- In the TOMHS and MRC trials, erectile dysfunction and impotence were more commonly observed with thiazide diuretics than with other antihypertensives.
- Others: thiazides rarely cause sulfonamide-type immune side effects, including rashes, dermatitis, eosinophilia, intra-hepatic cholestatic jaundice, necrotizing pancreatitis, blood dyscrasias, interstitial nephritis, and photosensitive dermatitis.

3. *Interactions*
   - Thiazides may potentiate the antihypertensive effects of other antihypertensive agents. The risk of postural hypotension may be exacerbated by alcohol, opioids, barbiturates, tricyclic antidepressants, MAOIs, baclofen, or tizanidine.
   - An excessive reduction in BP can be observed following the co-administration of ACEIs or ARBs in patients on thiazide diuretics. The risk of hypotension can be minimized by either discontinuing or reducing the dose of the diuretic, gradual titration of RAAS inhibitors, and careful monitoring of BP when starting the combined therapy.
   - The diuretic effects of thiazides are inhibited by NSAIDs (which additionally cause Na^+ retention and can predispose to functional renal insufficiency) and oestrogen-containing oral contraceptive pills.
   - The risk of hyponatraemia increases when used with carbamazepine and amphotericin.
   - Loop diuretics deliver a greater fraction of filtered Na^+ to the site of action of thiazides in the distal tubule, so that their combination produces a synergistic diuretic effect.
   - The risk of hypokalaemia increases in the elderly, malnourished or polymedicated patients, and patients with cirrhosis or HF, or those treated with loop diuretics, β-agonists, ACTH, corticosteroids, xanthines, acetazolamide, carbenoxolone, and reboxetine. In hepatic impairment, hypokalaemia induced by thiazides may precipitate coma, and so their use should be avoided. Monitor serum K^+ levels. Potassium-sparing diuretics exert adiditve diuretic effects and reduce the risk of hypokalaemia.
   - Hypokalaemia may increase the risk of ventricular proarrhythmia induced by AADs (e.g. amiodarone, digoxin, disopyramide, flecainide), increase the risk of ventricular arrhythmias when combining with QT-prolonging drugs, and antagonize the effects of some antiarrhythmics

(e.g. lidocaine, mexiletine). The risk of proarrhythmia increases in the elderly and in patients with cardiac hypertrophy, HF, or acute MI.
- Glucocorticoids and ACTH cause salt retention, hyperkalaemia, and hyperglycaemia and antagonize the antihypertensive effect of thiazides.
- Thiazides inhibit the release of insulin from the pancreas and may reduce the effectiveness of insulin and oral hypoglycaemic agents.
- Colestyramine and colestipol decrease their absorption; thiazides should be taken 1h before or 4h after a dose of the resin.
- Thiazides can precipitate hypercalcaemia in hyperparathyroid patients.
- Co-administration of thiazide diuretics with allopurinol increases the risk of severe allergic reactions in patients with CKD.
- The nephrotoxic effects of certain antibiotics (aminoglycosides) or cisplatin may be potentiated by thiazides.
- Thiazide diuretics decrease the renal excretion of lithium and increases the risk of lithium toxicity. Lithium levels should be monitored closely. Chronic lithium therapy causes nephrogenic diabetes insipidus, which is, at least partly, associated with a downregulation of aquaporin-2 (AQP2) in the collecting duct. Under these conditions, thiazide diuretics paradoxically decrease urine volume and increase urine osmolarity.
- Thiazides decrease renal Ca^{2+} excretion and increase the risk of hypercalcaemia when combined with calcium salts or vitamin D preparations.
- Thiazides may potentiate the effects of non-depolarizing neuromuscular blockers (e.g. tubocurarine).

4. *Cautions/notes*
   - During chronic thiazide therapy, electrolyte balance, blood glucose, uric acid levels, lipid levels, and BP should be monitored regularly, particularly when administered at high doses or in combination with other diuretics or in patients with renal impairment. During chronic therapy, a lipid-lowering diet is advisable.
   - If low doses of HCTZ (12.5–25mg/day) are insufficient to reduce BP, rather than increasing the dose, an ACEI or an ARB should be added to obtain a synergistic reduction in BP and reduce the risk of hypokalaemia.
   - Marked diuresis can produce hypovolaemia and postural hypotension, particularly in the elderly.
   - In older adults, excessive use of diuretics can lead to tiredness and fatigue.
   - Thiazides should be used with caution in patients with hypokalaemia, hyponatraemia, glucose intolerance, diabetes, symptomatic hyperuricaemia, and/or hypercalcaemia.
   - Long-term thiazide treatment can lead to insulin resistance, increase the risk of new-onset T2DM, and worsen diabetic control; the risk increases in patients with a family history of diabetes, abdominal obesity, or MetS. The risk increases when thiazides are combined with β-blockers, with carvedilol and nebivolol being the exceptions. In patients with MetS, thiazide diuretics should be avoided or given only in low doses (HCTZ 12.5mg or chlortalidone 15mg od).

- Patients treated with thiazides who consume large quantities of water can develop significant dilutional hyponatraemia.
- Potassium-sparing diuretics (spironolactone, eplerenone, amiloride, triamterene) attenuate the risk of hypokalaemia and reduce the risk of cardiac arrhythmias in patients treated with thiazides. Potassium-sparing diuretics are preferred to potassium supplements, as they correct both hypokalaemia and hypomagnesaemia. The spironolactone/HCTZ combination improves BP lowering and is particularly interesting in obese patients.
- Diuretic-induced hyperuricaemia rarely provokes gout, except in patients with a previous history of gout. In these patients, thiazides can be co-administered with allopurinol at a dose adjusted according to CrCl or with losartan, which is a uricosuric compound.
- With the exception of metolazone, thiazide diuretics become largely ineffective in patients with eGFR of <20–30mL/min or serum creatinine levels of >2mg/dL (180micromol/L). Thus, as CKD progresses to stages 4–5 during treatment, a thiazide should be substituted by a loop diuretic.
- Hypovolaemia, with a risk of prerenal azotaemia, can be lessened by reducing the starting dose of the diuretic.
- Thiazide-like diuretics should be avoided on the day of surgery to avoid a potential adverse interaction with surgery-dependent fluid depletion.
- Hypovolaemia and hyponatraemia stimulate renin secretion, leading to angiotensin II and aldosterone formation. This may limit the antihypertensive effect of thiazides.

5. *Pregnancy and lactation*
    - Thiazides cross the placental barrier, can cause fetal or neonatal abnormalities (thrombocytopenia, jaundice) and hypovolaemia, and decrease placental perfusion. Therefore, they should be avoided in pregnancy (Pregnancy category B). Amounts excreted in breast milk are likely to be too small to be harmful. Large doses may suppress lactation.
6. *Contraindications*
    - Refractory hypokalaemia, hyponatraemia, hypercalcaemia.
    - Symptomatic hyperuricaemia and gout.
    - Pre-existing hypovolaemia.
    - Untreated Addison's disease.
    - Severe renal or hepatic impairment.
    - Hypersensitivity to thiazides or sulfonamide.
    - Pregnancy and breastfeeding.

Thrombolytic agents

(See also ➔ Alteplase, pp. 440–1, ➔ Streptokinase, pp. 764–5, ➔ Tenecteplase, p. 767, and ➔ Urokinase, pp. 789–90.)

Fibrinolytic agents are most useful in the setting of acute arterial thrombosis and occlusion, such as STEMI and peripheral arterial thrombosis, especially when prompt mechanical revascularization (PPCI) is not feasible. However, fibrinolytic agents simultaneously exert clot-dissolving and procoagulant actions and produce serious side effects. Thus, they should not be used in NSTE-ACS (UA and NSTEMI) where they have no benefit and increase the risk of bleeding.

Mechanism of action

Thrombolytic agents are serine proteases that work by converting plasminogen to the natural fibrinolytic agent plasmin, which lyses clots by breaking down fibrinogen and fibrin contained in a clot. They can be divided into two categories: (1) fibrin-specific agents such as alteplase (tPA), reteplase (rtPA), and tenecteplase, which produce limited plasminogen conversion in the absence of fibrin; and (2) non-fibrin-specific agents like SK. tPA is more effective than SK in producing higher early patency of infarcted related vessels. Tenecteplase and alteplase are equivalent on 30-day mortality, but non-cerebral bleeding and blood transfusions are less with tenecteplase. Alteplase and reteplase are equivalent in both mortality and haemorrhage.

Pharmacodynamics

Thrombolytic (fibrinolytic) agents given within the first 4h of onset of symptoms in patients with suspected acute MI and STEMI, to produce lysis of intracoronary thrombi, reopen the occluded artery, increase myocardial salvage (reduces infarct size), preserve LV function, and reduce mortality. The benefit is greatest within the first 2h and then falls off dramatically after 4h. Thus, thrombolytic agents should be administered as soon as possible after an acute MI if no contraindication exists.

Practical points

1. *Side effects*
   - Bleeding is the most frequent adverse reaction and can be fatal. Minor (haematoma, epistaxis at puncture sites, including cardiac catheterization site) and major bleeding (in GI, genitourinary, retroperitoneal, and intracerebral sites) is frequent, and major bleeding can result in permanent disability (in patients who experience stroke) or death. The incidence of bleeding varies widely, depending on the indication, dose, route, and duration of administration and concomitant therapy. The incidence of haemorrhagic strokes increases with increasing age and with fibrin-specific agents. Minor bleeding can occur mainly at sites of external incisions and vascular puncture; if such bleeding occurs, local measures should be taken to control the bleeding. If major bleeding occurs, concomitant heparin and antiplatelet therapy should be discontinued.

- The incidence of bleeding events varies, depending upon the use of arterial catheterization or other invasive procedures. The risk for intracranial haemorrhage (leading to death and permanent disability) increases in patients with advanced age or with elevated BP. Death and permanent disability are not uncommonly reported in patients who have experienced stroke (including intracranial bleeding) and other serious bleeding episodes.
- If serious bleeding in a critical location (intracranial, GI, retroperitoneal, pericardial) occurs, the thrombolytic should be immediately discontinued (as well as concomitant heparin) and haemorrhage can be treated with tranexamic acid, fresh plasma, or coagulation factors.
- CV: arrhythmias associated with reperfusion, cardiogenic shock, AVB, pulmonary oedema, HF, cardiac arrest, recurrent myocardial ischaemia, myocardial reinfarction, myocardial rupture, cardiac tamponade, pericarditis, pericardial effusion, thrombosis, embolism, and electromechanical dissociation.
- Others: nausea, vomiting, hypotension and allergic reactions (e.g. anaphylaxis, angio-oedema, laryngeal oedema, rash, urticaria) are more frequent with SK. Allergic reactions usually respond to antihistamine and/or corticosteroid therapy. Severe allergic reactions (anaphylaxis, angio-oedema) require immediate drug discontinuation.

2. *Interactions*
   - The risk of bleeding increases when thrombolytics are co-administered with anticoagulants, platelet anti-aggregants (aspirin, other non-steroidal anti-inflammatory agents, dipyridamole, and GPIIb/IIIa inhibitors), NSAIDs, and dextran solutions. In these patients, careful monitoring for bleeding (especially at arterial puncture sites) is recommended.
3. *Cautions/notes*
   - Before treatment, it is desirable to obtain a TT, aPTT, haematocrit, and platelet count to obtain the basal haemostatic status of the patient.
   - Heparin therapy without a loading dose can be initiated when the TT or aPTT is less than twice the normal control value.
   - As fibrin is lysed during thrombolytic therapy, bleeding from recent puncture sites may occur.
   - Thrombolytics should be administered using a programmable infusion pump only.
   - Treatment should be instituted soon after onset of acute MI or PE. Delay in starting therapy may decrease the potential for optimal efficacy.
   - IM injections and non-essential handling of the patient should be avoided during treatment.
   - BP should be closely monitored during treatment and during management of acute ischaemic/haemorrhagic stroke.
   - In the following conditions, the risk of haemorrhage may be increased and should be weighed against the anticipated benefits:
     —Recent major surgery (CABG, obstetric delivery, organ biopsy, previous puncture of non-compressible vessels).

—Cerebrovascular disease.
—Haemostatic defects.
—Recent GI or genitourinary bleeding. Any other condition in which bleeding constitutes a significant hazard or would be particularly difficult to manage because of its location.
—Recent trauma.
—Uncontrolled hypertension.
—High likelihood of a left heart thrombus (ex. MS with AF).
—Acute pericarditis, subacute bacterial endocarditis, suspected aortic dissection.
—Severe hepatic or renal dysfunction.
—Severe anaemia.
—Pregnancy.
—Diabetic proliferative retinopathy, haemorrhagic retinopathy, or other haemorrhagic ophthalmic conditions.
—Septic thrombophlebitis.
—Occluded AV cannula at a seriously infected site.
—Advanced age (>75 years) with suspicion of cerebral arteriosclerotic vascular degeneration, agitation, or confusion.
—Patients currently receiving oral anticoagulants or platelet anti-aggregants.

4. *Pregnancy and lactation*
    - There are no adequate and well-controlled studies in pregnant women (Pregnancy category C). Breast milk should be discarded within the first 24h after thrombolytic therapy.
5. *Contraindications*
    - Absolute contraindications:

—Active bleeding, known bleeding diathesis.
—Previous intracranial haemorrhage or stroke of unknown origin at any time.
—Intracranial conditions (damage, neoplasms, arteriovenous malformations, or aneurysms) that may increase the risk of bleeding. Current intracranial haemorrhage or suspicion of subarachnoid haemorrhage on pre-treatment evaluation. Ischaemic stroke in the preceding 6 months. Recent intracranial or intraspinal surgery or serious head trauma (within the preceding 3 weeks).
—Non-compressible punctures in the past 24h (e.g. liver biopsy, lumbar puncture).
—GI bleeding within the past month.

- Relative contraindications: current uncontrolled hypertension (SBP/DBP >180/110mmHg), prolonged or traumatic resuscitation, pregnancy or within 1 week postpartum, active peptic ulcer, oral anticoagulant therapy, TIA in the preceding 6 months, advanced liver disease, and infective endocarditis.

Ticagrelor

Oral, reversible, non-competitive platelet P2Y12 receptor antagonist.

Indications

Co-administration with aspirin is indicated for the prevention of atherothrombotic events in adult patients with ACS or a history of MI and a high risk of developing an atherothrombotic event.

Mechanism of action

Ticagrelor and its major metabolite reversibly interact with the platelet P2Y12 ADP receptor to inhibit platelet activation and aggregation. Ticagrelor does not prevent ADP binding but, when bound to the P2Y12 receptor, prevents ADP-induced signal transduction. Ticagrelor and its active metabolite are almost equipotent.

Pharmacodynamics

Ticagrelor has a faster onset of action and provides stronger and more consistent platelet inhibition than clopidogrel. Maximum inhibition of ADP-induced platelet aggregation (IPA) produced by ticagrelor (180mg) is reached at around 2h and is maintained for at least 8h. After 5 days, IPA in the ticagrelor group was similar to IPA in the placebo group.

Pharmacokinetics

Ticagrelor is metabolized via CYP3A4 (to a lesser extent by CYP3A5) to its major active metabolite AR-C124910XX, which reaches its peak plasma levels after 2.5 (1.5–5) h. Ticagrelor and the active metabolite are extensively bound to human plasma proteins (>99%), present a Vd of 88L, and are eliminated in the faeces (58%) and urine (26%, but ticagrelor in the urine is <1% of the dose). The mean t½ is approximately 7–10h for ticagrelor, and 9h for the active metabolite. The effects of age, gender, ethnicity, renal impairment, and mild hepatic impairment are modest and do not require dose adjustment. (See Table 8.1.7.)

Practical points

1. *Doses*
   - *ACS*: single 180mg loading dose; continued at 90mg bd. Treatment is recommended for 12 months in ACS patients, unless discontinuation is indicated.
   - History of MI: 60mg bd for at least 1 year.

   Prasugrel is administered with aspirin (75–100mg/day). No dose adjustment is required in the elderly or in patients with renal impairment.
2. *Side effects*
   - Bleeding is the more frequent side effect.
   - Dyspnoea (up to 14% in the first week of treatment), dizziness, vertigo, hypotension, diarrhoea, and bradycardia or asymptomatic ventricular pauses of 3s. The Study of Platelet Inhibition and Patient Outcomes (PLATO) and Prevention of Cardiovascular Events in Patients with Prior Heart Attack Using Ticagrelor Compared to Placebo on a Background of Aspirin (PEGASUS) trials excluded patients at an increased risk of bradycardic events (e.g. patients with

sinus syndrome, second- or third-degree AVB, or bradycardia-related syncope) if not protected with a pacemaker.
- Ticagrelor increases serum uric acid levels and serum creatinine levels, but these changes decreased after treatment was stopped.
- Rash, hypersensitivity reactions, including angio-oedema.

3. *Interactions*
   - Ticagrelor and its active metabolite are weak inhibitors of CYP3A4 and P-gp.
   - Strong CYP3A inhibitors (see Table 8.1.2) increase ticagrelor exposure and the risk of dyspnoea, bleeding, and other adverse events. This combination should be avoided. There was no effect of ticagrelor on the plasma levels of diltiazem.
   - Strong CYP3A inducers (see Table 8.1.2) substantially reduce ticagrelor exposure. This combination should be avoided.
   - Ciclosporin (P-gp and CYP3A inhibitor) should be administered with caution in patients treated with ticagrelor.
   - Doses of aspirin of >100mg/day reduce the effectiveness of ticagrelor.
   - Ticagrelor increases exposure of simvastatin and lovastatin; thus, doses of both statins should not exceed 40mg daily. No interaction with other statins.
   - Ticagrelor increases the plasma levels of digoxin; monitor these levels.
   - Heparins, enoxaparin, and ASA or products that alter haemostasis should be used with caution in combination with ticagrelor.
   - SSRIs (e.g. paroxetine, sertraline, and citalopram) may increase the risk of bleeding.
4. *Cautions/notes*
   - Ticagrelor inhibits hepatic CYP3A, increasing plasma levels of drugs metabolized through CYP3A (amlodipine, simvastatin, and atorvastatin). Moderate CYP3A inhibitors (diltiazem, verapamil, and amlodipine) increase the levels of ticagrelor and reduce the speed of its offset.
   - Do not administer ticagrelor with another oral P2Y12 platelet inhibitor.
   - Caution when ticagrelor is co-administered with medicinal products known to induce bradycardia.
   - Ticagrelor-treated patients requiring surgery warrant a minimum of a 5-day washout period to minimize bleeding complications.
5. *Pregnancy and lactation*
   - There are limited data in pregnant women (Pregnancy category C). Women of childbearing potential should use appropriate contraceptive measures to avoid pregnancy during ticagrelor therapy. A risk to newborns/infants cannot be excluded.
6. *Contraindications*
   - History of intracranial haemorrhage.
   - Active pathological bleeding.
   - Severe hepatic dysfunction.
   - Strong CYP3A4 inhibitors/inducers.
   - Hypersensitivity to ticagrelor or any component of the product.

Tirofiban

Non-peptide reversible antagonist of the platelet GPIIb/IIIa receptor (see ➲ Glycoprotein IIb/IIIa receptor antagonists, pp. 613–15).

CV indications

Tirofiban (combined with aspirin and UFH) is indicated for the:

- Prevention of early MI in adult patients presenting with NSTE-ACS, with the last episode of chest pain occurring within 12h and with ECG changes and/or elevated cardiac enzymes.
- Reduction of major CV events in patients with acute MI (STEMI) intended for PPCI.

Pharmacodynamics

Patients most likely to benefit are those at high risk of developing MI within the first 3–4 days after the onset of acute angina symptoms, including those who are likely to undergo an early PCI.

Pharmacokinetics

Tirofiban rapidly inhibits ADP-induced platelet aggregation, but platelet function returns to baseline 4–8h after discontinuation. It binds to plasma proteins (35%), presents a Vd of 0.18–0.25L/kg and a t½ of 1.5–2h, and is cleared via the renal (65%) and biliary (25%) routes, mainly as unchanged tirofiban. Drug clearance is not affected by hepatic impairment, but it is reduced by approximately 40% in subjects with CrCl of <60mL/min and by >50% in patients with CrCl of <30mL/min.

Practical points

1. *Doses*
    - Initial IV infusion: 0.4mcg/kg/min for 30min and then 0.1mcg/kg/min (0.075mcg/kg/min for patients with serum creatinine levels of ≤60mL/min), for up to 18h. Tirofiban is administered in combination with aspirin and UFH (50–60U/kg simultaneously with the start of tirofiban therapy; then approximately 1000U/h, titrated on the basis of an aPTT about twice the normal value).
    - In NSTE-ACS patients planned to undergo PCI within the first 4h of diagnosis or in patients with acute MI intended for primary PCI: an initial bolus of 25mcg/kg over 3min, followed by a continuous IV infusion of 0.15mcg/kg/min for 12–24h (up to 48h).
    - No dosage adjustment is necessary for the elderly.
2. *Side effects* (see ➲ Glycoprotein IIb/IIIa receptor antagonists, pp. 613–15)
3. *Interactions* (see ➲ Glycoprotein IIb/IIIa receptor antagonists, pp. 613–15)
4. *Cautions/notes* (see ➲ Glycoprotein IIb/IIIa receptor antagonists, pp. 613–15)
5. *Contraindications* (see ➲ Glycoprotein IIb/IIIa receptor antagonists, pp. 613–15)

Tolvaptan

Selective vasopressin V2 receptor antagonist.

CV indications

- Treatment of hospitalized adults with clinically significant euvolaemic or hypervolaemic hyponatraemia (serum Na^+ ≤125mEq/L) that is symptomatic and persists after fluid restriction, including patients with HF, cirrhosis, and syndrome of inappropriate antidiuretic hormone (SIADH).
- To slow the progression of cyst development and renal insufficiency of autosomal dominant polycystic kidney disease (ADPKD) in adults with CKD stages 1–3 at initiation of treatment with evidence of rapidly progressing disease.

Mechanism of action

Arginine vasopressin is a nonapeptide hormone released from the neurohypophysis in response to increases in plasma osmolarity, hypovolaemia, hypotension, and angiotensin II. Stimulation of V2 receptors, expressed on the basolateral membrane of the renal collecting ducts, increases the synthesis of AQP2 water channel-containing vesicles that increase water reabsorption. This water reabsorption decreases serum osmolarity, contributing to the development of dilutional hyponatraemia (serum Na^+ concentration) and increases in LV end-diastolic volume and pressure. Elevated levels of AVP are present in HF and contribute to the development of fluid retention and hyponatraemia.

Pharmacodynamics

Tolvaptan increases solute-free water excretion (i.e. produces aquaresis), decreases urine osmolality, and increases serum Na^+ concentrations in patients with acute HF and hyponatraemia. Unlike thiazide and loop diuretics, V2 receptor antagonists did not activate the RAAS.

Pharmacokinetics

Tolvaptan presents good oral availability (55%), reaching peak plasma concentrations after 2–3h. Co-administration of tolvaptan with a high-fat meal increases peak drug plasma levels up to 2-fold. Tolvaptan binds (99%) to plasma proteins, presents a Vd of 3L/kg, and is extensively metabolized in the liver via CYP3A4 (renal excretion is <1%). The terminal t½ is 6–12h.

Practical points

1. *Doses*
   - *SIADH*: starting dose of 15mg od, up to 60mg od. Treatment continues until the underlying disease is adequately treated or hyponatraemia is no longer a clinical issue.
   - *ADPKD*: twice daily in split dose regimens of 45mg + 15mg, 60mg + 30mg, or 90mg + 30mg. The morning dose is to be taken at least 30min before the morning meal. The second daily dose can be taken with or without food.

   Tolvaptan has not been studied in patients with severe renal failure or severe hepatic impairment. No dose adjustment is needed in elderly patients.

2. *Side effects*
   - Very common: nausea, thirst, fatigue, dry mouth, pollakiuria, nocturia, polydipsia, headache, dizziness.
   - Common: weakness, palpitations, dyspnoea, dyspepsia, constipation, anorexia, increase in liver transaminases.
3. *Interactions*
   - Moderate or strong CYP3A inhibitors increase tolvaptan exposure, while plasma concentrations decrease after the administration of CYP3A4 inducers (see Table 8.1.2). Avoid co-administration with strong CYP3A inhibitors or inducers.
   - Tolvaptan increases the plasma levels of dabigatran, digoxin, and lovastatin. Monitor plasma levels of digoxin.
   - Tolvaptan can block V2 receptors involved in the release of coagulation factors (e.g. von Willebrand factor) from endothelial cells. Avoid its combination with vasopressin analogues (i.e. desmopressin).
   - No interaction with warfarin, rosuvastatin, pitavastatin, or amiodarone.
4. *Cautions/notes*
   - Treatment should be initiated in patients only in hospital where serum Na^+ levels and volume status can be monitored closely. Avoid fluid restriction during the first 24h of therapy.
   - Too rapid correction of hyponatraemia (e.g. >12mEq/L over 24h) can cause osmotic demyelination, resulting in dysarthria, mutism, dysphagia, lethargy, affective changes, spastic quadriparesis, seizures, coma, and death.
   - If dehydration or renal dysfunction occurs, it can be necessary to interrupt or reduce the doses of tolvaptan and/or diuretics, increase fluid intake, and evaluate and address other potential causes of renal dysfunction or dehydration.
5. *Pregnancy and lactation*
   - Safety in pregnancy and breastfeeding have not been established (Pregnancy category C). Use in these situations is not recommended.
6. *Contraindications*
   - Hypersensitivity to tolvaptan and any of the other components.
   - Anuria, volume depletion, hypovolaemic hyponatraemia.
   - Hypernatraemia.
   - Concomitant use of strong CYP3A4 inhibitors.
   - Pregnancy and breastfeeding.
   - Elevated liver enzymes and/or signs or symptoms of liver injury prior to initiation of treatment.

Torasemide

Long-acting loop diuretic (see ➲ Loop diuretics, pp. 645–50).

CV indications

- Treatment of hypertension, alone or in combination with other antihypertensives.
- Oedema due to CHF and hepatic, pulmonary, or renal oedema.

Pharmacodynamics

(See ➲ Loop diuretics, pp. 645–50.)

Torasemide 20mg gives approximately the same degree of natriuresis as does furosemide 80mg, but absorption is much higher and constant. Torasemide inhibits aldosterone secretion and the binding of aldosterone to its receptor, which may explain why it produces less renal K^+ excretion than other loop diuretics in patients with chronic HF.

Pharmacokinetics

After IV administration, diuresis appears within 10min and peaks at 1h. Elimination t½ is 3.5h (cirrhosis 7–8h), but diuresis lasts approximately 6–8h. Because of its higher bioavailability and longer duration of action, the effects of torasemide are more predictable than those of furosemide. In the presence of renal failure, the t½ remains unaltered, probably because hepatic clearance increases. (See Table 8.1.5.)

Practical points

1. *Doses*
   - *Hypertension*: 5–10mg od; maximal effect after 4–6 weeks. At 2.5mg, it does not change plasma K^+ or glucose levels.
   - *HF*: 5–10mg od, up to 10–20mg od.
   - *Oedema*: 5mg od, up to a maximum of 40mg od.
   - *Oedema of hepatic cirrhosis*: 5–10mg od, titrated to 200mg od, given with an aldosterone antagonist.
2. *Common side effects* (see ➲ Loop diuretics, pp. 645–50)
3. *Interactions* (see ➲ Loop diuretics, pp. 645–50)
4. *Cautions/notes* (see ➲ Loop diuretics, pp. 645–50)
5. *Contraindications* (see ➲ Loop diuretics, pp. 645–50)

Trandolapril

Orally active ACEI (see ➔ Angiotensin-converting enzyme inhibitors, pp. 459–64).

Indications

- Treatment of hypertension.
- Treatment of LV dysfunction after acute MI.

Pharmacodynamics

In patients with reduced LV function, trandolapril administered 3–7 days post-MI significantly reduces the risk of overall mortality, mortality from CV causes, sudden death, and the development of severe HF. In patients with T2DM, hypertension, and normoalbuminuria, trandolapril decreased the development of persistent microalbuminuria.

Pharmacokinetics

Trandolapril is a prodrug rapidly absorbed after oral administration that is hydrolysed to trandolaprilat, a specific ACEI, reaching peak plasma concentrations after 3–8h. (See Table 8.1.10.)

Practical points

1. *Doses*
   - *Hypertension*: initial dose is 0.5–1mg daily. Most patients require 2–4mg od. Treatment should be initiated at 0.5mg in hepatic impairment, under close supervision. Maximum doses should be reduced also in patients with renal impairment (CrCl <10mL/min: a dose of 2mg/day under close supervision).
   - *LV dysfunction after acute MI*: initial dose 0.5mg od going up to 4mg od. In patients with chronic renal failure, despite the predominant biliary excretion, there is some accumulation of trandolaprilat. Thus, initial dose should be reduced to 0.5mg daily when CrCl of <30mL/min or in hepatic cirrhosis.
3. *Common side effects* (see ➔ Angiotensin-converting enzyme inhibitors, pp. 459–64)
4. *Interactions* (see ➔ Angiotensin-converting enzyme inhibitors, pp. 459–64)
5. *Cautions/notes* (see ➔ Angiotensin-converting enzyme inhibitors, pp. 459–64)
6. *Contraindications* (see ➔ Angiotensin-converting enzyme inhibitors, pp. 459–64)

Treprostinil

Synthetic analogue of prostacyclin (PGI2) with sufficient chemical stability to be administered at ambient temperature.

CV indications

- Treatment of PAH in patients with NYHA class II–IV symptoms to diminish symptoms associated with exercise.
- In patients with PAH requiring transition from epoprostenol to diminish the rate of clinical deterioration.

Mechanism of action

(See ➔ Epoprostenol, pp. 577–9.)

Pharmacodynamics

Treprostinil is chemically stable at room temperature and has a longer t½, permitting continuous SC infusion, rather than continuous IV infusion, avoiding the risks of severe infection and thrombosis. Treprostinil causes a dose-related negative inotropic and lusitropic effects. No major effects on cardiac conduction have been observed.

Treprostinil reduces RV and LV afterload and improves symptoms, exercise capacity (6MWT), and haemodynamics (increases CO and stroke volume) in patients with NYHA functional class II–IV symptoms and aetiologies of idiopathic or heritable PAH, PAH associated with congenital systemic-to-pulmonary shunts, or PAH associated with connective tissue diseases. The greatest exercise improvement is observed in patients who are more compromised at baseline and who could tolerate the upper-quartile dose (>13.8ng/kg/min). Benefit was maintained in patients who completed the transition from IV epoprostenol to IV treprostinil.

Pharmacokinetics

Treprostinil is relatively rapidly and completely absorbed after SC infusion (bioavailability 100%), reaching steady-state levels after 10h, following the administration of 10ng/kg/min for 72h. It binds to plasma proteins (91%); its Vd is 0.2L/kg, and it is highly metabolized in the liver by CYP2C8 and excreted in the urine (79%; only 4% of the dose is excreted unchanged) and faeces (13%). Its elimination t½ is 4.5h, following IV and SC administration. Thus, both SC and IV administration of treprostinil are bioequivalent at steady state at a dose of 10ng/kg/min. In patients with moderate hepatic insufficiency, the C_{max} of treprostinil (10ng/kg/min SC for 150min) increased 2- and 4-fold, respectively, and the clearance was reduced by up to 80%, as compared to healthy subjects. No studies have been performed in patients with renal insufficiency or severe hepatic insufficiency.

Practical points

1. *Doses.*
   - *Oral*: 0.25mg PO bd, with food. Mean dose: 3.5mg bd. Maximum dose: 21mg bd.
   - *Infusion*: 1.25ng/kg/min by continuous SC or IV infusion. If the initial dose is not tolerated, decrease to 0.625ng/kg/min. The SC route is preferred, but the drug may be administered by a central IV line

if the SC route is not tolerated. Doses are increased by 1.25ng/kg/min weekly for the first 4 weeks, and thereafter 2.5ng/kg/min every week. IV dosing is similar to that used in SC delivery. The optimal dose varies between individual patients, between 20 and 80ng/kg/min. Do not discontinue abruptly (potential for severe rebound PAH and death). In patients with mild to moderate hepatic insufficiency, the initial dose should be decreased to 0.625ng/kg/min; doses should be increased cautiously.

- *Inhalation*. Initial dosage: three breaths (18mcg) per treatment session (1–2 breaths, if not tolerated). Administer in four separate treatment sessions each day, approximately 4h apart, during waking hours. Maintenance dose: dosage should be increased by an additional three breaths at approximately 1- to 2-week intervals, if tolerated. Titrate to target maintenance dosage of nine breaths (54mcg) per treatment session, as tolerated. Avoid in patients with moderate hepatic impairment (Child–Pugh class B). Severe hepatic impairment: contraindicated.
- No dose adjustments in patients with renal impairment.

2. *Side effects*
   - Infusion site reactions (pain, irritation, erythema, pruritus, or rash) appear in 85% of patients. Infusion site pain leads to discontinuation in 8% of patients. Headache, flushing, nausea, emesis, pain in jaws, arms, or legs, dry mouth, restlessness, anxiety, unusual tiredness, or weakness.
   - Others: diarrhoea, oedema, vasodilatation, hypotension, dyspnoea, fatigue, chest pain, RV HF, and pallor.
   - Adverse events attributable to IV administration: arm swelling, paraesthesiae, haematoma, thrombophlebitis, systemic infections, bone pain, pruritus, dizziness, rash (macular or papular), cellulitis, and drug delivery system malfunction. Thus, continuous IV infusion should be reserved for patients who are intolerant of the SC route or in whom these risks are considered warranted.
   - SC infusion: severe infusion site pain, reaction, bleeding, and bruising.
   - Inhaled: cough, throat irritation, pharyngolaryngeal pain, gastric ulcer.
3. *Interactions* (see ➲ Epoprostenol, pp. 577–9)
   - Gemfibrozil (a CYP2C8 inhibitor) increases, while rifampicin, a CYP2C8 enzyme inducer, decreases exposure to treprostinil.
   - No interactions have been found between treprostinil and paracetamol, fluconazole, sildenafil, or warfarin.
4. *Cautions/notes* (see ➲ Epoprostenol, pp. 577–9)
   - Oral doses: take with food. Swallow tablets whole. Do not chew, break, or crush.
   - Treprostinil inhibits platelet aggregation and increases risk of bleeding, particularly in patients receiving concurrent anticoagulant/antiplatelet therapy.
   - In patients with diverticulosis, tablets can become lodged in a diverticulum.
   - In patients with low arterial BP it may produce symptomatic hypotension.

- Treprostinil SC injection is indicated for continuous infusion administration only. Patients should have the ability to use an SC catheter and infusion pump for a prolonged period of time.
- Treprostinil injection is preferably administered via a self-inserted SC catheter, using an ambulatory SC infusion pump.
- Treprostinil can be administered as supplied or diluted for IV infusion with sterile water for injection, 0.9% sodium chloride injection, a sterile diluent for epoprostenol prior to administration.
- Given the complexity of administration of both IV and SC treprostinil, initiation of therapy should be in a setting with equipment and personnel for monitoring and emergency treatment.
- Because of the risks associated with chronic indwelling CVCs, including serious bloodstream infections, continuous IV infusion should be reserved for patients who are intolerant of the SC route or in whom these risks are considered warranted.
- The overall infection rate is significantly greater than that of epoprostenol, with a higher rate of Gram-negative bacteraemia.
- Abrupt interruption of the treprostinil infusion can lead to severe rebound PAH and death and should be avoided. Restarting the infusion within a few hours after an interruption can be done using the same dose rate. Interruptions for longer periods may require retitrating the dose of treprostinil.

5. *Pregnancy and lactation*
   - Caution is advised when administering this medication to pregnant women (Pregnancy category B). It is not known whether treprostinil is excreted in breast milk.
6. *Contraindications* (see ➔ Epoprostenol, pp. 577–9)
   - Severe hepatic impairment.

Triamterene

Potassium-sparing diuretic (see ➔ Amiloride, pp. 443–5).

Indications

- Treatment of oedematous conditions in HF, liver cirrhosis, or nephrotic syndrome, and in conditions associated with corticosteroid treatment.

Mechanism of action

In contrast to MRAs, K^+ retention induced by triamterene is independent of aldosterone.

Pharmacokinetics

(See Table 8.1.5.)

Practical points

1. *Doses*
   - *Starting dose*: 50mg bd, after meals, increased to 200mg daily. When combined with another diuretic or antihypertensive agent, doses should be adjusted according to the patient's response. Reduce the dose when combined with an ACEI/ARB.
2. *Side effects*
   - Hyperkalaemia, hypokalaemia, weakness, dizziness, headache, hyperglycaemia, thrombocytopenia, megaloblastic anaemia, dry mouth, rash, photosensitivity, nausea and vomiting, diarrhoea. Rare cases of jaundice and/or liver enzyme abnormalities have been reported.
3. *Interactions* (see ➔ Amiloride, pp. 443–5)
   - The combination of indometacin and triamterene can precipitate acute renal failure.
   - Triamterene can potentiate the effects of antihypertensives, other diuretics, pre-anaesthetic and anaesthetic agents, and skeletal muscle relaxants (non-depolarizing).
   - In diabetics, dosage adjustments of hypoglycaemic agents may be necessary.
4. *Cautions/notes* (see ➔ Amiloride, pp. 443–5)
   - Hepatic failure and renal failure both slow the elimination of triamterene.
5. *Pregnancy and lactation*
   - Triamterene can cross the placental barrier and should be avoided in pregnant women due to the risk of feminization of the fetus observed in animal studies and during lactation (Pregnancy category C).
6. *Contraindications* (see ➔ Amiloride, pp. 443–5)

Trimetazidine

Metabolic modulator acting as a 3-ketoacyl CoA thiolase inhibitor.

CV indications

- Symptomatic treatment of patients with stable angina pectoris who are inadequately controlled by, or intolerant to, first-line anti-anginal therapies (i.e. β-blockers and CCBs).

Mechanism of action

Trimetazidine improves myocardial glucose utilization through the inhibition of long-chain 3-ketoacyl CoA thiolase activity, the last enzyme involved in mitochondrial fatty acid β-oxidation, which results in a reduction in fatty acid oxidation and a stimulation of glucose oxidation. Unlike conventional anti-anginal agents, its anti-anginal and anti-ischaemic effects are not associated with changes in heart rate, BP, or myocardial blood flow.

Pharmacodynamics

Trimetazidine reduces the frequency of weekly angina attacks, improves exercise time, and reduces glyceryl trinitrate usage and time to 1-mm ST-segment depression, when compared to placebo. In diabetic persons, trimetazidine improves HbA1c, increases forearm glucose uptake, and improves endothelial function. Trimetazidine has not been evaluated in large-outcome studies in stable CAD (SCAD) patients.

Pharmacokinetics

(See Table 8.1.11.)

Practical points

1. *Dose*
   - 20mg tds (35mg bd for modified-release formulation) during meals. Moderate renal impairment (CrCl 30–65mL/min) or in the elderly: 35mg in the morning after breakfast.
2. *Side effects*
   - Heartburn, nausea, vomiting, dry mouth, hot flushes, diarrhoea, weakness, muscular cramps, dizziness, depression, sedation, drowsiness, palpitations, visual disturbances, anorexia.
   - A recent EMA evaluation found cases of Parkinsonian (or extrapyramidal) symptoms (such as tremor, rigidity, akinesia, and hypertonia), gait instability, restless leg syndrome, and other related movement disorders, reversible after treatment discontinuation.
3. *Interactions*
   - There are no interactions between trimetazidine and β-blockers, CCBs, nitrates, heparin, hypolipidaemic agents, or digoxin.
4. *Cautions/notes*
   - Dose reduction may be required with renal impairment.
5. *Pregnancy and lactation*
   - Safety in pregnancy and during breastfeeding has not been sufficiently evaluated. Therefore, its use is not recommended under these circumstances.
6. *Contraindications*
   - Parkinson's disease and motion disorders [such as tremor (shaking), muscle rigidity, walking disorders, and restless leg syndrome].
   - Severe renal impairment.
   - Pregnancy and breastfeeding.

Urokinase

A highly purified form of naturally occurring human urokinase obtained from human neonatal kidney cells (see ➲ Thrombolytic agents, pp. 774–6).

Indications

Intravascular lysis of blood clots in the following conditions:

- Extensive acute proximal DVT.
- Acute massive PE.
- Acute occlusive PAD with limb-threatening ischaemia.
- Thrombosed arteriovenous haemodialysis shunts.
- Thrombosed CVCs.

Mechanism of action

Urokinase is an enzyme produced by the kidney and found in the urine. It consist of an A chain of 2000Da, linked by a sulfhydryl bond to a B chain of 30,400Da. It converts plasminogen to plasmin, which degrades fibrin clots, as well as fibrinogen. Urokinase produces an increased circulatory fibrinolytic activity, which disappears within a few hours after discontinuation, while the decrease in plasma levels of fibrinogen and plasminogen and the increase in the amount of circulating fibrin and fibrinogen degradation products can persist for 12–24h.

Pharmacodynamics

(See ➲ Thrombolytic agents, pp. 774–6).

Pharmacokinetics

Urokinase administered IV presents a Vd of 11.5L, is metabolized in the liver, and is excreted in the bile and urine. It presents an elimination t½ for biologic activity of 12 (10–20) min. The inactive degradation products are excreted via the bile and primarily via the kidneys. Plasma levels increased 2- to 4-fold in patients with moderate to severe cirrhosis and impaired kidney function.

Practical points

1. *Dose*
    - *DVT*: IV infusion using an initial dose of 4400IU/kg over 10–20min, followed by a maintenance dose of 100,000IU/h for 2–3 days.
    - *PE*: IV infusion using an initial dose of 4400IU/kg over 10–20min, followed by a maintenance dose of 4400IU/kg/h for 12h.
    - *Occlusive PAD*: local intra-arterial catheter-directed graded infusion using 4000IU/min (i.e. 240,000IU/h) for 2–4h or until restoration of antegrade flow, followed by a dose of 1000–2000IU/min until complete lysis or a maximum of 48h.
    - *Thrombosed arteriovenous haemodialysis shunts*: local forced periodic infusion (pulse spray) into both branches of the shunt at a concentration of 5000–25,000IU/mL, up to a total dose of 250,000IU. If necessary, the application can be repeated every 30–45min, up to a maximum of 2h.

- *Thrombosed CVCs*: urokinase dissolved in physiological saline at a concentration of 5000IU/mL. A volume sufficient to completely fill the lumen of the occluded catheter should be instilled and either locked for a duration of 20–60min or pushed with aliquots of saline before the lysate is aspirated. The procedure may be repeated, if necessary

2. *Side effects* (see ➔ Thrombolytic agents, pp. 774–6)
3. *Interactions* (see ➔ Thrombolytic agents, pp. 774–6)
4. *Cautions/notes* (see ➔ Thrombolytic agents, pp. 774–6)
5. *Pregnancy and lactation*
   - Pregnancy category B. It is not known whether this drug is excreted in human milk.
6. *Contraindications* (see ➔ Thrombolytic agents, pp. 774–6)
   - Hypersensitivity to the active substance or any of the excipients.

Valsartan

ARB (see ➔ Angiotensin II AT1 receptor blockers, pp. 456–8).

Indications

- Treatment of hypertension.
- Treatment of clinically stable adult patients with symptomatic HF or asymptomatic LV systolic dysfunction after a recent (12h to 10 days) MI to reduce CV mortality.
- Treatment of adult patients with symptomatic HF when ACEIs are not tolerated or in β-blocker-intolerant patients as add-on therapy to ACEIs when MRAs cannot be used.

Pharmacokinetics

(See Table 8.1.9.)

Practical points

1. *Doses*
   - *Hypertension*: 40–80mg od (titrated to a maximum of 320mg od). No dose adjustment is required in renal impairment where CrCl is >10mL/L or mild to moderate hepatic impairment.
   - *HF*: starting dose of 40mg bd, uptitrated to 80mg and 160mg bd, as tolerated by the patient.
   - *Post-MI*: it can be started as early as 12h after an MI at the dose of 20mg bd. The dose may be uptitrated within 7 days to 40mg bd, with subsequent titrations to a target maintenance dose of 160mg bd. If symptomatic hypotension or renal dysfunction occurs, consider a dosage reduction.
2. *Side effects* (see ➔ Angiotensin II AT1 receptor blockers, pp. 456–8)
3. *Interactions* (see ➔ Angiotensin II AT1 receptor blockers, pp. 456–8)
   - Valsartan is a substrate of the hepatic uptake transporter OATP1B1/OATP1B3 and the hepatic efflux transporter MRP2. Thus, co-administration of inhibitors of the uptake transporter (e.g. rifampicin, ciclosporin) or efflux transporter (e.g. ritonavir) may increase the systemic exposure to valsartan.
4. *Cautions/notes* (see ➔ Angiotensin II AT1 receptor blockers, pp. 456–8)
5. *Pregnancy and lactation* (see ➔ Angiotensin II AT1 receptor blockers, pp. 456–8)
6. *Contraindications* (see ➔ Angiotensin II AT1 receptor blockers, pp. 456–8)
   - Severe hepatic impairment, biliary cirrhosis, cholestasis.
   - Hypersensitivity to active substances, other sulfonamide-derived medicinal products, or any of the excipients.
   - Co-administration with aliskiren in patients with diabetes mellitus or renal impairment (GFR <60mL/min/1.73m^2).

Verapamil

Non-dihydropyridine CCB with class IV antiarrhythmic activity (see ➲ Calcium channel blockers, pp. 504–9).

CV indications

(See ➲ Calcium channel blockers, pp. 504–9.)

- Treatment of hypertension, alone or in combination with other antihypertensives.
- Treatment and prophylaxis of angina pectoris (including effort, vasospastic, and unstable angina).
- Treatment and prophylaxis of PSVT and control of ventricular rate in atrial flutter/AF.
- Secondary prevention of reinfarction after an acute MI in patients without HF not receiving diuretics (apart from low-dose diuretics when used for indications other than HF) when β-blockers are not appropriate.
- LV fascicular tachycardia, symptomatic patients with idiopathic left VT and mitral and tricuspid annular tachycardia, and/or papillary muscle tachycardia.

Mechanism of action

(See ➲ Calcium channel blockers, pp. 504–9.)

Pharmacodynamics

(See ➲ Calcium channel blockers, pp. 504–9.)

Verapamil produces antihypertensive, anti-anginal, and antiarrhythmic effects.

Some patients with exercise-induced VT caused by triggered automaticity may respond to verapamil. Verapamil is also a drug of choice in drug-induced TdP, and it can be an alternative to β-blockers in CPVT. In short-coupled TdP, IV verapamil should be considered to acutely suppress/prevent an electrical storm or recurrent ICD discharges. In all other ventricular arrhythmias, verapamil is contraindicated because of its negative inotropic effects; occasionally, verapamil can suppress ventricular arrhythmias associated with myocardial ischaemia.

In patients with *HCM*, verapamil reduces afterload, symptoms, and the outflow tract gradient, improves diastolic function, enhances exercise performance, and decreases sudden death. However, in patients with severe LV dysfunction (e.g. PCWP >20mmHg, LVEF <30%), verapamil can deteriorate ventricular function, and patients on long-term verapamil develop severe side effects, including SA and AV nodal dysfunction and occasionally overt HF.

Pharmacokinetics

Pharmacokinetic properties of different modified-release preparations may differ. It presents poor oral bioavailability because of the extensive first-pass metabolism. It is extensively metabolized in the liver via CYP3A4; norverapamil is a long-acting active metabolite that has 20% of the effect of verapamil. The t½ of verapamil is approximately 3–7h but increases during chronic administration, in the elderly, and in patients with renal or hepatic insufficiency (up to 14h). After IV administration, verapamil acts within 5min. (See Tables 8.1.3 and 8.1.6.)

Practical points

1. *Doses*
   - Dosing varies, depending on the type of preparation and the manufacturer.
   - *Hypertension*: PO 120mg/day (maximum dose 480mg/day), given od or bd (sustained-release formulations) or tds for standard short-acting preparations. Lower doses are required in older patients or those with advanced renal or hepatic disease or when there is concurrent β-blockade. Verapamil is also available in combination with trandolapril.
   - *Angina*: 240–360mg/day (maximum dose 480mg daily).
   - *SVTs*. IV: 5–10mg slow IV bolus dose (over 2–3min); a 5–10mg dose can be repeated 5–15min later, if necessary. PO: 40–120mg tds.
   - *Rate control in patients with atrial flutter/AF*: 5–10mg (0.075–0.15mg/kg) IV bolus over 2min monitoring BP and ECG; a further 5mg may be given after 5–10 min. Maintenance dose: 120–360mg/day in divided doses.
   - *Secondary prevention of reinfarction*: 120mg tds or verapamil sustained-release 240mg od. Treatment starts 7–15 days after an MI in patients without a history of HF and no signs of CHF.
2. *Side effects* (see ➔ Calcium channel blockers, pp. 504–9)
   - Frequent: constipation (particularly in the elderly).
   - Negative inotropism (especially in patients with reduced LVEF).
   - Rare: gynaecomastia, erythromelalgia, hyperprolactinaemia, pain in the gums, facial pain, and transient mental confusion. In older adults, verapamil may predispose to GI bleeding.
3. *Interactions* (see ➔ Calcium channel blockers, pp. 504–9)
   - Verapamil acts as a CYP3A4 and P-gp inhibitor, which explains the multiple possible drug interactions of these drugs.
   - Avoid co-administration with potent CYP3A4 inhibitors or inducers (see Table 8.1.2). It can be administered with caution with less potent CYP3A4 inhibitors or inducers.
   - Verapamil inhibits CYP3A and potentially increases plasma levels of atorvastatin, simvastatin, and lovastatin. Thus, these statins should be administered with caution at low doses. The 10mg dose of simvastatin should not be exceeded in patients taking verapamil. Fluvastatin, pravastatin, and rosuvastatin are not metabolized by CYP3A4 and are less likely to interact with verapamil.
   - Verapamil may increase the plasma concentrations of almotriptan, ciclosporin, dabigatran, doxorubicin, everolimus, glibenclamide, ketoconazole, prazosin, sildenafil, sirolimus, tacrolimus, theophylline, and terazosin.
   - Verapamil decreases the clearance and increases the plasma levels of digoxin; thus, plasma digoxin levels should be monitored and the dose reduced to avoid the risk of bradycardia or AVB. In digitalis toxicity, rapid IV verapamil is absolutely contraindicated.

- β-blockers: the combination of verapamil with β-blockers is effective in some patients with chronic stable angina but increases the risk of bradycardia, AVB, hypotension, or HF, and therefore, it should be used under close supervision. To avoid pharmacokinetic interactions, verapamil should be combined with hydrophilic β-blockers (atenolol, nadolol). IV β-blockers should not be given to patients treated with verapamil.
  —Verapamil may increase the plasma concentrations of metoprolol and propranolol.
- Antiarrhythmics: concomitant use of verapamil and antiarrhythmics may lead to additive CV effects (e.g. AVB, bradycardia, hypotension, HF) and should be avoided. Verapamil may decrease the clearance of flecainide and increases plasma quinidine levels. Co-administration of verapamil with either disopyramide or flecainide increases the risk of myocardial depression and asystole.
- Co-administration with ivabradine is contraindicated due to the additional heart rate-lowering effect.
- *CNS*: verapamil increases the risk of lithium toxicity and may increase the plasma levels of imipramine, carbamazepine, and phenytoin. Verapamil increases the elimination time of buspirone, midazolam, and triazolam. Thus, dose adjustments are needed.
- Concomitant use of verapamil with aspirin may increase the risk of bleeding.
- Hypotension and bradycardia have been described in patients treated with verapamil receiving telithromycin.
- Verapamil may increase blood alcohol concentrations and prolong its effects.
- Verapamil can potentiate the activity of some muscular-blocking agents (decrease the dose of verapamil and/or of the neuromuscular-blocking agent).
- The combination of verapamil with inhaled anaesthetics may increase the risk of AVB, bradycardia, hypotension, or HF and should be avoided.
- Sulfinpyrazone may reduce the plasma concentrations of verapamil and antagonizes its antihyprertensive effect.
- Verapamil increases exposure to colchicine. This combination is not recommended.
- The combination with IV dantrolene may cause hypotension, myocardial depression, and hyperkalaemia and is contraindicated.

4. *Cautions/notes* (see ➔ Calcium channel blockers, pp. 504–9)
   - Diltiazem and verapamil are not recommended to reduce BP in patients with HFrEF because of their negative inotropic action. Verapamil increases the risk of HF worsening and HF hospitalizations.
   - Co-administration with β-blockers, antiarrhythmics, or cardiac glycosides may increase the risk of bradycardia, AVB, and hypotension and should be avoided.
   - Verapamil should be used with caution in patients with reduced LV function, mild bradycardia, first-degree AVB, or prolonged PR interval.

- Verapamil is extensively metabolized in the liver, and the dose should be reduced and carefully titrated in patients with hepatic dysfunction and in the elderly.
- Patients with HCM on long-term verapamil can develop severe side effects, including SA and AV nodal dysfunction and occasionally HF.
- Abrupt withdrawal of verapamil may produce rebound angina.

5. *Pregnancy and lactation* (see ➔ Calcium channel blockers, pp. 504–9)
6. *Contraindications* (see ➔ Interactions, pp. 793–5) (see ➔ Calcium channel blockers, pp. 504–9)
   - In wide QRS complex VT, especially when given IV. Verapamil-induced hypotension, which may lead to CV collapse, VF, and death.
   - For ventricular rate control in patients with WPW syndrome.

Vernakalant

It is a multiple ion channel blocker with atrial-selective blocking properties.

Indications

- Rapid conversion of recent-onset AF to sinus rhythm in adults: (1) for non-surgery patients: AF of ≤7 days' duration; and (2) for post-cardiac surgery patients: AF of ≤3 days' duration.

Mechanism of action

Vernakalant is a mixed Na^+ (I_{Na} and $I_{Na,late}$) and atria-preferred K^+ channel blocker. It blocks the ultrarapid delayed rectifier K^+ current (I_{Kur}), the transient outward current (I_{to}), and the acetylcholine-sensitive K^+ current (I_{KACh}). It binds with high affinity to the inactivated state of the Na^+ channels and presents fast-onset/fast-offset kinetics, decreasing cardiac excitability and conduction velocity in a voltage- and frequency-dependent manner, so that its potency increases in depolarized tissues (–70mV) and at high heart rates. Because of its fast offset kinetics, vernakalant is not expected to cause disturbances in conduction or proarrhythmia once the heart rate slows and the I_{Na} blockade is no longer required. Blockade of the I_{NaL} may counteract the prolongation of the ventricular APD and prevent or reduce early afterdepolarizations (EADs) underlying LQTS arrhythmias such as TdP.

Pharmacodynamics

Vernakalant prolongs atrial APD and refractoriness which favours termination of AF but has no effect on ventricular or AV nodal refractoriness, heart rate, or BP and produced small changes in the PR, QRS, and QT intervals.

Vernakalant is a fast, safe, and effective alternative to class IC AADs and amiodarone, leading to the cardioversion of recent-onset AF (<7 days) to sinus rhythm within 8 and 14min. Vernakalant can eliminate the need for conscious sedation or anaesthesia that is necessary for electric conversion and the risk of proarrhythmic effects seen with other AADs. Vernakalant, however, is not effective in converting atrial flutter to sinus rhythm.

Pharmacokinetics

Its rapid and extensive redistribution decreases plasma drug concentrations by >40% within 5min after the end of an infusion, so that drug pharmacokinetics are not influenced by the CP2D6 genotype. Acute exposure is not significantly influenced by age, gender, history of CHF, or renal or hepatic impairment. (See Table 8.1.3.)

Practical points

1. *Doses*
   - The initial IV dose is 3mg/kg infused over 10min; a second 10min infusion of 2mg/kg may be administered after 15min if conversion to sinus rhythm did not occur. If conversion to sinus rhythm occurs during the infusion, vernakalant should be continued to completion.

2. *Side effects*
   - The commonest side effects within the first 2h after IV infusion are: dysgeusia, sneezing, paraesthesiae, nausea, cough, pruritus, bradycardia, complete AVB, hypotension, atrial flutter, AF, VPBs, symptomatic monomorphic NSVT, and cardiogenic shock. These effects are mild and transient in duration, leading to drug withdrawal in 1.3% of patients (0.9% in placebo). BP return to baseline after 15–20min.
3. *Interactions*
   - Because vernakalant is not highly bound to serum proteins and its short t½, competition is not expected between vernakalant and other highly protein-bound drugs (amiodarone, digoxin, diltiazem, furosemide, propranolol, verapamil, warfarin).
   - Vernakalant is a substrate and a moderate inhibitor of CYP2D6. However, acute IV administration of vernakalant does not modify the pharmacokinetics of chronically administered 2D6 substrates.
4. *Cautions/notes*
   - The incidence of transient hypotension and NSVT increases in patients with HF; the risk of ventricular proarrhythmia increases in patients with VHD. The incidence of hypotension is reduced when patients are adequately hydrated.
   - In patients with AF, vernakalant (3mg/kg, 10min infusion) prolongs the QRS and QTc intervals, but values returned to normal within 2h.
   - Oral AAD therapy can start 2h after the administration of vernakalant.
   - Vernakalant should be administered with caution in patients with hypertrophic obstructive or restrictive cardiomyopathies, constrictive pericarditis, advanced hepatic impairment, or NYHA class I or II due to the higher risk of hypotension and ventricular arrhythmias.
5. *Pregnancy and lactation*
   - There are no data on the use of vernakalant hydrochloride in pregnant women, and it is unknown whether vernakalant/metabolites are excreted in human milk.
6. *Contraindications*
   - Severe AS, SBP <100mmHg, and advanced HF (NYHA classes III–IV).
   - QT >440ms.
   - Severe bradycardia, sinus node dysfunction, or second- or third-degree AVB in the absence of a pacemaker.
   - ACS (including MI) within the last 30 days.
   - Patients who received IV class I or III AADs within 4h prior to vernakalant.
   - Hypersensitivity to the active substance or any of the excipients.

Vorapaxar

Reversible antagonist of the platelet protease-activated receptor-1 (PAR-1).

Indications

- Reduce thrombotic CV events in patients with a history of MI or with PAD. Vorapaxar is co-administered with aspirin (and, where appropriate, clopidogrel).

Mechanism of action

Thrombin is an essential component of the coagulation cascade and also a potent agonist for platelet activation. Vorapaxar inhibits thrombin-induced and thrombin receptor agonist peptide (TRAP)-induced platelet aggregation in *in vitro* studies but does not inhibit platelet aggregation induced by ADP, collagen, or thromboxane A2 and does not affect coagulation parameters *ex vivo* (TT, PT, aPTT, ACT, ECT).

Pharmacodynamics

Vorapaxar achieves ≥80% inhibition of TRAP-induced platelet aggregation within 1 week of treatment, and because of the long terminal elimination t½, inhibition of TRAP-induced platelet aggregation at a level of 50% persisted 4 weeks after drug discontinuation. Vorapaxar does not modify P-selectin, sCD40L, or hs-CRP concentrations. In patients with MI or PAD, it reduced the rate of a combined endpoint of CV death, MI, stroke, and urgent coronary revascularization.

Pharmacokinetics

Vorapaxar is biotransformed via CYP3A4 and CYP2J2, leading to a major active circulating metabolite (M20). The systemic exposure of M20 is approximately 20% of the exposure to vorapaxar. Vorapaxar and M20 are highly bound to plasma proteins (≥99%), present a Vd of approximately 6L/kg, and are eliminated in the faeces (56%) and urine (25%), but no unchanged vorapaxar is detected in the urine. No dose adjustment is needed, based on age, race, gender, weight, and mild to moderate hepatic or renal impairment. (See Table 8.1.7.)

Practical points

1. *Doses*
   - The dose is 2.08mg PO od, with or without food.
2. *Side effects*
   - The commonest is bleeding. Patients with a history of ischaemic stroke had a higher rate for intracranial haemorrhage on vorapaxar than on placebo.
   - Others: anaemia, iron deficiency, depression, retinopathy, diplopia and related oculomotor disturbances, rash, eruptions.
3. *Interactions*
   - Co-administration with strong CYP3A inhibitors/inducers (see Table 8.1.2) should be avoided.
   - Co-administration of weak or moderate CYP3A inhibitors with vorapaxar does not increase the bleeding risk or modify the efficacy of vorapaxar (see Table 8.1.2).

- There are no pharmacokinetic or pharmacodynamic interactions between vorapaxar and warfarin or prasugrel.
- There is no experience with vorapaxar as the only administered antiplatelet agent; it has been studied only as an addition to aspirin and/or clopidogrel. The combination of aspirin, vorapaxar, and clopidogrel significantly prolongs the bleeding time.

4. *Cautions/notes*
   - Discontinue in patients who experience a stroke, TIA, or intracranial haemorrhage.
5. *Pregnancy and lactation*
   - There are no adequate and well-controlled studies of the use of this drug in pregnant women (Pregnancy category B).
6. *Contraindications*
   - History of stroke, TIA, or intracranial haemorrhage.
   - Active pathological bleeding such as intracranial haemorrhage or peptic ulcer.

Warfarin

Oral coumarin anticoagulant.

CV indications

- Prophylaxis of systemic embolism in patients with rheumatic heart disease and AF.
- Prophylaxis after insertion of prosthetic heart valves.
- Prophylaxis and treatment of venous thrombosis and PE.
- Transient attacks of cerebral ischaemia.

Mechanism of action

Warfarin inhibits the vitamin K-dependent synthesis of biologically active forms of the Ca^{2+}-dependent clotting factors II, VII, IX, and X, as well as the anticoagulant proteins C and S. The precursors of these factors require the carboxylation of their glutamic acid residues by γ-carboxyglutamic acid residues to allow the coagulation factors to bind to the phospholipid surfaces on the vascular endothelium, thereby accelerating blood coagulation. Reduced vitamin K acts as a cofactor for γ-carboxylation. This reaction requires reduced vitamin K and is catalysed by γ-glutamyl carboxylase. This carboxylation is coupled to the oxidation of vitamin K to its epoxide. Vitamin K epoxide is regenerated to vitamin K reduced by vitamin K epoxide reductase complex-1 (VKORC-1).

Warfarin directly inhibits the C1 subunit of VKORC-1, reduces the levels of reduced vitamin K, and induces the hepatic synthesis of partially decarboxylated proteins, with reduced coagulant activity. After a loading dose of warfarin, the appearance of its anticoagulant effect requires the degradation of functional clotting factors and the synthesis of non-functioning factors. The factor with the shortest t½ is factor VII (4–6h), and that with the longest t½ is factor II (approximately 60h). The t½ of proteins C and S are approximately 8h and 30 h, respectively. The anticoagulant effect of warfarin can be overcome by low doses of vitamin K1 (phytomenadione).

Warfarin has no direct effect on an established thrombus; once thrombus formation has occurred, the goals of anticoagulant treatment are to prevent further extension of the formed clot and to prevent secondary thromboembolic complications.

Pharmacodynamics

The anticoagulant effect of warfarin is dose-dependent. It occurs within 24h after drug administration but peaks after 72–96h and persists for 2–5 days. Large loading doses do not shorten the time to achieve a full therapeutic effect but cause rapid falls in protein C levels, which may precipitate paradoxical thrombosis in the first few days of warfarin therapy.

Monitoring. The risk-to-benefit ratio of the treatment should be periodically assessed by monitoring of the INR in each individual patient. The INR should be determined daily or on alternate days in the early days of treatment. Once the INR has stabilized in the target range, it can be determined at longer intervals. The INR should be monitored more frequently in patients at an increased risk of overcoagulation, e.g. patients with severe hypertension or liver or renal disease, or patients with poor adherence. An INR of 2–3 is appropriate for patients with DVT/PE, post-MI, or AF, while for patients with prosthetic heart valves, the recommended INR range is from 2 to 3.5, with lower values for those with bioprosthetic valves and mechanical aortic, rather than mitral, valves. Efficacy in reducing the risk of clot formation and embolism (e.g. prevention of stroke in AF) diminishes sharply with an INR of <2 and is absent with an INR of <1.5. Conversely, the risk of bleeding (e.g. intracranial bleeding) increases significantly when the INR is >4 and in patients aged >75 years. Once the steady-state warfarin requirement is reached, the INR needs only be checked once every 4–6 weeks. Variations in INR control and warfarin requirements may be influenced by dietary changes and drug interactions.

AF. In patients with AF, adjusted-dose warfarin and antiplatelet agents reduce stroke by 64% and 22%, respectively, in patients with AF, but warfarin is substantially more efficacious (by approximately 40%) than antiplatelet therapy. Furthermore, warfarin therapy prevents stroke, systemic embolism, MI, and vascular death better than single or dual antiplatelet therapy with aspirin and clopidogrel; greater benefits were seen in patients with a high time in therapeutic range (TTR). Warfarin is recommended for stroke prevention in patients with: (a) AF and moderate to severe MS or mechanical heart valves (target INR 2.0–3.0 or 2.5–3.5), based on the type and location of the prosthesis; (b) prior stroke, TIA, or a CHA2DS2-VASc score of ≥2; (c) NVAF with a CHA2DS2-VASc score of ≥2 and end-stage CKD (CrCl <15mL/min) or on haemodialysis (INR 2.0–3.0), although warfarin was associated either with a neutral or an increased risk of stroke in database analyses of patients on dialysis; and (d) in male AF patients with a CHA2DS2-VASc score of 1 or female AF patients with a CHA2DS2-VASc score of 2, considering individual characteristics and patient preferences. When patients are treated with warfarin, the TTR should be kept as high as possible and closely monitored. However, NOACs have a favourable balance between efficacy and safety, compared with warfarin, for the prevention of stroke/systemic embolism in NVAF and are recommended in preference to warfarin in patients who are eligible for a NOAC.

MI. Long-term therapy with warfarin after MI reduces the risk of total mortality (24%) and CVAs (55%), compared with placebo. Warfarin (INR 2–2.5), in combination with aspirin (75mg/day), was superior to aspirin alone in reducing the incidence of death, non-fatal reinfarction, thromboembolic events, and stroke in patients with STEMI. However, major non-fatal bleeding was more frequent in patients receiving warfarin.

Pharmacokinetics

Warfarin is a racemic mixture of R- and S-enantiomers. The S-enantiomer has 2–5 times the anticoagulation activity of the R-enantiomer, but its clearance is faster. The elimination of warfarin is almost entirely by hepatic metabolism (mainly via CYP2C9, 2C19, 2C8, 1A2, and 34A); metabolites are principally excreted into the urine (92%) and, to a lesser extent, into bile. S-warfarin is mainly metabolized by CYP2C9, a polymorphic enzyme; R-warfarin is metabolized by CYP1A2 and 3A4 to inactive hydroxylated metabolites, and by vitamin K epoxide reductase (VKORC-1) to metabolites with minimal anticoagulant activity. The t½ of R-warfarin ranges from 37 to 89h, and that of S-warfarin from 21 to 43h. The efficacy of warfarin is affected primarily when the metabolism of S-warfarin is altered. (See Table 8.1.1.)

Carriers of CYP2C9*2 and *3 alleles (11% and 7% in Caucasians, respectively) encoding the enzyme present with decreased S-warfarin clearance, require lower maintenance doses, and are at a higher risk of serious and life-threatening bleeding complications. Some variants of VKROC (VKORC1*2), which can lead to reduced susceptibility to warfarin, may explain up to 30% of the variation in warfarin doses and also the relative resistance to warfarin in some individuals. Comorbidities such as hepatic dysfunction, severe renal insufficiency, thyroid dysfunction, acute concomitant diseases (fever, sepsis, heart failure, diarrhoea), and concomitant therapies may influence warfarin pharmacokinetics.

Practical notes

1. *Doses*
   - Therapy can be initiated with a dose of 2–5mg/day for 5 days, monitoring the INR daily until it reaches the therapeutic range, but the dose should be tailored to individual requirements, then three times weekly for 2 weeks. Most patients are satisfactorily maintained at a dose of 2–10mg daily, taken at the same time each day (mean 4–5mg daily, but this may vary from 1mg to 20mg daily). This wide range confirms that doses must be individualized according to the INR. Genetic-based testing is available to identify patients very low warfarin requirements. Elderly and patients with hepatic or renal insufficiency, HF, malnutrition (leading to vitamin K deficiency), hyperthyroidism (enhances the catabolism of vitamin K), or an increased risk of bleeding require lower doses; myxoedema has the opposite effect. CKD is associated with both a lower warfarin maintenance dose and decreased stability of anticoagulation and an increased bleeding risk, requiring tighter anticoagulation monitoring. Asians require lower doses, while African-Americans require higher doses. The dosage of warfarin which may be used in children has not yet been established.
   - In patients with DVT, warfarin should be initiated concurrently with IV heparin or LMWH. Thereafter, oral anticoagulation alone should be continued for at least 3 months. For documented PE, either LMWH or UFH should be given, followed by oral warfarin continued for approximately 6 months in the absence of recurrences. If recurrences appear, indefinite therapy should be considered.
   - For the transitioning from parenteral anticoagulation, warfarin should be started at least 4 days before UFH is discontinued to allow for the inactivation of circulating vitamin K-dependent coagulation factors; UFH can be discontinued once the INR has been in the therapeutic range for 2 days.
2. *Side effects*
   - The most frequently reported side effect is bleeding; thus, all patients treated with warfarin should have the INR monitored regularly and the dose adjusted to the desired INR. Bleeding from any tissue or organ can occur, even when the INR is within the therapeutic range, particularly in older adults. Risk factors for bleeding include high intensity of anticoagulation (INR >4.0), age ≥65, highly variable INR, history of GI bleeding, uncontrolled hypertension, cerebrovascular

disease, serious heart disease, risk of falling, anaemia, malignancy, trauma, renal insufficiency, and concomitant drugs.

- Haemorrhagic necrosis, systemic atheroemboli, and cholesterol microemboli, including purple toe syndrome.
- *Others*: skin disorders (alopecia, urticaria, rash, dermatitis), GI (nausea, vomiting, flatulence, diarrhoea), hepatic dysfunction (jaundice, cholestatic hepatitis, elevated liver enzymes), pancreatitis, fall in haematocrit, agranulocytosis. Chronic warfarin (>1 year) may produce osteoporotic fractures, more frequently in males.
- *Skin necrosis* may occur in patients treated with high doses of warfarin after cardiopulmonary bypass, particularly in patients with protein C deficiency. Due to the shorter t½ of proteins S and C (8h and 30h, respectively), relative to vitamin K-dependent clotting factors, warfarin can promote an initial prothrombotic state, which may be exaggerated with deficiencies in the underlying levels of protein S or C and can lead to thrombosis in small vessels in adipose tissue. To avoid this adverse effect, start with lower doses under the cover of heparin. Treatment is fresh frozen plasma (providing protein C), IV heparin, and temporary discontinuation of warfarin.
- *Warfarin-related nephropathy* (a type of AKI) is caused by excessive anticoagulation with warfarin; this nephropathy can be associated in some patients with irreversible kidney injury and with an increased risk of mortality.
- *Treatment of bleeding*: if bleeding appears within 1h of ingestion of >0.25mg/kg, consider activated charcoal (50g for adults; 1g/kg for children), although the benefit is uncertain.
- *Non-life-threatening haemorrhage*: vitamin K1 (phytomenadione, 10–20mg IV over 30min). In patients unresponsive to vitamin K or with life-threatening bleeding or when rapid re-anticoagulation is desirable (e.g. valve replacements), give prothrombin complex concentrate (factors II, VII, IX, and X) 30–50U/kg or (if no concentrate available) fresh frozen plasma (15mL/kg). Monitor the INR for at least 48h to determine when to restart normal therapy.
- In patients with an INR of >8.0, but no bleeding or minor bleeding: stop warfarin, and give vitamin K1 (0.5–1mg for adults; 15–30mcg/kg for children) by slow IV injection or 5mg by mouth. For partial reversal of anticoagulation, give smaller oral doses of vitamin K1 (0.5–2.5mg IV); repeat the dose if the INR is still too high after 24h. Large doses of phytomenadione may completely reverse the effects of warfarin and make re-establishment of anticoagulation difficult. If the INR is 5.0–8.0, with no bleeding or minor bleeding: stop warfarin, restart when the INR is <5.0.

3. *Interactions*

Warfarin presents multiple drug interactions. The INR should be monitored closely when CYP2C9 inducers/inhibitors are initiated or discontinued (see Table 8.1.2).

- *Drugs which are contraindicated*: drugs used in the treatment or prophylaxis of thrombosis, or other drugs with adverse effects on haemostasis by increasing the risk of bleeding. Fibrinolytic drugs (SK and alteplase) are contraindicated in patients receiving warfarin.

- *Drugs that are substrates for the enzymes that metabolize warfarin or inhibit their activity*. They may increase the plasma concentrations of warfarin and the INR, potentially increasing the risk of bleeding. When these drugs are administered, warfarin dosage may need to be reduced and INR monitoring increased.
  —Antiarrhythmics: amiodarone, propafenone, quinidine.
  —Antiepileptics: phenytoin, sodium valproate.
  —Azole antifungals: fluconazole, itraconazole, ketoconazole.
  —Anti-ulcer drugs: cimetidine, lansoprazole, omeprazole.
  —β-blocker: check the INR if propranolol is prescribed.
  —Broad-spectrum antibiotics may potentiate the effect of warfarin by reducing the gut flora which produce vitamin K: cephalosporins, chloramphenicol, clarithromycin, ciprofloxacin, co-trimoxazole, erythromycin, mofloxacin, latamoxef, metronidazole, penicillins, sulfamethoxazole, sulfonamides, trimethoprim.
  —Chemotherapy drugs: with caution in patients treated with carbozantinib, etoposide+carboplatine, erlotinib, gefitinib, ifosfamide or paclitaxel. Avoid the combination with capecitabine, fluorouracil, imatinib, or tamoxifen (CYP2C9 inhibitors). Carbozantinib, ceritinib, regorafenib, rucaparib, and vemurafenib inhibit the metabolism of warfarin. Monitor the INR.
  —Hormone antagonists: bicalutamide, toremifene, tamoxifen, and flutamide. Enzalutamide decreases warfarin exposure by 65%; avoid this combination.
  —Leucotriene antagonists: zafirlukast, zileuton.
  —Lipid-lowering agents: statins (rosuvastatin, simvastatin) and fibrates.
  —Uricosuric agents: allopurinol, sulfinpyrazone.
  —Others: alcohol (acute ingestion), capecitabine, chondroitin, disulfiram, glucosamine, tamoxifen, thyroid hormones, tramadol, and vitamin E.
- Drugs that can enhance the effects of warfarin when used concomitantly due, in part, to the respective mechanisms include:
  —Additive effects: heparins and heparin derivatives, LMWHs, NSAIDs, factor Xa and thrombin inhibitors, platelet anti-aggregants, dipyridamole, or epoprostenol.
  —Low-dose aspirin with warfarin increases the risk of GI bleeding. Warfarin may be given initially with UFH in the initial treatment of thrombosis, until the INR is in the correct range.
  —NSAIDs inhibit the synthesis of prothrombin and platelet aggregation, exert pro-ulcerogenic effects, and displace warfarin from plasma proteins.
  —Serotonin and serotonin and noradrenaline reuptake inhibitors (citalopram, desvenlafaxine, duloxetine, escitalopram, fluoxetine, fluvoxamine, levomilnacipran, milnacipran, paroxetine, sertraline, venlafaxine, vilazodone). Monitor the INR in patients receiving such combinations.
  —Chemotherapy drugs: carboplatin, dasatinib, doxorubicin, erlotinib, gefitinib, ibrutinib, ibritumomab, nintedanib, obinutuzumab, romidepsin, vincristine increase the risk of bleeding. Monitor the INR.

—Others: anabolic steroids, clofibrate, entacapone, fluorouracil, ifosfamide, imatinib, bicalutamide, flutamide, fluvastatin, iloprost, testosterone, tricyclic antidepressants. Fish oils and flax seed oil increase the risk of bleeding.

- Drugs that can induce the metabolism, and so diminish the effects, of warfarin, and hence necessary to increase the dose:

  —Inducers of CYP2C9, 1A2, and/or 3A4 (see Table 8.1.2) have the potential to decrease warfarin exposure, being necessary to increase the dose.

  —Resins, laxatives, sucralfate, and orlistat may reduce the absorption of warfarin.

  —Other drugs: azathioprine, griseofulvin, mercaptopurine, aminoglutethimide, danazol, oestrogens, progestogens, retinoids, and vitamin C.
- Protein-bound drugs can increase the effects of warfarin by interfering with its protein binding and include: NSAIDs, sulfonamides, and sulfonylureas.
- Warfarin can increase the plasma levels of chlorpropamide, tolbutamide, and anticonvulsants (phenytoin and phenobarbital).
- Food. Because the amount of vitamin K in food may affect the response to warfarin, patients taking warfarin should avoid drastic changes in dietary habits. Ingestion of vitamin K and foods rich in vitamin K (e.g. liver, Brussels sprouts, spinach, chickpeas, broccoli, watercress) can antagonize the anticoagulant effect of warfarin, and it may be necessary to increase the dosage of warfarin. Grapefruit and cranberry juice enhance the anticoagulant effect of warfarin and should be avoided.

  —Acute ingestion of a large amount of alcohol may inhibit the metabolism of warfarin and increase the INR. Conversely, chronic heavy alcohol intake may induce the metabolism of warfarin. Moderate alcohol intake can be permitted.
- Herbal medicines. Some herbal products can increase the effect of warfarin: agrimony, alfalfa, aniseed, bilberry, dandelion, danshen, devil´s claw, dong quai (*Angelica sinensis*), evening primrose oil, feverfew, garlic, ginger, garlic, ginkgo biloba, ginseng, liquorice, nettle, papain, parsley, passion flower, red clover, tonka beans. Conversely, boldo may reduce the anticoagulant effects.

4. *Cautions/notes*
   - Warfarin presents a narrow therapeutic index, slow 'onset' and 'offset' of action, and multiple interactions with drugs, food, and herbal medicines. Thus, the dosage of warfarin must be individualized according to the patient's INR response, clinical factors (age, race, body weight, gender, concomitant medications, and comorbidities), drug therapy (including over-the-counter medications), or intercurrent illness.
   - Potent CYP2C9 and CYP3A4 inhibitors and inducers alter the metabolic clearance of warfarin and should be avoided if possible.
   - Vitamin K antagonists (acenocoumarol and warfarin) represent an alternative to LMWHs and DOACs when they are contraindicated in patients with severe renal impairment.

- All patients treated with warfarin should have the INR monitored regularly. Those at high risk of bleeding may benefit from more frequent INR monitoring, careful dose adjustment to the desired INR, and a shorter duration of therapy. Unexpected bleeding at therapeutic levels should always be investigated and the INR monitored.
- Patients should be instructed on measures to minimize the risk of bleeding and to report immediately to physicians signs and symptoms of bleeding. The safest rule is to tell patients on oral anticoagulation not to take any over-the-counter medications nor any new drugs without consultation, and for the physician to checklist any new drug that is used. This is also necessary when dietary changes are anticipated, as during travel.
- Warfarin should be given with caution to patients where there is a risk of serious haemorrhage (e.g. concomitant NSAID use, recent ischaemic stroke, bacterial endocarditis, previous GI bleeding). Warfarin with low-dose aspirin increases the risk risk of GI bleeding. Monitor closely.
- UFH may affect the INR. Thus, when warfarin is administered in patients treated with heparin, baseline and subsequent INR determinations must be determined at a time when UFH activity is too low to affect the PT, i.e. at least 5h after the last IV bolus of UFH, 4h after cessation of a continuous IV infusion of heparin, or 24h after the last SC heparin injection. If continuous IV UFH infusion is used, the PT can be measured at any time.
- Warfarin may increase the aPTT test, even in the absence of UFH. A marked elevation (>50s) in the aPTT, with an INR in the desired range, is an indication of an increased risk of post-operative haemorrhage.
- In patients wth AF presenting with an acute embolic stroke, warfarin is indicated if cerebral haemorrhage is excluded. In large strokes, warfarin should be delayed for 1 week to allow full evolution to occur. In patients with a recent TIA, warfarin is only recommended when symptoms persist despite aspirin or clopidogrel therapy or when there is a major cardiac source of embolism.
- Patients with protein C deficiency are at risk of developing skin necrosis. For these patients, it is advisable to introduce warfarin therapy slowly, without a loading dose.
- Rare cases of calciphylaxis have been reported in patients taking warfarin. If calciphylaxis is diagnosed, appropriate treatment should be started and stopping treatment with warfarin should be considered.
- Surgery. When there is no risk of severe bleeding, surgery can be performed with an INR of <2.5. Warfarin need not be stopped before routine dental surgery, e.g. tooth extraction.
  —When there is a risk of severe bleeding, warfarin should be stopped 3 days prior to surgery; if warfarin cannot be stopped 3 days beforehand, anticoagulation should be reversed with low-dose vitamin K.
  —Patients with hyper- or hypothyroidism should be closely monitored on starting warfarin therapy.

—Acquired or inherited warfarin resistance should be suspected if larger-than-usual daily doses of warfarin are required to achieve the desired anticoagulant effect.
—Genetic variability in CYP2C9 and VKORC-1 can significantly affect dose requirements for warfarin. If familial polymorphisms are known, extra care is warranted.
—Patients with rare hereditary problems of galactose intolerance, Lapp lactase deficiency, or glucose–galactose malabsorption should avoid warfarin.

5. *Pregnancy and lactation*
   - Warfarin is contraindicated in women who are, or may become, pregnant because it passes through the placenta, is teratogenic, and may cause fatal fetal haemorrhage *in utero* (Pregnancy category X). The teratogenic effect is greatest in the first trimester, and the risk of fetal bleeding in the last trimester. Thus, women of childbearing age who are taking warfarin should use effective contraception during treatment. If the patient becomes pregnant, use UFH or LMWH in the first trimester, monitoring regularly the aPTT or anti-Xa levels, respectively; they should be discontinued 12h before labour induction and restarted postpartum, together with warfarin, for 4–5 days. Warfarin is excreted into breast milk at low concentrations and is considered compatible with breastfeeding.
6. *Contraindications*
   - Hypersensitivity to warfarin or to any other components.
   - Clinically significant bleeding tendencies associated with: active ulceration of the GI, genitourinary, or respiratory tract, cerebrovascular haemorrhage, cerebral aneurysms, dissecting aorta, pericarditis, bacterial endocarditis.
   - Pregnancy (first and third trimesters), within 48h postpartum.
   - Within 72h of major surgery with a risk of severe bleeding.
   - Drugs where interactions may lead to a significantly increased risk of bleeding.
   - Severe hepatic impairment.

Xipamide

Thiazide-like diuretic drug (see ➔ Thiazide and related diuretics, pp. 768–73).

Indications

- Treatment of hypertension, alone or combined with other antihypertensive drugs.

Pharmacodynamics

Unlike thiazides, only terminal renal failure renders xipamide ineffective.

Pharmacokinetics

The diuretic effect starts about an 1h after administration, reaches its peak effect after 3–6h, and lasts for nearly 24h. (See Table 8.1.5.)

Practical points

1. *Doses*
   - *Hypertension*: 5–20mg as a single early morning dose.
   - *Use as a diuretic*: initial dose of 40mg daily in a single early morning dose. Higher doses, of up to 80mg, may be employed in resistant cases.
2. *Side effects* (see ➔ Thiazide and related diuretics, pp. 768–73)
3. *Interactions* (see ➔ Thiazide and related diuretics, pp. 768–73)
4. *Cautions/notes* (see ➔ Thiazide and related diuretics, pp. 768–73)
5. *Pregnancy and lactation* (see ➔ Thiazide and related diuretics, pp. 768–73)
6. *Contraindications* (see ➔ Thiazide and related diuretics, pp. 768–73)

Further reading

Al-Khazaali A, Arora R. P-glycoprotein: a focus on characterizing variability in cardiovascular pharmacotherapeutics. *Am J Ther* 2014;21:2–9.

Brunton L, Knollmann B, Hilal-Dandan R (eds). *Goodman and Gilman's. The Pharmacological Basis of Therapeutics*, 13th ed. McGraw-Hill Education: New York, NY; 2018.

Catapano AL, Graham I, De Backer G, *et al.*; ESC Scientific Document Group. 2016 ESC/EAS guidelines for the management of dyslipidaemias. *Eur Heart J* 2016;37:2999–3058.

Chatzizisis YS, Koskinas KC, Misirli G, Vaklavas C, Hatzitolios A, Giannoglou GD. Risk factors and drug interactions predisposing to statin-induced myopathy: implications for risk assessment, prevention and treatment. *Drug Saf* 2010;33:171–87.

CredibleMeds®. *Combined list of drugs that prolong QT and/or cause torsades de pointes (TdP)*. Available from: https://crediblemeds.org/pdftemp/pdf/CombinedList.pdf [accessed 3 October 2018].

Dan GA, Martinez-Rubio A, Agewall S, *et al.*; ESC Scientific Document Group. Antiarrhythmic drugs: clinical use and clinical decision making: a consensus document from the European Heart Rhythm Association (EHRA) and European Society of Cardiology (ESC) Working Group on Cardiovascular Pharmacology, endorsed by the Heart Rhythm Society (HRS), Asia-Pacific Heart Rhythm Society (APHRS) and International Society of Cardiovascular Pharmacotherapy (ISCP). *Europace* 2018;20:731–2.

Divakaran S, Loscalzo J. The role of nitroglycerin and other nitrogen oxides in cardiovascular therapeutics. *J Am Coll Cardiol* 2017;70:2393–410.

Electronic Medicines Compendium (eMC). Available from: https://www.medicines.org.uk/emc/ [accessed 3 October 2018].

European Medicines Agency. Available from: https://www.ema.europa.eu/en/medicines [accessed 3 October 2018].

Galiè N, Humbert M, Vachiery JL, *et al.* 2015 ESC/ERS Guidelines for the diagnosis and treatment of pulmonary hypertension: The Joint Task Force for the Diagnosis and Treatment of Pulmonary

Hypertension of the European Society of Cardiology (ESC) and the European Respiratory Society (ERS): Endorsed by: Association for European Paediatric and Congenital Cardiology (AEPC), International Society for Heart and Lung Transplantation (ISHLT). *Eur Heart J* 2016;**37**:67–119.

Heidbuchel H, Verhamme P, Alings M, *et al.*; ESC Scientific Document Group. Updated European Heart Rhythm Association practical guide on the use of non-vitamin-K antagonist anticoagulants in patients with non-valvular atrial fibrillation: executive summary. *Eur Heart J* 2017;**38**:2137–49.

theheart.org Medscape. *Cardiology*. Available from: https://www.medscape.com/cardiology [accessed 3 October 2018].

Ibanez B, James S, Agewall S, *et al.*; ESC Scientific Document Group. 2017 ESC Guidelines for the management of acute myocardial infarction in patients presenting with ST-segment elevation: The Task Force for the management of acute myocardial infarction in patients presenting with ST-segment elevation of the European Society of Cardiology (ESC). *Eur Heart J* 2018;**39**:119–77.

Kaski JK, Haywood C, Mahida S, Baker S, Khong T, Tamargo J (eds). *Drugs in Cardiology*. Oxford University Press: Oxford; 2010.

Kirchhof P, Benussi S, Kotecha D, *et al.*; ESC Scientific Document Group. 2016 ESC Guidelines for the management of atrial fibrillation developed in collaboration with EACTS. *Eur Heart J* 2016;**37**:2893–962.

López-Sendón J, Swedberg K, MacMurray J, *et al.* Expert Consensus Document on β-adrenergic receptor blockers: The Task Force on beta-blockers of the European Society of Cardiology. *Eur Heart J* 2004;**25**:1341–62.

López-Sendón J, Swedberg K, MacMurray J, *et al.* Expert Consensus Document on angiotensin converting enzyme inhibitors in cardiovascular disease. The Task Force on ACE-inhibitors of the European Society of Cardiology. *Eur Heart J* 2004;**25**:1454–70.

Mega JL, Simon T. Pharmacology of antithrombotic drugs: an assessment of oral antiplatelet and anticoagulant treatments. *Lancet* 2015;**386**:281–91.

Aronson JK (ed). *Meyler's Side Effects of Drugs: The International Encyclopedia of Adverse Drug Reactions and Interactions*, 16th ed. Elsevier Science: Oxford; 2015.

Opie LH, Gersh BJ. *Drugs for the Heart*, 8th ed. Elsevier Saunders: Philadelphia, PA; 2013.

Preston CL (ed). *Stockley's Drug Interactions: A Source Book of Interactions, Their Mechanisms, Clinical Importance and Management*, 11th ed. Pharmaceutical Press: London; 2016.

Priori SG, Blomström-Lundqvist C, Mazzanti A, *et al.* 2015 ESC Guidelines for the management of patients with ventricular arrhythmias and the prevention of sudden cardiac death: The Task Force for the Management of Patients with Ventricular Arrhythmias and the Prevention of Sudden Cardiac Death of the European Society of Cardiology (ESC). Endorsed by: Association for European Paediatric and Congenital Cardiology (AEPC). *Eur Heart J* 2015;**36**:2793–867.

Roffi M, Patrono C, Collet JP, *et al.*; ESC Scientific Document Group. 2015 ESC Guidelines for the management of acute coronary syndromes in patients presenting without persistent ST-segment elevation: Task Force for the Management of Acute Coronary Syndromes in Patients Presenting without Persistent ST Segment Elevation of the European Society of Cardiology (ESC). *Eur Heart J* 2016;**37**:267–315.

RxList. Available from: https://www.rxlist.com/script/main/hp.asp [accessed 3 October 2018].

Tamargo J, Segura J, Ruilope LM. Diuretics in the treatment of hypertension. Part 1: thiazide and thiazide-like diuretics. *Expert Opin Pharmacother* 2014;**15**:527–47.

Tamargo J, Segura J, Ruilope LM. Diuretics in the treatment of hypertension. Part 2: loop diuretics and potassium-sparing agents. *Expert Opin Pharmacother* 2014;**15**:605–21.

Medscape. Available from: http://reference.medscape.com [accessed 3 October 2018].

Wiggins BS, Saseen JJ, Page RL 2nd, *et al.*; American Heart Association Clinical Pharmacology Committee of the Council on Clinical Cardiology; Council on Hypertension; Council on Quality of Care and Outcomes Research; and Council on Functional Genomics and Translational Biology. Recommendations for management of clinically significant drug–drug interactions with statins and select agents used in patients with cardiovascular disease: a scientific statement from the American Heart Association. *Circulation* 2016;**134**:e468–95.

Section 9

Non-cardiac drugs affecting the heart—from A to Z

Section editor

Juan Tamargo

Non-cardiac drugs affecting the heart—from A to Z

Eva Delpón and Juan Tamargo

Analgesics

Opioids and related drugs

- *Indications*: prolonged relief of severe pain.
- *Classification*: (1) pure agonists: codeine, etorphine, fentanyl (and analogues), hydromorphone, methadone, morphine, pethidine, tapentadol, tramadol; (2) partial/mixed agonists: buprenorphine, meptazinol, nalorphine, pentazocine; (3) antagonists: naloxone, naltrexone.
- *Mechanism of action*: opioid receptor agonists; μ receptors are responsible for most of the analgesic effects; δ receptors are important in the periphery, and κ receptors at the spinal level. Tramadol is a weak μ receptor agonist that inhibits noradrenaline and serotonin neuronal uptake; it is often combined with paracetamol.
- *Adverse effects*: class effect: hypotension, bradycardia, tachycardia, palpitations, orthostatic hypotension, syncope, respiratory depression. Uncommon: hypertension; circulatory depression, shock, and cardiac arrest reported after a severe overdose. Opioids produce addiction, abuse, and misuse and life-threatening respiratory depression.
- *Cautions*: patients with a recent MI due to increased heart rate and BP, those with arterial or pulmonary hypertension or cardiac arrhythmias. Morphine reduces absorption and decreases the plasma levels of clopidogrel, ticagrelor, and prasugrel.
- *Contraindications*: patients with respiratory depression, phaeochromocytoma, HF secondary to chronic lung disease, head injury, or raised intracranial pressure.

Fentanyl and analogues (alfentanil, lofentanil, remifentanil, sufentanil)

- *Indications*: breakthrough pain in adult patients using opioid therapy for chronic cancer pain; analgesic agents for use during induction and/or maintenance of general anaesthesia; analgesia in mechanically ventilated intensive care adult patients.
- *Mechanism of action*: μ-opioid receptor agonists. Their activity is antagonized by naloxone.
- *Adverse effects*: uncommon: hypotension, bradycardia, post-operative hypertension. Rare: asystole/cardiac arrest usually preceded by bradycardia. Unknown: AVB.
- *Cautions*: patients debilitated, with previous bradyarrhythmias, hypovolaemia, or hypotension; the elderly are more sensitive to their CV adverse effects. They are metabolized by CYP3A4, and potent inhibitors/inducers of CYP3A4 (see Table 8.1.2) may increase/reduce their effects, respectively.

Drugs used in opioid dependence

Lofexidine

- *Indications*: relieve symptoms in patients undergoing opioid detoxification.
- *Mechanism of action*: central α2A-adrenoceptor agonist.
- *Adverse effects*: very common: bradycardia, hypotension. Unknown: QT prolongation.

- *Cautions*: patients with CAD, bradycardia, and recent MI. Reduce the dose gradually (over 2–4 days or longer) to minimize BP elevation. Avoid lofexidine in patients at risk of QT prolongation (see Table 9.1.1). This medicine contains lactose. Avoid in patients with hereditary problems of fructose intolerance, glucose–galactose malabsorption, or sucrose–isomaltase insufficiency.

Methadone

- *Indications*: opioid drug addictions (as a narcotic abstinence syndrome suppressant); analgesic for moderate to severe pain.
- *Mechanism of action*: μ-opioid receptor agonist with much longer half-life (>24h) than morphine.
- *Adverse effects*: uncommon: facial flush, hypotension. Rare: bradycardia, palpitations, orthostatic hypotension, facial flushing, QT prolongation (TdP at high doses).
- *Cautions*: tolerance and dependence may occur. Abrupt cessation of treatment can lead to withdrawal symptoms (less intense, but more prolonged than with morphine). With caution in patients at risk for developing QT prolongation (see Table 9.1.1), cardiac conduction abnormalities, advanced heart disease, or CAD, family history of sudden death or treated with potent cytochrome P450 CYP3A4 inhibitors (see Table 8.1.2). ECG monitoring is recommended prior to, and during, treatment.

Naloxone

- *Indications*: reversal of opioid overdose and especially respiratory depression; diagnosis of suspected acute opioid overdose or intoxication.
- *Mechanism of action*: specific competitive antagonist at opioid receptors.
- *Adverse effects*: common: tachycardia, hypotension, hypertension. Uncommon: bradycardia, arrhythmia. Very rare: VT/VF cardiac arrest. Adverse effects are more frequent in post-operative patients with a pre-existing CV disease.
- *Cautions*: too sudden reversal can cause cardiac arrhythmias, hypertension, and cardiac arrest. If the duration of effect of the opioids is longer than that of naloxone, the patient must be kept under continuous supervision and repeated doses must be given, if necessary.

Table 9.1.1 Drugs that prolong the QTc interval and risk factors for QTc prolongation

Drugs that prolong the QT interval	• Antiarrhythmics: class IA (disopyramide, procainamide, quinidine), IC (flecainide, propafenone), and III (e.g. amiodarone, dofetilide, dronedarone, ibutilide, sotalol) • Antipsychotics: (1) first generation: cyamemazine, chlorpromazine, droperidol, haloperidol, levomepromazine, pimozide, promethazine, thioridazine, trifluoperazine; (2) atypical: amisulpride, aripiprazole, clozapine, iloperidone, olanzapine, quetiapine, risperidone, sertindole, sulpiride, sultopride, tiapride, ziprasidone • Antidepressants: (1) tricyclic/tetracyclic antidepressants: amitriptyline, clomipramine, desipramine, doxepin, imipramine, nortriptyline, protriptyline, trazodone, trimipramine; (2) other: bupropion, citalopram, escitalopram, fluoxetine, mirtazapine, moclobemide, paroxetine, pimozide, sertraline, sertindole, sultopride, venlafaxine • Antimicrobial agents: (1) macrolides (azithromycin, clarithromycin, erythromycin, roxithromycin, telithromycin); (2) quinolones (ciprofloxacin, gemifloxacin, levofloxacin, moxifloxacin, norfloxacin, ofloxacin, sparfloxacin); (3) antifungals: fluconazole, itraconazole, ketoconazole, posaconazole, voriconazole); (4) others: bedaquiline, pentamidine, trimethoprim + sulfamethoxazole, telavancin • Anticonvulsants: felbamate, fosphenytoin, pregabalin • Antimalarials: amantadine, chloroquine, dihydroartemisinin + piperaquine, halofantrine, lumefantrine, mefloquine, quinine • Anti-migraine: naratriptan, sumatriptan, zolmitriptan • Anti-protozoal: metronidazole • Antivirals: amantadine, foscarnet, non-nucleoside reverse transcriptase inhibitor (rilpivirine), HIV protease inhibitors (atazanavir, nelfinavir, saquinavir), • GI medicines: dolasetron, domperidone, granisetron, ondansetron • Chemotherapy drugs: abiratenone, arsenic trioxide, belinostat, bosutinib, bortezomib, capecitabine, crizotinib, cyclophosphamide, dasatinib, docetaxel, eribulin, fluorouracil, paclitaxel, tamoxifen, thalidomide, toremifene, TKIs (bosutinib, dasatinib, lapatinib, nilotinib, pazopanib, ponatinib, ribociclib, sorafenib, sunitinib, vemurafenib), vandetanib, vincamine, vorinostat • H1 antihistaminics: diphenhydramine, mequitazine, mizolastine

	• Hormonal therapy: anti-androgens, degarelix, goselerin, leuprolide, tamoxifen, toremifene • Others: anagrelide, apomorphine, bepridil, cocaine, dexmedetomidine, fingolimod, galantamine, levacetylmethadol, lithium, methadone, mifepristone, oxytocin, pasireotide, perfluten lipid microspheres, ranolazine, solifenacin, tacrolimus, tetrabenazine, tizanidine, tolterodine
Risk factors for QTc prolongation	• Correctable: nausea, vomiting, diarrhoea, potassium-wasting diuretics, bradyarrhythmias, recent conversion from AF, electrolyte disturbances [hypokalaemia (≤3.5 mEq/L), hypomagnesaemia (≤1.6mg/dL), hypocalcaemia (≤8.5mg/dL)], hypothyroidism, concurrent treatment with CYP450 inhibitors, and concurrent use of QT-prolonging drugs (http://www.crediblemeds.org) • Baseline QT prolongation (QTc >470ms in females, >450ms in males) confirmed by repeat ECG • Non-correctable: congenital or acquired QTc prolongation, family history of sudden death and/or syncope, female sex, advanced age, CV disease (LVH, CHF, CAD), MI, impaired renal or hepatic function leading to increased drug exposure • Cautions: do not start treatment in patients with uncorrectable electrolyte abnormalities, QTc >500ms, congenital or acquired long QT syndrome. Prior to and following treatment, evaluate ECG and electrolytes after 15 days and then as clinically indicated. Withhold drugs that prolong the QT interval in patients who develop QTc >500ms or a prolongation >60ms above the baseline (grade 3). Upon recovery to QTc ≤500ms (grade ≤ 2), restart at a reduced dose. Permanently discontinue treatment if the QTc interval remains >500ms and increased >60ms from pre-treatment values after controlling cardiac risk factors for QT prolongation. Frequency of monitoring should be individualized, depending on the patient's characteristics and the causative drug

Antibacterial drugs

Bedaquiline

- *Indications*: treatment of multidrug-resistant tuberculosis.
- *Mechanism of action*: inhibits ATP synthase in *Mycobacterium tuberculosis*, an essential enzyme required for cellular energy, leading to a bactericidal effect.
- *Adverse effects*: common: QT prolongation.
- *Cautions*: an ECG should be obtained before, and at least monthly after, starting treatment. CYP3A4 inhibitors/inducers increase/decrease drug exposure, respectively (see Table 8.1.2). In patients with risk factors for QT prolongation (see Table 9.1.1).

β-lactams (ertapenem)

- *Indications*: intra-abdominal infections, community-acquired pneumonia, acute gynaecological infections, and diabetic foot infections of the skin and soft tissue. Prophylaxis of surgical site infections following elective colorectal surgery.
- *Mechanism of action*: inhibits bacterial cell wall synthesis, following attachment to penicillin-binding proteins.
- *Adverse effects*: common: phlebitis/thrombophlebitis. Uncommon: sinus bradycardia, hypotension, hot flushes. Rare: arrhythmias, tachycardia, hypertension.
- *Contraindications*: severe hypersensitivity (e.g. anaphylactic reaction, severe skin reaction) to any other type of β-lactam antibacterial agent.

Daptomycin

- *Indications*: treatment of *Staphylococcus aureus* bacteraemia when complicated with skin and soft tissue infections, right-sided infective endocarditis. Daptomycin is active against Gram-positive bacteria only.
- *Mechanism of action*: inserts into the cell membrane of Gram-positive bacteria, causing cell wall depolarization, rapid inhibition of protein, DNA, and RNA synthesis, and bacterial cell death.
- *Adverse effects*: common: hypo-/hypertension. Uncommon: SVT, AF/flutter, extrasystoles, flushes. Daptomycin can produce anaphylaxis/hypersensitivity reactions and increases plasma creatine phosphokinase (CPK) levels, associated with muscular pain and/or weakness and cases of myositis.
- *Cautions*: plasma CPK should be measured at baseline and at regular intervals. Avoid daptomycin in patients taking other drugs associated with cardiomyopathy. False prolongation of prothrombin time (PT) and elevation of INR have been reported in patients on daptomycin when certain recombinant thromboplastin reagents are utilized for the assay.

Macrolides (azithromycin, clarithromycin, erythromycin, roxithromycin, spiramycin, telithromycin)

- *Indications*: infections caused by Gram-positive (e.g. *Streptococcus pneumoniae*) and limited Gram-negative bacteria (e.g. *Neisseria gonorrhoeae, Haemophilus influenzae, Mycoplasma pneumoniae, Legionella*, and some *Chlamydia*).

- *Mechanism of action*: reversible binding to the P site on the 50S subunit of the bacterial ribosome, preventing RNA-dependent protein synthesis in sensitive organisms.
- *General adverse effects*: macrolides prolong the QT interval and can produce ventricular tachyarrhythmias, including VT and TdP. Uncommon: palpitations, hot flushes. Unknown: hypotension
- *Cautions*: erythromycin and clarithromycin prolong the QT interval; caution when co-administered with QT-prolonging drugs (see Table 9.1.1). Some macrolides (clarithromycin and erythromycin, not azithromycin) are potent inhibitors of the cytochrome P450 system, particularly CYP3A4. Thus, they increase exposure of drugs metabolized by the cytochrome P450 system and increase the risk of myopathy when co-administered with statins extensively metabolized by CYP3A4. Inhibition of P-gp by clarithromycin may increase exposure to digoxin. Macrolides increase the anticoagulant effect of warfarin and colchicine toxicity.
- *Contraindications*: avoid clarithromycin and erythromycin in patients with congenital or acquired QT prolongation or ventricular cardiac arrhythmia, including TdP. Co-administration of clarithromycin with ticagrelor or ranolazine is contraindicated.

Quinupristin with dalfopristin

- *Indications*: vancomycin-resistant *Enterococcus faecium* and complicated skin infections caused by *Staphylococcus aureus* (meticillin-susceptible) or *Streptococcus pyogenes*.
- *Mechanism of action*: dalfopristin binds to the 23S portion of the 50S ribosomal subunit, enhancing the binding of quinupristin by a factor of about 100. In addition, it inhibits peptidyl transferase. Quinupristin binds to a nearby site on the 50S ribosomal subunit and prevents elongation of the polypeptide.
- *Adverse effects*: uncommon: chest pain, palpitations, tachycardia, hypotension, thrombophlebitis.
- *Cautions*: quinupristin/dalfopristin significantly inhibit P450 3A4, leading to potential multiple drug interactions.

Quinolones (ciprofloxacin, gemifloxacin, levofloxacin, lomefloxacin, moxifloxacin, norfloxacin, oxofloxacin)

- *Indications*: broad-spectrum antibiotics effective against both Gram-negative and Gram-positive bacteria.
- *Mechanism of action*: they inhibit bacterial topoisomerases II (a bacterial DNA gyrase) and IV.
- *Adverse effects*: prolong the QTc interval and can produce ventricular arrhythmias, including TdP in patients at risk. Uncommon: palpitations, tachycardia, AF, hypotension, phlebitis (IV route).
- *Cautions*: the risk of TdP increases in patients with known risk factors for prolonged QT interval (see Table 9.1.1). Some quinolones (not levofloxacin) inhibit CYP1A2 and increase the plasma concentrations of drugs primarily metabolized by CYP1A2 (theophylline, tacrine, clozapine). PT/INR should be monitored frequently during and shortly after co-administration of quinolones and a VKA.
- *Contraindications*: patients with congenital and acquired prolonged QT interval or previous symptomatic arrhythmias.

Rifampicin

- *Indications*: treatment of all forms of tuberculosis and multibacillary and paucibacillary leprosy. Treatment of asymptomatic carriers of *Neisseria meningitidis* or *Haemophilus influenzae*.
- *Mechanism of action*: inhibits DNA-dependent RNA polymerase activity.
- *Adverse effects*: in overdose: hypotension, sinus tachycardia, ventricular arrhythmias. Seizures and fatal cardiac arrest have been reported.
- *Cautions*: rifampicin is a potent inducer of certain CYP1A2, 2C9, 2C19, 2D6, and 3A4, increasing the metabolism and reducing the activity of multiple drugs (see Table 8.1.2). Dosages of drugs metabolized by these enzymes may require adjustment when starting or stopping concomitantly administered rifampicin.

Telavancin

- *Indications*: adults with nosocomial pneumonia, including ventilator-associated pneumonia, known or suspected to be caused by meticillin-resistant *Staphylococcus aureus*.
- *Mechanism of action*: inhibits cell wall biosynthesis and exerts bactericidal activity against susceptible Gram-positive bacteria.
- *Adverse effects*: uncommon: angina pectoris, AF, bradycardia, CHF, QTc prolongation, palpitations, sinus tachycardia, supraventricular/ventricular extrasystoles, flushing, hypertension, hypotension, phlebitis.

Vancomycin

- *Indications*: serious infections caused by meticillin-resistant *Staphylococcus aureus*. Orally for the treatment of staphylococcal enterocolitis and pseudomembranous colitis due to *Clostridium difficile*.
- *Mechanism of action*: inhibits cell wall biosynthesis in Gram-positive bacteria. It can also alter bacterial cell membrane permeability and RNA synthesis.
- *Adverse effects*: vancomycin is very irritating, producing local phlebitis, chills, and rare cases of vasculitis. It should be infused IV in a dilute solution over ≥60min to avoid rapid infusion-related reactions (i.e. exaggerated hypotension, including shock and rarely cardiac arrest). Care must be taken to avoid extravasation.
- *Cautions*: co-administration of vancomycin and anaesthetic agents has been associated with erythema, histamine-like flushing, and anaphylactoid reactions. Concurrent and/or sequential use of potentially neurotoxic and/or nephrotoxic drugs (amphotericin, aminoglycosides, bacitracin, polymyxin B, colistin, viomycin, or cisplatin) requires careful monitoring.

Antidiabetics drugs

- *Indications*: to improve glycaemic control in diabetic patients when diet, weight reduction, and exercise do not provide adequate glycaemic control.
- *Adverse effects*: CV effects of hypoglycaemia include tachycardia, hypertension, palpitations, angina pectoris, and cardiac arrhythmias.
- *Drug interactions*: many drugs can modify glucose blood levels.
  - Some drugs can produce hyperglycaemia and may lead to loss of glycaemic control and/or increase the patient's insulin requirements: bortezomib, CCBs, corticosteroids, danazol, diazoxide, oestrogens and oral contraceptives, glucagon, isoniazid, phenothiazines, phenytoin, rifampicin, sympathomimetics, thiazide diuretics, thyroid-stimulating agents. In patients taking these drugs, perform more frequent blood glucose monitoring and adjust the dosage of the antidiabetic drug during therapy and upon its discontinuation.
  - The following drugs may enhance the hypoglycaemic effect of antidiabetic drugs: allopurinol, anabolic steroids and male sex hormones, ACEIs, coumarin anticoagulants, fenfluramine, fibrates, monoamine oxidase inhibitors (MAOIs), NSAIDs, some antibacterial agents (chloramphenicol, certain long-acting sulfonamides, tetracyclines, quinolone antibiotics, and clarithyromycin). Non-selective β-blockers may mask the symptoms of hypoglycaemia.
  - Non-selective β-adrenergic blockers can produce hypo-/hyperglycaemia. Use a β1-selective blocker.
  - Antidiabetic treatment should be closely monitored in T2DM obese patients taking orlistat.
- In patients treated with these drugs, it is necessary to monitor glucose blood levels periodically during the treatment.

Alpha-glucosidase inhibitors (acarbose, miglitol)

- *Indications*: T2DM as an adjunct to diet and exercise to improve glycaemic control.
- *Mechanism of action*: oligosaccharides that competitively inhibit pancreatic α-amylase and membrane-bound intestinal α-glucoside hydrolase enzymes.
- *Adverse effects*: oedema, thrombocytopenia.
- *Cautions*: acarbose decreases digoxin plasma levels; increase the dose of digoxin, and monitor digoxin plasma levels. Colestyramine may enhance the effects of acarbose.
- *Contraindications*: diabetic ketoacidosis, inflammatory bowel disease, colonic ulceration, or partial intestinal obstruction.

Biguanides: metformin

- *Indications*: first-line treatment of T2DM in adults, particularly in overweight patients. Orphan designation for treatment of paediatric polycystic ovary syndrome.
- *Mechanism of action*: it reduces hepatic glucose production (inhibits gluconeogenesis and glycogenolysis) and increases glucose uptake and

utilization by skeletal muscle and intestinal glucose absorption. It also decreases plasma glucagon levels.

- *Adverse effects*: flushing, palpitations
- *Cautions*: alcohol, diuretics, especially loop diuretics, NSAIDs (including COX-2 inhibitors), ACEIs, and ARBs may increase the risk of lactic acidosis.
  - Metformin should be temporarily suspended in patients undergoing surgical procedures (except minor procedures) and radiological studies involving intravascular administration of iodinated contrast materials which may result in acute alteration of renal function; metformin should be restarted when the renal function is stable.
  - Caution in older patients with CHF and renal or hepatic insufficiency.
- *Contraindications*: patients with HF, renal (CrCl <30mL/min) or respiratory failure (hypoxic pulmonary disease), recent MI, or shock. Patients with metabolic or diabetic acidosis, dehydration, and/or prerenal azotaemia.

Dipeptidyl peptidase 4 (DPP-4) inhibitors (alogliptin, linagliptin, saxagliptin, sitagliptin, vildagliptin)

- *Indications*: T2DM as: (1) monotherapy in patients for whom metformin is inappropriate; (2) dual oral therapy in combination with metformin, a sulfonylurea, or pioglitazone; (3) triple oral therapy in combination with a sulfonylurea and metformin or pioglitazone and metformin. As an add-on to insulin (with or without metformin).
- *Mechanism of action*: selective inhibitors of DPP-4 that increase the levels of glucagon-like peptide-1 (GLP-1) and glucose-dependent insulinotropic polypeptide (GIP). They stimulate glucose-dependent insulin release and inhibit glucagon secretion. In cardiovascular outcome trials DPP-4 inhibitors neither increased nor decreased cardiovascular events.
- *Adverse effects*: DPP-4 inhibitors have been associated with a risk of developing acute pancreatitis. Serious hypersensitivity reactions. Assessment of renal function is recommended prior to initiating therapy and periodically thereafter. Alogliptin and saxagliptin increase hospitalizations for HF.
- *Cautions*: CYP3A4/5 inducers (see Table 8.1.2) may reduce the glycaemic-lowering effect of saxagliptin.
- *Contraindications*: previous history of a serious hypersensitivity reaction.

Drugs acting on the sulfonylurea receptor: insulin secretagogues

- *Mechanism of action*: they inhibit ATP-dependent potassium channels in the membrane of pancreatic β-cells. This results in membrane depolarization, activation of voltage-gated calcium channels, increase in calcium ion influx, and release of insulin via exocytosis. They also reduce glucagon secretion and increase insulin binding to its receptors.
- These drugs require functioning β-cells in the pancreatic islets, being ineffective in T1DM.

Sulfonylureas: glibenclamide, gliclazide, glimepiride, glipizide, glyburide

- *Indications*: adjunct to diet and exercise to improve glycaemic control in adults with T2DM.
- *Adverse effects*: weight gain. CV mortality, non-fatal MI, and risk of mortality are increased in monotherapy with glimepiride, glibenclamide, gliclazide, and tolbutamide, compared with metformin. Sulfonylureas may prevent protective ischaemic cardiac preconditioning after MI.
- *Cautions*: they exhibit multiple drug interactions. Allopurinol and azole antifungals (itraconazole, ketoconazole) increase exposure to sulfonylureas. The combination of bosentan and sulfonylureas decreases the plasma levels of both drugs. Sulfonylureas increase the plasma levels and adverse effects of ciclosporin. Cimetidine, heparin, and tricyclic antidepressants can potentiate the hypoglycaemic effects of sulfonylureas. Colesevelam binds to glimepiride and reduces its GI absorption; glimepiride should be administered at least 4h prior to colesevelam. Sulfonylureas can potentiate the effects of warfarin; adjustment of the anticoagulant may be necessary.
    - Co-administration of sulfonylureas with other antidiabetics increases the risk of hypoglycaemia.
    - Gemfibrozil and maprotiline may increase the effects of glibenclamide.
    - Glimepiride is metabolized by CYP2C9; its plasma levels are influenced by concomitant CYP2C9 inducers or inhibitors (see Table 8.1.2).
    - They should be replaced by insulin for a few days after MI.
- *Contraindications*: T1DM, diabetic coma, ketoacidosis.

Meglitinides: nateglinide, repaglinide

- *Indications*: for combination therapy with metformin in T2DM inadequately controlled on metformin alone.
- *Adverse effects*: they may increase ischaemic events and LV dysfunction in patients with underlying severe CAD. No effect on reducing CV outcomes.
- *Cautions*: CYP2C9 and CYP3A4 inhibitors (see Table 8.1.2) may potentiate their hypoglycaemic effect.
- *Contraindications*: T1DM, diabetic ketoacidosis, with or without coma.

GLP-1 analogues (albiglutide, dulaglutide, exenatide, liraglutide, lixisenatide)

➲ See Chapter 8.1, Glucagon-like peptide 1 receptor agonists (GLP-1RAs), pp. 605–8.

Pioglitazone

- *Indications*: second- or third-line treatment of T2DM (in combination with sulfonylureas, metformin, or insulin). Monotherapy in adults (particularly overweight patients) in whom metformin is contraindicated or not tolerated.
- *Mechanism of action*: nuclear receptor peroxisome proliferator-activated receptor (PPAR) gamma agonist in target tissues for insulin action (adipose tissue, skeletal muscle, and liver). Improves insulin sensitivity. Maximum glucose-lowering effect is observed after 2 months.

- *Adverse effects*: very common: oedema (the risk increases when co-administered with insulin). Common: weight gain, HF. Possible CHF exacerbation in older patients with underlying CAD.
- *Cautions*: patients should be observed for signs and symptoms of HF. Pioglitazone should be discontinued if any deterioration in cardiac status occurs. Because of an increased risk of bladder cancer, fractures, and HF, the risk/benefit ratio should be considered carefully before and during treatment in the elderly.
- *Contraindications*: patients with HF, T1DM, diabetic ketoacidosis, or a history of bladder cancer.

Sodium–glucose co-transporter 2 inhibitors: canaglifozin, dapagliflozin, empagliflozin

➲ See Chapter 8.1, Sodium–glucose co-transporter 2 inhibitors (SGLT2Is), pp. 746–9.

Insulins

- *Indications*: diabetes mellitus in adults, adolescents, and children aged 1 year and above.
- *Mechanism of action*: they lower blood glucose levels by stimulating peripheral glucose uptake (in skeletal muscle and fat) and inhibiting hepatic glucose production.
- *Types of insulins*: (1) ultra-short-acting: recombinant insulins (lispro, aspart, glulisine); (2) short-acting: regular zinc insulin; (3) intermediate-acting: insulin NPH; (4) long-acting: insulin glargine, detemir, and degludec.
- *Adverse effects*: weight gain, peripheral oedema. Insulin stimulates the sympathetic nervous system, hypokalaemia, promotes renal sodium retention, and/or stimulates vascular smooth muscle hypertrophy.
- *Cautions/contraindications*: the possible risk of HF due to fluid retention has not been associated to an increase in the risk of mortality or hospitalization for HF. Alcohol may increase or reduce the hypoglycaemic effect of insulin.

Antiemetic drugs

Cannabinoids (nabilone)

- *Indications*: control of nausea and vomiting caused by chemotherapeutic agents.
- *Mechanism of action*: binds to cannabinoid receptors to block emetic mechanisms.
- *Adverse effects*: hypotension, orthostatic hypotension, tachycardia, palpitations, flushing.
- *Cautions*: in elderly, hypertension and heart disease. Nabilone is an abusable substance.

5-HT3 antagonists (dolasetron, granisetron, ondansetron, palonosetron, ramosetron)

- *Indications*: prevention and treatment of nausea and vomiting associated with chemotherapy, radiotherapy, or post-operatively.
- *Mechanism of action*: selective serotonin 5-HT3 receptor antagonists.
- *Adverse effects*: uncommon: prolongation of PR and QT intervals, arrhythmias.
  - Dolasetron: very common: hypotension, oedema. Common: bradycardia, palpitations, T-wave and ST–T wave changes, Mobitz I AVB, atrial flutter/AF.
  - Ondansetron: uncommon: chest pain with or without ST-segment depression, bradycardia, cardiac arrhythmias.
  - Palonosetron: uncommon: AVB.
- *Cautions*: in patients with underlying cardiac disease, bradycardia, bundle branch block, CHF, and QT prolongation or those treated with QT-prolonging drugs (see Table 9.1.1); ECG monitoring is recommended.
  - Dolasetron: severe hypotension, bradycardia, and syncope have been reported closely following IV administration.
- *Contraindications*:
  - Dolasetron: in patients with QT prolongation, second- and third-degree AVB, co-administration of class II/III antiarrhythmic agents. IV administration is not indicated because of risk for QT prolongation.

Receptor antagonists (cyclizine, domperidone, metoclopramide)

- *Indications*: prevention and treatment of nausea and vomiting associated with motion sickness, surgery, acute migraine, chemotherapy, or radiotherapy. Metoclopramide: restores normal coordination and tone to the upper GI tract.
- *Mechanism of action*: cyclizine: histamine H1 and muscarinic receptor antagonist. Domperidone: dopamine D2/D3 receptor antagonist at the gastric level and in the chemoreceptor trigger zone, which lies outside the blood–brain barrier in the area postrema. Metoclopramide: dopamine D2 antagonist in the chemoreceptor trigger zone and muscarinic M1 receptor agonist in the upper GI tract.

- *Adverse effects*:
  - Cyclizine: very common: palpitations, tachycardia (IV), hypertension/hypotension, arrhythmias.
  - Metoclopramide: uncommon: hypotension, bradycardia, and sinus arrest (particularly IV). Unknown: bradycardia (IV), QT prolongation, TdP, AVB, hypertension.
  - Domperidone: prolongs the QTc interval, ventricular arrhythmias (TdP), and SCD.
- *Cautions*:
  - Cyclizine: in patients with severe HF or acute MI, because it may cause a fall in CO, associated with an increase in heart rate, mean BP, and PCWP.
  - Domperidone: its main metabolic pathway is CYP3A4; potent CYP3A4 inhibitors (see Table 8.1.2) increase domperidone plasma levels.
  - Metoclopramide (IV) in patients with cardiac conduction disturbances, QTc prolongation, bradycardia, or electrolyte disturbances or those taking drugs known to prolong the QT interval. Drug exposure levels increase when co-administered with strong CYP2D6 inhibitors.
- *Contraindications*: avoid domperidone in patients treated with potent CY3A4 inhibitors; those with QT prolongation, treated with QT-prolonging drugs or with risk factors for TdP (see Table 9.1.1); those with underlying cardiac diseases (CHF) due to an increased risk of proarrhythmia.

Substance P antagonist (aprepitant)

- *Indications*: prevention of nausea and vomiting associated with cancer chemotherapy.
- *Mechanism of action*: selective high-affinity antagonist at human substance P neurokinin 1 (NK1) receptors.
- *Adverse effects*: uncommon: palpitations, flushing. Rare: bradycardia.
- *Cautions*: in patients receiving drugs with a narrow therapeutic index metabolized primarily through CYP3A4. In patients on warfarin therapy, monitor PT/INR closely. Avoid the combination with DOACs.

Antifungal drugs

Amphotericin

- *Indications*: severe systemic and/or deep mycoses (disseminated candidiasis, aspergillosis, mucormycosis, chronic mycetoma, cryptococcal meningitis) and mucocutaneous and visceral leishmaniasis.
- *Mechanism of action*: it binds to ergosterol, a fungal membrane sterol not found in animal cells, resulting in the formation of pores that cause the rapid leakage of a variety of intracellular components.
- *Adverse effects*: very common: hypotension, hypokalaemia, hypomagnesaemia. Common: chest pain/tightness, tachycardia, vasodilatation, flushing, thrombophlebitis (by IV route). Not known: cardiac arrest, ventricular arrhythmias (VT).
- *Cautions*: co-administration with other nephrotoxic agents (ciclosporin, aminoglycosides, polymyxins, tacrolimus, pentamidine) enhances the risk of drug-induced renal toxicity; regular monitoring of renal function is recommended. Corticosteroids and diuretics (loop and thiazide) may potentiate hypokalaemia. Amphotericin-induced hypokalaemia may potentiate digitalis toxicity.

Antimetabolites (flucytosine)

- *Indications*: systemic yeast and fungal infections (cryptococcosis, candidiasis, chromomycosis, and infections due to *Torulopsis glabrata* and *hansenul*)
- *Mechanism of action*: it is converted into fluorouracil in fungal, but not human, cells. Fluorouracil inhibits thymidylate synthetase and DNA synthesis.
- *Adverse effects*: uncommon: myocardial toxicity, cardiac arrest, ventricular dysfunction, and VF due to coronary spasm.
- *Cautions*: monitor serum potassium levels. The solution is physically incompatible with other drugs.

Azoles

- *Classification*: (1) imidazoles: clotrimazole, ketoconazole (use other more effective, less toxic drugs), miconazole; (2) triazoles: fluconazole, itraconazole, posaconazole, voriconazole.
- *Indications*: candidiasis, dermatophytosis, and onychomycosis. Fluconazole: cryptococcal meningitis, coccidioidomycosis. Itraconazole: histoplasmosis, blastomycosis, and aspergillosis. Posaconazole: aspergillosis or candidiasis, chromoblastomycosis, and mycetoma. Voriconazole: aspergillosis, infections caused by *Scedosporium* and *Fusarium* species.
- *Mechanism of action*: inhibit 14-α-sterol-demethylase, the enzyme responsible for converting lanosterol to ergosterol, the main sterol in fungal cell membranes.
- *Adverse effects*: common: tachycardia, supraventricular arrhythmias, QT prolongation, hypotension, hypertension, phlebitis. Rare: hypotension, oedema, hypokalaemia, TdP. Unknown: CHF, ventricular extrasystoles, VT, VF, AVB, bundle branch block, thrombophlebitis.

- *Cautions/contraindications*: they inhibit CYP3A4, 2C9, and 2C19, increasing the plasma levels of multiple drugs metabolized by these enzymes. Drug interactions occur less often with fluconazole. With caution in patients with QT prolongation (see Table 9.1.1), symptomatic arrhythmias, or HF. Close monitoring of PT/INR and dose adjustment in patients treated with warfarin. Avoid their use in patients treated with potent CYP450 inducers (see Table 8.1.2), since these drugs are likely to decrease their plasma levels.

Anti-inflammatory and immunosuppressant drugs

Anakinra

- *Indications*: recurrent pericarditis. Treatment of RA in combination with methotrexate and cryopyrin-associated periodic syndromes.
- *Mechanism of action*: recombinant IL-1β receptor antagonist.
- *Adverse effects*: very common: headache, injection site reactions (erythema, ecchymosis, inflammation, and pain), hypercholesterolaemia. Common: serious infections, neutropenia, thrombocytopenia.
- *Contraindications*: in patients with CrCl of <30mL/min or neutropenia (absolute neutrophil count $<1.5 \times 10^9$/L).

Azathioprine

- *Indications*: recurrent pericarditis, autoimmune chronic active hepatitis, severe RA, SLE, chronic refractory idiopathic thrombocytopenic purpura, autoimmune haemolytic anaemia, pemphigus vulgaris, polyarteritis nodosa, dermatomyositis, and polymyositis; to improve the survival of organ transplants, including renal, cardiac, and hepatic transplants, and to reduce the requirement for corticosteroids in renal transplant recipients.
- *Mechanism of action*: it is metabolized into 6-mercaptopurine and purine thio-analogues acting as a purine antimetabolite.
- *Adverse effects*: rare, but life-threatening, hepatic veno-occlusive disease and reversible pneumonitis have been described.
- *Cautions*: allopurinol inhibits xanthine oxidase, the enzyme that breaks down azathioprine, thus increasing its toxicity. Inhibits the effect of warfarin.

Gold salts (sodium aurothiomalate)

- *Indications*: active progressive RA and progressive juvenile chronic arthritis, especially if polyarticular or seropositive.
- *Mechanism of action*: inhibits the synthesis of prostaglandins, modulates phagocytic cells, and inhibits MHC class II–peptide interactions. Presents immunosuppressive anti-rheumatic effects.
- *Adverse effects*: anaphylactoid reactions with hypotension, tachycardia, flushing, dyspnoea, palpitations, and collapse.

Interferon gamma-1B

- *Indications*: chronic granulomatous disease or severe malignant osteopetrosis.
- *Mechanism of action*: possesses both antiviral and immunoregulatory activities.
- *Adverse effects*: unknown: HF, MI, tachyarrhythmia, AVB, hypotension, DVT, PE.
- *Cautions*: patients with pre-existing cardiac disease may experience an acute, self-limiting exacerbation of their condition.

Non-steroidal anti-inflammatory drugs

- *Indications*: acute pericarditis (ibuprofen, indometacin). Relief of mild to moderate pain. Symptomatic relief of rheumatic diseases (RA, osteoarthritis), musculoskeletal, traumatic, and post-operative pain, headache and migraine, and dysmenorrhoea.
- *Mechanism of action*: inhibit COX-1 and COX-2 and the synthesis of prostaglandins and thromboxanes. Exert analgesic (especially inflammatory pain), anti-inflammatory, and antipyretic properties.
- *General adverse effects*: very common to common: hypertension, peripheral oedema, palpitations, CHF. COX-2 inhibitors (coxibs) and some NSAIDs (particularly at high doses and in long-term treatment) may increase the risk of arterial thrombotic events (i.e. MI or stroke) and cardiac arrest. Vasculitis and eosinophilic pneumonitis have been reported.
- *Cautions*: NSAIDs (particularly diclofenac and indometacin) and COX-2-selective inhibitors increase CV events. NSAIDs increase the risk of developing HF in patients with hypertension, diabetes, or renal failure. Avoid NSAIDs, if possible, in patients with CHF; if needed, use COX-1-selective drugs at low doses and for a short period of time. High doses and long-term treatment with NSAIDs may increase the risk of arterial thrombotic events (MI or stroke).
  - Naproxen seems associated with lower CV risk than COX-2 inhibitors and other NSAIDs; high doses of ibuprofen may be associated with an increased risk of thrombotic events.
  - NSAIDs and coxibs can lead to new-onset hypertension or worsening of pre-existing hypertension, which may contribute to an increased incidence of CV events.
  - Patients with a history of hypertension, CAD, PAD, and/or cerebrovascular disease. NSAIDs may cause renal failure (and analgesic nephropathy on chronic consumption), particularly in the elderly, patients with impaired renal, cardiac, or hepatic dysfunction, and in those on ACEIs; monitor renal function in these patients.
  - NSAIDs may decrease the effects of antihypertensives and loop diuretics and increase the plasma levels of digitalis, lithium, or methotrexate and the effects of anticoagulants and antiplatelets. Monitor blood plasma levels of digoxin and lithium, as well as PT/INR. Co-administration with ciclosporin or tacrolimus increases the risk of nephrotoxicity; monitor renal function. Co-administration with potassium-sparing diuretics increases the risk of hyperkalaemia. The combination of NSAIDs (or with aspirin and coxibs) is not recommended because of the cumulative risk of adverse events.
- *Contraindications*: patients with uncontrolled hypertension, CHF, CAD or MI, TIA, severe kidney disease, or a history of allergic-type NSAID hypersensitivity reactions (aspirin-induced asthma). Third trimester of pregnancy. Preterm infants with congenital heart disease in whom patency of the patent ductus arteriosus is necessary for satisfactory pulmonary or systemic blood flow (e.g. pulmonary atresia, severe tetralogy of Fallot, severe coarctation of the aorta).
  - In the setting of CABG surgery and in patients with suspected or confirmed cerebrovascular bleeding, haemorrhagic diathesis, and incomplete haemostasis, and those at high risk of bleeding.

COX-1-selective inhibitors (aspirin, flurbiprofen, ibuprofen, indometacin, ketoprofen, ketorolac, naproxen, tolmetin)

- *Adverse effects*: bradycardia, chest pain, flushing, palpitations.
- *Cautions*: naproxen attenuates aspirin's ability to irreversibly inhibit thromboxane production and its antiplatelet effect. Regular NSAIDs plus aspirin use is associated with an increase in MI relative risk, compared to aspirin alone.

COX-2-selective inhibitors (celecoxib, etoricoxib, parecoxib)

- *Indications*: symptomatic relief of osteoarthritis, RA, and ankylosing spondylitis; post-operative pain; pain and signs of inflammation associated with acute gout.
- *Mechanism of action*: selective COX-2 inhibitors. They reduce prostacyclin production by the vascular endothelium but do not block thromboxane A2 production by platelets.
- *Adverse effects*: common: hypertension. Uncommon: CHF, palpitations, tachycardia, aggravation of hypertension. Unknown: arrhythmia. COX-2 inhibitors increase the risk of thrombotic events (especially MI and stroke), relative to placebo and some NSAIDs. An increased number of serious CV events, mainly MI, has been found in subjects with sporadic adenomatous polyps treated with celecoxib.
- *Cautions*: patients with significant CV risk factors should be treated with a selective COX-2 inhibitor only after careful consideration. Monitor BP, as they can reduce the effect of most antihypertensives. Patients with a history of HF, LV dysfunction, or pre-existing oedema, since inhibition of prostaglandin synthesis may result in deterioration of renal function and fluid retention. Coxibs are not a substitute for aspirin (or antiplatelet therapy) for the prophylaxis of CV thromboembolic diseases, because of their lack of antiplatelet effects. Patients receiving oral anticoagulants should be closely monitored (PT/INR). Celecoxib is an inhibitor of CYP2D6.
- *Contraindications*: CHF (NYHA classes II–IV), uncontrolled hypertension, established CAD, PAD, and/or cerebrovascular disease, post-operative pain following CABG surgery. Pregnancy and breastfeeding. Patients with a history of allergy to aspirin or NSAIDs.

Tocilizumab

- *Indications*: active RA, active systemic juvenile idiopathic arthritis, juvenile idiopathic polyarthritis.
- *Mechanism of action*: recombinant humanized anti-human interleukin 6 (IL-6) receptor monoclonal antibody that binds specifically to soluble and membrane-bound IL-6 receptors (sIL-6R and mIL-6R).
- *Adverse effects*: hypercholesterolaemia, hypertriglyceridaemia.
- *Cautions*: patients with an increased risk for CV disorders and CV risk factors (e.g. hypertension, hyperlipidaemia). In patients taking medicinal products metabolized via CYP450 3A4, 1A2, or 2C9 (e.g. atorvastatin, CCBs, theophylline, warfarin, ciclosporin), doses may need to be increased to maintain a therapeutic effect.

Tumour necrosis factor alpha inhibitors

Adalimumab

- *Indications*: treatment of active RA, polyarticular juvenile idiopathic arthritis, severely active ankylosing spondylitis, active and progressive psoriatic arthritis, chronic plaque psoriasis, severe hidradenitis suppurativa, severe Crohn's disease, severely active ulcerative colitis, and uveitis.
- *Mechanism of action*: it binds specifically to TNF-α and neutralizes the biological function of TNF-α by blocking its interaction with p55 and p75 cell surface TNF receptors.
- *Adverse effects*: common: tachycardia, hypertension, flushing, haematoma. Uncommon: MI, arrhythmia, CHF, aortic aneurysm, vascular arterial occlusion, thrombophlebitis, PE, pleural effusion. Rare: cardiac arrest, pulmonary fibrosis.
- *Cautions*: patients with mild HF (NYHA classes I/II).
- *Contraindications*: CHF and new-onset CHF have been reported with TNF-α blockers. Avoid in patients with moderate to severe heart failure (NYHA classes III–IV), active tuberculosis, or other severe infections.

Certolizumab pegol

- *Indications*: treatment of adult patients with moderately to severely active RA, axial spondyloarthritis, and psoriatic arthritis.
- *Mechanism of action*: recombinant Fab antibody fragment against TNF-α which is conjugated to an approximately 40-kDa polyethylene glycol to delay the metabolism and elimination of the drugs. It binds to free and membrane-bound human TNF-α and neutralizes its activity.
- *Adverse effects*: common: hypertension. Uncommon: arrhythmias (AF, palpitations), ischaemic coronary artery disorders, CHF (new onset or worsening), oedema, bleeding. Rare: pericarditis, AVB, CVA, arteriosclerosis, Raynaud's phenomenon.
- *Cautions*: CHF and new-onset CHF have been reported with TNF-α blockers. Avoid in patients with moderate to severe HF (NYHA classes III–IV), active tuberculosis, or other severe infections.

Etanercept

- *Indications*: RA, juvenile idiopathic arthritis, psoriatic arthritis, axial spondyloarthritis, ankylosing spondylitis, non-radiographic axial spondyloarthritis, plaque psoriasis, and paediatric plaque psoriasis.
- *Mechanism of action*: dimeric human TNF-α receptor (TNFR) p75–Fc fusion protein made up of two extracellular domains of the human 75-kDa (p75) TNFR linked to the Fc portion of human IgG1.
- *Adverse effects*: rare: worsening of CHF, rare reports of new-onset CHF in patients without known pre-existing CV disease, interstitial lung disease (pneumonitis, pulmonary fibrosis), injection site reactions.
- *Contraindications*: patients with serious infections.

Golimumab

- *Indications*: adult patients with moderately to severely active RA, psoriatic arthritis, or ankylosing spondylitis. Treatment of moderately to severely active ulcerative colitis.
- *Mechanism of action*: human monoclonal antibody that forms high-affinity, stable complexes with both the soluble and transmembrane bioactive forms of human TNF-α, preventing the binding of TNF-α to its receptors.
- *Adverse effects*: common: hypertension. Uncommon: arrhythmia, ischaemic coronary artery disorders, thrombosis, flushing, interstitial lung disease. Rare: new-onset or worsening of HF.
- *Cautions*: CHF and new-onset CHF have been reported with TNF-α blockers. Avoid in patients with moderate to severe HF (NYHA classes III–IV), active tuberculosis, or other severe infections.

Immunosuppressant drugs: calcineurin inhibitors (ciclosporin, tacrolimus) and mTOR inhibitors (everolimus, sirolimus)

- *Indications*: (1) ciclosporin: prevention of graft rejection following solid organ, allogeneic bone marrow, and stem cell transplantation; treatment of transplant cellular rejection in patients previously receiving other immunosuppressive agents; prevention or treatment of graft-versus-host disease; (2) everolimus: treatment of hormone receptor-positive, HER2/neu-negative advanced breast cancer, unresectable or metastatic, well- or moderately differentiated neuroendocrine tumours of pancreatic origin, neuroendocrine tumours of GI or lung origin, and advanced renal cell carcinoma; (3) sirolimus: prophylaxis of organ rejection in patients receiving a renal transplant; (4) tacrolimus: prophylaxis of transplant rejection in liver, kidney, or heart allograft recipients and treatment of allograft rejection resistant to treatment with other immunosuppressants.
- *Mechanism of action*: ciclosporin and tacrolimus bind to cyclophilin; the complex binds to calcineurin and inhibits its phosphatase activity, the formation of lymphokines, and T-lymphocyte activation (i.e. immunosuppression). Everolimus and sirolimus bind to FK506 binding protein-12 (FKBP-12), and the FKPB-12–drug complex inhibits the activation of mTOR, leading to a reduction in cell proliferation and angiogenesis.
- *Adverse effects*: very common: hypertension. Common/rare: pericardial effusion.
  - Ciclosporin: very common: flushing.
  - Everolimus: very common: VTE. Common: tachycardia, epistasis, renal graft thrombosis, lymphocele.
  - Sirolimus: very common: tachycardia, lymphocele. Common: VTE (DVT).
  - Tacrolimus: common: CAD, tachycardia, thromboembolic and ischaemic events, peripheral vascular disorders. Uncommon: SVT, ventricular arrhythmias, palpitations, cardiac arrest, HF, cardiomyopathies, ventricular hypertrophy. Very rare: QT prolongation and TdP.
- *Cautions*: these drugs present multiple drug interactions. Ciclosporin inhibits CYP3A4, P-gp, and organic anion transporter proteins (OATPs) and may increase plasma levels of many medication substrates of these enzymes/transporters. Everolimus and sirolimus are extensively metabolized by CYP3A4; caution when given with strong CYP3A4 inhibitors and inducers (see Table 8.1.2). Sirolimus is also a substrate of P-gp.
  - *Tacrolimus*: regular ECG and echocardiography are recommended pre- and post-transplant. Increased risk of cardiac complications in patients with CV risk factors, pre-existing heart disease, or corticosteroid usage. Most cases of cardiac hypertrophy are reversible and occur at higher doses. Caution in patients with risk factors for QT prolongation (see Table 9.1.1).

Anti-obesity drugs

- *Indications*: as an adjunct to diet and increased physical activity for long-term weight management in adults with an initial BMI of ≥30kg/m² (obese) or ≥27kg/m² (overweight) in the presence of at least one weight-related comorbidity (e.g. hypertension, T2DM, or dyslipidaemia).

Lorcaserin

- *Mechanism of action*: selectively activates 5-HT2C receptors on anorexigenic pro-opiomelanocortin (POMC) neurons located in the hypothalamus.
- *Adverse effects*: hypertension, bradycardia, regurgitant cardiac valve (aortic/mitral) disease.
- *Cautions*: patients with regurgitant cardiac valvular (mitral and/or aortic) disease, CHF, bradycardia, or a history of heart block greater than first-degree. In patients who develop signs or symptoms of VHD, drug discontinuation should be considered. Monitor plasma glucose levels in diabetics, as weight loss increases the tendency of precipitating hypoglycaemia. The effect of lorcaserin on CV morbidity and mortality has not been established.

Naltrexone/bupropion

- *Mechanism of action*: bupropion reduces appetite and increases energy expenditure by increasing the activity of POMC neurons. Naltrexone blocks opioid receptors on POMC neurons, further increasing POMC activity.
- *Adverse effects*: common: hot flushes, hypertension, palpitations. Uncommon: tachycardia, MI.
- *Cautions*: monitor BP, heart rate, and blood glucose levels prior to and regularly during treatment. Patients with a history of heart attack or stroke in the previous 6 months, life-threatening arrhythmias, or CHF were excluded from clinical trials.
- *Contraindications*: uncontrolled hypertension.

Anti-migraine drugs

Cyproheptadine

- *Indications*: anti-allergic and antipruritic activity; patients with vascular types of headache.
- *Mechanism of action*: serotonin and histamine antagonist with anticholinergic and sedative properties.
- *Adverse effects*: hypotension, palpitations, extrasystoles, tachycardia.
- *Cautions/contraindications*: cyproheptadine may cause a false-positive test result for tricyclic antidepressant drugs. Avoid in patients with galactose intolerance, Lapp lactase deficiency, or glucose–galactose malabsorption.

Ergot alkaloids (ergotamine)

(See ➔ Bromocriptine, p. 886; ➔ Ergometrine, p. 888.)

- *Indications*: abort or prevent acute migraine attacks.
- *Mechanism of action*: activate 5-HT1D receptors on: (1) intracranial blood vessels, leading to vasoconstriction and relief of migraine headache; and (2) sensory nerve endings of the trigeminal system, inhibiting pro-inflammatory neuropeptide release.
- *Adverse effects*: rare: hypertension, vasoconstrictive complications (ischaemia, coldness and whiteness of the extremities, paraesthesiae), palpitations, bradycardia, or tachycardia. Very rare: myocardial ischaemia and MI, often associated with coronary artery spasm. Overdose causes intense arterial vasoconstriction ('ergotism'). Rare reports of retroperitoneal and/or pleuropulmonary fibrosis and fibrotic thickening of the heart valves.
- *Cautions*: co-administration with potent CYP3A4 inhibitors (see Table 8.1.2) has been associated with vasospasm, leading to cerebral ischaemia and/or ischaemia of the extremities. Propranolol potentiates the vasoconstriction of ergotamine.
- *Contraindications*: pre-existing vascular diseases (CAD, obliterative vascular disease, angina, claudication, peripheral ischaemia, Raynaud's or Buerger's syndromes) and hypertension.

Triptans (almotriptan, eletriptan, frovatriptan, naratriptan, rizatriptan, sumatriptan, zolmitriptan)

- *Indications*: acute treatment of migraine attacks, with or without aura.
- *Mechanism of action*: 5-HT1B and 1D receptor agonists that produce: (1) direct vasoconstriction of intracranial extracerebral vessels (sumatriptan and rizatriptan cause vasoconstriction of the middle meningeal arteries); (2) inhibition of vasoactive neuropeptide release by trigeminal terminals innervating intracranial vessels and the dura mater; (3) inhibition of nociceptive neurotransmission within the trigemino–cervical complex in the brainstem and the upper cervical spinal column.
- *Adverse effects*: common: palpitations, tachycardia, hot flushes. Triptans are associated with coronary vasospasm and angina pectoris with ischaemic ECG changes. Uncommon: peripheral vascular ischaemia.

Rare: bradycardia, syncope, transient increases in BP, cases of MI—even in patients without any underlying CV disease. Patients with hypersensitivity to sulfonamides may exhibit an allergic reactions following the administration of sumatriptan.

- *Cautions*: patients with mild controlled hypertension. Concomitant use of triptans with ergotamine or its derivatives or other triptans increases the risk of coronary artery vasospasm and transient increase in BP after treatment. Wait at least 24h following the use of ergotamine-containing preparations before administering a triptan. Propranolol (not nadolol or metoprolol) increases the plasma levels of rizatriptan.
- *Contraindications*: patients with moderate or severe hypertension, CAD, coronary vasospasm, Raynaud's disease, peripheral vascular disease, and a history of serious neurological conditions (CVA or TIA).

Anti-protozoal drugs

Antimalarial drugs

Artemether with lumefantrine

- *Indications*: treatment of acute, uncomplicated *Plasmodium falciparum* malaria.
- *Mechanism of action*: interferes with parasite transport proteins, produces disruption of mitochondrial function, inhibits angiogenesis, and modulates host immune function.
- *Adverse effects*: very common: palpitations. Common: QT prolongation.
- *Cautions*. CYP3A4 inhibitors/inducers (see Table 8.1.2) should be used with caution. Lumefantrine inhibits CYP2D6 and can increase the plasma concentrations of drugs metabolized by CYP2D6 that prolong the QT interval (e.g. flecainide, imipramine, amitriptyline, clomipramine); avoid the combination.
- *Contraindications*: patients with QT prolongation or treated with QT-prolonging drugs (see Table 9.1.1). History of symptomatic cardiac arrhythmias, bradycardia, or CHF.

Chloroquine (and hydroxychloroquine)

- *Indications*: prophylaxis and treatment of malaria. Treatment of amoebic hepatitis and abscess, treatment of discoid and systemic lupus erythematosus, and treatment of RA.
- *Mechanism of action*: inhibits heme polymerase activity, leading to the accumulation of free heme inside red cells; the heme–chloroquine complex is highly toxic to the cell and disrupts membrane function.
- *Adverse effects*: uncommon: cardiomyopathy leading to HF, sometimes with fatal outcomes. Rare: hypotension, QT prolongation, arrhythmias, including VT, TdP, and VF, have been reported at therapeutic doses.
- *Cautions/contraindications*: chloroquine increases plasma ciclosporin and digoxin levels. It should be used with caution in patients receiving QT-prolonging drugs (see Table 9.1.1). Concomitant use of amiodarone is contraindicated.

Halofantrine

- *Indications*: treatment of *Plasmodium falciparum* or *Plasmodium vivax* malaria.
- *Mechanism of action*: inhibits the polymerization of heme molecules (by the parasite enzyme 'heme polymerase') and forms toxic complexes with ferriprotoporphyrin IX that damage the membrane of the parasite. It blocks HERG cardiac channels.
- *Adverse effects*: chest pain, palpitations, postural hypotension, QT prolongation, TdP, cardiac arrhythmias.
- *Cautions*: ECG (QTc) monitoring recommended before and during treatment. Avoid its combination with QT-prolonging drugs or in conditions that prolong the QT interval (see Table 9.1.1). With caution in patients with a history of cardiac arrhythmias.

Mefloquine

- *Indications*: prophylaxis and treatment of *Plasmodium falciparum* malaria.
- *Mechanism of action*: forms toxic complexes with ferriprotoporphyrin IX that damage the membrane of the parasite.
- *Adverse effects*: unknown: hypotension, syncope, flushing, hypertension, tachycardia/palpitations, bradycardia, AVB, and cardiac conduction disturbances.
- *Cautions*: patients with cardiac conduction disorders or treated with drugs that alter intra-cardiac conduction. Co-administration with quinine and/or chloroquine may produce ECG abnormalities and arrhythmias.
- *Contraindications*: halofantrine should not be used with mefloquine or within 15 weeks after the last dose of mefloquine due to potentially fatal QTc prolongation. Avoid combinations with QT-prolonging drugs (see Table 9.1.1).

Proguanil/atovaquone

- *Indications*: prophylaxis and treatment of *Plasmodium falciparum* malaria.
- *Mechanism of action*: atovaquone is a selective inhibitor of the cytochrome bc1 complex in the parasitic electron transport chain. Proguanil is metabolized into its active metabolite cycloguanil, which inhibits dihydrofolate reductase and disrupts the parasitic deoxythymidylate synthesis.
- *Adverse effects*: uncommon: palpitations. Unknown: tachycardia.
- *Cautions*: metoclopramide reduces the plasma levels of atovaquone (use another antiemetic). Proguanil may potentiate the effect of warfarin; the dose should be adjusted, based on the INR.

Quinine

- *Indications*: prophylaxis and treatment of *Plasmodium falciparum* malaria.
- *Mechanism of action*: it may interfere with lysosome function or nucleic acid synthesis in the malaria parasite.
- *Adverse effects*: hypotension, ECG changes (PR, QRS, and QT prolongation, T-wave flattening), AVB, ventricular tachyarrhythmias (including VT, VF, and TdP), and cardiac arrest.
- *Cautions*: in patients with AF, heart block, other cardiac conduction defects, or other serious heart disease. Quinine has the potential to inhibit the metabolism of CYP3A4 and CYP2D6 substrates (see Table 8.1.2), increasing their plasma levels. Quinine increases the plasma levels of digoxin and flecainide and may enhance the effect of warfarin (monitor the INR/PT).
- *Contraindications*: patients with acute or acquired QT prolongation (see Table 9.1.1).

Trypanosomicidal and leishmanicidal drugs

Pentamidine isetionate

- *Indications*: treatment of pneumonia due to *Pneumocystis carinii*, cutaneous leishmaniasis, and sleeping sickness caused by *Trypanosoma gambiense*. Prevention of *P. carinii* pneumonia in patients with HIV infection.
- *Mechanism of action*: interferes with microbial nuclear metabolism by inhibition of DNA, RNA, phospholipid, and protein synthesis.
- *Adverse effects*: common: hypotension, flushing. Rare: QT prolongation, cardiac arrhythmias, CVA, vasculitis, phlebitis. Unknown: TdP, bradycardia. Fatalities due to severe hypotension and cardiac arrhythmias have been reported.
- *Cautions*: in patients with CV disease, ventricular arrhythmias, bradycardia (<50bpm), or QT prolongation. Monitor the QTc before and during treatment (see Table 9.1.1). Concurrent use of other nephrotoxic medications may increase the potential for nephrotoxicity.

Sodium stibogluconate

- *Indications*: treatment of visceral and cutaneous leishmaniasis.
- *Mechanism of action*: reduces DNA, RNA, protein, and purine nucleoside triphosphate levels. The reduction in ATP and GTP synthesis contributes to decreased macromolecular synthesis.
- *Adverse effects*: ECG changes (QT prolongation, reduction in T-wave amplitude, T-wave inversion), bradycardia. Fatal cardiac arrhythmias at higher doses.
- *Cautions*: in patients with CV disease, monitor the ECG. Avoid its combination with QT-prolonging drugs or in known conditions that prolong the QT interval (see Table 9.1.1).

Trimethoprim/sulfamethoxazole (co-trimoxazole)

- *Indications*: treatment and prevention of *Pneumocystis jiroveci* (*Pneumocystis carinii*) pneumonitis and toxoplasmosis. Treatment of nocardiosis, acute urinary and respiratory tract infections, acute otitis media, and travellers' diarrhoea.
- *Mechanism of action*: sulfamethoxazole competitively inhibits the utilization of para-aminobenzoic acid in the synthesis of dihydrofolate by the bacterial cell, resulting in bacteriostasis. Trimethoprim is a competitive inhibitor of bacterial dihydrofolate reductase and blocks the production of tetrahydrofolate.
- *Adverse effects*: common: headache, hyperkalaemia, skin rashes. Cough, shortness of breath, and pulmonary infiltrates may be early signs of respiratory hypersensitivity.
- *Cautions*: co-trimoxazole potentiates the effect of warfarin and sulfonylureas and can increase digoxin plasma levels. Close monitoring of serum potassium levels in patients taking other drugs that produce hyperkalaemia. Combination with thiazides increases the risk of thrombocytopenia.

Antiviral drugs

Antiretroviral treatment

- *Classification*: (1) nucleoside reverse transcriptase inhibitors (NRTIs): abacavir, didanosine, lamivudine, stavudine, tenofovir, zidovudine; (2) non-nucleoside reverse transcriptase inhibitors (NNRTIs): delavirdine, efavirenz, etravirine, nevirapine; (3) integrase inhibitors (INSTIs): delavirdine, nevirapine, etravirine; (4) protease inhibitors (PIs): amprenavir, atazanavir, darunavir, fosamprenavir, indinavir, lopinavir, nelfinavir, ritonavir, saquinavir, tipranavir—they inhibit HIV-1 and HIV-2 proteases, which prevents the cleavage of viral polyproteins, resulting in the production of immature non-infectious virus particles; (5) entry inhibitors: enfuvirtide, maraviroc; (6) integrase inhibitor: raltegravir.
- *Indications*: treatment of HIV-1.
- *Adverse effects*: general: lipodystrophy (NRTIs, PIs), insulin resistance, increases in cholesterol or triglycerides (NNRTIs, PIs), decrease in bone density, lactic acidosis (NRTIs), PR and QT prolongation (PIs). Etravirine and raltegravir presents with a low frequency of dyslipidaemia.
  - Atazanavir: uncommon: hypertension, TdP. Rare: oedema, palpitations.
  - Darunavir: uncommon: MI, angina pectoris, sinus bradycardia, tachycardia, palpitations.
  - Lopinavir and ritonavir: common: hypertension. Uncommon: DVT, MI, AVB (in patients with structural heart disease), tricuspid valve incompetence. Rare: second- and third-degree heart block in patients with structural heart disease. Unknown: palpitations, pulmonary oedema, MI.
  - Saquinavir/ritonavir: PR and QT prolongation (TdP reported rarely). An ECG should be performed prior to, and during, treatment.
  - Zidovudine: rare: cardiomyopathy.
- *Cautions*: most PIs inhibit CYP3A; they can increase the plasma levels of medicinal products that are substrates of this isoform, while CYP3A4 inducers may reduce their plasma levels (see Table 8.1.2). With caution when co-administered with medicinal products that induce PR or QT prolongation (see Table 9.1.1) and in patients with pre-existing AVB or bundle branch block. Lopinavir and ritonavir may increase plasma digoxin levels. Co-administration with simvastatin or lovastatin may increase the risk of myopathy. Saquinavir interacts with other drug substrates for CYP3A4 and/or P-gp and should be used with caution.
  - Efavirenz and nevirapine are inducers of CYP3A, and potentially CYP2B6, and reduce the plasma levels of substrates of both isoenzymes.
- *Contraindications*: PIs (amprenavir, atazanavir, indinavir, and ritonavir) should not be administered concurrently with medicinal products with a narrow therapeutic window which are substrates of CYP3A4. Avoid ritonavir or saquinavir in patients with congenital/acquired QT prolongation (see Table 9.1.1), bradycardia, HFrEF, and a previous history of symptomatic arrhythmias. Atazanavir: avoid co-administration with simvastatin, lovastatin, or sildenafil.

DNA polymerase inhibitors (aciclovir, ganciclovir, foscarnet, valganciclovir)

- *Indications*: aciclovir: treatment of herpes simplex virus (HSV) and varicella-zoster virus (VZV) infections. Ganciclovir/valganciclovir: CMV in immunocompromised patients. Foscarnet: CMV and HSV.
- *Mechanism of action*: inhibit viral DNA polymerase and DNA replication.
- *Adverse effects*: uncommon: hypotension, palpitations, cardiac arrhythmias.
  - Foscarnet: common: palpitations, hypertension, thrombophlebitis. Unknown: QT prolongation.
- *Cautions*: patients with risk factors for QT prolongation (see Table 9.1.1).

Maraviroc

- *Indications*: treatment of C–C chemokine receptor type 5 (CCR5)-tropic human HIV-1 infection.
- *Mechanism of action*: selectively binds to the human chemokine receptor CCR5, preventing CCR5-tropic HIV-1 from entering cells.
- *Adverse effects*: common: postural hypotension. Rare: angina, MI.
- *Cautions*: patients with CV disease. Maraviroc is a substrate of CYP3A4; CYP3A4 inducers reduce maraviroc exposure and its therapeutic effects (see Table 8.1.2).

Treatment of hepatitis C virus (HCV) infection

Daclatasvir, elbasvir/grazoprevir, ledipasvir/sofosbuvir, simeprevir, telaprevir

- *Indications*: chronic HCV infection. Daclatasvir: genotype 1, 3, or 4 infections; elbasvir/grazoprevir and simeprevir: genotype 1 and 4 infections; ledipasvir/sofosbuvir: genotypes 1, 4, 5, or 6 infections; telaprevir: genotype 1 infection.
- *Mechanism of action*: daclatasvir, elbasvir, ledipasvir: inhibit HCV NS5A serine protease essential for viral RNA replication and virion assembly. Grazoprevir: inhibits HCV NS3/4A serine protease, necessary for the proteolytic cleavage of the HCV-encoded polyprotein and essential for viral replication. Paritaprevir: NS3/4A serine protease inhibitor. Simeprevir: inhibits HCV NS3/4A protease needed for viral replication. Telaprevir: HCV NS3/4A serine protease inhibitor. Sofosbuvir: inhibitor of HCV NS5B RNA-dependent polymerase.
- *Adverse effects*: cases of symptomatic bradycardia requiring pacemaker intervention, particularly when combined with amiodarone and sofosbuvir. Due to amiodarone's long half-life (up to 90 days), patients discontinuing amiodarone just prior to starting combination therapy to treat HCV infections should undergo cardiac monitoring for at least the first 2 weeks. Patients who develop signs and symptoms of bradycardia should seek medical evaluation immediately.
- *Cautions*: multiple, sometimes serious, drug interactions. Daclastavir and paritaprevir are substrates of CYP3A; inhibitors/inducers of CYP3A increase/decrease their plasma levels and therapeutic effects. Daclatasvir inhibits P-gp, OATP1B1 and B3 and BCRP. Telaprevir inhibits CYP3A; potent CYP3A inducers reduce telaprevir plasma concentrations and drug efficacy. Elbasvir/grazoprevir: strong CYP3A inducers; avoid co-administration with drugs that are metabolized via CYP3A and present a narrow therapeutic index. Ledipasvir and sofosbuvir are substrates of P-gp and BCRP. Caution if administered with bradycardic agents.
- *Contraindications*: avoid their use with strong CYP3A4 and P-gp inducers (see Table 8.1.2). Telaprevir is contraindicated during pregnancy.

Ribavirin

- *Indications*: treatment of chronic hepatitis C.
- *Mechanism of action*: guanosine analogue used to stop viral RNA synthesis and viral messenger RNA capping.
- *Adverse effects*: common: tachycardia, palpitations, hypotension, flushing. Uncommon: MI. Rare: cardiomyopathy, arrhythmias, vasculitis. Very rare: myocardial and peripheral ischaemia, pericardial effusion, pericarditis.
- *Cautions*: patients with pre-existing cardiac disease (MI, CHF, arrhythmias) should be closely monitored. Recommend ECG prior to treatment.

Bone disorders

Bisphosphonates (alendronic acid, disodium pamidronate, risedronate, zoledronic acid)

- *Indications*: post-menopausal osteoporosis, Paget's disease, tumour-induced hypercalcaemia, osteolytic lesions, and bone pain in patients with bone metastases associated with breast cancer or multiple myeloma (MM).
- *Mechanism of action*: inhibit bone reabsorption by inhibiting osteoclast activity and promoting osteoclast apoptosis.
- *Adverse effects*: uncommon: hypertension, hypokalaemia, tachycardia, CHF due to fluid overload, hypotension, AF (alendronic acid, zoledronic acid).
- *Cautions*: the risk of AF increases in patients with HF, CAD, or diabetes.

Selective oestrogen receptor modulators: raloxifene, lasofoxifene

- *Indications*: treatment and prevention of osteoporosis in post-menopausal women.
- *Mechanism of action*: selective oestrogen receptor modulators (SERMs) with oestrogenic actions on bone and anti-oestrogenic actions on the uterus and breast.
- *Adverse effects*: very common: vasodilation (hot flushes), hypertension. Common: peripheral oedema. Uncommon: VTE (DVT, PE, arterial thromboembolic reactions), thrombocytopenia, fatal strokes.
- *Cautions*: the risk–benefit balance should be considered in patients at risk of VTE of any aetiology. Thus, they should not be used in primary/secondary prevention of CV diseases in women.
- *Contraindications*: history of VTE, including DVT, PE, and retinal vein thrombosis.

Teriparatide

- *Indications*: osteoporosis in post-menopausal women and in men at increased risk of fracture.
- *Mechanism of action*: recombinant form of endogenous human parathyroid hormone consisting of the first (*N*-terminus) 34 amino acids, i.e. rhPTH[1–34]. It increases the apposition of new bone on trabecular and cortical bone surfaces by increasing the number/activity of osteoblasts. It also increases blood calcium levels by increasing renal calcium resorption and phosphate excretion and converting 25-hydroxyvitamin D to its most active metabolite (1,25-dihydroxyvitamin D3).
- *Adverse effects*: common: hypotension, palpitations, dyspnoea, hypercholesterolaemia. Uncommon: tachycardia.
- *Cautions*: the risk of AF increases in patients with HF, CAD, or diabetes.

Tibolone

- *Indications*: oestrogen deficiency symptoms and prevention of osteoporosis in post-menopausal women.
- *Mechanism of action*: synthetic steroid drug with oestrogenic, progestogenic, and weak androgenic activity.
- *Adverse effects*: VTE (DVT and PE). Increases the risk of ischaemic stroke from the first year of treatment.
- *Contraindications*: previous or current VTE (DVT, PE), known thrombophilic disorders (e.g. protein C, protein S, or antithrombin deficiency), or a history of arterial thromboembolic disease (e.g. angina, MI, stroke, or TIA).

Cancer chemotherapy

Alkylating agents (busulfan, cyclophosphamide, ifosfamide, melphalan, platinum compounds)

- *Indications*: different types of cancer.
- *Mechanism of action*: they interfere with DNA replication by cross-linking of DNA strands, DNA strand breaking, and abnormal base pairing.
- *General adverse effects*: CHF, myocarditis, pericarditis, hypotension, and hypertension. Risk factors include total bolus dose, older age, combination therapy with other anticancer drugs, and mediastinal irradiation. Cisplatin and ifosfamide may cause HF due to myocardial ischaemia. Alkylating agents contribute to the development of pulmonary veno-occlusive disease.
  - Bulsulfan: very common: tachycardia, thrombosis, vasodilatation. Common: arrhythmia, AF, cardiomegaly, pericardial effusion, pericarditis. Uncommon: ventricular extrasystoles, bradycardia, femoral artery thrombosis, capillary leak syndrome.
  - Cyclophosphamide: ST–T wave changes, QT prolongation, pericardial effusion and cardiac tamponade, supraventricular (AF) and ventricular arrhythmias.
  - Estramustine. IHD, MI, thromboembolism.
  - Melphalan: AF.
- *Cautions*: patients with risk factors for cardiotoxicity and the elderly, patients with pre-existing cardiac diseases (CAD, CHF) and those with previous radiation. Patients with QT prolongation or risk factors for QT prolongation (see Table 9.1.1).

Platinum compounds (cisplatin, carboplatin, oxaliplatin)

- *Indications*: multiple cancers (testes, ovary). Carboplatin: ovarian carcinoma of epithelial origin and small cell lung cancer (SCLC).
- *Mechanism of action*: inhibit DNA synthesis by producing intrastrand and interstrand cross-links in DNA. Protein and RNA synthesis are also inhibited, to a lesser extent.
- *Adverse effects*: common: arrhythmias, bradycardia, tachycardia, arterial thrombosis (CAD), thromboembolism. Rare: AF, myocardial/cerebrovascular ischaemia, MI. Unknown: thrombotic microangiopathy, Raynaud's phenomenon. Very rare: cardiac arrest.
- *Cautions*: cisplatin produces severe cumulative nephrotoxicity, ototoxicity, and neuropathies.

Angiogenesis inhibitors (lenalidomide and thalidomide)

They slow/stop the growth of new blood vessels, which a tumour needs to grow and survive.

- *Indications*: lenalidomide: MM, myelodysplastic syndromes, mantle cell lymphoma. Thalidomide: MM.
- *Mechanism of action*: stimulate T-cell, IL-2, and interferon-γ production; inhibit the production of TNF-α; modulate the expression of cell surface adhesion molecules; inhibit the secretion of VEGF. Thalidomide inhibits the proliferation of endothelial cells.

- *Adverse effects*: common: bradycardia, AF, MI, CHF, tachycardia, hypertension, hypotension, venous and arterial thromboembolic events (DVT, PE), vasculitis. Uncommon: arrhythmias, atrial flutter, QT prolongation, peripheral ischaemia.
- *Cautions*: MI and stroke have been described in patients with risk factors (prior thrombosis); the risk is greatest during the first 5 months of therapy. Patients should be closely monitored, requiring mandatory thromboprophylaxis with aspirin or anticoagulation. Lenalidomide: monitor digoxin plasma levels.

Anthracyclines (doxorubicin, daunorubicin, epirubicin, idarubicin, mitoxantrone)

- *Indications*: acute leukaemias, Hodgkin's and non-Hodgkin's lymphomas, paediatric malignancies, and various solid tumours.
  - Doxorubicin: metastatic breast cancer, advanced ovarian cancer, progressive MM, and acquired immune deficiency syndrome (AIDS)-related Kaposi's sarcoma in patients with low CD4 counts and extensive mucocutaneous or visceral disease.
  - Daunorubicin: acute myeloid leukaemia and acute lymphocytic leukaemia.
  - Epirubicin: breast and bladder carcinoma, advanced ovarian cancer, gastric cancer, SCLC.
  - Idarubicin: acute non-lymphocytic leukaemia, breast cancer.
  - Mitoxantrone: metastatic breast cancer, non-Hodgkin's lymphoma, and adult acute non-lymphocytic leukaemia.
- *Mechanism of action*: (1) intercalation into DNA strands, thus preventing replication; (2) inhibition of topoisomerase II, blocking DNA transcription and replication; (3) generation of free oxygen radicals.
- *General adverse effects*: common: LV dysfunction, ventricular arrhythmias, hypotension, flushing, hypertension, phlebitis (IV). ECG changes: non-specific ST-changes, T-wave flattening, reduction of the QRS complex, QTc prolongation. Rare: bradycardia, AF, extrasystoles, supraventricular and ventricular arrhythmias, sinoatrial block, AVB and bundle branch block, and ventricular asystole requiring pacemaker implantation, acute pericarditis, angina pectoris, and MI. Uncommon: SVT, vasculitis, VTE, thrombophlebitis, DVT, and PE.
  - Cardiotoxicity can be seen acutely (during administration), soon after administration (days to weeks) and months to years later: (1) acute toxicity (i.e. supraventricular arrhythmia, transient LV dysfunction, and pericarditis/myocarditis with ECG changes) is usually reversible, but it can eventually lead to cardiotoxicity later; (2) early toxicity: ECG changes, cardiac arrhythmias, reduction of LVEF, CHF, hypotension, pericardial effusion, fibrinous pericarditis, and epicardial fibrosis; (3) late toxicity: HF, non-ischaemic DCM.
  - Risk factors for cardiotoxicity: extremes of age (<15 and >65 years), female gender, schedule (risk is reduced by weekly low-dose administration), total cumulative doses (doxorubicin >400mg/m^2; epirubicin >900mg/m^2; idarubicin 400mg/m^2; mitoxantrone >120mg/m^2), pre-existing CV disease (LV dysfunction, hypertension, CAD,

VHD), diabetes mellitus, concomitant use of cancer chemotherapy (in particular, paclitaxel and trastuzumab), and prior mediastinal/pericardial irradiation.

- *Cautions*: evaluate cardiac function [ECG, echocardiography, or preferably multigated acquisition (MUGA) scan] and biomarkers (troponin, natriuretic peptides) before, and periodically during, treatment, particularly in patients receiving high cumulative doses and with risk factors. Evaluation of LVEF is mandatory before each additional administration of anthracyclines that exceeds the recommended dose. If cardiomyopathy appears, the benefit of continued therapy must be carefully evaluated.
    - Strategies to reduce cardiotoxicity: select alternative non-cardiotoxic chemotherapy; use analogues (epirubicin, pixantrone) or preparations with lower cardiotoxicity (e.g. liposomal doxorubicin); reduce the cumulative dose, and use continuous infusions (up to 48–96h) to decrease the peak plasma levels, and cardioprotective drugs (dexrazoxane in women with breast cancer who received a cumulative dose of >300mg/m^2 of doxorubicin or >540mg/m^2 of epirubicin). ACEIs, ARBs, and β-blockers are effective in the prevention of anthracycline-induced cardiotoxicity (LV dysfunction or development of symptomatic HF) in patients with normal cardiac function and low risk before treatment.
    - Avoid concomitant use of trastuzumab; if used, should be 24 weeks apart. Paclitaxel used in combination with anthracyclines enhances their cardiotoxicity; it is recommended to administer anthracyclines before paclitaxel, to separate the infusions, and/or to limit the cumulative doxorubicin dose to 360mg/m^2.
- *Contraindications*: HF, recent MI, severe arrhythmias, unstable angina pectoris, or myocardiopathy.

Antimetabolites

- *Classification*: (1) folate antagonists: methotrexate, pemetrexed, raltitrexed. They inhibit dihydrofolate reductase and interfere with DNA synthesis, repair, and cellular replication. Pemetrexed also inhibits thymidylate synthase and glycinamide ribonucleotide formyltransferase, enzymes used in purine and pyrimidine synthesis; (2) purine analogues: cladribine, fludarabine, mercaptopurine, tioguanine; and (3) pyrimidine analogues: AZA, capecitabine, cytarabine, fluorouracil, gemcitabine.
- *Indications*:
    - Capecitabine: metastatic colorectal cancer, advanced gastric cancer, locally advanced or metastatic breast cancer.
    - Cladribine: hairy cell leukaemia (HCL) and B-cell chronic lymphocytic leukaemia (CLL).
    - Clofarabine: acute lymphoblastic leukaemia (ALL) in paediatric patients.
    - Cytarabine: acute myeloid leukemia, ALL, and lymphomas.
    - Gemcitabine: locally advanced or metastatic bladder cancer, adenocarcinoma of the pancreas, non-small cell lung cancer (NSCLC), ovarian carcinoma, and breast cancer.

    - Fludarabine: B-cell CLL.
    - Fluorouracil: several cancers, particularly colon and breast cancer.
    - Methotrexate: acute leukaemias, non-Hodgkin's lymphoma, soft tissue and osteogenic sarcomas, and solid tumours (breast, lung, head and neck, bladder, cervical, ovarian, and testicular carcinoma). Treatment of severe psoriasis.
    - Pemetrexed: malignant pleural mesothelioma and NSCLC.
- *Mechanism of action*: block the synthesis and use of nucleic acids required for DNA replication.
- *Adverse effects*: chest pain, angina pectoris, ischaemia-related ECG abnormalities, arrhythmias, MI (even with normal coronary arteries), thrombophlebitis. Other: CHF, cardiac arrhythmias.
    - Capecitabine: uncommon: DVT, hypo-/hypertension, hot flushes, palpitations, cardiac arrhythmias (including sinus tachycardia, AF, VF, TdP, and bradycardia).
    - Clofarabine: very common: flushing. Common: tachycardia, pericardial effusion and pericarditis, hypotension, capillary leak syndrome, haematoma.
    - Cytarabine: fatal cases of acute pericarditis and cardiomyopathy have been reported with cytarabine in combination with cyclophosphamide.
    - Gemcitabine: rare: AF, peripheral vasculitis and gangrene, hypotension. Gemcitabine should be discontinued if capillary leak syndrome develops during therapy.
    - Fluorouracil: rare: cerebral, intestinal, and peripheral ischaemia, Raynaud's syndrome, thromboembolism, thrombophlebitis. Very rare: cardiac arrest and SCD.
    - Methotrexate: pericarditis, pericardial effusion, hypotension, and arterial/venous thromboembolic events. Some NSAIDs increase serum methotrexate levels.
    - Pemetrexed: uncommon: CV and cerebrovascular events, MI, angina, TIA, stroke.
- *Cautions*: patients with a history of heart disease or with pre-existing CAD should be closely monitored. Prophylactic administration of anti-anginal drugs may not be effective. Pyrimidine analogues should be withheld if myocardial ischaemia occurs.
    - Capecitabine: when co-administered with VKAs, monitor INR/PT regularly.
    - Monitor digoxin plasma levels in patients treated with cytarabine.

Antimicrotubule agents

Docetaxel, paclitaxel

- *Indications*: breast, NSCLC, head and neck and ovarian cancer.
- *Mechanism of action*: stabilize the microtubule structure and inhibit mitosis.
- *Adverse effects*: common: tachycardia, SVT, hot flushes, hypertension, lymphoedema. Rare: sinus node dysfunction, bradyarrhythmias, AVB, AF, LV dysfunction, and CHF. Uncommon: hypotension, peripheral coldness, orthostatic hypotension. Rare cases of MI and thromboembolic events.
- *Cautions*: HF in combination with or after anthracyclines, cyclophosphamide, or trastuzumab. Cardiac assessment should be performed before and every 3 months during treatment.

Eribulin

- *Indications*: locally advanced or metastatic breast cancer and unresectable liposarcoma.
- *Mechanism of action*: inhibits the growth phase of microtubules and sequesters tubulin into non-productive aggregates.
- *Adverse effects*: uncommon: tachycardia, QT prolongation, hypotension, hot flushes, PE. Rare: DVT.
- *Cautions/contraindications*: ECG monitoring is recommended in patients with CHF, bradyarrhythmias, or concomitant treatment with QT-prolonging drugs (see Table 9.1.1). Eribulin should be avoided in patients with congenital LQTS.

Arsenic trioxide

- *Indications*: relapsed/refractory acute promyelocytic leukaemia.
- *Mechanism of action*: it causes: (1) morphological changes and DNA fragmentation, characteristic of apoptosis, in NB4 human promyelocytic leukaemia cells; and (2) damage or degradation of the fusion protein Pro-Myelocytic Leukaemia/Retinoic Acid Receptor-alpha (PML/RAR alpha).
- *Adverse effects*: very common: QT prolongation (and TdP sometimes fatal), tachycardia, complete AVB, palpitations. Common: hypokalaemia, vasculitis, hypotension, hyperglycaemia. Uncommon: HF, chest pain, AF/flutter, VT. Acute promyelocytic leukaemia differentiation syndrome characterized by fever, dyspnoea, weight gain, pulmonary infiltrate, and pleural or pericardial effusion.
- *Cautions/contraindications*: prior to and during therapy, monitor the ECG and correct risk factors for QT prolongation (see Table 9.1.1). If syncope or a rapid or irregular heartbeat develops, immediate hospitalization and monitoring are required. With QTc prolongation, drug discontinuation is indicated until the QTc is <460ms. Avoid drugs that prolong the QT interval.

Epidermal growth factor receptor (ErbB-1, or HER1) inhibitors (cetuximab, erlotinib, gefitinib, lapatinib, pertuzumab, trastuzumab)

- *Indications*: HER2-positive breast tumours overexpressing HER2 (ErbB2). Erlotinib: NSCLC and pancreatic cancer.
- *Mechanism of action*: (1) humanized monoclonal antibodies against HER2: pertuzumab, trastuzumab, trastuzumab emtansine (T-DM1); (2) erlotinib and lapatinib inhibit the tyrosine kinase of epidermal growth factor receptor type 1.
- *General adverse effects*: they should be administered sequentially after treatment with other therapies, mainly anthacyclines.
    - Monoclonal antibodies: very common: hypotension/hypertension, palpitations, atrial flutter, hot flushes, decreased LVEF (including HF). Common: SVT, cardiomyopathy, vasodilatation. Uncommon: bradycardia, pericardial effusion. Unknown: bradycardia, pericarditis, cardiogenic shock.
    - Lapatinib: very common: hot flushes, dyspnoea. Common: decreased LVEF. Potential risk of TdP and SCD due to QTc prolongation. Uncommon: interstitial lung disease/pneumonitis.
- *Cautions*:
    - Cardiotoxicity: careful cardiac assessment (history, examination, ECG, echocardiography ± MRI) prior to, and at regular intervals during, treatment. In contrast to anthracyclines, trastuzumab-induced cardiotoxicity is frequently reversible after drug interruption and/or treatment with ACEIs and β-blockers.
    - Risk factors: age (>65 years), BMI >30kg/mg^2, LV dysfunction, hypertension, CAD, CHF, co-treatment with paclitaxel, docetaxel, or anthracyclines, or previous chest radiotherapy. Because trastuzumab may persist for several months after drug withdrawal; avoid anthracyclines for up to 7 months after stopping trastuzumab.
    - If LVEF is <45% or is 45–50% associated with ≥10% below the baseline, treatment should be suspended and LVEF assessment repeated within 3 weeks. If LVEF has not improved or has declined further, or symptomatic CHF has developed, drug discontinuation should be considered, unless the benefits for the patient are deemed to outweigh the risks. Close BP monitoring, discontinuation of drugs known to raise BP, and aggressive management of hypertension are recommended.
    - Erlotinib: potent inhibitor of CYP1A1; moderate inhibitor of CYP3A4 and CYP2C8. Potent CYP3A4 inducers significantly decrease erlotinib plasma concentrations (see Table 8.1.2).
    - Lapatinib: monitor the QT interval (see Table 9.1.1). Concomitant treatment with inducers of CYP3A4 should be avoided.

Histone deacetylase inhibitors (belinostat, panobinostat, romidepsin, vorinostat)

- *Indications*: belinostat: peripheral T-cell lymphoma. Panobinostat: relapsed and/or refractory MM. Romidepsin, vorinostat: cutaneous T-cell lymphoma (CTCL).
- *Mechanism of action*: potent inducers of cell cycle arrest, re-differentiation, and apoptosis through an accumulation of hyperacetylated histone proteins.
- *Adverse effects*: belinostat: hypotension, phlebitis, QT prolongation. Romidepsin: tachycardia, ventricular arrhythmia. Vorinostat: thromboembolism, DVT, QT prolongation.
    - Panobinostat: very common: hypotension. Common: bradycardia AF, sinus tachycardia, tachycardia, hypertension. Uncommon: MI, haemorrhagic shock.
- *Cautions*: panobinostat: avoid if QTcF is ≥480ms or above 60ms from the baseline (see Table 9.1.1). Reduce the dose in patients taking strong CYP3A and/or P-gp inhibitors. Vorinostat: prior history of thromboembolic disease, drugs/conditions that prolong the QT interval. It prolongs the INR in patients treated with coumarin derivatives.

Immune checkpoint inhibitors (atezolizumab, avelumab, durvalumab, ipilimumab, nivolumab, pembrolizumab)

- They help the body to recognize and destroy cancer cells escaping from the native immune system.
- *Indications*: atezolizumab: locally advanced or metastatic urothelial carcinoma. Avelumab: metastatic Merkel cell carcinoma. Durvalumab: locally advanced or metastatic urothelial carcinoma. Ipilimumab: advanced melanoma. Natalizumab: highly active relapsing–remitting multiple sclerosis. Nivolumab: melanoma, NSCLC, renal cell carcinoma, squamous cell cancer of the head and neck, and Hodgkin's lymphoma. Pembrolizumab: advanced melanoma, metastatic NSCLC, and relapsed or refractory classical Hodgkin's lymphoma.
- *Mechanism of action*: atezolizumab: Fc-engineered, humanized IgG1 monoclonal antibody that directly binds to programmed death-ligand 1 (PD-L1) and provides dual blockade of the PD-1 and B7.1 receptors. Avelumab: human IgG1 monoclonal antibody directed against PD-L1. Durvalumab: human IgG1 κ monoclonal antibody that blocks the interaction of PD-L1 with PD-1 and CD80 (B7.1) molecules. Ipilimumab: cytotoxic T-lymphocyte antigen 4 (CTLA-4) immune checkpoint inhibitor that blocks T-cell inhibitory signals induced by the CTLA-4 pathway. Nivolumab: human IgG4 monoclonal antibody, which binds to the programmed cell death-1 (PD-1) receptor and blocks its interaction with PD-L1 and PD-L2. Pembrolizumab: humanized monoclonal antibody which binds to the PD-1 receptor and blocks its interaction with PD-L1 and PD-L2 ligands.
- *Adverse effects*:
    - Atezolizumab: common: hypotension.
    - Avelumab: very common: peripheral oedema. Common: hypotension, hypertension, pneumonitis. Rare: myocarditis.

- Ipilimumab: common: hypotension, flushing. Uncommon: arrhythmia, AF, vasculitis, peripheral ischaemia, orthostatic hypotension. Unknown: temporal arteritis.
- Nivolumab: common: hypertension. Uncommon: tachycardia. Rare: ventricular arrhythmias, AF, myocarditis, vasculitis.
- Pembrolizumab: common: hypertension.

- *Cautions*: nivolumab: patients should be monitored for cardiac and pulmonary adverse reactions, electrolyte disturbances, and dehydration prior to, and periodically during, treatment. New-onset arrhythmias and conduction blocks may be the initial presentation for myocarditis.

Inhibitors of mammalian target of rapamycin (everolimus, pimecrolimus, sirolimus, temsirolimus)

- *Indications*: (1) everolimus: kidney, liver, and heart transplantation; renal angiomyolipoma associated with tuberous sclerosis complex, subependymal giant cell astrocytoma, or refractory seizures associated with tuberous sclerosis complex; hormone receptor-positive, HER2/neu-negative advanced breast cancer; neuroendocrine tumours of pancreatic origin or of GI or lung origin, renal cell carcinoma; (2) pimecrolimus: atopic dermatitis where treatment with topical corticosteroids is not possible; (3) sirolimus: prophylaxis of organ rejection in adults at low to moderate immunological risk receiving a renal transplant; (4) temsirolimus: renal cell carcinoma, mantle cell lymphoma.
- *Mechanism of action*: they bind to the intracellular protein FKBP-12, and the FKBP–drug complex binds to and inhibits the activity of mTOR.
- *Adverse effects*: common: tachycardia, CHF, hypertension, VTE (DVT, venous thrombosis), thrombophlebitis. Hypercholesterolaemia, hypertriglyceridaemia, hyperglycaemia.
  - Everolimus: common: haemorrhage. Uncommon: CHF, flushing.
  - Sirolimus/temsirolimus: uncommon: pericardial effusion.
- *Cautions*: patients with diabetes or lipid disorders. They are metabolized by CYP3A4; avoid the use of strong CYP3A4 inhibitors/inducers (see Table 8.1.2). Everolimus and sirolimus are substrates and inhibitors of P-gp; avoid potent P-gp inhibitors. Patients with CNS tumours receiving anticoagulants and temsirolimus may be at an increased risk of developing intracerebral bleeding.

Inhibitors of poly (ADP-ribose) polymerase (PARP) enzymes (olaparib, rucaparib)

- *Indications*: deleterious *BRCA* mutation (germline and/or somatic), associated advanced ovarian cancer.
- *Mechanism of action*: inhibit PARP-1, PARP-2, and PARP-3 required for DNA transcription, cell cycle regulation, and DNA repair.
- *Adverse effects*: hypercholesterolaemia.
- *Cautions*: olaparib co-administration with strong or moderate CYP3A inhibitors is not recommended (see Table 8.1.2). Rucaparib is metabolized by CYP2D6.

Interferons

They are inducible cytokines released by host cells in response to the presence of several pathogens, such as viruses, bacteria, and parasites, and also tumour cells. They exhibit antiviral, antiproliferative, and immunomodulatory activities. Present minimal drug interactions.

Interferon alfa-2A

- *Indications*: HCL, Philadelphia chromosome-positive chronic myelogenous leukaemia (CML), CTCL, chronic hepatitis B and C, follicular non-Hodgkin's lymphoma, advanced renal cell carcinoma, and AJCC (American Joint Committee on Cancer) stage II malignant melanoma.
- *Mechanism of action*: inhibits DNA, RNA, and protein synthesis. Induces the innate antiviral immune response.
- *Adverse effects*: common: arrhythmia, palpitations, cyanosis. Uncommon: hyper-/hypotension. Rare: CHF, MI, pulmonary oedema, cardiorespiratory arrest, vasculitis.
- *Contraindications*: severe pre-existing cardiac disease (HF, MI, hypertension, or arrhythmias) must be closely monitored.

Interferon alfa-2B

- *Indications*: chronic hepatitis B and C, HCL, CML, MM, follicular lymphoma, carcinoid tumours, malignant melanoma.
- *Mechanism of action*: inhibits viral replication.
- *Adverse effects*: common: palpitations, tachycardia, hypertension. Rare: cardiomyopathy. Very rare: MI, cardiac ischaemia, peripheral oedema, hypotension. Unknown: CHF, pericardial effusion, arrhythmia.
- *Contraindications*: pre-existing cardiac disease, e.g. uncontrolled CHF, recent MI, severe arrhythmic disorders.

Interleukin-2 (aldesleukin)

- *Indications*: treatment of metastatic renal cell carcinoma.
- *Mechanism of action*: recombinant IL-2 that regulates the activities of white blood cells.
- *Adverse effects*: very common: tachycardia, arrhythmias (AF, SVT), chest pain, hypotension. Common: cyanosis, phlebitis, transient ECG changes, myocardial ischaemia, palpitations, CV disorders including HF, hypertension. Uncommon: thrombosis, thrombophlebitis, haemorrhage.
- *Cautions*: it has been associated with capillary leak syndrome. Monitor BP and ECG.

Monoclonal antibodies (alemtuzumab, daclizumab, dinutuximab, rituximab)

- *Indications*: (1) alemtuzumab: resistant CLL, relapsing forms of multiple sclerosis; (2) daclizumab: relapsing forms of multiple sclerosis; (3) dinutuximab: paediatric patients with high-risk neuroblastoma; (4) rituximab: RA, non-Hodgkin's lymphoma, follicular lymphoma.
- *Mechanism of action*: (1) alemtuzumab: humanized monoclonal antibody directed against the cell surface glycoprotein CD52; (2) daclizumab: humanized IgG1 monoclonal antibody that binds to CD25 (IL-2Rα) and prevents IL-2 from binding to

CD25; (3) dinutuximab: chimeric monoclonal antibody that binds to the glycolipid antigen disialoganglioside expressed on the surface of neuroblastoma cells; (4) rituximab: anti-CD20 monoclonal antibody.

- *Adverse effects*:
    - Alemtuzumab: very common: hypotension, flushing. Common: bradycardia, tachycardia, palpitations, abnormal ECG. Uncommon: CHF, cardiomyopathy, decreased LVEF.
    - Daclizumab: common: peripheral oedema, hypertension, hypotension, tachycardia.
    - Dinutuximab: hypotension, capillary leak syndrome, haemorrhage, hypertension, tachycardia, hyponatraemia, hypokalaemia, hyperglycaemia, hypertriglyceridaemia.
    - Rituximab: common: MI, AF, atrial flutter, tachycardia, hypertension, hypotension, orthostatic hypertension. Uncommon: LV failure, SVT, VT, bradycardia, angina, myocardial ischaemia. Rare: HF, severe cardiac events, CHF, vasculitis.
- *Cautions*: hypotension during infusion may require antihypertensives being withheld 12h prior to infusion. Monitor closely patients with a history of cardiac disease and/or on cardiotoxic chemotherapy.
    - Dinutuximab: serious and potentially life-threatening infusion reactions. Monitor BP and electrolyte disturbances during treatment; immediately interrupt therapy in patients with symptomatic hypotension.

Proteasome inhibitors (bortezomib, carfilzomib, ixazomib)

- *Indications*: MM and mantle cell lymphoma.
- *Mechanism of action*: bind to the catalytic site of the 26S proteasome, a large protein complex that degrades ubiquitinated proteins.
- *Adverse effects*: common: hypotension or hypertension. Uncommon: new or worsening HF, pericarditis, angina and MI, AF, tachycardia/bradycardia, CVA, thrombophlebitis, haemorrhage, DVT. Rare: CVA, VTE (DVT and PE with fatal outcomes), venous insufficiency, AVB, QT prolongation and TdP (bortezomib), cardiac arrest.
    - Ixazomib: produces minimal CV adverse effects. Thrombocytopenia, oedema.
- *Cautions*: in patients treated with antihypertensive drugs and HF. Bortezomib is a substrate of CYP3A4, 2C19, and 1A2. Monitor the patients and consider a dose reduction when co-administered with strong CYP3A4 inhibitors (see Table 8.1.2). Bortezomib: concomitant use with QT-prolonging drugs (see Table 9.1.1).
- *Contraindications*: bortezomib in patients with acute diffuse infiltrative pulmonary and pericardial disease.

Topoisomerase inhibitors (etoposide, teniposide)

- *Indications*: refractory testicular tumours, SCLC, acute monoblastic (AML M5), and acute myelomonoblastic leukaemia (AML M4).
- *Mechanism of action*: cause breaks in DNA by either an interaction with DNA topoisomerase II or the formation of free radicals.
- *Adverse effects*: common: MI, arrhythmias, transient hypotension following rapid IV administration, hypertension.

Tyrosine kinase inhibitors

Bcr-Abl tyrosine kinase inhibitors (bosutinib, dasatinib, imatinib, nilotinib, ponatinib)

- *Indications*: Philadelphia chromosome-positive (Ph+) CML and Ph+ ALL and lymphoid blast CML. Imatinib: myelodysplastic/myeloproliferative diseases associated with platelet-derived growth factor receptor gene rearrangements; hypereosinophilic syndrome and/or chronic eosinophilic leukaemia with FIP1L1–PDGFRα rearrangement.
- *General adverse effects*: common: flushing, haemorrhage, CHF, LV dysfunction, arrhythmias (including AVB, tachycardia, ventricular extrasystoles, bradycardia), hypertension, angina, MI, QT prolongation, peripheral arterial occlusive disease, venous thrombosis, and embolisms. Occasionally peripheral and pulmonary oedema and serious fluid retention (e.g. pleural effusion, pericardial effusion, pulmonary oedema, ascites). Unknown: pericarditis.
    - Dasatinib: uncommon: cardiomegaly, T-wave abnormal. Rare: myocarditis, ACS, cardiac arrest, DVT, embolism, livedo reticularis, severe precapillary PAH. Unknown: AF.
    - Imatinib: uncommon: subdural haematoma, peripheral coldness, hypotension, Raynaud's phenomenon. Rare: arrhythmia, SCD, pericardial or pleural effusion, pulmonary hypertension. Not known: pericarditis, cardiac tamponade, thrombosis/embolism.
    - Nilotinib: uncommon: AF, cyanosis, intermittent claudication, peripheral arterial occlusive disease. SCD in patients with a history of cardiac disease or significant cardiac risk factors. Potential risk of TdP and SCD due to QTc prolongation.
    - Ponatinib: occlusions in coronary, retinal, cerebral, peripheral, and renal arteries, leading to fatal MI, stroke, permanent visual impairment, and urgent revascularization procedures. Consider drug discontinuation in patients who develop HF. Unknown: AF.
- *Cautions*: before treatment, the CV status of patients should be evaluated and CV risk factors monitored and actively managed during therapy, according to standard guidelines. Patients with cardiac disease or risk factors for HF should be monitored carefully for signs and symptoms of fluid retention. CHF and LV dysfunction are more frequent in patients with advanced age, risk factors (e.g. hypertension, hyperlipidaemia, diabetes), or CV comorbidities (documented CAD). Stop the drug if PAH develops.
    - Dasatinib and nilotinib prolong the QT interval; close ECG monitoring is advisable. With caution to patients who develop or may develop QT prolongation. Avoid QT-prolonging drugs (see Table 9.1.1).
    - Bosutinib, dasatinib, imatinib, and ponatinib are metabolized by CYP3A4; co-administration with strong CYP3A4 inducers/inhibitors may reduce/increase their plasma levels (see Table 8.1.2). Avoid this combination.
    - Avoid the combination of imatinib with DOACs; use with caution the combination of nilotinib with DOACs.

BRAF serine–threonine kinase inhibitors (dabrafenib, trametinib, vemurafenib)

- *Indications*: adult patients with unresectable or metastatic melanoma with a *BRAF V600* mutation.
- *Mechanism of action*: BRAF serine–threonine kinase inhibitors. Vemurafenib and dabrafenib: inhibit BRAF proteins containing the *V600E* or *V600K* mutation. Trametinib: allosteric inhibitor of mitogen-activated extracellular signal-regulated kinase (MEK).
- *Adverse effects*: very common: hypotension. Common: hypertension, LVEF reduction/LV dysfunction, bradycardia, haemorrhagic events. Unknown: myocarditis, QT prolongation, vasculitis.
- *Cautions*: dabrafenib and vemurafenib are substrates of CYP3A4; co-administration of strong CYP3A4 inhibitors or inducers may alter drug exposure (see Table 8.1.2). Vemurafenib increases digoxin plasma levels. Vemurafenib: potential risk of TdP and SCD due to QTc prolongation. Treatment not recommended when baseline QTc >500ms.

Crizotinib

- *Indications*: anaplastic lymphoma kinase (ALK)-positive advanced NSCLC; ROS1-positive advanced NSCLC.
- *Mechanism of action*: selective inhibitor of receptor tyrosine kinases, including ALK, hepatocyte growth factor receptor (HGFR, c-Met), ROS1 (c-ros), and Recepteur d'Origine Nantais (RON).
- *Adverse effects*: very common: bradycardia, dizziness. Common: QT prolongation, HF, syncope.
- *Cautions*: monitor the ECG before and during treatment, and avoid concomitant use with QT-prolonging drugs (see Table 9.1.1). Risk of excessive bradycardia when used in combination with other bradycardic agents. Co-administration of crizotinib with strong CYP3A inhibitors/ inducers (see Table 8.1.2) may increase/decrease crizotinib plasma levels.

Ibrutinib

- *Indications*: relapsed/refractory mantle cell lymphoma (MCL), CLL, or Waldenström's macroglobulinaemia.
- *Mechanism of action*: inhibitor of Bruton's tyrosine kinase.
- *Adverse effects*: very common: haemorrhage, bruising. Common: minor (contusion, epistaxis, petechiae) and major haemorrhagic events (GI, intracranial, haematuria), AF, arrhythmias, hypertension.
- *Cautions*: co-administration of strong or moderate CYP3A4 inhibitors increase ibrutinib exposure (see Table 8.1.2). AF affects patients with a prior history of AF and age ≥65 years.

Vascular endothelial growth factor/vascular endothelial growth factor receptor inhibitors (aflibercept, axitinib, bevacizumab, cabozantinib, lenvatinib, pazopanib, ponatinib, ramucirumab, regorafenib, sorafenib, sunitinib, vandetanib)

- *Indications*:
  - Aflibercept: metastatic colorectal cancer.
  - Axitinib: renal cell carcinoma and several other tumour types.
  - Bevacizumab: breast, colorectal, non-small cell lung, non-squamous non-small cell lung, renal, epithelial ovarian, Fallopian tube, cervix, and primary peritoneal cancers.

- Cabozantinib: advanced renal cell carcinoma.
- Lenvatinib: locally advanced or metastatic, differentiated (papillary/follicular/Hürthle cell) thyroid carcinoma refractory to radioactive iodine.
- Pazopanib: advanced renal cell carcinoma and advanced soft tissue sarcoma.
- Ponatinib: CML and Ph+ ALL.
- Ramucirumab: advanced gastric cancer or gastro-oesophageal junction adenocarcinoma.
- Regorafenib: metastatic colorectal cancer and advanced GI stromal tumours (GISTs).
- Sorafenib: renal cell carcinoma, hepatocellular carcinoma, and differentiated thyroid carcinoma.
- Sunitinib: GIST, metastatic renal cell carcinoma and pancreatic neuroendocrine tumours.
- Vandetanib: non-resectable, locally advanced, or metastatic medullary thyroid cancer in adult patients.

- *Mechanism of action*: inhibit the activity of VEGF and VEGF receptors (VEGFRs) which modulate angiogenesis. Some can also inhibit multiple receptor tyrosine kinases (RTKs) implicated in growth, neoangiogenesis, and metastatic progression of cancer: (1) antibodies: bevacizumab, ramucirumab; (2) multi-target tyrosine kinase inhibitors (TKIs): afatinib, axitinib, cabozantinib, pazopanib, ponatinib, sorafenib, sunitinib, vandetanib; (3) ramucirumab: human receptor-targeted antibody anti-VEGFR2; (4) aflibercept: recombinant fusion protein consisting of portions of human VEGFR 1 and 2 extracellular domains fused to the Fc portion of human IgG1.
- *Adverse effects*: very common: hypertension. Common: hot flushes, VTE, and serious, sometimes fatal, arterial thromboembolic events (ATEs) (including MI, CVA, and cerebral ischaemia). Uncommon: bradycardia, LV dysfunction, myocardial ischaemia, HFrEF, hypertensive crisis, haemorrhage. Pazopanib, sorafenib, sunitinib, and vandetanib: potential risk of TdP and SCD due to QTc prolongation. Sorafenib, sunitinib: AF. Risk factors for cardiac dysfunction: age ≥65 years, prior thromboembolic events, pre-existing HF, significant CAD, diabetes, left-sided VHD (e.g. MR), prior radiotherapy to left chest wall, or previous anthracycline treatment.
  - Bevacizumab: common: LV dysfunction, CHF, SVT, venous thromboembolic reactions including PE. Very rare: renal thrombotic microangiopathy.
  - Pazopanib: common: VTE, LV dysfunction. Uncommon: bradycardia, MI, hypertension, haemorrhage.
  - Sorafenib: very common: haemorrhage (including GI, respiratory, cerebral). Common: CHF, myocardial ischaemia. Uncommon: hypertensive crisis. Patients with unstable CAD or recent MI were excluded from clinical trials.
  - Sunitinib: common: CHF, MI, cardiomyopathy, pericardial effusion, DVT, hot flushes, flushing. Uncommon: CHF, MI, cardiomyopathy, pericardial effusion.

- *Cautions*: careful assessment of CV factors at baseline, close BP monitoring, and discontinuation of drugs known to raise BP. ACEIs and β-blockers are the preferred antihypertensive drugs in patients with HF or LV dysfunction. Temporary suspension is recommended in patients with severe uncontrolled hypertension. Caution in patients with clinically significant CV disease (pre-existing CAD or HF) treated with bevacizumab.
  - Strong inhibitors of CYP3A4 (see Table 9.1.1) increases pazopanib and sunitinib plasma concentrations and should be avoided. Avoid the combination of axitinib, sunitinib, or vandetanib with DOACs.
- *Contraindications*: patients who experience a severe ATE. Pazopanib, sorafenib, sunitinib, and vandetanib: monitor the QT interval; avoid in patients with QT prolongation (see Table 9.1.1). Patients with life-threatening thromboembolic reactions or thrombotic microangiopathy and those with thromboembolic reactions ≤ grade 3 should be closely monitored.

Vinca alkaloids (vinblastine, vincristine, vindesine, vinorelbin)

- *Indications*: acute leukaemia, rhabdomyosarcoma, neuroblastoma, Wilm's tumour, Hodgkin's disease, and other lymphomas.
- *Mechanism of action*: they bind to tubulin and inhibit its polymerization into microtubules, directly causing metaphase arrest.
- *Adverse effects*: uncommon: coronary vasospasm, chest pain, and acute myocardial ischaemia and MI (particularly if previous mediastinal radiotherapy). Other: acute pulmonary effects, Raynaud's phenomenon, and hand–foot syndrome.
- *Cautions*: avoid the combination of vinblastine with DOACs.

Other

Abiraterone

- *Indications*: high-risk metastatic hormone-sensitive prostate cancer in adult men, in combination with androgen deprivation therapy (ADT); after failure of ADT when chemotherapy is not yet clinically indicated; when the disease has progressed on or after a docetaxel-based chemotherapy regimen.
- *Mechanism of action*: selective inhibitor of CYP17, an enzyme expressed in, and required for, androgen biosynthesis in testicular, adrenal, and prostatic tumour tissues.
- *Adverse effects*: very common: hypertension. Common: HF, angina pectoris, AF, hypokalaemia, and fluid retention due to increased mineralocorticoid levels. Uncommon: other arrhythmias. Other: MI, QT prolongation.
- *Cautions*: it should be used with caution in patients with a history of CV disease. Phase III studies excluded patients with uncontrolled hypertension and clinically significant heart disease (MI or ATEs in the past 6 months, severe or unstable angina, or class III–IV HF). Monitor BP, serum potassium levels, ECG (QT prolongation in patients experiencing hypokalaemia), fluid retention, and other signs and symptoms of CHF. Avoid the combination with DOACs.

Ribociclib

- *Indications*: in combination with an aromatase inhibitor in post-menopausal women with hormone receptor (HR)-positive, HER2-negative locally advanced or metastatic breast cancer.
- *Mechanism of action*: selective inhibitor of cyclin-dependent kinase (CDK) 4 and 6.
- *Adverse effects*: very common: dyspnoea. Common: syncope, epistaxis. Potential risk of TdP and SCD due to QTc prolongation.
- *Cautions*: concomitant use of strong CYP3A4 inhibitors should be avoided (see Table 8.1.2).
- *Contraindications*: patients at significant risk of developing QTc prolongation.

Central nervous system

Alzheimer's disease

Cholinesterase inhibitors (donezepil, galantamine, rivastigmine)

- *Indications*: mild to moderately severe dementia of the Alzheimer's type.
- *Mechanism of action*: selective, competitive, and reversible inhibitors of acetylcholinesterase that facilitate cholinergic neurotransmission.
- *Adverse effects*: uncommon/rare: hypertension, bradycardia, sinoatrial block, AVB, supraventricular arrhythmias, AF, palpitations, flushing, hypotension.
- *Cautions*: in patients with bradycardia (a risk factor for TdP), sick sinus syndrome, or supraventricular cardiac conduction disturbances. Digoxin, AADs, verapamil, diltiazem, and β-blockers cause additive bradycardic effects.

Memantine

- *Indications*: treatment of Alzheimer's disease.
- *Mechanism of action*: non-competitive *N*-methyl-*D*-aspartate (NMDA) receptor antagonist binding preferentially to NMDA receptor-operated cation channels and blocking the effects of excessive levels of glutamate, resulting in neuronal degeneration.
- *Adverse effects*: common: hypertension. Uncommon: HF, venous thrombosis/thromboembolism.
- *Cautions*: patients with recent MI, uncompensated CHF, or uncontrolled hypertension were excluded in most clinical trials.

Antidepressants

Tricyclic/tetracyclic antidepressants: amitriptyline, doxepin, duloxetine, imipramine, maprotiline, mianserin, mirtazapine, nortriptyline)

- *Indications*: symptoms of depressive illness, treatment of moderate to severe stress urinary incontinence, relief of nocturnal enuresis in children.
- *Mechanism of action*: SNRIs; sodium and L-type CCBs; antagonists or inverse agonists of 5-HT1A/2A, α1/α2-adrenergic and D2 dopaminergic [muscarinic, histaminergic, gamma-aminobutyric acid (GABA)] receptors.
- *Adverse effects*: common: hypotension, orthostatic hypotension, sinus tachycardia, palpitations. Occasionally: ECG changes (QRS, QT, and PR prolongation), arrhythmias (including VT/VF), bundle branch block, hypertension. Very rare: conduction disorders (bundle branch block), TdP, and fatal cardiac arrhythmias. SCD in patients with CV disease.
- *Cautions*: avoid co-administration of medications that prolong the QT interval or with risk factors for QT prolongation (see Table 9.1.1). Supervise closely patients with CV disorders. Diltiazem, labetalol, propranolol, and verapamil increase the plasma levels of imipramine. Increased risk of ventricular arrhythmias with AADs. They may potentiate the CV effects of sympathomimetic drugs. Increased risk of hypotension when co-administered with antihypertensives and vasodilators.
- *Contraindications*: history of MI, heart block, or cardiac arrhythmias, CHF, CAD.

Selective serotonin reuptake inhibitors (citalopram, escitalopram, fluoxetine, fluvoxamine, paroxetine, sertraline)

- *Indications*: major depressive episodes; panic, social anxiety, generalized anxiety, obsessive–compulsive and post-traumatic stress disorders.
- *Adverse effects*: common: palpitations, flushing. Uncommon/ rare: hypotension, palpitations, tachycardia/bradycardia, ECG abnormalities (QRS and QT prolongation), vasculitis.
- *Cautions*: consider an ECG before and during treatment in patients with CV disease. Caution in patients with QT prolongation or taking medications that prolong the QT interval (see Table 9.1.1). Sertraline and citalopram are the preferred SSRIs post-MI. SSRIs may increase the risk of bleeding when co-administered with oral anticoagulants, antiplatelets agents, and aspirin/NSAIDs. Monitor the PT/INR.
    - Fluoxetine is a strong inhibitor of CYP2D6; administer with caution with CYP2D6 substrates. Potent CYP3A4 inhibitors may increase serum trazodone levels (see Table 8.1.2).
- *Contraindications*: citalopram and escitalopram in patients with QT prolongation. Trazodone in patients with acute MI.

Serotonin noradrenaline reuptake inhibitors (desvenlafaxine, duloxetine, venlafaxine)

- *Indications*: prevention and treatment of major depressive episodes and seasonal affective disorder (SAD). Duloxetine: treatment of severe stress urinary incontinence and diabetic peripheral neuropathic pain.
- *Adverse effects*: common: hypertension, flushing, palpitations. Uncommon: tachycardia, supraventricular arrhythmias (AF with duloxetine). Rare: supraventricular arrhythmias (AF), hypertensive crisis. Venlafaxine: QT prolongation, VT (including TdP), VF, hypercholesterolaemia.
- *Cautions*: venlafaxine: caution in patients with recent MI, unstable heart disease, or risk factors for QT prolongation (see Table 9.1.1). Increased risk of bleeding when SNRIs are combined with oral anticoagulants or antiplatelet agents. Caution if a duloxetine capsule is co-administered with medicinal products predominantly metabolized by CYP2D6 (see Table 8.1.2).
- *Contraindications*: duloxetine in patients with uncontrolled hypertension.

Selective noradrenaline reuptake inhibitors (reboxetine)

- *Indications*: acute treatment of depressive illness/major depression.
- *Adverse effects*: common: tachycardia, palpitations, hypo-/hypertension.
- *Cautions*: potent inhibitors/inducers of CYP3A4 increase/decrease drug plasma levels (see Table 8.1.2).

Serotonin antagonist and reuptake inhibitors (SARIs) (trazodone)

- *Indications*: anxiety and depression.
- *Adverse effects*: very common: hypotension, orthostatic hypotension. Common/uncommon: ECG changes (QT prolongation), cardiac arrhythmias (including TdP).

- *Cautions*: in patients with QT prolongation or taking QT-prolonging drugs (see Table 9.1.1). Potent inhibitors/inducers of CYP3A4 increase/decrease drug plasma levels (see Table 8.1.2).
- *Contraindications*: acute MI.

Monoamine oxidase inhibitors (isocarboxazid, moclobemide, phenelzine, tranylcypromine)

- *Indications*: major depressive episodes, treatment of social phobia.
- *Mechanism of action*: inhibit monoamine oxidase (MAO) type A that preferentially deaminates serotonin, melatonin, dopamine, noradrenaline, and adrenaline.
- *Adverse effects*: common: hypotension, flushing, arrhythmias, palpitations, ventricular extrasystoles, and VT. Hypertensive episodes when co-administered with tricyclic antidepressants. Moclobemide can cause QT interval prolongation.
- *Cautions*: they present multiple interactions with other drugs and foods. Marked hypertension when combined with sympathomimetics. Moclobemide in patients with risk factors for QT prolongation (see Table 9.1.1).
- *Contraindications*: patients with severe CV disease.

Antiepileptic drugs

- *Mechanisms of action*: (1) sodium channel blockers: carbamazepine, eslicarbazepine, lacosamide, lamotrigine, oxcarbazepine, phenytoin, rufinamide, topiramate; (2) GABA receptor agonists: benzodiazepines (clobazam, clonazepam), phenobarbital, primidone, topiramate; (3) GABA reuptake inhibitors: tiagabine; (4) glutamate receptor blockers: felbamate (NMDA), perampanel [α-amino-3-hydroxy-5-methyl-4-isoxazolepropionic acid (AMPA)]; (5) potentiate GABA action: valproate; (6) neuronal potassium channel openers: retigabine; (7) binding to the α2δ (alpha-2-delta) subunit of voltage-gated calcium channels: gabapentin, pregabalin; (8) sodium and T-type CCBs: zonisamide; (9) T-type CCBs: ethosuximide; (10) binding to the synaptic vesicle protein 2A: levetiracetam, brivaracetam.
- *Adverse effects*:
  - Carbamazepine: rare: cardiac conduction disorders (QRS widening), hypertension, hypotension. Very rare: bradycardia, palpitations, arrhythmias, AVB, CHF, aggravation of CAD, thrombophlebitis, embolism (e.g. PE), hyponatraemia.
  - Felbamate: frequent: palpitations, tachycardia. Rare: SVT, QT prolongation, TdP.
  - Gabapentin: common: hypertension. Uncommon: palpitations.
  - Lacosamide: uncommon: bradycardia, AVB, AF, atrial flutter.
  - Oxcarbazepine: very rare: arrhythmias, AVB. Unknown: hypertension.
  - Pregabalin: uncommon: tachycardia, AVB, sinus tachycardia, CHF, hypotension, hypertension, flushing. Rare: QT prolongation, sinus tachycardia. Reports of CHF in elderly patients with neuropathic pain.
  - Phenobarbital: bradycardia, hypotension, syncope.

- Phenytoin: hypotension, bradycardia, intra-cardiac conduction blockade, arrhythmias including VF.
- Topiramate: uncommon: bradycardia, palpitations, hypotension. Rare: Raynaud's phenomenon. Monitor serum digoxin levels.
- Valproate: adverse effects: haemorrhage; uncommon: vasculitis.

- *Cautions*: antiepileptic drugs present multiple drug interactions.
  - Carbamazepine is a potent inducer of CYP3A4, 1A2, 2B6, and 2C9/19 and may reduce plasma concentrations of many drugs metabolized by these isoforms. Monitor serum sodium levels, particularly if co-administered with furosemide.
  - Phenobarbital is a potent inducer of CYP3A4 and 2C isoforms and may reduce plasma concentrations of many drugs metabolized by these isoforms.
  - Phenytoin is metabolized by CYP2C9 and CYP2C19 and presents multiple drug interactions because it is subject to saturable metabolism. Phenytoin plasma levels increase in patients treated with amiodarone, dicoumarol, diltiazem, nifedipine, and ticlopidine. Phenytoin increases the metabolism of warfarin, digoxin, nifedipine, nimodipine, nisoldipine, simvastatin, and verapamil.
- *Contraindications*:
  - Carbamazepine: patients with conduction disturbances (AVB, arrhythmia).
  - Phenytoin: bradycardia, sinoatrial block, second-/third-degree AVB, Stokes–Adams syndrome.

Antipsychotic drugs

- *General indications*: psychosis, principally schizophrenia and bipolar disorder.
- *General adverse effects*: common: hypotension and orthostatic hypotension. Uncommon: some drugs cause weight gain and hypercholesterolaemia and may increase the risk of diabetes. VTE (including PE and DVT), MI, and stroke have been reported. QT prolongation is common but is more frequent with amisulpride, pimozide, thioridazine, and ziprasidone. They are associated with an increased risk of death, mainly due to HF, SCD, and cerebrovascular events in elderly patients with dementia-related psychosis.

Typical antipsychotic drugs (chlorpromazine, haloperidol, pimozide, sulpiride, thioridazine, trifluoperazine)

- *Mechanism of action*: dopamine D2 receptor antagonists. They may also affect cholinergic, α-adrenergic, histaminergic, and serotonergic receptors.
- *Adverse effects*:
  - Class effects: rare to very rare (depending on specific drugs): atrial and ventricular arrhythmias (including VF and VT), bradycardia, AVB, QT prolongation, TdP, sudden death (possibly related to TdP). ECG changes: QRS widening, ST-depression, U-waves, and T-wave changes.
- *Cautions*: patients with CV disease, hypotension, bradycardia, AVB, QT prolongation, or a family history of sudden death. Risk factors for VTE should be identified before and during treatment. Patients on antipsychotic drugs should have an ECG prior to and during treatment.

Avoid drugs that prolong the QTc interval, and correct risk factors for QT prolongation (see Table 9.1.1).
- *Contraindications*: patients with cardiac diseases, QT prolongation, history of ventricular arrhythmias or TdP, bradycardia, or second-/third-degree heart block.

Atypical antipsychotic drugs (amisulpride, aripiprazole, clozapine, olanzapine, paliperidone, pimavanserin, quetiapine, risperidone, ziprasidone)
- *Indications*: acute and chronic schizophrenia.
- *General adverse effects*: orthostatic hypotension, syncope and reflex tachycardia, bradycardia, AVB, palpitations, ventricular arrhythmias, QT prolongation and TdP, cardiac arrest, and sudden unexplained death. ECG changes: QT prolongation, ST-segment depression and flattening or inversion of T-waves.
  - Clozapine: myocarditis or cardiomyopathy (some cases fatal), agranulocytosis. Myocarditis or cardiomyopathy should be suspected in patients who experience tachycardia at rest, especially in the first 2 months of treatment, arrhythmias, chest pain, and other signs and symptoms of HF. Patients who develop clozapine-induced myocarditis or cardiomyopathy should not be re-exposed to clozapine.
  - Risperidone: common: hypertension. Uncommon: AF, bradycardia.
- *Cautions*: ECG monitoring is recommended before and during treatment. Although not all atypical antipsychotics prolong the QT interval, they should all be used with caution in patients with QT prolongation or taking QT-prolonging drugs (see Table 9.1.1). Patients with known CV disease (history of MI or CAD, HF, or conduction abnormalities), cerebrovascular disease, conditions which would predispose patients to hypotension (dehydration, hypovolaemia, antihypertensive medications), or hypertension. Patients treated with antipsychotics often present risk factors for VTE; they should be identified and preventative measures taken.
- *Contraindications*: significant CV disease, CHF, cardiac hypertrophy, arrhythmias, or bradycardia (<50bpm).

Anxiolitic and hypnotic drugs

Benzodiazepines (alprazolam, chlordiazepoxide, diazepam, lorazepam, midazolam, oxazepam, temazepam)
- *General indications*: acute anxiety states, acute excitement or acute mania; anxiety associated with depression; control of status epilepticus; conscious sedation before and during diagnostic or therapeutic procedures; short-term treatment of insomnia. Anaesthesia: pre-medication before induction of anaesthesia, induction of anaesthesia, or as a sedative component in combined anaesthesia.
- *Mechanism of action*: they bind to a specific regulatory site in the GABA-A receptor, increase the neuronal membrane permeability to chloride ions, and enhance the inhibitory effect of GABA.
- *Adverse effects*: uncommon: bradycardia, hypotension, vasodilatation, cardiac arrest. Life-threatening reactions (respiratory depression, apnoea, respiratory and/or cardiac arrest) are more likely in the elderly and chronically ill or debilitated patients. Severe anaphylactic/anaphylactoid reactions.

- *Cautions*: extreme care when administering benzodiazepines (mainly IV) to very ill elderly patients or patients with limited pulmonary reserve or compromised respiratory function. Caution in patients in whom a drop in BP might lead to CV or cerebrovascular complications. Verapamil/diltiazem increase the plasma levels and half-life of midazolam.
  - Benzodiazepines produce additive depressant effects when co-administered with alcohol or other drugs that depress the CNS.
  - Use of benzodiazepines may lead to tolerance and dependence (patients with a medical history of alcohol and/or medicinal product abuse). Rapid withdrawal of prolonged therapy can lead to withdrawal symptoms (tachycardia, palpitations, mild hypertension, and orthostatic hypotension).
- *Contraindications*: severe respiratory insufficiency or acute respiratory depression.

Drugs for bipolar disorders/mania (lithium)

- *Indications*: treatment of acute manic or hypomanic episodes and recurrent depressive disorders; prophylaxis against bipolar affective disorders; control of aggressive or self-mutilating behaviour.
- *Adverse effects*: rare: ECG changes (flattening or inversion of T-waves, QT prolongation), bradycardia, sinus node dysfunction, AVB, oedema, hypotension, peripheral circulatory collapse, cardiomyopathy.
- *Cautions*: cardiac, thyroid, and renal function should be assessed before treatment. Avoid the use of QT-prolonging drugs (see Table 9.1.1). Lithium presents a narrow therapeutic index and can interact with multiple drugs; monitor drug plasma levels. NSAIDs, COX-2 inhibitors, thiazides, ACEIs, and ARBs decrease lithium clearance and increase its plasma levels.
- *Contraindications*: cardiac disease, HF, and patients with LQTS or Brugada syndrome.

Drugs for attention-deficit/hyperactivity disorder (atomoxetine, methylphenidate, dexamfetamine, modafinil)

- *Indications*: treatment of attention-deficit/hyperactivity disorder (ADHD). Modafinil: excessive sleepiness associated with narcolepsy.
- *Mechanism of action*: (1) atomoxetine: highly selective and potent inhibitor of the presynaptic noradrenaline transporter; (2) methylphenidate: blocks the reuptake of noradrenaline and dopamine into the presynaptic neuron; (3) dexamfetamine: sympathomimetic amine with CNS stimulant and anorectic activity; (4) modafinil: inhibits dopamine reuptake.
- *Adverse effects*: sudden death has been reported in patients with structural cardiac abnormalities.
  - Atomoxetine: uncommon: hypertension, QT prolongation, tachycardia, palpitations. Rare: Raynaud's phenomenon.
  - Dextroamphetamine: common: palpitations, tachycardia, hypertension, vasculitis. Very rare: cardiac arrest, cardiomyopathy, MI.
  - Methylphenidate: common: hypertension. Rare; chest pain, angina. Very rare: MI, SVT, bradycardia, ventricular extrasystoles, cardiac arrest, cerebral arteritis, Raynaud´s phenomenon.
  - Modafinil: common vasodilatation. Uncommon: bradycardia, hypo-/hypertension.

- *Cautions*: an ECG is recommended before treatment. Heart rate and BP should be regularly monitored.
  - Atomoxetine: CYP2D6 inhibitors increase drug plasma levels. Atomoxetine may decrease the effectiveness of antihypertensive drugs. Risk of QT prolongation when administered with other QT-prolonging drugs (see Table 9.1.1).
  - Modafinil: PT/INR should be monitored regularly during modafinil use. Modafinil decreases the elimination of drugs that are substrates for CYP2C19 (see Table 8.1.2).
- *Contraindications*: patients with severe CV or cerebrovascular disorders, advanced arteriosclerosis, or potentially life-threatening arrhythmias.

Huntington's chorea

Tetrabenazine

- *Indications*: hyperkinetic motor disorders associated with Huntington's chorea.
- *Mechanism of action*: inhibits the reuptake and facilitates the depletion of monoamines (dopamine, serotonin, noradrenaline, and histamine) from nerve terminals.
- *Adverse effects*: common: hypotension. Unknown: bradycardia, QTc prolongation, orthostatic hypotension.
- *Cautions*: patients with QT prolongation or risk factors for QT prolongation (see Table 9.1.1) or receiving CYP2D6 inhibitors (see Table 8.1.2).

Multiple sclerosis

Glatiramer acetate

- *Indications*: relapsing forms of multiple sclerosis.
- *Mechanism of action*: affects various levels of the innate and adaptive immune response, generating deviation from the pro-inflammatory to the anti-inflammatory pathway.
- *Adverse effects*: very common: vasodilatation. Common: palpitations, tachycardia. Uncommon: extrasystoles, sinus bradycardia, tachycardia, varicose vein.
- *Cautions*: flushing, chest pain, dyspnoea, and palpitations/tachycardia may occur within minutes of drug injection. Symptoms are transient and resolve spontaneously.

Fingolimod

- *Indications*: highly active relapsing–remitting multiple sclerosis.
- *Mechanism of action*: sphingosine 1-phosphate receptor modulator.
- *Adverse effects*: common: bradycardia, AVB, hypertension. Very rare: T-wave inversion.
- *Cautions*: all patients should have an ECG and BP measurement performed prior to, and 6h after, the first dose.
- *Contraindications*: patients with hypertension, sick sinus syndrome, or sinoatrial heart block, symptomatic bradycardia, second-degree Mobitz type II or higher AVB, recurrent syncope, or QT prolongation.

Interferon beta-1A

- *Indications*: relapsing multiple sclerosis; patients with a single demyelinating event with an active inflammatory process, if it is severe enough to warrant treatment with IV corticosteroids.
- *Mechanism of action*: reduces neuronal inflammation, increases the production of nerve growth factor, and improves neuronal survival.
- *Adverse effects*: common: flushing. Unknown: vasodilatation, cardiomyopathy, CHF, palpitations, arrhythmia, tachycardia.
- *Cautions*: fatal cases of thrombotic microangiopathy, manifested as thrombotic thrombocytopenic purpura or haemolytic uraemic syndrome, have been described.

Interferon beta-1B

- *Indications*: patients with a single demyelinating event with an active inflammatory process, relapsing–remitting multiple sclerosis, or secondary progressive multiple sclerosis with active disease.
- *Mechanism of action*: possesses both antiviral and immunoregulatory activities.
- *Adverse effects*: common: palpitations, hypertension. Fatal cases of thrombotic microangiopathy, manifested as thrombotic thrombocytopenic purpura or haemolytic uraemic syndrome, have been described.
- *Cautions*: patients with pre-existing cardiac disorders (CHF, CAD, or arrhythmia) should be monitored for worsening of their cardiac condition.

Ocrelizumab

- *Indications*: relapsing or primary progressive forms of multiple sclerosis.
- *Mechanism of action*: humanized monoclonal antibody designed to selectively target CD20, a cell surface antigen present on pre-B and mature B-lymphocytes.
- *Adverse effects*: common: tachycardia, oedema.
- *Cautions*: monitor for infusion-related reactions (including dyspnoea, flushing, hypotension, fatigue, headache, and tachycardia).

Tizanidine

- *Indications*: spasticity associated with multiple sclerosis or with spinal cord injury or disease.
- *Mechanism of action*: central $\alpha 2$-adrenergic receptor agonist that increases presynaptic inhibition of motor neurons.
- *Adverse effects*: common: hypotension, rebound hypertension, bradycardia, tachycardia. Unknown: QTc prolongation.
- *Cautions*: patients with CV disease or CAD. ECG monitoring is recommended during treatment.
- *Contraindications*: congenital or acquired prolonged LQTS, history of cardiac arrhythmias. Co-administration with strong inhibitors of CYP1A2 (see Table 8.1.2).

Parkinson's disease

Amantadine

- *Indications*: Parkinson's disease; prophylaxis and treatment of influenza A infection.
- *Mechanism of action*: weak antagonist of the NMDA-type glutamate receptor; increases dopamine release and blocks dopamine reuptake. Specifically inhibits the replication of influenza A viruses.
- *Adverse effects*: very common: ankle oedema, livedo reticularis. Common: palpitations, orthostatic hypotension. Very rare: HF, QT prolongation, and possible risk of ventricular arrhythmias.
- *Cautions*: in patients with CHF, amantadine may exacerbate oedema. Patients with QT prolongation or risk factors for QT prolongation (see Table 9.1.1).

Anticholinergic drugs (benztropine, orphenadrine, procyclidine, trihexyphenidyl)

- *Indications*: parkinsonism, including drug-induced extrapyramidal symptoms.
- *Mechanism of action*: antimuscarinic drugs.
- *Adverse effects*: tachycardia.
- *Cautions*: patients with hypertension, cardiac diseases, glaucoma, or prostatic hypertrophy.

Catechol-O-methyltransferase (COMT) inhibitors (entacapone, opicapone, tolcapone)

- *Indications*: an adjunct to standard preparations of levodopa/benserazide or carbidopa for use in adult patients with Parkinson's disease.
- *Adverse effects*: common: hypotension, orthostatic hypotension, angina. Uncommon: MI, palpitations.
- *Cautions*: isoprenaline, adrenaline, noradrenaline, dopamine, and dobutamine should be administered with caution.

Dopamine agonists (apomorphine, bromocriptine, cabergoline, lisuride, pergolide, pramipexole, ropinirole, rotigotine)

- *Indications*: idiopathic Parkinson's disease and early treatment of the motor symptoms of the disease.
- *Mechanism of action*: apomorphine: D1 and D2 receptor agonist. Bromocriptine, cabergoline, and pramipexole: dopamine D2 receptor agonists. Lisuride: D2–D4 and 5-HT1A and 5-HT2A/C receptor agonist. Ropinirole: D2/D3 dopamine agonist. Rotigotine: non-selective (D1–D3) receptor agonist.
- *Adverse effects*: uncommon: hypotension, postural hypotension. Unknown: palpitations, AF, SVT. Cases of retroperitoneal fibrosis, pulmonary infiltrates, pleural effusion, pleural thickening, pericarditis, and cardiac valvulopathy have been reported in some patients treated with ergot-derived agents (bromocriptine, cabergoline, lisuride, pergolide).
    - Cabergolide: common: angina pectoris. Very rare: erythromelalgia. Unknown: digital vasospasm.
    - Rotigotine: common: hypertension. Unknown: palpitations, AF, SVT.

- *Cautions*: in patients with pre-existing hypotension or treated with vasodilator or antihypertensives. Ergot derivatives: pre-treatment echocardiography to discard pulmonary, pleural, pericardial, or valvular diseases.
- *Contraindications*: cabergoline: patients with valvulopathy, those with a history of pulmonary, pericardial, and retroperitoneal fibrotic disorders. Rotigotine: MRI or cardioversion.

Levodopa

- *Indications*: idiopathic Parkinson's disease.
- *Mechanism of action*: levodopa is the metabolic precursor of dopamine. It can be given with dopa-decarboxylase inhibitors (benserazide or carbidopa).
- *Adverse effects*: common: palpitations, orthostatic hypotension, syncope. Uncommon: hypertension, cardiac arrhythmias. Rare: phlebitis.
- *Cautions*: patients with severe CV or pulmonary diseases, recent MI, and a history of cardiac arrhythmias. In these patients, cardiac function should be carefully monitored during the initial dosage administration and titration.
- *Contraindications*: patients with severe HF, severe cardiac arrhythmia, and acute stroke.

Monoamine oxidase B inhibitors (rasagiline, safinamide, selegiline)

- *Indications*: Parkinson's disease in combination with levodopa; symptomatic parkinsonism.
- *Mechanism of action*: irreversible MAO-B selective inhibitors. Safinamide also blocks sodium channels.
- *Adverse effects*: common: hypotension, bradycardia. Uncommon: arrhythmias, palpitations, angina, SVT, postural hypotension. Rare: hypertensive crisis, MI, arterial vasospasm.
- *Contraindications*: in combination with levodopa in patients with severe CV disease, arterial hypertension, hyperthyroidism, phaeochromocytoma, tachycardia, arrhythmias, severe angina pectoris. They should not be used with sympathomimetics. Safinamide is contraindicated in patients with retinopathy.

Diagnostic imaging agents

Perfluten

- *Indications*: contrast enhancement of the endocardial borders during echocardiography.
- *Mechanism of action*: suspension of microspheres of human serum albumin with perfluten.
- *Adverse effects*: common: QT prolongation. Other: headache, nausea, vomiting, dizziness, altered taste, dyspnoea, malaise, injection site reactions.
- *Cautions*: fatal cardiac arrests and other serious non-fatal adverse reactions (cardiac or respiratory arrest, hypotension, supraventricular and ventricular arrhythmias, respiratory distress, anaphylactoid reactions, and loss of consciousness are uncommonly reported). Always have cardiopulmonary resuscitation personnel/equipment readily available prior to administration, and monitor all patients for acute reactions. Concomitant use with QT-prolonging drugs (see Table 9.1.1); monitor the QT interval.

Endocrinology

Levothyroxine sodium

- *Indications*: hypothyroidism; pituitary thyroid-stimulating hormone suppression.
- *Mechanism of action*: synthetic 3,3',5,5'- tetraiodothyronine used for replacement or supplemental therapy in congenital or acquired hypothyroidism of any aetiology.
- *Adverse effects*: tachycardia, palpitations, cardiac arrhythmias, angina, MI, cardiac hypertrophy, and cardiac arrest.
- *Cautions*: levothyroxine has a narrow therapeutic index. In patients with CV disorders and in the elderly, levothyroxine should be initiated at lower doses and titrated up slowly. An ECG before starting treatment with levothyroxine is advised. In patients with CAD, levothyroxine should be monitored closely because of an increased risk of arrhythmias. Co-administration of levothyroxine and sympathomimetics may precipitate angina pectoris in patients with CAD.

Glucocorticoids (dexamethasone, prednisolone)

- *Oral/parenteral use*: beclometasone, betamethasone, dexamethasone, methylprednisolone, prednisone, prednisolone, triamcinolone.
- *Topical use*: clobetasol, fluocinolone acetonide, fluticasone, mometasone, prebnicarbate.
- *Indications*: treatment of acute pericarditis in patients with contraindications to, or failure of, aspirin/NSAIDs and colchicine. Potent anti-inflammatory effects against multiple endocrine, rheumatic (RA), collagen, and dermatological disorders. Control of cerebral oedema.
- *Mechanism of action*: immediate anti-inflammatory and antiproliferative effects and delayed immunosuppressive effects. They inhibit chemotaxis, the activity of immune cells, and the release and effect of mediators of inflammatory and immune reactions.
- *Adverse effects*: unknown: palpitations, tachycardia, hypertension, oedema, CHF in predisposed patients, hypokalaemia. At high doses: hypercoagulability, raised intracranial pressure.
- *Cautions*: patients with hypertension, CHF, or recent MI (ventricular rupture reported). Glucocorticoids increase the hypokalaemic effects of other drugs. Hypokalaemia increases the toxicity of cardiac glycosides and predisposes to cardiac arrhythmias, especially TdP. Hypokalaemia should be corrected before corticosteroid treatment initiation. The blood glucose-lowering effect of antidiabetic agents is reduced. Glucocorticoids increase the risk of GI haemorrhages induced by NSAIDs. The blood levels and effects of ciclosporin and cyclophosphamide are increased. Co-treatment with CYP3A inhibitors may increase the risk of adverse effects, while CYP3A4 inducers decrease their efficacy (see Table 8.1.2); these combinations should be avoided, when possible. They may increase or inhibit the response to warfarin. Systemic formulations of prednisolone/prednisone containing medicinal products in doses that provide a systemic concentration equivalent to ≥15mg prednisolone daily may increase the incidence

of (possibly fatal) scleroderma renal crisis with hypertension and decreased urinary output in patients with scleroderma. Monitor blood pressure and renal function.
- *Contraindications*: acute and chronic bacterial or viral infections, uncontrolled hypertension.

Inhibitors of adrenocortical steroid synthesis

Aminoglutethimide

- *Indications*: treatment of Cushing's syndrome and metastatic breast cancer.
- *Mechanism of action*: it inhibits the conversion of cholesterol to D5-pregnenolone (and C-11, C-18 and C-21 hydroxylations), decreasing the production of adrenal glucocorticoids, mineralocorticoids, oestrogens, and androgens (medical adrenalectomy). It also blocks the conversion of androgens to oestrogens.
- *Adverse effects*: uncommon: hypotension/orthostatic hypotension, dizziness, tachycardia.

Ketoconazole

(See ➔ Azoles, pp. 827–8.)
- Strongly inhibits gonadal and adrenal steroid hormone synthesis. Used in the treatment of Cushing's syndrome.

Metyrapone

- *Indications*: diagnosis and treatment of patients with Cushing's syndrome.
- *Mechanism of action*: competitive inhibitor of steroid 11β-hydroxylase in the adrenal cortex.
- *Adverse effects*: salt and water retention, dizziness, hypo-/hypertension, hyponatraemia, hyperkalaemia.

Pasireotide

- *Indications*: adults with Cushing's disease for whom pituitary surgery is not an option or has not been curative.
- *Mechanism of action*: somatostatin analogue.
- *Adverse effects*: common: QT prolongation, bradycardia, hypotension, hyperglycaemia.
- *Cautions*: patients treated with QT-prolonging drugs (see Table 9.1.1) or with bradycardic drugs [β-blockers, acetylcholinesterase inhibitors (e.g. rivastigmine, physostigmine), verapamil, diltiazem, certain antiarrhythmics].

Somatomedins (mecasermin)

- *Indications*: children and adolescents from 2 to 18 years with severe primary insulin-like growth factor-1 deficiency.
- *Mechanism of action*: recombinant human insulin-like growth factor-1.
- *Adverse effects*: common: cardiac murmur, tachycardia.
  Uncommon: cardiomegaly, LVH, mitral/tricuspid valve incompetence, chest discomfort, increased intracranial pressure.
- *Cautions*: CV examination, ECG, and echocardiography pre- and post-treatment recommended.

Somatostatin analogues (lanreotide, octreotide)

- *Indications*: acromegaly, vasoactive intestinal peptide tumours, thyrotropic adenomas, gastro-entero-pancreatic (particularly carcinoid) tumours, GI haemorrhage (including bleeding from oesophageal varices). Octreotide: treatment of TSH-secreting pituitary adenomas.
- *Mechanism of action*: long-acting somatostatin analogues that decrease the secretion of growth hormone (GH), gastrin, vasoactive intestinal polypeptide, glucagon, secretin, serotonin, and pancreatic polypeptide.
- *Adverse effects*: common: sinus bradycardia (<50bpm), ECG changes, hot flushes, hypoglycaemia or hyperglycaemia. Uncommon: tachycardia.
- *Cautions*: because of the risk of bradycardia, dose adjustment of β-blockers, diltiazem, and verapamil may be necessary. Dose adjustments of insulin and antidiabetic medicinal products may be required.

Vasopressin agonists (desmopressin, terlipressin, vasopressin)

- *Indications*: (1) desmopressin: vasopressin-sensitive cranial diabetes insipidus and post-hypophysectomy polyuria/polydipsia; primary nocturnal enuresis; to increase factor VIII:C and factor VIII:Ag in patients with mild to moderate haemophilia or von Willebrand's disease undergoing surgery or following trauma; (2) terlipressin: bleeding oesophageal varices; (3) vasopressin: to increase BP in adults with vasodilatory shock (e.g. post-cardiotomy or sepsis) who remain hypotensive despite fluids and catecholamines.
- *Mechanism of action*: desmopressin and terlipressin: synthetic analogues of vasopressin. Vasopressin binds to vascular V1 receptors, leading to vasoconstriction, and to V2 receptors in the distal or collecting tubules of the kidney and promotes reabsorption of water (antidiuresis).
- *Adverse effects*: (1) desmopressin: water retention/hyponatraemia; (2) terlipressin: common: bradycardia, signs of ischaemia in the ECG, hypertension, peripheral vasoconstriction, facial pallor, QT prolongation, and ventricular arrhythmias, including TdP. Uncommon: AF, ventricular extrasystoles, tachycardia, chest pain, MI, fluid overload with pulmonary oedema; (3) vasopressin: peripheral vasoconstriction, bradycardia, AF, myocardial ischaemia.
- *Cautions*: patients with hypertension, recognized heart disease, and fluid and/or electrolyte imbalance. Terlipressin: caution patients with uncontrolled hypertension, cerebral or peripheral vascular diseases, cardiac arrhythmias, or CAD. Monitor BP, heart rate, and fluid balance.
- *Contraindications*: desmopressin: unstable angina, decompensated HF. Terlipressin: patients with septic shock with a low CO.

General anaesthetics

Inhalational anaesthetics (desflurane, isoflurane, sevoflurane)

- *Indications*: induction and maintenance of general anaesthesia for inpatient and outpatient surgery.
- *Mechanism of action*: enhance the function of inhibitory GABA-A and glycine receptors. They also activate 2P potassium channels and inhibit a variety of excitatory cation channels.
- *Adverse effects*: inhalation agents cause a dose-dependent cardiorespiratory depression. Very common: bradycardia, hypotension. Common: tachycardia, hypertension. Unknown: QT prolongation (rarely associated with TdP), AVB, AF, extrasystoles, cardiac arrest. Hypotension and respiratory depression increase, as anaesthesia is deepened. Increases in serum potassium levels leading to cardiac arrhythmias, particularly during the post-operative period, in paediatric patients receiving suxamethonium.
- *Cautions*: co-administration with β-blockers increases the risk of hypotension and depressed cardiac contractility. β-sympathomimetic agents increase the risk of ventricular arrhythmias. Co-administered with calcium antagonists: marked hypotension with dihydropyridines; bradycardia and AVB with diltiazem or verapamil. Caution when administered in patients at risk for QT prolongation (see Table 9.1.1).

Intravenous anaesthetics

Etomidate

- *Indications*: IV induction of general anaesthesia. Hypnotic drug without analgesic activity.
- *Mechanism of action*: it binds at GABA-A receptors and prolongs the inhibitory effect of GABA.
- *Adverse effects*: common: vein pain, hypotension. Uncommon: bradycardia, ventricular extrasystoles, phlebitis, hypertension. Very rare: cardiac arrest, AVB, shock, thrombophlebitis (including superficial thrombophlebitis and DVT).
- *Cautions*: etomidate suppresses the production of adrenal steroids; avoid in patients with adrenal insufficiency.

Ketamine

- *Indications*: diagnostic and surgical procedures that do not require skeletal muscle relaxation, induction of anaesthesia, and to supplement low-potency agents.
- *Mechanism of action*: NMDA receptor antagonist; it also acts on opioid receptors and monoamine transporters.
- *Adverse effects*: common: tachycardia (>100bpm), hypertension, increased cerebral blood flow, and myocardial and cerebral oxygen consumption due to increased sympathetic tone. Uncommon: bradycardia, arrhythmias, hypotension.

- *Cautions*: patients with hypertension and cardiac diseases. Ketamine increases myocardial oxygen consumption and should be used in caution in patients with cardiac diseases (e.g. CHF, myocardial ischaemia, MI), mild to moderate hypertension, and tachyarrhythmias.
- *Contraindications*: in patients with hypertension, severe coronary or myocardial disease, CVA, or cerebral trauma.

Propofol

- *Indications*: induction and maintenance of general anaesthesia; sedation for diagnostic and surgical procedures, alone or in combination with local or regional anaesthesia; sedation of ventilated patients aged >16 years in the ICU.
- *Mechanism of action*: potentiates the inhibitory effect of GABA via GABA-A receptors.
- *Adverse effects*: common: bradycardia, hypotension, apnoea. Very rare: pulmonary oedema, arrhythmias, decreases CO. Uncommon: venous thrombosis or phlebitis.
- *Cautions*: patients with cardiac or respiratory impairment, those who are hypovolaemic or debilitated. Occasionally, hypotension may require use of IV fluids and reduction of the rate of administration of propofol.

Thiopental

- *Indications*: (1) induction of general anaesthesia and as an adjunct to provide hypnosis during balanced anaesthesia with other anaesthetics, including analgesics and muscle relaxants; (2) adjunct for control of convulsive disorders; (3) to reduce intracranial pressure, if controlled ventilation is provided.
- *Mechanism of action*: barbiturates potentiate the effect of GABA through binding to a site on the GABA-A receptor, particularly in the mesencephalic reticular activating system.
- *Adverse effects*: myocardial depression, tachycardia, and venodilation, leading to hypotension and reduced CO; cardiac arrhythmias.
- *Cautions*: patients with severe CVD, hypertension, hypovolaemia, and severe respiratory diseases. Antihypertensives and vasodilators increase the risk of hypotension.

The haematopoietic system

Drugs used in platelet disorders (anagrelide)

- *Indications*: essential thrombocytosis or overproduction of blood platelets.
- *Mechanism of action*: inhibition of PDE-2 and -3 and phospholipase A2.
- *Adverse effects*: common: palpitations, tachycardia. Uncommon: CHF, hypertension, arrhythmias (AF, SVT, VT), syncope. Rare: angina, MI, cardiomyopathy, pericardial effusion, vasodilatation, postural hypotension, and pulmonary hypertension. Unknown: TdP.
- *Cautions*: because of their positive inotropic and chronotropic effects, they should be used with caution in patients with known or suspected heart disease. A pre-treatment CV examination (ECG and echocardiography) and close monitoring of the QTc interval and risk factors for prolongation of the QT interval are recommended (see Table 9.1.1).

Erythropoiesis-stimulating agents (ESAs) (human recombinant erythropoietin, darbepoetin alfa, epoetin alfa and beta, methoxy polyethylene glycol-epoetin beta)

- *Indications*: symptomatic anaemia associated with CKD or in cancer patients with non-myeloid malignancies receiving chemotherapy.
- *Mechanism of action*: erythropoietin binds to the erythropoietin receptor on the erythroid progenitor cells in the bone marrow, increasing erythropoiesis.
- *Adverse effects*: hypertension (especially during the early phase of treatment or when the haematocrit rises too rapidly), thromboembolic events (including PE). A few cases of hypertensive encephalopathy occurred in patients with uncontrolled BP.
- *Cautions*: serious CV events and significant risk of VTE when the haemoglobin level is >12g/dL. BP should also be monitored regularly while on ESAs.
- *Contraindications*: uncontrolled hypertension, CV disease, coronary, carotid, and peripheral arterial disease, recent MI.

Iron salts (ferrous sulfate, carbonyl iron, ferric citrate, iron dextran complex, iron sucrose, ferric carboxymaltose)

- *Indications*: prophylaxis and treatment of iron deficiency anaemia. Oral ferrous iron salts are the most economical and effective agents for the treatment of iron deficiency anaemia. Reserve parenteral iron for patients who are either unable to absorb oral iron, who have increasing anaemia despite adequate doses of oral iron, and when there is a clinical need to deliver iron rapidly to iron stores. IV ferric carboxymaltose in symptomatic patients (serum ferritin <100mcg/L, or ferritin between 100 and 299mcg/L and transferrin saturation <20%) in order to alleviate HF symptoms and to improve exercise capacity and quality of life.
- *Mechanism of action*: replacement therapy for iron deficiency.
- *Adverse effects*: rare: tachycardia, hypertension or hypotension, flushing.

- *Cautions*: serious hypersensitivity reactions (hypotension, loss of consciousness, and/or collapse); drug administration must be stopped immediately if observed.
- *Contraindications*: anaemia without iron deficiency, iron malabsorption, repeated blood transfusions, regional enteritis, and ulcerative colitis.

Granulocyte colony-stimulating factor (G-CSF) (filgrastim, lenograstim, pegfilgrastim)

- *Indications*: reduction in the duration of neutropenia and the incidence of febrile neutropenia in adult patients treated with cytotoxic chemotherapy.
- *Mechanism of action*: G-CSF is a glycoprotein, which regulates the production and release of neutrophils from the bone marrow.
- *Adverse effects*: uncommon: capillary leak syndrome. Hypersensitivity-type reactions, including skin rash, urticaria, angio-oedema, dyspnoea, erythema, flushing, and hypotension. Rare: pulmonary oedema, infiltrates, and fibrosis.

Recombinant human granulocyte–macrophage colony-stimulating factors (rhuGM-CSF) (sargramostim)

- *Indications*: neutropenia induced by chemotherapy during the treatment of acute myeloid leukaemia; mobilization of haematopoietic progenitor cells; post-stem cell transplantation; myeloid reconstitution following autologous or allogeneic bone marrow transplantation.
- *Adverse effects*: pericardial effusion, arrhythmia, tachycardia, hypotension, peripheral oedema, thrombosis.
- *Cautions*: patients with fluid retention, cardiac diseases, CHF, pulmonary infiltrates, lung disease.
- *Contraindications*: concomitant use with chemotherapy and radiotherapy.

Thrombopoietin receptor agonists (eltrombopag)

- *Indications*: patients with chronic immune (idiopathic) thrombocytopenia.
- *Mechanism of action*: thrombopoietin (TPO) receptor agonist that induces the proliferation and differentiation of bone marrow progenitor cells.
- *Adverse effects*: uncommon: DVT, superficial thrombophlebitis, flushing, palpitations, tachycardia, MI, QT prolongation.
- *Cautions*: thrombotic/thromboembolic complications may result from increases in platelet counts, particularly patients with known risk factors for thromboembolism (e.g. factor V Leiden, antithrombin III deficiency, antiphospholipid syndrome, chronic liver disease). The drug should be taken 2h before or 4h after food, antacids, or mineral supplements.

Histamine H1 receptor antagonists

First generation (alimemazine, chlorphenamine, clemastine, cyproheptadine, diphenhydramine, promethazine)

- *Indications*: symptomatic relief of allergy, hay fever, urticaria, pruritus, and cold. Cyproheptadine: prophylaxis of migraine. Diphenhydramine: prophylaxis of motion sickness, parkinsonism, night-time sleep aid.
- *Mechanism of action*: H1 receptor antagonists. Cyproheptadine: serotonin and histamine antagonist with anticholinergic and sedative properties.
- *Adverse effects*: palpitations, extrasystoles, tachycardia, hypotension.
  - Alimemazine: ECG changes (widened QT interval, ST-depression, U-waves and T-wave changes), atrial and ventricular arrhythmias (VT, VF), AVB.
- *Cautions*: in patients with severe CAD. Antihistamine overdosage may lead respiratory and cardiac arrest and death. Phenothiazines can increase the hypotensive effect of most antihypertensive drugs, especially α-adrenergic-blocking agents.
- *Contraindications*: diphenhydramine contains lactose.

Second generation (cetirizine, desloratadine, fexofenadine, loratadine, mequitazine, mizolastine)

- *Indications*: relief of nasal and ocular symptoms of seasonal and perennial allergic rhinitis and chronic idiopathic urticaria.
- *Adverse effects*: rare: hypotension, tachycardia, palpitations. Mizolastine: bradycardia, QT prolongation not associated with cardiac arrhythmias. Mequitazine: QT prolongation.
- *Cautions*: patients with QT prolongation (see Table 9.1.1).
- *Contraindications*: CYP3A4 or CYP2D6 inhibitors increase loratadine plasma levels (see Table 8.1.2). Mequitazine and mizolastine: patients with QT prolongation or electrolyte imbalance, in particular hypokalaemia.

Overactive bladder

- *Indications*: urge incontinence and/or increased urinary frequency and urgency, as may occur in patients with overactive bladder syndrome.

Mirabegron

- *Mechanism of action*: β3-adrenergic agonist.
- *Adverse effects*: common: tachycardia, AF, hypertension, QT prolongation. In some cases, angio-oedema occurred after the first dose.
- *Cautions*: mirabegron is a moderate CYP2D6 inhibitor that increases the systemic exposure of drugs metabolized by this isoform. Monitor serum digoxin levels. Patients with risk factors for QT prolongation (see Table 9.1.1).

Solifenacin

- *Mechanism of action*: competitive inhibitor of the muscarinic M3 subtype receptors.
- *Adverse effects*: unknown: QT prolongation, TdP, AF, palpitations, tachycardia.
- *Cautions*: in patients with risk factors for QT prolongation (see Table 9.1.1), severe renal impairment, moderate hepatic impairment, or concomitant use of potent CYP3A4 inhibitors (see Table 8.1.2).

Tolterodine

- *Mechanism of action*: competitive, specific muscarinic receptor antagonist with a selectivity for the urinary bladder over salivary glands.
- *Adverse effects*: common: palpitations. Uncommon: tachycardia, HF, QT prolongation, arrhythmias, flushing.
- *Cautions*: in patients with risk factors for QT prolongation (see Table 9.1.1). Concomitant systemic medication with potent CYP3A4 inhibitors is not recommended (see Table 8.1.2).

Peripheral nervous system

Alpha-adrenoceptor antagonists (alfuzosin, tamsulosin)

- *Indications*: functional symptoms of benign prostatic hypertrophy.
- *Mechanism of action*: α1A-adrenoceptor antagonists at the prostate, bladder base, and prostatic urethra.
- *Adverse effects*: common: hypotension, orthostatic hypotension, palpitations. Very rare: tachycardia, flushing.
- *Cautions*: potentiates the vasodilator effect of antihypertensives and nitrates.
- *Contraindications*: history of orthostatic hypotension.

Neuromuscular-blocking drugs (atracuronium, pancuronium, pipecuronium, suxamethonium, vecuronium)

- *Indications*: skeletal muscle relaxation to facilitate endotracheal intubation, mechanical ventilation, and a wide range of surgical and obstetric procedures.
- *Mechanism of action*: they block neuromuscular transmission, causing paralysis of the muscle. (1) Non-depolarizing: atracuronium, pancuronium, pipecuronium, vecuronium—they act as competitive antagonists at the post-synaptic nicotinic receptors of the motor endplate; (2) depolarizing: suxamethonium—they depolarize the skeletal muscle cell membrane.
- *Adverse effects*: non-depolarizing drugs: tachycardia, transient hypotension (it may be due to the release of histamine; no hypotension with pancuronium and pipecuronium), skin flushing. Suxamethonium: bradycardia, potassium release from skeletal muscle, potentially resulting in ventricular arrhythmias and cardiac arrest.
- *Cautions*: suxamethonium injection should not be mixed with any other drug prior to its administration. Monitor for the potential for hyperkalaemia. Patients on digitalis are more susceptible to the effects of hyperkalaemia.

Local anaesthetics (bupivacaine, lidocaine, prilocaine, tetracaine)

- *Indications*: reversible absence of local or regional pain sensation (analgesia).
- *Mechanism of action*: block voltage-gated sodium channels in the neuronal membrane that are responsible for the generation and propagation of nerve impulses.
- *Adverse effects*: very common: hypotension. Common: bradycardia, intra-cardiac conduction disturbances, hypertension. Rare: complete heart block, cardiac arrhythmias, cardiac arrest. Decreased myocardial contractility and vasodilatation lead to hypotension and CV collapse. Bupivacaine presents greater cardiotoxicity.
- *Cautions*: avoid accidental intravascular injection. Careful monitoring is required during the first 30min after injection. They should be used with caution in patients receiving class I AADs.

Proton pump inhibitors (PPIs)

Dexlansoprazole, esomeprazole, lansoprazole, omeprazole, pantoprazole, rabeprazole

- *Indications:* treatment and prevention of oesophageal duodenal and stomach ulcers, NSAID-associated gastric and duodenal ulcers, gastroesophageal reflux disease, reflux oesophagitis, and Zollinger-Ellison syndrome. In combination with appropriate antibiotics, *Helicobacter pylori* eradication in peptic ulcer disease.
- *Mechanism of action:* bind and irreversibly block the H^+ K^+-ATPase (proton pump) in gastric parietal cells, and inhibit both basal acid secretion and stimulated acid secretion, irrespective of stimulus.
- *Adverse effects:* headache, peripheral oedema. Possible link between PPIs and cardiac. It has been suggested that chronic use of PPIs might be associated with an increased risk of stroke and death.
- *Cautions:* the decrease in intragastric acidity might increase or decrease the absorption of medicinal products where gastric pH is an important determinant of oral bioavailability (i.e. HIV protease inhibitors). They increase plasma concentrations of drugs that are metabolized by CYP3A4. They increase the plasma concentration of digoxin; monitor digoxin plasma levels. PPIs can decrease exposure to the active metabolite of clopidogrel; the combination should be discouraged. They can reduce the plasma levels of theophylline and increase the INR and prothrombin time in patients receiving warfarin concomitantly (monitor INR). CYP2C19 and CYP3A4 inhibitors/inducers can markedly increase/reduce plasma levels of PPIs. CYP2C19 inhibitors may increase the systemic exposure of PPIs.

  PPIs are often overprescribed, rarely deprescribed, and frequently started inappropriately during a hospital stay with use extended for a long duration without appropriate medical indication.
- *Contraindications.* Avoid the combination with erlotinib, nelfinavir, and methotrexate.

The reproductive system

Anti-androgens and related drugs

Androgen receptor antagonists (apalutamide, bicalutamide, enzalutamide, flutamide, nilutamide)

- *Indications*: treatment of metastatic prostate cancer.
- *Mechanism of action*: non-steroidal anti-androgens. Competitively bind androgen receptors and inhibit testosterone stimulation of cell growth in prostate cancer.
- *Adverse effects*: common: hot flushes, hypertension. Bicalutamide and enzalutamide prolong the QT interval. Enzalutamide: increases the risk of CAD; monitor for signs and symptoms of CAD and optimize management of cardiovascular risk factors. Nilutamide: interstitial pneumonitis, pulmonary fibrosis.
- *Cautions*: bicalutamide inhibits CYP3A4; caution when co-administered with drugs metabolized predominantly by CYP3A4 (see Table 8.1.2). Apalutamide and enzalutamide: avoid if possible, concomitant strong CYP2D8 and 3A4 inducers. Androgen deprivation therapy may prolong the QT/QTc interval; caution in patients with a history of, or risk factors for, TdP (see Table 9.1.1). Periodic monitoring of cardiac function is recommended in patients with heart disease. Avoid the combination of enzalutamide with DOACs.

5α reductase inhibitors (finasteride, dutasteride)

- *Indications*: treatment of benign prostatic hyperplasia. Finasteride: treatment of androgenetic alopecia.
- *Mechanism of action*: block the conversion of testosterone to dihydrotestosterone.
- *Adverse effects*: palpitations. Rare: dutasteride increases the risk of HF.
- *Cautions*: CYP3A4 inhibitors may increase the plasma levels of dutasteride.

Cyproterone

- *Indications*: treatment of prostatic cancer or hot flushes in patients treated with luteinizing hormone-releasing hormone (LHRH) analogues or who have had orchidectomy.
- *Mechanism of action*: it blocks androgen receptors and suppresses the release of luteinizing hormone (LH) (which, in turn, reduces testosterone levels). With LHRH analogues, it reduces the initial increase of testosterone.
- *Adverse effects*: hot flushes, hypertension, thromboembolic events, MI.
- *Cautions*: patients with previous arterial or venous thrombotic/thromboembolic events (e.g. DVT, PE, MI), a history of CVAs, or advanced malignancies are at an increased risk of further thromboembolic events.

Selective oestrogen receptor modulators and anti-oestrogens

Selective oestrogen receptor modulators (bazedoxifene, ospemifene, raloxifene, tamoxifen, toremifene)

- *Indications*: bazedoxifene: oestrogen deficiency symptoms in post-menopausal women with a uterus for whom treatment with progestin-containing therapy is not appropriate. Ospemifene: treatment of dyspareunia in women. Raloxifene: reduce the risk of breast cancer in high-risk post-menopausal women. Tamoxifen: hormone-dependent metastatic breast cancer in post-menopausal patients; anovulatory infertility. Toremifene: hormone-dependent metastatic breast cancer in post-menopausal women.

- *Mechanism of action*: they bind to oestrogen receptors, acting either as agonists or as antagonists in different tissues. They act as anti-oestrogens in breast and endometrium; beneficial oestrogenic actions in bone, liver, and brain during post-menopausal hormone therapy. Tamoxifen: stimulates ovulation in anovulatory infertility. Toremifene binds specifically to oestrogen receptors, competitively with oestradiol.
- *General adverse effects*: very common: hot flushes, vasodilatation. Uncommon: oedema, VTE events, ischaemic cerebrovascular events. Increase in the risk of thromboembolic events (VTE, stroke, thrombophlebitis, and PE), MI, palpitations.
  - Tamoxifen, toremifene: QT prolongation (see Table 9.1.1).
- *Cautions*: if a patient presents with VTE, tamoxifen should be stopped immediately and appropriate antithrombosis measures initiated. Tamoxifen, toremifene: avoid in patients with QT prolongation, treated with drugs known to prolong QT interval or uncorrected hypokalaemia/hypomagnesaemia (see Table 9.1.1). Tamoxifen increases the anticoagulant effect of coumarin-type anticoagulants; careful monitoring (INR/PT) is recommended. The metabolism of toremifene is inhibited by CYP3A inhibitors (see Table 8.1.2).
- *Contraindications*: women with active or past history of VTE (DVT, arterial thromboembolic disease, PE, and retinal vein thrombosis).
  - Raloxifene: increased risk of fatal stroke occurred in post-menopausal women with documented CAD or at increased risk for major coronary events.
  - Tamoxifen: potent inhibitors of CYP2D6 (see Table 8.1.2) should, whenever possible, be avoided during tamoxifen treatment, as they reduce the plasma level of an active metabolite. Tamoxifen and toremifene: patients with QT prolongation (QTc >500ms), those treated with QT-prolonging drugs, symptomatic bradycardia, HFrEF, or a previous history of symptomatic arrhythmias.

Anti-oestrogens (clomifene, fulvestrant)

- *Indications*: clomifene: treatment of infertility in anovulatory women. Fulvestrant: treatment of hormone receptor positive metastatic breast cancer in post-menopausal women or previously treated with endocrine therapy or with disease progression after tamoxifen; women with resistance to aromatase inhibitors.
- *Mechanism of action:* clomifene: increases output of pituitary gonadotrophins, which stimulates the maturation and endocrine activity of the ovarian follicle. Fulvestrant: competitive oestrogen receptor (ER) antagonist that binds to the ER with an affinity comparable to that of oestradiol; downregulates the ER protein in human breast cancer cells and inhibits breast tumour growth.
- *General adverse effects:* clomifene: flushes, palpitations, tachycardia. Fulvestrant: very common: flushing peripheral oedema. Common: VTE.
- *Cautions*: patients with bleeding diatheses, thrombocytopenia, or those taking anticoagulant treatment.

Oestrogen synthesis inhibitors

Non-steroidal (anastrozole, letrozole) and steroidal inhibitors (exemestrane, formestane).

- *Indications*: hormone-dependent metastatic breast cancer in post-menopausal patients.
- *Mechanism of action*: inhibit the aromatase enzyme and prevent the conversion of androstenedione to oestrone and oestradiol in all peripheral tissues.
- *General adverse effects:* very common: hot flushes, hypertension. Uncommon: oedema, VTE events, ischaemic cerebrovascular events.
    - Anastrozole: uncommon: thrombophlebitis (including superficial and deep vein thrombophlebitis), palpitations, tachycardia, ischaemic cardiac events (angina, MI). Rare: PE, arterial thrombosis, cerebrovascular infarction.
- *Cautions*: uncontrolled hypertension. Increased risk of ischaemic cardiovascular events in women with pre-existing CAD; use only if benefits greatly outweigh risks.

Diagnosis and treatment of gonadal disorders

Gonadotrophin-releasing hormone (GnRH) analogues (buserelin, goserelin, histrelin, leuprolide, nafarelin, triptorelin)

- *Indications*: endometriosis, diagnosis and treatment of precocious puberty, palliative treatment of advanced prostate or breast cancer, uterine leiomyomata.
- *Mechanism of action*: after an initial increase in gonadotrophin secretion, they downregulate the GnRH receptor and inhibit the pituitary–gonadal axis.
- *Adverse effects*: very common: hot flushes, oedema. Common: palpitations, tachycardia, hypertension. MI and CHF are observed in males with prostate cancer. The risk appears to be increased when used in combination with anti-androgens. QT prolongation with risk of TdP and SCD.
- *Cautions*: hypertensive patients and those treated with medicinal products known to prolong the QT interval (see Table 9.1.1) should be carefully evaluated. Hypercalcaemia has been reported in cancer patients with bone metastases after starting treatment with goserelin.

Hyperglycaemia and an increased risk of developing diabetes, MI, sudden cardiac death, and stroke have been reported in men receiving GnRH analogues for prostate cancer. Evaluate cardiovascular risk before and routinely during therapy.

Gonadotrophin-releasing hormone (GnRH) antagonists (cetrorelix, degarelix, ganirelix)

- *Indications*: suppression of gonadotropin secretion and used with exogenous gonadotropins for assisted reproduction. Degarelix: treatment of advanced hormone-dependent prostate cancer. Cetrorelix, ganirelix: prevention of premature luteinising hormone (LH) surges in women undergoing controlled ovarian hyperstimulation for assisted reproduction techniques (ART).

- *Mechanism of action*: suppress testosterone production by decreasing LH and FSH. Delay LH surge, which in turn prevent ovulation until follicles are of adequate size.
- *Adverse effects*: common: hot flushes, headache.
- *Cautions*: CV (stroke and MI) and QT prolongation have been reported in patients on androgen deprivation therapy. Therefore, cardiovascular risk factors should be taken into account. Avoid the combination with drugs that prolong the QTc interval (see Table 9.1.1.). Long-term androgen deprivation may cause obesity and insulin resistance increasing the risk for diabetes.

Bromocriptine

- *Indications*: prevention/suppression of postpartum physiological lactation; hyperprolactinaemia; menstrual cycle disorders and female infertility: amenorrhoea and oligomenorrhoea, with or without galactorrhoea, drug-induced hyperprolactinaemic disorders, polycystic ovary syndrome; prolactinomas; premenstrual symptoms and benign breast disease; acromegaly; Parkinson's disease.
- *Mechanism of action*: potent agonist at dopamine D2 receptors and various serotonin receptors. It also inhibits prolactin release.
- *Adverse effects*: uncommon: hypotension, orthostatic hypotension. Rare: tachycardia, bradycardia, arrhythmia, pleural and pulmonary fibrosis, pleuritis, dyspnoea. Very rare: pallor of fingers and toes induced by cold, cardiac valve fibrosis, pericarditis, and pericardial effusion. Retroperitoneal fibrosis has been reported on long-term and high-dose treatment.
- *Cautions*: periodic monitoring of BP during the first weeks of therapy; caution in patients treated with drugs that can alter BP. HF can be a presentation of constrictive pericarditis and valvular fibrosis. Patients with unexplained pleuropulmonary disorders should be examined, and drug discontinuation should be contemplated.
- *Contraindications*: patients with uncontrolled hypertension during pregnancy or postpartum or evidence of cardiac valvulopathy.

Hormone replacement therapy (HRT)

- *Indications*: relieves symptoms of the menopause. Prevention and treatment of osteoporosis.
- *Forms of HRT*: oestrogen alone, combined oestrogen and progestagen, SERMs and/or tibolone, a synthetic steroid drug with oestrogenic, progestogenic, and weak androgenic effects.
- *Adverse effects*: hypertension, oedema, palpitations, thromboembolic disease (VTE, PE), ischaemic stroke, and MI.
- *Cautions*: HRT increases the risk of VTE in women with risk factors for arterial disease and VTE. Increased risk of CAD when HRT started >10 years after the menopause.
- *Contraindications*: patients with CAD, DVT, and PE. Stop treatment in patients with sudden severe chest pain or breathlessness, SBP/DBP >160/100mmHg, and unexplained leg swelling. HRT should not be used as either primary or secondary prevention of CV disease in women.

Steroids

Anabolic steroids (nandrolone)

- *Indications*: osteoporosis in post-menopausal women.
- *Mechanism of action*: semi-synthetic steroids with enhanced anabolic and reduced androgenic activities.
- *Adverse effects*: hypertension, oedema, cardiac hypertrophy, arrhythmias, CHF, hypercholesterolaemia.
- *Cautions*: nandrolone enhances the action of coumarin-type agents.

Danazol

- *Indications*: endometriosis, fibrocystic breast disease, and hereditary angio-oedema.
- *Mechanism of action*: synthetic steroid derived from ethisterone that suppresses the pituitary–ovarian axis.
- *Adverse effects*: oedema, hypertension, palpitations, tachycardia, thrombotic events, MI, insulin resistance.
- *Cautions*: danazol can potentiate the action of warfarin, increases the risk of myopathy when co-administered with statins metabolized by CYP3A4 (simvastatin, atorvastatin, lovastatin), and reduces the effect of antihypertensive drugs.
- *Contraindications*: active thrombosis or thromboembolic disease and a history of such events.

Ethinylestradiol

- *Indications*: oral contraception; HRT in menopause.
- *Mechanism of action*: semi-synthetic derivative of oestradiol used as the oestrogenic component in oral contraceptives.
- *Adverse effects*: uncommon: hypertension. Rare: venous and arterial thromboembolism, varicose veins. Use of any combined hormonal contraceptive increases the risk of VTE. Uncommon: hypertension.
- *Cautions*: in women with risk factors for VTE. CYP3A4 inhibitors can decrease its plasma levels (see Table 8.1.2).
- *Contraindications*: presence of VTE, a history of DVT or PE, predisposition for VTE, major surgery with prolonged immobilization, or a history of arterial thromboembolism (e.g. angina, MI, stroke, or TIA).

Testosterone

- *Indications*: replacement therapy for male hypogonadism when testosterone deficiency has been confirmed.
- *Mechanism of action*: primary male sex hormone and an anabolic steroid.
- *Adverse effects*: common: flushing. Uncommon: hypertension, oedema.
- *Cautions*: androgens cause sodium, potassium, calcium, and water retention, leading to oedema; caution in patients predisposed to oedema (i.e. severe cardiac, hepatic, or renal insufficiency) or CAD. Testosterone increases the activity of VKAs (monitor the INR). The hypoglycaemic effect of antidiabetics may be enhanced.

Drugs acting on the uterus

Carbetocin

- *Indications*: controls postpartum haemorrhage, particularly following a Caesarean section under epidural/spinal anaesthesia.
- *Mechanism of action*: long-acting synthetic analogue of oxytocin receptors on the uterine smooth muscle.
- *Adverse effects*: very common: hypotension, flushing. Common: chest pain, dyspnoea, tachycardia.
- *Contraindications*: serious CV disorders.

Ergometrine

- *Indications*: management of the third stage of labour and treatment of postpartum haemorrhage.
- *Mechanism of action*: partial agonist of myometrial 5-HT2 receptors and α-adrenergic receptors.
- *Adverse effects*: cardiac arrhythmias, palpitations, bradycardia, chest pain, coronary vasospasm, with very rare reports of MI. Hypertension, vasoconstriction, dyspnoea, and pulmonary oedema.
- *Cautions*: strong CYP3A4 inhibitors may raise the levels of ergot derivatives (see Table 8.1.2).
- *Contraindications*: hypertension, occlusive vascular disorders. Patients with CAD or Prinzmetal's angina can develop angina and MI due to coronary vasospasm.

Mifepristone

- *Indications*: termination of pregnancy, softening and dilatation of the cervix, labour induction in fetal death *in utero*.
- *Mechanism of action*: synthetic steroid with anti-progestational action as a result of competition with progesterone at the progesterone receptors. It also increases prostaglandins by inhibiting prostaglandin dehydrogenase.
- *Adverse effects/cautions*: very common: hypertension.
  Uncommon: hypotension, postural hypotension, palpitations, hot flushes, dizziness, chills. Rare: MI, Adam–Stokes syndrome, superficial thrombophlebitis. Life-threatening vaginal bleeding and infections may occur. Mifepristone may increase serum levels of drugs that are CYP3A4 substrates (see Table 8.1.2).
- *Contraindications*: haemorrhagic disorders, concurrent anticoagulant therapy.

Myometrial relaxants (atosiban)

- *Indications*: delay imminent preterm birth in pregnant adult women.
- *Mechanism of action*: competitive antagonist of human oxytocin at the receptor level.
- *Adverse effects*: common: tachycardia, hot flushes, hypotension, injection site reactions.
- *Contraindications*: abnormal fetal heart rate.

Oxytocin

- *Indications*: induction of labour for medical reasons; control of postpartum bleeding.
- *Mechanism of action*: oxytocin stimulates its receptors in the myometrium.

- *Adverse effects*: common: hypotension, tachycardia, bradycardia. Uncommon: arrhythmias. Unknown: myocardial ischaemia, QT prolongation.
- *Cautions*: oxytocin can produce cardiac arrhythmias in patients with QT prolongation or risk factors for TdP (see Table 9.1.1). Patients with a predisposition for myocardial ischaemia (i.e. HCM, VHD, and/or CAD, including coronary artery vasospasm).

Prostaglandin derivatives

- Very rare, potentially fatal CVAs (MI, coronary artery spasm, severe hypotension) have been reported in patients taking prostaglandins.

Carboprost

- *Indications*: treatment of postpartum haemorrhage due to uterine atony.
- *Mechanism of action*: synthetic analogue of PGF2α (15-methyl-PGF2α) with potent oxytocic properties.
- *Adverse effects*: common: hot flushes. Uncommon: hypertension, tachycardia, palpitations, vasovagal syndrome, hot flushes.
- *Cautions*: carboprost can decrease maternal arterial oxygen content. Caution in patients with active cardiac, pulmonary, renal, or hepatic disease. It should be used only in centres with specialized obstetric units.

Dinoprostone

- *Indications*: therapeutic termination of pregnancy, missed abortion, and hydatidiform mole by the IV route.
- *Mechanism of action*: prostaglandin E2 induces contraction of the uterine muscle at any stage of pregnancy.
- *Adverse effects*: hypertension, transient vasovagal symptoms, cardiac arrest, and anaphylactic reactions including anaphylactic shock.
- *Cautions*: it should be used in specialized obstetric units.
- *Contraindications*: patients with asthma, hypertension/hypotension, or CV disease. Rare cases of CV collapse reported with prostaglandins.

Gemeprost

- *Indications*: softening and dilatation of the cervix, therapeutic termination of pregnancy during the second trimester of pregnancy.
- *Mechanism of action*: prostaglandin E1 analogue (16,16-dimethyl-trans-δ2 PGE1 methyl ester).
- *Adverse effects*: chest pain, palpitations. Serious, potentially fatal CV adverse effects (MI and/or spasm of the coronary arteries and severe hypotension) have been reported with prostaglandins.
- *Cautions*: patients with CV insufficiency.

Drugs for erectile dysfunction

Phosphodiesterase inhibitors (sildenafil, tadalafil, vardenafil)

- *Indications*: treatment of erectile dysfunction in adult men. Tadalafil: treatment of signs and symptoms of benign prostatic hyperplasia.
- *Mechanism of action*: potent and selective PDE-5 inhibitors. With sexual stimulation, they increase cGMP levels, leading to smooth muscle relaxation in the corpus cavernosum, inflow of blood into the penile tissues, and erection.

- *Adverse effects*: common: flushing, headache. Uncommon: palpitations, tachycardia. Rare: ventricular arrhythmias, MI, angina, hypotension.
- *Cautions*: prior to treatment, evaluate the CV status of the patient, since there is a degree of cardiac risk associated with sexual activity. Patients with LV outflow obstruction, e.g. aortic stenosis and idiopathic hypertrophic subaortic stenosis, can be sensitive to the action of PDE-5 inhibitors. Guanylate cyclase stimulators (riociguat), antihypertensives, and vasodilators potentiate the hypotensive effects of PDE-5 inhibitors. In patients taking strong CYP3A4 inhibitors, the maximum dose of tadalafil is 10mg.
- *Contraindications*: hypotension (BP <90/50mmHg), a recent history of stroke or MI (within the last 6 months), or unstable angina. Sildenafil: in patients using any form of organic nitrate, either regularly and/or intermittently, PDE-5 inhibitors are contraindicated.

The respiratory system

Anti-asthmatic drugs

Selective beta 2-adrenoceptor agonists (e.g. formoterol, salbutamol, salmeterol, terbutaline)

- *Indications*: management of bronchospasm in patients suffering from asthma or COPD.
- *Mechanism of action*: dilate the bronchi by direct stimulation of β2-receptors, increase mucus clearance by acting on the cilia, and inhibit the release of mediators from mast cells and of TNF-α from monocytes.
- *Adverse effects*: very common: tremor, headache. Common: palpitations, tachycardia. Rare: arrhythmias including AF, SVT, extrasystoles, vasodilatation, hypokalaemia. Unknown: myocardial ischaemia, peripheral vasodilatation. At high doses: ventricular tachyarrhythmias, SCD. New use of long-acting β2-agonists increases the early risk for CVD (CAD, cardiac arrhythmia, HF, or ischaemic stroke) in people with COPD.
- *Cautions/contraindications*: patients with severe heart disease (CAD, tachyarrhythmias, or HF), use of cardiac glycosides, or diabetes mellitus. Due to their positive inotropic effect, β2-agonists should not be used in patients with HCM. They should not be co-administered with non-selective β-blockers. The risk of hypokalaemia increases by xanthines, steroids, diuretics, and long-term laxatives. Because they produce a hyperglycaemic effect, additional blood glucose controls are recommended initially in diabetic patients.

Antimuscarinic bronchodilators (ipratropium, tiotropium)

- *Indications*: reversible bronchospasm associated with COPD. Concomitantly with inhaled β2-agonists for the treatment of reversible airways obstruction as in acute and chronic asthma.
- *Mechanism of action*: long-acting muscarinic receptor antagonists.
- *Adverse effects*: uncommon: tachycardia, palpitations. Unknown: SVT, AF. New use of long-acting muscarinic antagonists increases the early risk for CVD (CAD, cardiac arrhythmia, HF, or ischaemic stroke) in people with COPD.
- *Cautions*: patients with recent MI (<6 months), unstable or life-threatening cardiac arrhythmias, hospitalization of HF within the past year.

Leukotriene antagonists (montelukast)

- *Indications*: prophylaxis and chronic treatment of asthma in adults and paediatric patients aged 12 months and older. Relief of symptoms of seasonal allergic rhinitis. Prophylaxis of exercise-induced bronchoconstriction.
- *Mechanism of action*: blocks the action of leukotriene D4 on the cysteinyl leukotriene receptor CysLT1 in the lungs and bronchial tubes.
- *Adverse effects*: rare: palpitations.
- *Cautions*: montelukast is metabolized by CYP3A4, 2C8, and 2C9.

5-lipo-oxygenase inhibitors (zileuton)

- *Indications*: prophylaxis and chronic treatment of asthma in adults and children aged 12 years and older.
- *Mechanism of action*: inhibitor of 5-lipo-oxygenase, the enzyme that catalyses the formation of leukotrienes from arachidonic acid.

- *Adverse effects*: headache.
- *Cautions*: zileuton doubles serum theophylline concentrations; reduce the dose and monitor serum theophylline concentrations closely. Zileuton increases the PT in patients treated with warfarin; monitor the PT closely.

Omalizumab

- *Indications*: patients with convincing immunoglobulin E (IgE)-mediated asthma; chronic idiopathic urticaria. It is not indicated for the treatment of acute asthma exacerbations, acute bronchospasm, or status asthmaticus.
- *Mechanism of action*: recombinant DNA-derived humanized monoclonal antibody that selectively binds to human IgE.
- *Adverse effects*: uncommon: postural hypotension, flushing. Systemic allergic reactions, including anaphylaxis and anaphylactic shock, have been reported within 2h after the injection of omalizumab.

Roflumilast

- *Indications*: severe COPD associated with chronic bronchitis in patients with a history of frequent exacerbations, as an add-on to bronchodilator treatment.
- *Mechanism of action*: selective inhibitor of PDE-4, a major cAMP-metabolizing enzyme, with anti-inflammatory activity.
- *Adverse effects*: nausea, diarrhoea, headaches, insomnia, palpitations.

Theophylline

- *Indications*: prophylaxis and treatment of reversible bronchospasm associated with asthma and COPD.
- *Mechanism of action*: competitive non-selective PDE-3 and -4 inhibitor, which raises intracellular cAMP. Non-selective adenosine (A1, A2, A3) receptor antagonist. Restores the reduced histone deacetylase activity induced by oxidative stress. Theophylline stimulates the myocardium and reduces venous pressure in CHF, increasing CO.
- *Adverse effects*: theophylline has a narrow therapeutic window. Nausea, diarrhoea, abdominal pain, ectopic beats, supraventricular and ventricular tachycardia, and CNS excitation (headaches, insomnia, dizziness, irritability, restlessness, nervousness). In overdose, life-threatening arrhythmias can develop.
- *Cautions*: in patients with cardiac arrhythmias and other CV disease. Plasma theophylline concentrations increase in HF, pulmonary oedema, and cor pulmonale. β-blockers antagonize bronchodilation. Theophylline can potentiate hypokalaemia resulting from β2-agonist therapy, steroids, and diuretics.

Respiratory stimulants (doxapram)

- *Indications*: stimulate respiration in patients with drug-induced post-anaesthesia respiratory depression or apnoea, drug-induced CNS depression, chronic pulmonary disease associated with acute hypercapnia.
- *Mechanism of action*: respiratory stimulation mediated through peripheral carotid chemoreceptors; at higher doses, stimulate central respiratory centres in the medulla.
- *Adverse effects*: sinus tachycardia, bradycardia, extrasystoles, VT and VF, hypertension, phlebitis, chest pain, and chest tightness.
- *Cautions/contraindications*: monitor BP and heart rate. Avoid in patients with CAD, CVAs, severe hypertension, and proven/suspected PE.

Syndrome of Fabry (agalsidase alfa/beta)

- *Indications*: recombinant human protein α-galactosidase A; patients with Fabry disease (α-galactosidase A deficiency).
- *Mechanism of action*: agalsidase provides α-galactosidase A and limits the accumulation of glycosphingolipids, predominantly GL-3, in many body tissues.
- *Adverse effects*: very common: flushing. Common: tachycardia, palpitations, hypertension. Uncommon: bradycardia, chest pain, dyspnoea, fatigue. Serious infusion reactions (headache, nausea, pyrexia, flushing, fatigue). Many patients developed immunoglobulin G (IgG) antibodies (some develop IgE) to agalsidase alfa within the first 3 months.
- *Interactions*: avoid drugs (chloroquine, amiodarone, gentamicin) that potentially inhibit intracellular galactosidase A activity.
- *Cautions*: because of the potential for severe infusion reactions, appropriate medical support measures should be readily available. Patients with advanced Fabry disease or who develop antibodies to the protein may have a higher risk of severe complications from infusion-associated reactions.

Tobaccco smoking cessation (nicotine, varenicline, bupropion)

- *Indications*: relieve and/or prevent cravings and nicotine withdrawal symptoms associated with tobacco dependence.

Nicotine

- *Mechanism of action*: stimulates cholinergic nicotinic receptors in the peripheral and central nervous systems; weak inhibitor of neuronal reuptake of noradrenaline and dopamine.
- *Adverse effects*: uncommon: palpitations, hypertension, hot flushes. Rare: chest pain, dyspnoea, and arrhythmias.
- *Cautions*: monitor more closely blood glucose levels in diabetic patients.

Varenicline

- *Mechanism of action*: partial agonist at $\alpha4\beta2$ neuronal nicotinic receptors.
- *Adverse effects*: uncommon: MI, angina, tachycardia, palpitations, hypertension, hot flushes. Rare: AF, ECG changes (ST-segment depression, decreased T-wave amplitude).

Bupropion

- *Mechanism of action*: selective inhibitor of neuronal reuptake of noradrenaline and dopamine.
- *Adverse effects*: uncommon: tachycardia, hypertension, flushing. Rare: palpitations, vasodilatation, postural hypotension.
- *Cautions*: bupropion inhibits the CYP2D6 pathway. Decrease the starting dose of drugs with narrow therapeutic indices predominantly metabolized by CYP2D6 (see Table 8.1.2). Bupropion may decrease digoxin plasma levels. Monitor patients with neuropsychiatric diseases.

Vitamins

Vitamin D (ergocalciferol)

- *Indications*: treatment of vitamin D deficiency and maintenance of vitamin D levels.
- *Mechanism of action*: provitamin D2. It stimulates intestinal calcium absorption, the incorporation of calcium into the osteoid, and release of calcium from bone tissue.
- *Adverse effects*: rare: signs of hypercalcaemia; hypertension, tachyarrhythmias.
- *Cautions*: with thiazide diuretics, may cause hypercalcaemia. Patients treated with cardiac glycosides are more susceptible to cardiac arrhythmias.

Further reading

CredibleMeds®. *Combined list of drugs that prolong QT and/or cause torsades de pointes (TDP)*. Available from: https://crediblemeds.org/pdftemp/pdf/CombinedList.pdf [accessed 10 September 2018].

Electronic Medicines Compendium (eMC). Available from: https://www.medicines.org.uk/emc [accessed 10 September 2018].

European Medicines Agency. *European public assessment reports*. Available from: http://www.ema.europa.eu/ema/index.jsp?curl=pages/medicines/landing/epar_search.jsp&mid=WC0b01ac058001d124 [accessed 10 September 2018].

Brunton L, Knollmann B, Hilal-Dandan R (eds). *Goodman and Gilman's The Pharmacological Basis of Therapeutics*, 13th ed. McGraw-Hill Education: New York, NY; 2018.

Indiana University. *Drug interactions: Flockhart Table*™. Available from: http://medicine.iupui.edu/clinpharm/ddis/main-table/ [accessed 10 September 2018].

Kaski JK, Haywood C, Mahida S, Baker S, Khong T, Tamargo J (eds). *Oxford Handbook of Drugs in Cardiology*. Oxford University Press: Oxford; 2010.

Aronson JK (ed). *Meyler's Side Effects of Drugs, 16th ed. The International Encyclopedia of Adverse Drug Reactions and Interactions*. Elsevier Science: Oxford; 2015.

Opie LH, Gersh BJ. *Drugs for the heart*, 8th ed. Elsevier Saunders: Philadelphia, PA; 2013.

RxList. Available from: https://www.rxlist.com/script/main/hp.asp [accessed 10 September 2018].

Schmidt M, Lamberts M, Olsen AM, *et al*. Cardiovascular safety of non-aspirin non-steroidal anti-inflammatory drugs: review and position paper by the working group for Cardiovascular Pharmacotherapy of the European Society of Cardiology. *Eur Heart J* 2016;**37**:1015–23.

Preston CL (ed). *Stockley's Drug Interactions*, 11th ed. Pharmaceutical Press: London; 2016.

The heart.org Medscape. Available from: https://www.medscape.com/cardiology [accessed 10 September 2018].

Zamorano JL, Lancellotti P, Rodriguez Muñoz D, *et al*.; Authors/Task Force Members; ESC Committee for Practice Guidelines (CPG); Document Reviewers. 2016 ESC Position Paper on cancer treatments and cardiovascular toxicity developed under the auspices of the ESC Committee for Practice Guidelines: The Task Force for cancer treatments and cardiovascular toxicity of the European Society of Cardiology (ESC). *Eur J Heart Fail* 2017;**19**:9–42.

Index

Note: *b*, *f*, and *t* after locators denote boxes, figures and tables.

C

F

G

H

I

J

K

L

N

S

T

U

V